Handbook of Psychiatry in Palliative Medicine

Handbook of Psychiatry in Palliative Medicine

Psychosocial Care of the Terminally Ill

THIRD EDITION

EDITED BY

Harvey Max Chochinov, MD, PhD

*Distinguished Professor of Psychiatry, University of Manitoba;
Senior Scientist, CancerCare Manitoba Research Institute
Department of Psychiatry University of Manitoba
Winnipeg, MB, Canada*

William Breitbart, MD

*Chairman, Jimmie C. Holland Chair in Psychiatric Oncology
Department of Psychiatry and Behavioral Sciences
Memorial Sloan Kettering Cancer Center
New York, NY, USA*

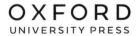

OXFORD
UNIVERSITY PRESS

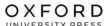

Oxford University Press is a department of the University of Oxford. It furthers
the University's objective of excellence in research, scholarship, and education
by publishing worldwide. Oxford is a registered trade mark of Oxford University
Press in the UK and certain other countries.

Published in the United States of America by Oxford University Press
198 Madison Avenue, New York, NY 10016, United States of America.

© Oxford University Press 2023

First Edition published in 2000
Second Edition published in 2009
Third Edition published in 2023

Library of Congress Cataloging-in-Publication Data
Names: Chochinov, Harvey Max, editor. | Breitbart, William, 1951– editor.
Title: Handbook of psychiatry in palliative medicine : psychosocial care of
the terminally ill / [edited by] Harvey Max Chochinov, William Breitbart.
Description: 3rd edition. | New York, NY : Oxford University Press, [2023] |
Includes bibliographical references and index.
Identifiers: LCCN 2022027367 (print) | LCCN 2022027368 (ebook) |
ISBN 9780197583838 (hardback) | ISBN 9780197583852 (epub) |
ISBN 9780197583869
Subjects: MESH: Palliative Care—psychology | Terminally Ill—psychology |
Psychotherapy—methods | Pain Management | Holistic Health
Classification: LCC RC451.4.T47 (print) | LCC RC451.4.T47 (ebook) |
NLM WB 310 | DDC 362.17/5—dc23/eng/20220826
LC record available at https://lccn.loc.gov/2022027367
LC ebook record available at https://lccn.loc.gov/2022027368

DOI: 10.1093/med/9780197583838.001.0001

9 8 7 6 5 4 3 2 1

Printed by Sheridan Books, Inc., United States of America

To my wife Michelle and our remarkable children, Lauren, Rachel, and our soon to be son-in-law Cam.
In memory of my dear mother Shirley Chochinov, sister Ellen Chochinov and Joyce Basman—never to be forgotten.
—Harvey Max Chochinov

To my son Samuel Benjamin Breitbart.
Never forget how much I love you and how proud I am to be your father.
I tried to live my life and learn some "wisdom" to pass on to you (and hopefully to my patients, colleagues, and the world).
I hope you keep this book to remember after I am gone.
I hope you have learned that "passing love along is what we were born to do."
—William Breitbart

Contents

PART IV   Ethical, Existential, and Spiritual Issues in Palliative Care

PART V   Understanding and Managing Symptoms

PART VI   Psychotherapeutic Interventions in Palliative Care

PART VII Life Cycle Considerations in Palliative Care

Foreword I

Kathleen M. Foley

This third edition of the *Handbook of Psychiatry in Palliative Medicine: Psychosocial Care of the Terminally Ill*, with its expansive 45 chapters, stands as an extraordinary example of the exponential growth of our knowledge and understanding of the physical, psychological, social, spiritual, and ethical dimensions of palliative care for patients, families, and caregivers. This new publication serves as an up-to-date compilation of the new and expanding evidence base for palliative care interventions for physical and psychological distress, coming at a time when a range of national and international policy initiatives are supporting the integration of palliative care into national health strategies.

In the 11 years since the *Handbook*'s last edition, a range of new national and international studies and policy initiatives have identified palliative care as a serious public health challenge. Access to pain relief and palliative care is recognized as a human right and is recognized as a fundamental component of national health systems and as an essential service within universal health coverage reform. The World Health Organization (WHO) 2014 Resolution on Palliative Care called on Member States to integrate palliative care into national health systems and provide resources for the education and training of healthcare professionals to implement palliative care. The 2021 second edition of the *Global Atlas for Palliative Care* now estimates that 56.8 million people globally need palliative care, including 31.1 million prior to and 25.7 million near the end of life. Sixty-seven percent of those in need are adults over the age of 50 and 7% are children; 76% of those in need live in low- and middle-income countries, with noncommunicable diseases accounting for 69% of the adult need. The 2018 Lancet Commission Report on Palliative Care and Pain Relief has created a metric, "health-related suffering," to help national governments assess their palliative care needs to estimate the economic costs for service delivery, and this measure is now being widely used. To assess the implementation of palliative care services, the WHO has identified 10 core indicators to assess palliative care integration. Thus, a strong palliative care policy agenda now exists and parallels the increasing research evidence on the effectiveness of palliative care interventions. In both resource-rich and resource-limited countries, numerous studies demonstrate that palliative care improves patients' and caregivers' quality of life, mood, and symptom control and facilitates decision-making on goals of care. Several studies have demonstrated that palliative care is associated with earlier referral to hospice, has a survival advantage, and is cost effective.

In this evolving palliative care landscape, with palliative care recognized as a medical subspecialty, the demand for credible, authoritative, comprehensive information on the domains of palliative care has never been greater and particularly for educational information on the psychiatric and psychological needs of patients and families.

This new edition meets that challenge in a uniquely important way, with the majority of chapters focused on a range of psychological, existential, social, and spiritual symptoms of patients and families. Each chapter stands alone as an authoritative discussion on a specific topic, but together the text represents an encyclopedic resource of essential information that healthcare professionals need to know about the psychosocial and ethical issues that challenge the provision of expert care for those with serious illness and facing death. Like its earlier editions, this text continues to excel as a compendium of the most current theoretical and practical aspects of assessing patients', families', and caregivers' distress and existential suffering and providing information on evidence-based therapeutic interventions for challenging psychiatric complaints and syndromes. Healthcare professionals, trainees, students, and those who care for the seriously ill and dying will benefit enormously from the opportunity to readily access the clinically relevant content written by expert clinicians and researchers and adapt it, in turn, to their own teaching in core palliative care curricula and clinical practice. The chapters reinforce the need for expertise in psychiatry and psychology to provide comprehensive generalized or specialized palliative care.

The *Handbook*'s editors, Drs. Chochinov and Breitbart, are exceptionally gifted clinicians, educators, and researchers and have assembled a cadre of experts to describe and define the psychiatric aspects of palliative care, a field they have pioneered, enriched, and expanded, mentored by the late Dr. Jimmie Holland. This *Handbook*'s third edition serves as a testament to their scholarship, engagement, and persistence in advocating for understanding and improving the psychiatric needs of the seriously ill and dying, their families, and their caregivers.

Foreword II

Eduardo Bruera

Palliative medicine emerged during the late 1980s and had its origins in the hospice move-ment. Initially practiced in the community, it later became adopted by acute care and academic settings, and it became a subspecialty. Psychosocial oncology emerged from consultation-liaison psychiatry in a small number of cancer centers and rapidly expanded nationally and globally. Both disciplines were practiced by clinical teams with independent structures and processes, and they both had different scientific organizations, journals, and annual meetings for many years. Over time it became progressively clear that the two dis-ciplines are making great efforts toward the alleviation of suffering due to the loss of "per-sonhood" in an otherwise disease-oriented healthcare world.

Drs. Chochinov and Breitbart are true pioneers of a field they termed "psychiatric pal-liative medicine." They understood the common purpose of the efforts of psycho-oncology and palliative medicine and the great opportunity for cross-fertilization and mutual sup-port. They are two giant and revered leaders with a unique characteristic: they are clinically and academically comfortable and claimed as theirs by both fields!

This third edition of the *Handbook of Psychiatry in Palliative Medicine* captures, more successfully than any other publication, the progress in our fields and the multiple areas of successful clinical and academic collaboration. The 45 chapters in this volume are written by the most prominent experts in the field and are loaded with a harmony of evidence and clinical pearls. The chapters are truly a revelation and impeccably edited. This third edition includes new chapters and sections, and it is the most comprehensive text on the subject of psychosocial care of the terminally ill. I am grateful for the opportunity to have con-tributed to all three editions of the volume, and, in my view, this third edition is by far the best. This volume should be mandatory reading for all clinicians in psycho-oncology and palliative medicine and for those involved in the care of patients with cancer and other serious chronic diseases.

We have come to expect excellence from Drs. Chochinov and Breitbart in all aspects of their work, including their lectures, publications, and books. I started reading this volume with great expectations, and, from the very first chapters, I realized it exceeded all my expectations. This work will bring together these two complementary aspects of person-centered care, and, in the process, it will not only help thousands of patients, but it will also help us rethink structures and processes within healthcare institutions and universities.

I am grateful to the editors and authors for all I have learned and enjoyed while reading this amazing volume.

Preface

Harvey Max Chochinov and William Breitbart

In March 2020, the World Health Organization declared COVID-19 a worldwide pandemic. Our lives were suddenly turned topsy-turvy, with each of us grappling with the vagaries of a virus intent on wreaking global havoc. How we lived, by necessity, suddenly changed, and, for those working in palliative care, tending to the dying and how people died changed as well. Strict public health measures, forced isolation, restricted family access, healthcare provider distress, people dying alone, and prohibitions on community rituals of mourning all led to a mounting sense of helplessness, disbelief, and gnawing grief. It was within this context that we decided the time was right to again gather the world leaders in psychosocial palliative care and give them an impeccable platform to declare the state of the art and once again raise the bar on palliative care in the aftermath of this dreadful pandemic.

Thirteen years have passed since the second edition of *The Handbook of Psychiatry in Palliative Medicine* was published. Since the first edition was released in 2000, *The Handbook* has come to occupy an important and distinctive niche within the literary anthology of palliative medicine. Worldwide sales affirm that this volume has attracted a broad readership, transcending culture, race, politics, and geography. The message this implies is one worth highlighting: while individual circumstances, local traditions, and cultural practices may vary, many of the issues facing people approaching death are universal. That is to say, encountering illness, facing vulnerability, and confronting personal mortality is part of the human condition. Hence, the scope of palliative care is global and its mandate as compelling and multifaceted as is the breadth of human suffering.

Unlike the previous two editions, this one has a subtitle: *Psychosocial Care of the Terminally Ill.* This revised title was chosen with purpose and intent, declaring an expanded mandate reaching across multiple disciplines with a vested interest in psychosocial care of the terminally ill. This echoes the teachings of Dame Cicely Saunders, founder of the modern hospice movement, who well understood the complexities of dying and that the human body, as well as the human psyche and the human spirit, all have the capacity to suffer. While a focus on somatic issues has sometimes overshadowed attention to psychological, existential, and spiritual end-of-life challenges, the past two decades have seen an all-encompassing, multidisciplinary approach to care for the dying beginning to take hold. *The Handbook of Psychiatry in Palliative Medicine: Psychosocial Care of the Terminally Ill* is our attempt to affirm the importance of this approach.

A textbook can only serve as a placeholder or landmark for the status of a field at a particular point in time. Since its initial publication in 2000, psychosocial palliative care has evolved and the net effect on palliative medicine has been transformative. Palliation that neglects psychosocial dimensions of patient and family experience de facto fails to meet contemporary standards of comprehensive palliative care. Such is the context and rationale for embarking on this third edition. To do justice to this daunting task, we have again enlisted the world's foremost experts in palliative medicine. Like the first and second edition, the third edition of the *Handbook of Psychiatry in Palliative Medicine: Psychosocial Care of the Terminally Ill*, features a cadre of authors considered international leaders in the field. Without their expertise, wisdom, and generous contribution to this project, this volume would simply not have been possible.

The volume is divided into 45 chapters (12 more than the previous edition) and seven distinct sections, including Psychiatric and Psychosocial Palliative Care: Overview; Psychiatric Complications of Terminal Illness; Psychosocial Issues in Palliative Care; Ethical, Existential, and Spiritual Issues in Palliative Care; Understanding and Managing Symptoms; Psychotherapeutic Interventions in Palliative Care; and Life Cycle Considerations in Palliative Care. While some of the chapters from the second edition have been included in this third edition, each has been updated and, in some instances, new authors brought on board to reflect recent innovations and insights, along with reflections on the state of research and research opportunities within those subject areas.

There are also many new chapters that have been added to this third edition. In the section on Psychiatric and Psychosocial Palliative Care, Tom and Nora Hutchinson have provided a new chapter entitled "Healing and Whole-Person Care." In the section on Psychiatric Complications of Terminal Illness, Madeline Li and colleagues have authored a new chapter on "Medical Assistance in Dying," while John Wynn has provided a chapter on "Difficult Personality Traits and Disorders in Palliative Care."

The section on Psychosocial Issues in Palliative Care has several significant changes. In addition to the excellent updated chapters by Patricia Parker, Jaroslava Salman, Ayla Pelleg, Wendy Lichtenthal, David Kissane, Talia Zaider, Daniel McFarland, Mary Vachon, and a group of extraordinary co-authors, there are several noteworthy new chapters. Gary Rodin and colleagues have written a chapter entitled "Screening for Psychological Distress in the Palliative Care Setting," and Carrie Wu and colleagues have authored a chapter addressing the "Psychosocial Benefits of Early Palliative Care Intervention." In addition, Allison Applebaum and Hannah-Rose Mitchell have written a chapter entitled "Cancer Caregivers," while Laura Polacek and colleagues have authored a new chapter on "Prognostic Understanding in the Terminally Ill."

In Ethical, Existential, and Spiritual Issues in Palliative Care, there are several exciting new chapters, including a chapter on "Palliative Aesthetics," by B. J. Miller and colleagues; a chapter on "Compassion," by Daranne Harris and Shane Sinclair; and a chapter on "Demoralization in Palliative Care" by David Kissane and colleagues.

The section on Understanding and Managing Symptoms contains two new chapters, by Jane Hopkinson and colleagues on "Eating Issues in Palliative Cancer Patients," and Meredith Hays and colleagues on "Fatigue at End of Life." All 11 chapters in Psychotherapeutic Interventions in Palliative Care are new, featuring the world's leading authorities on various psychotherapeutic approaches targeting distress in patients approaching end of life. The emergence of these therapeutic interventions is a strong signal of how the field of psychosocial palliative care has exponentially grown over the past decade. Finally, the section Life Cycle Considerations in Palliative Care contains a new chapter on "Psychiatry in Multidisciplinary Pediatric Palliative Care" by Julia Kearney and Megan Gilman.

The authors of every chapter deserve special and sincere thanks. The "ripple" effects of any publication are often intangible. If, however, someday, somewhere, the knowledge contained within these pages leads to a gentler touch, a more insightful approach, and a better death, it is hard to imagine more gratifying recompense.

There are many people who helped make this volume a reality. We begin with Dr. Jimmie Holland, who died in December 2017. In the Foreword she wrote for the second edition, she stated that if all the work of the two editors were erased, "the size of the gap in our knowledge of the psychological care of dying patients would be gigantic." In truth, she was being overly kind. Having founded the field of psycho-oncology, *she* was the giant. We are proud of all the ways Jimmie touched both our lives, how she helped shape us as clinicians and researchers. Jimmie challenged us to reach higher and inspired us by way of her example. Her career provided the foundation for the entirety of our lifetime of work. Her imprint on us personally—and the field of psychiatry, psycho-oncology, and palliative care—is indelible and undeniable. Without her, this volume would never have happened.

We are, of course, indebted to the editorial staff at Oxford University Press, especially Andrea Knobloch. We are also indebted to our colleagues, trainees, and staff at the University of Manitoba, Department of Psychiatry, CancerCare Manitoba, and at Memorial Sloan Kettering Cancer Center, Department of Psychiatry and Behavioral Sciences, and the Department of Neurology, Pain and Palliative Care Service.

Special mention must be made of our managing editor at Memorial Sloan Kettering Cancer Center, Laurie Schulman. Without her extraordinary organizational skills, tenacity, and guidance, this project would not have gotten off the ground. While the two co-editors are well intentioned, enthusiastic, with lofty goals, both lack the organizational ability to keep track of the myriad details of such a mammoth undertaking. Laurie, thank you for making this possible, for keeping it fun, and for being the calm and steady hand on the tiller of this project.

We are, of course, eternally indebted to our many patients and their families who have taught us so much over the years.

This Preface would be incomplete without acknowledging one another. We first met in 1986 as mentor (W. B.) and mentee (H. M. C.). Over the ensuing decades, life has often moved us along similar academic pathways, with the third edition of the *Handbook of Psychiatry in Palliative Medicine: Psychosocial Care of the Terminally Ill* being but one tangible output of our many collaborations. The blessing of our friendship, which is now well into its fourth decade, is simply beyond measure. We are proud to have shepherded three editions of this extraordinary *Handbook*, which we hope will live on as a testament, not only to the knowledge we aspire to share, but also to a friendship we hope will endure two lifetimes.

—H. M. C.
Winnipeg, Manitoba, Canada

—W. B.
New York, NY, USA

Contributors

Yesne Alici, MD, FAPA, FACLP
Attending Psychiatrist and Associate
Professor of Clinical Psychiatry
Department of Psychiatry and Behavioral
Sciences
Memorial Sloan Kettering Cancer Center
New York, NY, USA

Koji Amano, MD
Assistant Chief
Department of Palliative Medicine
National Cancer Center Hospital
Chuo-ku, Tokyo, Japan

Jaya S. Amaram-Davila, MD
Assistant Professor
Department of Palliative Care
Rehabilitation and Integrative Medicine
University of Texas MD Anderson
Cancer Center
Houston, TX, USA

Allison J. Applebaum, PhD
Associate Attending Psychologist and
Director, Caregivers Clinic
Department of Psychiatry and Behavioral
Sciences
Memorial Sloan Kettering Cancer Center
New York, NY, USA

Joseph A. Arthur, MD
Associate Professor
Department of Palliative Care and
Rehabilitation Medicine; Division of
Cancer Medicine
The University of Texas MD Anderson
Cancer Center
Houston, TX, USA

Smita C. Banerjee, PhD
Associate Attending Behavioral Scientist
Department of Psychiatry and Behavioral
Sciences
Memorial Sloan Kettering Cancer Center
New York, NY, USA

Vickie E. Baracos, PhD
Professor
Department of Oncology
University of Alberta
Edmonton, AB, Canada

Alan Bates, MD, PhD
Acting Program Medical Director
Supportive Care
BC Cancer
Vancouver, BC, Canada

Vanessa Battista, DNP, MBA, RN, MS, CPNP-PC, CHPPN, FPCN
Senior Nursing Director, Palliative Care
Department of Psychosocial Oncology and Palliative Care
Dana Farber Cancer Institute
Boston, MA, USA

Richard W. Bauer, MDiv, MSW
Board Certified Chaplain
George Washington University Institute for Spirituality and Health
George Washington University
Washington, DC, USA

Mohamad Baydoun, RN, PhD
Assistant Professor
Faculty of Nursing
University of Regina
Regina, SK, Canada

Leslie Blackhall, MD, MTS
Associate Professor of Medicine
Department of Palliative Care
University of Virginia School of Medicine
Charlottesville, VA, USA

Irene Bobevski, PhD, DPsych(Clin)
Senior Research Fellow
Department of Medicine
University of Notre Dame Australia
Sydney, Australia

Anna E. Bone, BA, MPH, PhD
Lecturer in Epidemiology and Palliative Care
Cicely Saunders Institute of Palliative Care, Policy, and Rehabilitation
King's College London
London, UK

Anthony P. Bossis, PhD
Clinical Assistant Professor
Department of Psychiatry
NYU Grossman School of Medicine
New York, NY, USA

William Breitbart, MD
Chairman, Jimmie C. Holland Chair in Psychiatric Oncology and Attending Psychiatrist
Department of Psychiatry and Behavioral Sciences
Memorial Sloan Kettering Cancer Center
New York, NY, USA

Stephanie Brody, PsyD
Lecturer in Psychiatry, Department of Psychiatry (part-time), Harvard Medical School; Clinical Associate in Psychology/Attending Psychologist, McLean Hospital
Department of Psychiatry
McLean Hospital/Harvard Medical School
Belmont, MA, USA

Eduardo Bruera, MD
Professor and Chair
Department of Palliative, Rehabilitation and Integrative Medicine
The University of Texas MD Anderson Cancer Center
Houston, TX, USA

Justin Burke, DPhil
Executive Director
Institute for Advanced Dialectical Research
Seattle, WA, USA

Ira Byock, MD, FAAHPM
Founder and Senior Vice President for Strategic Innovation
Providence St. Joseph Health Institute for Human Caring
Gardena, CA, USA

Linda E. Carlson, PhD
Professor
Department of Oncology
University of Calgary
Calgary, AB, Canada

Nathan I. Cherny, AM, MBBS, FRACP, FRCP, LLD
Department of Oncology and
Palliative Care
Shaare Zedek Medical Center
Jerusalem, Israel

Martin S. Chin, MD
Attending Psychiatrist
Department of Psychiatry and Behavioral
Sciences
Memorial Sloan Kettering Cancer Center
New York, NY, USA

Harvey Max Chochinov, MD, PhD
Distinguished Professor of Psychiatry,
University of Manitoba; Senior Scientist,
Cancer Care Manitoba Research Institute
Department of Psychiatry
University of Manitoba
Winnipeg, MB, Canada

Melissa M. Duva, PhD
Licensed Clinical Psychologist
Bee Well NYC
New York, NY, USA

Linda Emanuel, PhD, MD, FABPA
Psychoanalyst
Mongan Institute
Massachusetts General Hospital
Boston, MA, USA

Andrew S. Epstein, MD, FAAHPM
Associate Attending
Gastrointestinal Oncology and Supportive
Care Services, Department of Medicine
Memorial Sloan Kettering Cancer Center
New York, NY, USA

Kari L. Esbensen, MD, PhD
Assistant Professor of Medicine and
Senior Faculty Fellow
Department of Medicine, Division of
Hospital Medicine, and Emory Center
for Ethics
Emory University
Atlanta, GA, USA

Carol Fadalla
Clinical Psychology PhD Candidate and
BA in Psychology
Clinical Psychology PhD Candidate and
Research Assistant
Department of Clinical Psychology
Texas Tech University
Lubbock, TX, USA

Nathan Fairman, MD, MPH
Associate Clinical Professor
Department of Psychiatry and Behavioral
Sciences
University of California Davis School of
Medicine
Sacramento, CA, USA

Alexandra Farag, MD, CCFP (PC)
Assistant Clinical Professor
Division of Palliative Care, Department of
Family Medicine
McMaster University
Hamilton, ON, Canada

Betty R. Ferrell, PhD, MA, CHPN, FAAN, FPCN
Professor
Division of Nursing Research and
Education
City of Hope
Duarte, CA, USA

Kathleen M. Foley, MD
Member Emeritus, Memorial Sloan
Kettering Cancer Center
Professor Emeritus of Neurology,
Neuroscience and Pharmacology, Weill
Medical College Cornell University
New York, NY, USA

David Fudge, MD, BSc(H), FRCP(c)
Psychiatrist
Department of Psychiatry and Behavioural
Neurosciences
St. Joseph's Healthcare Hamilton
Hamilton, ON, Canada

Bryan Gascon, MSc
Medical Student
Temerty Faculty of Medicine
University of Toronto
Toronto, ON, Canada

Login S. George, PhD
Assistant Professor
Institute for Health; School of Nursing
Rutgers University
New Brunswick, NJ, USA

Megan Gilman, MD
Assistant Attending Psychiatrist
Department of Psychiatry and Behavioral Sciences
Memorial Sloan Kettering Cancer Center
New York, NY, USA

Johanna Glaser, MD
Resident Physician
Division of General Internal Medicine
University of California, San Francisco
San Francisco, CA, USA

Barbara Gomes, PhD
Coordinating Researcher
Faculty of Medicine
University of Coimbra
Coimbra, Portugal

Luigi Grassi, MD
Chair and Professor of Psychiatry
Department of Neuroscience and Rehabilitation
University of Ferrara
Ferrara, Italy

Sarah Hales, MD, PhD
Psychiatrist
Department of Supportive Care
Princess Margaret Cancer Centre
Toronto, ON, Canada

Daranne Harris, MDiv
Faculty of Nursing
University of Calgary
Calgary, AB, Canada

Meredith Hays, DO, MPH
Palliative Care Physician
Department of Palliative Care
Sacred Heart Medical Center
Spokane, WA, USA

Marjorie Heule, MS
Department of Psychology
Wayne State University
Detroit, MI, USA

Irene J. Higginson, BMedSci, BMBS, PhD, FMedSci, FRCP, FFPHM
Professor of Palliative Care and Policy
Cicely Saunders Institute
King's College London
London, UK

Jane B. Hopkinson, PhD, RN
Velindre Professor of Nursing and Interdisciplinary Cancer Care
School of Healthcare Sciences
Cardiff University
Cardiff, UK

Lee Hulbert-Williams, PhD
Associate Professor
School of Psychology
University of Chester
Chester, UK

Nicholas J. Hulbert-Williams, PhD, CPsychol
Professor & Head of the Department of Psychology
Department of Psychology
Edge Hill University
Ormskirk, UK

Nora Hutchinson, MD, CM, MPhil
Instructor
Hospital Medicine Unit
Massachusetts General Hospital
Boston, MA, USA

Tom A. Hutchinson, MB
Professor and Director of McGill Programs
in Whole Person Care
Department of Medicine
McGill University
Montreal, PQ, Canada

Scott A. Irwin, MD, PhD
Director Patient and Family Support
Program; Professor of Psychiatry and
Behavioral Neurosciences
Cedars-Sinai Cancer and the Department
of Psychiatry and Behavioral Neurosciences
Cedars-Sinai Health System
Los Angeles, CA, USA

Julia A. Kearney, MD
Associate Attending Psychiatrist and
Clinical Director
Department of Psychiatry and Behavioral
Sciences
Memorial Sloan Kettering Cancer Center
New York, NY, USA

R. Garrett Key, MD
Assistant Professor
Department of Psychiatry and Behavioral
Sciences
University of Texas at Austin Dell
Medical School
Austin, TX, USA

**David W. Kissane, MBBS, MPM, MD,
FRANZCP, FAChPM, FACLP**
Chair of Palliative Medicine Research,
University of Notre Dame Australia;
Emeritus Professor of Psychiatry, Monash
University, Victoria, Australia
School of Medicine
University of Notre Dame Australia
Sydney, New South Wales, Australia

Manuela Kogon, MD
Clinical Professor
Stanford Center for Integrative Medicine,
Department of Psychiatry and Behavioral
Sciences
Stanford University School of Medicine
Stanford, CA, USA

Juee Kotwal, MBS
Senior Business Manager
Department of Supportive Care Medicine
City of Hope
Duarte, CA, USA

Elissa Kozlov, PhD
Assistant Professor
Department of Health Behavior, Society
and Policy
Rutgers School of Public Health
Piscataway, NJ, USA

Han Le Santisi, DO
Attending Physician
Department of Medicine, Division of
Palliative Medicine
Cooper Healthcare
Camden, NJ, USA

Madeline Li, MD, PhD
Psychiatrist
Department of Supportive Care
Princess Margaret Cancer Centre
Toronto, ON, Canada

Wendy G. Lichtenthal, PhD
Director, Bereavement Clinic; Associate
Attending Psychologist
Department of Psychiatry and Behavioral
Sciences
Memorial Sloan Kettering Cancer Center
New York, NY, USA

Matthew Loscalzo, LCSW
Executive Director
People and Enterprise Transformation
Emeritus Professor Supportive Care
Medicine Professor Population Sciences
City of Hope
Duarte, CA, USA

Margaret M. Mahon, PhD, CRNP, FAAN, FPCN
Nurse Practitioner
Pain & Palliative Care
National Institutes of Health
Bethesda, MD, USA

Carmine Malfitano, PhD, MSW, RSW
Clinician Specialist
Department of Supportive Care
Princess Margaret Cancer Centre,
University Health Network
Toronto, ON, Canada

Christopher Manschreck, MD
Attending Psychiatrist, Assistant Professor
Department of Psychiatry and Behavioral
Sciences
University of New Mexico
Albuquerque, NM, USA

Konstantina Matsoukas, MLIS
Research Informationist
Medical Library
Memorial Sloan Kettering Cancer Center
New York, NY, USA

Meghan McDarby, PhD
Postdoctoral Research Fellow
Department of Psychiatry and Behavioral
Sciences
Memorial Sloan Kettering Cancer Center
New York, NY, USA

Daniel C. McFarland, DO
Associate Professor and Director of
Psycho-Oncology
Department of Psychiatry
University of Rochester
Rochester, NY, USA

Diane E. Meier, MD
Professor
Department of Geriatrics and Palliative
Medicine
Icahn School of Medicine at Mount Sinai
New York, NY, USA

B. J. Miller, MD
Founder
Mettle Health
Mill Valley, CA, USA

Hannah-Rose Mitchell, PhD, MPH
Postdoctoral Research Fellow
Department of Psychiatry and Behavioral
Sciences
Memorial Sloan Kettering Cancer Center
New York, NY, USA

Chelsea Moran, MA
PhD Candidate
Department of Psychology
University of Calgary
Calgary, AB, Canada

R. Sean Morrison, MD
Ellen and Howard C. Katz Professor
and Chair
Brookdale Department of Geriatrics and
Palliative Medicine
Icahn School of Medicine at Mount Sinai
New York, NY, USA

Robert A. Neimeyer, PhD
Director
Portland Institute for Loss and Transition
Portland, OR, USA

John-Jose Nunez, MD, MSc, FRCPC
Clinical Research Fellow
Department of Psychiatry
University of British Columbia
Vancouver, BC, Canada

Timothy O'Shea, MD, MPH
Associate Professor
Department of Medicine
McMaster University
Hamilton, ON, Canada

Aliza A. Panjwani, PhD
Psychologist
Department of Supportive Care
Princess Margaret Cancer Centre,
University Health Network
Toronto, ON, Canada

Patricia A. Parker, PhD
Attending Psychologist and Director,
Communication Skills Training and
Research Program
Department of Psychiatry and Behavioral
Sciences
Memorial Sloan Kettering Cancer Center
New York, NY, USA

Ayla Pelleg, MD
Assistant Professor
Brookdale Department of Geriatrics and
Palliative Medicine
The Icahn School of Medicine at
Mount Sinai
New York, NY, USA

Hayley Pessin, PhD
Research Associate
Department of Psychiatry and Behavioral
Sciences
Memorial Sloan Kettering Cancer Center
New York, NY, USA

William Pirl, MD, MPH
Vice Chair for Psychosocial Oncology
Department of Psychosocial Oncology and
Palliative Care
Dana-Farber Cancer Institute
Boston, MA, USA

Laura C. Polacek, MA
Graduate Student
Department of Psychology
Fordham University
Bronx, NY, USA

Russell K. Portenoy, MD
Professor of Neurology and Family and
Social Medicine
Albert Einstein College of Medicine
Bronx, NY, USA

Holly G. Prigerson, PhD
Professor and Director, Cornell Center for
Research on End-of-Life Care
Department of Medicine
Weill Cornell Medicine
New York, NY, USA

**Christina Puchalski, MD, MS,
FACP, FAAHPM**
Professor of Medicine
Department of Medicine
George Washington University School of
Medicine
Washington, DC, USA

Anna K. L. Reyners, MD, PhD
Professor
Department of Medical Oncology
University Medical Center Groningen
Groningen, Netherlands

Kailey E. Roberts, PhD
Assistant Professor
Adult Clinical Psychology, Ferkauf
Graduate School of Psychology
Yeshiva University
Bronx, NY, USA

Gary Rodin, MD
Professor
Department of Psychiatry
Princess Margaret Cancer Centre,
University Health Network, University of
Toronto
Toronto, ON, Canada

Madeline Rogers, MSW
Research Program
Coordinator-Interventionist
Department of Medicine
Weill Cornell Medicine
New York, NY, USA

William E. Rosa, PhD, MBE, NP-BC
Assistant Attending Behavioral Scientist
Department of Psychiatry and Behavioral
Sciences
Memorial Sloan Kettering Cancer Center
New York, NY, USA

Barry Rosenfeld, PhD
Professor
Department of Psychology
Fordham University
New York, NY, USA

Stephen Ross, MD
Research Associate Professor of Psychiatry
Department of Psychiatry
NYU Grossman School of Medicine
New York, NY, USA

Andrew J. Roth, MD
Attending Psychiatrist at Memorial
Sloan Kettering Cancer Center, Professor
of Clinical Psychiatry at Weill Cornell
Medical College
Department of Psychiatry and Behavioral
Sciences
Memorial Sloan Kettering Cancer Center
New York, NY, USA

Jaroslava Salman, MD, FACLP
Assistant Professor of Psychiatry
Department of Supportive Care Medicine
City of Hope
Duarte, CA, USA

Tasha Mari Schoppee, PhD
Director of Nursing, Respite Services
Community Hospice & Palliative Care
University of Florida
Jacksonville, FL, USA

Shane Sinclair, PhD
Professor and Director, Compassion
Research Lab
Faculty of Nursing
University of Calgary
Calgary, AB, Canada

Jonathan Singer, PhD
Assistant Professor
Department of Psychological Science
Texas Tech University
Lubbock, TX, USA

Cardinale B. Smith, MD, PhD
Professor
Division of Hematology and Medical
Oncology and Brookdale Department of
Geriatrics and Palliative Medicine
Icahn School of Medicine at Mount Sinai
New York, NY, USA

David Spiegel, MD
Jack, Lulu, and Sam Willson Professor in
the School of Medicine and Associate Chair
Department of Psychiatry and Behavioral
Sciences
Stanford University
Stanford, CA, USA

Karen E. Steinhauser, PhD
Professor, Health Scientist
Department of Population Health Sciences,
Medicine, Research Health Scientist
Duke University School of Medicine and
Durham VA Health Care System, Health
Services Research and Development,
Center of Innovation to Accelerate
Discovery and Practice Transformation
(ADAPT)
Durham, NC, USA

Daniel P. Sulmasy, MD, PhD
Hellegers Professor of Biomedical Ethics
and Director
Kennedy Institute of Ethics
Georgetown University
Washington, DC, USA

Jennifer Temel, MD
Professor of Medicine
Department of Medicine/Division of
Hematology/Oncology
Harvard Medical School/Massachusetts
General Hospital
Boston, MA, USA

Kelly Trevino, PhD
Associate Attending Psychologist
Department of Psychiatry and Behavioral
Sciences
Memorial Sloan Kettering Cancer Center
New York, NY, USA

Mary L. S. Vachon, RN, RP, PhD
Psychotherapist in Private Practice,
Adjunct Professor
Department of Psychiatry and Dalla Lana
School of Public health
Temerty Faculty of Medicine, University of
Toronto
Toronto, ON, Canada

Elisha Waldman, MD, FAAHPM
Associate Professor of Pediatrics
Division of Palliative Care
Lurie Children's Hospital of Chicago
Chicago, IL, USA

Leah E. Walsh, MS
Predoctoral Research Fellow
Department of Psychiatry and Behavioral
Sciences
Memorial Sloan Kettering Cancer Center
New York, NY, USA

Amanda Watsula, MA
Clinical Research Supervisor
Department of Psychiatry and Behavioral
Sciences
Memorial Sloan Kettering Cancer Center
New York, NY, USA

**Kathleen Baba Willison, RN, MSc,
CHPCN(c)**
Clinical Nurse Specialist—Palliative Care;
Assistant Clinical Professor
School of Nursing; Division of Palliative
Care, Department of Family Medicine
McMaster University
Hamilton, ON, Canada

Joseph G. Winger, PhD
Assistant Professor
Department of Psychiatry and Behavioral
Sciences
Duke University
Durham, NC, USA

**Anne Woods, BA, RN, MDiv, MD,
CCFP, FCFP**
Assistant Clinical Professor; Co-Head of
Service
Division of Palliative Care, Department of
Family Medicine; Palliative Care Service,
Department of Medicine
McMaster University; St. Joseph's
Healthcare Hamilton
Hamilton, ON, Canada

Carrie C. Wu, MD
Instructor
Department of Psychosocial Oncology and
Palliative Care
Dana-Farber Cancer Institute
Boston, MA, USA

John Wynn MD, DLFAPA
Clinical Professor
Department of Psychiatry and Behavioral
Sciences
University of Washington School of
Medicine
Seattle, WA, USA

Talia I. Zaider, PhD
Assistant Attending Psychologist
Department of Psychiatry and Behavioral
Sciences
Memorial Sloan Kettering Cancer Center
New York, NY, USA

Camilla Zimmermann, MD, PhD
Professor and Department Head
Department of Supportive Care
Princess Margaret Cancer Centre
Toronto, ON, Canada

PART I

Psychiatric and Psychosocial Palliative Care

Overview

Hospice and Palliative Care
Putting Those Affected Before Their Disease

Irene J. Higginson, Barbara Gomes, and Anna E. Bone

Introduction: Whole-Person Approaches in Hospice and Palliative Care

From its origins, with leaders such as Dame Cicely Saunders, Eric Wilkes, Colin Murray Parkes, and James Hanratty in the United Kingdom; Balfour Mount in Canada; Vittorio Ventafridda in Italy; and Elizabeth Kubler-Ross and Avery Weisman in the United States, hospice and palliative care has always embraced the "whole" person, in the context of their family. From her observations of people with advanced and progressive illness, Dame Cicely Saunders introduced the concept of *total pain*. Pain had physical, emotional, social, and spiritual components, all of which needed to be addressed. Of course, excellent control of pain and other symptoms is vital, but the role of the palliative care team, including the physicians, is much more than this. It also extends beyond expertise in the management of physical and psychiatric symptoms. Effective symptom control may be necessary before other goals of hospice and palliative care can be achieved. But, equally, failure to address emotional, social, or spiritual components of symptoms may lead to inadequate symptom control. Physicians can and should contribute to this holistic assessment and care. This is why palliative medicine is a rewarding field for physicians: there is much opportunity to practice comprehensive whole-person care.

As described in detail throughout this text, mental disorders and psychological distress are among the most common and troublesome complications of advanced illness. The roles, therefore, of psychiatrists, psychologists, social workers, and all variety of psychosocial professionals in palliative care are critical. The prevalence of psychological symptoms and distress in advanced illness is not well described due to a lack of longitudinal research and varied definitions. However, systematic review of symptom prevalence in five advanced conditions—cancer, HIV/AIDS, heart failure, chronic obstructive pulmonary disease, and renal disease—found that the point prevalence of depression ranged up to 80%, depending on the definitions and criteria used (see Figure 1.1).[1,2] A more recent review found similar levels of depression and anxiety in up to 74%.[3] Relief of suffering in the psychological domain is a priority in palliative care and provides the psychiatrist, nurses, and related psychosocial professionals with opportunities to contribute to the care of patients in this setting through direct patient care, liaison with other clinicians on the palliative care team, education, and research.

The psychological, social, and spiritual concerns of patients and their families are highly individual and vary according to personality and circumstances. For some it is coming to terms with the reality of their situation, articulating and achieving specific life goals, planning for the remaining time, and getting their affairs in order. Hospice and palliative care teams can facilitate this, and, in some instances, forgiveness and reconciliation to heal broken relationships help patients and families express their love for one another and say their goodbyes.[4,5] With help and encouragement, some patients and families can construct and share meaning and savor stories that have knit their lives together. Hope can be preserved and directed toward achievable goals, such as family events and special occasions, and dignity maintained and respected. Families can be supported in their caregiving and losses and throughout their grieving.

Early descriptions of palliative and hospice care recognized the need to integrate physical, psychological, social, and spiritual care of patients and their families.[5,6] Indeed, most widely accepted definitions of hospice and palliative care emphasize the integration of these domains of care. For example, in its definition of hospice, the National Hospice and Palliative Care Organization (NHPCO) of the United States explicitly states that social, spiritual, and emotional care are provided along with physical care.[4] The NHPCO definition also includes declarations that hospice care serves both patients and their families,

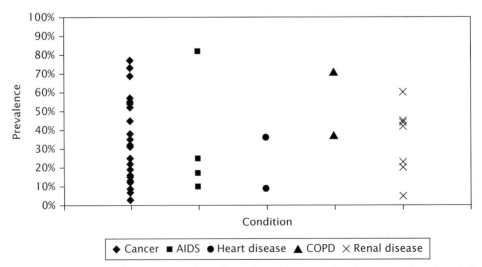

FIGURE 1.1 Prevalence of depression in five advanced conditions: results of a systematic review of 33 studies. *Source*: Solano JP, Gomes B, Higginson IJ. *J Pain Symptom Manage*. 2006;31(1):58–69.

emphasizes quality of life, works to preserve and promote opportunities for growth at this stage of life, aims to assist patients in preparation for death, and offers care for bereaved survivors.[4] Similarly, the World Health Organization's (WHO) definition of palliative care states that the control of psychological, social, and spiritual problems for patients and their families is integral to care and deserving of attention equal to that given in addressing the patient's physical problems.[7]

Among physicians, these aspects of palliative care align closely with the training and expertise of psychiatrists and some other specialties such as old age medicine or geriatrics and pediatrics. Nurses play critical roles in providing psychosocial assessment and care, and many have additional psychological, counseling, or communications training. Mental health professionals, social workers, and other psychosocial workers are sometimes integrated into hospice and palliative care teams, but the reality is that hospice programs have highly varied access to psychiatrists or psychologists for consultations or participation in the work of the interdisciplinary team.[8] Despite their modest numbers, psychiatrists are making significant contributions to advance the field of palliative medicine and have done so from the very inception of the field, both in palliative care and through cancer care, in the field of psycho-oncology.

Multiprofessional Contributions to Hospice and Palliative Care: The Role of Key Individuals and Groups

Cicely Saunders

Dame Cicely Saunders represents the multiprofessional team within one person. She began training as a ward nurse in 1941, at St. Thomas Hospital in London, England, and later retrained as a social worker. Witnessing the pain and suffering of patients at the end of life, she began to seek solutions. She worked as a volunteer in the early homes for the "terminally ill," where she witnessed the regular administration of pain relief (then the "Brompton's cocktail"). Because she wanted to change practice, she retrained again, now in medicine. She pioneered and encouraged others to test drug treatments for pain relief, and she also collected detailed observations and tape-recorded interviews with patients and families. It was through this that she recognized the "total" nature of pain. As Saunders explained, "It soon became clear that each death was as individual as the life that preceded it and that the whole experience of that life was reflected in a patient's dying. This led to the concept of 'total pain,' which was presented as a complex of physical, emotional, social, and spiritual elements. The whole experience for a patient includes anxiety, depression, and fear; concern for the family who will become bereaved; and often a need to find some meaning in the situation, some deeper reality in which to trust."[9]

Through her work Saunders made contact with Professor Colin Murray Parkes and Professor John Hinton, both psychiatrists. Later she persuaded both of them to work within the hospice she went on to found, St. Christopher's Hospice, setting the trend for UK hospices to develop links and integration with psychiatric services. In 2002, she founded Cicely

Saunders International, a charity whose purpose is to address the lack of evidence in palliative care and to provide better care for patients and families, through research.

Elizabeth Kubler-Ross

A Swiss-born psychiatrist who moved to the United States with her husband, Dr. Elisabeth Kubler-Ross changed Western cultural resistance to dealing with death and the teaching of how to accept it. Shocked by indifference to dying that she witnessed in a Chicago hospital, Kubler-Ross generated a large body of work in *thanatology*, a field she had helped to create, in particular on the stages that dying people go through.[10] Although now considered overly rigid and simplistic, her five-stage model helped to put death and dying on the medical map and, in particular, helped health professionals to deal with a factor they had long refused to acknowledge. Her major output was in books, magazine articles, and open lectures, rather than in academic journals. She reached a large public, as well as influencing nursing, medical, and psychosocial professionals.

Avery D. Weisman

Dr. Weisman was a North American psychiatrist who did much early work in the area of thanatology. He wrote several books based on his observations and coined the term "appropriate death," which "means dying the best possible way, not only retaining vestiges of what made life important and valuable, but surviving with personal significance and self-esteem, with minimal distress and few symptoms, for as long as possible." He proposed four helpful goals for an "appropriate" death: (1) reducing but not necessarily eliminating internal conflict, such as fears about dying; (2) making dying people's dying compatible with their own views of themselves and their achievements; (3) preserving or restoring relationships as much as possible; and (4) setting and fulfilling some of the dying person's realistic and expressed aims, such as seeing a birth or a family event. These goals underpin much of palliative care practice today as well as several of the new interventions being tested.[11–13]

John Hinton

Professor John Hinton qualified in medicine from King's College Hospital, London, in 1949 and specialized in psychiatry across the road, at the Maudsley Hospital (1955–1961). Although he had general psychiatric interests, an interest in the experiences of dying patients was his main research theme. Perhaps the first most seminal work was his report in 1963 of the distress experienced by people dying in hospital,[14,15] coming 4 years before the opening of St. Christopher's Hospice and Ann Cartwright's population-based survey of life before death.[16] Hinton's work drew attention to the mental distress and other symptoms encountered at the end of life for people affected by cancer and other terminal conditions, then to care in different settings,[17] the awareness of dying and communication,[18–20] and quality home care.[21–23]

Colin Murray Parkes

Professor Colin Murray Parkes turned his attentions toward psychiatry and in particular the mind–body relationship, recognizing the limitations of a heroic and mechanistic approach to medicine. Similar to Hinton, he trained at the Maudsley Hospital, London, focusing increasingly on stress and trauma and, through this, bereavement. His MD thesis in 1962 examined "normal grief."[24] This work brought him into contact with Dame Cicely Saunders, who invited him to become Honorary Consultant Psychiatrist at St. Christopher's Hospice; James Hanratty, medical director at St. Joseph's Hospice also invited him to become Honorary Consultant, and Parkes began to work with both hospices. Parkes further developed his ideas of "loss and change," not only in the loss of a spouse but also in other losses, such as loss of a limb or sight;[25] factors determining phantom limb pain;[26] and, most recently, the after-effects of major disasters.[27] His work on factors determining the outcomes of bereavement[28] led to the development of risk assessment tools that are still used today. He also made a major contribution to evidence on the effectiveness of hospice and palliative care programs: he published the first UK evaluations of inpatient and community hospice and palliative care.[29] Although quasi-experimental in nature, Parkes compared bereaved spouses' reports about patients receiving hospice and routine care and quantified for the first time the benefits of hospices,[30–32] not only for patients but also for the bereaved spouse.[33] He is Life President of Cruse Bereavement Care, the UK's leading national charity for bereaved people.

Peter Maguire

Professor Peter Maguire's work has caused a complete change in the way that communication occurs with patients and families facing life-threatening illness and thus is worthy of mention. Trained in Psychiatry in the United Kingdom, his early research showed that many patients in a medical ward had anxiety or depressive illnesses that added to their suffering; these patients were not receiving any help with their psychological distress because their doctors were unaware of it. Over the next 30 years, Maguire devoted his professional life to overcoming this problem, especially in the field of cancer. He researched the various ways that doctors and nurses might block patients from expressing their worries during clinical interviews, focusing especially on the highly charged situations of breaking bad news and death and dying, when most blocking occurs. Then he developed and evaluated training programs in communication skills for doctors and nurses, producing a model that underpins current best practice in supportive and palliative care.[34,35]

Jimmie Holland

In the United States and across the globe, Professor Jimmie Holland has spearheaded the field of psycho-oncology, with her research focusing on the psychological impact of cancer on individuals and their families, studying how cancer affects patients, their families, and caregivers and how psychological and behavioral factors affect the risk of cancer and survival. Holland is credited with putting psychosocial and behavioral research on the agenda of the American Cancer Society in the early 1980s, leading to the creation of the Society's scientific advisory committee on psychosocial and behavioral research. She is also the founding President of the International Psycho-Oncology Society (IPOS) and the American Psychosocial Oncology Society (APOS). From her base at Memorial Sloan-Kettering Cancer Center in New York, she has pioneered the study of the ways in which counseling, complementary therapies, and medication can reduce the distress experienced by cancer patients and their families, including among neglected groups, such as those from different cultures and older patients.[36–39]

Mary Vachon

Dr. Mary Vachon trained in nursing and took a master's degree in sociology; her PhD thesis studied widowhood.[40] Her research developed awareness of grief as a psychological phenomenon, and she also demonstrated adaptation over time and the effect of supportive and self-help interventions,[41] improving on the earlier models of factors affecting bereavement outcomes[42] and also bringing to the fore the role of social support.[43] She also pioneered the study of stress among patients and caregivers. Her work on caregivers extended not only to the family but also to the nursing and medical professionals, for whom she advocated methods to reduce and control stress.[44–46]

Sheila Payne

Professor Sheila Payne contributed greatly to multidisciplinary work in palliative care, helping find ways to achieve a shared vision within teams in different contexts and cultures.[47] A health psychologist with background in nursing, she worked in several specialist research units focused on palliative and end of life care in the United Kingdom, collaborating extensively with colleagues abroad. Her research focused on the experiences and needs of older people approaching the end of life and of the family caregivers supporting them, helping shed light on the life restrictions, strain, and emotional distress related to caregiving and the limited support available to them.[48] Recognized as an influential leader and champion of psychosocial care at the end of life, she was president of the European Association for Palliative Care from 2011 to 2015 (the first non-medical person so elected) and holds an Emeritus Chair at the International Observatory on End of Life Care at Lancaster University.

Psychosocial Organizations and Initiatives Across the Globe

Scholarship in the field of psychiatric and psychological aspects of first cancer and latterly palliative care has been nurtured within several organizations. Multiprofessionals from oncology, psychiatry, psychology, palliative medicine, nursing, social work, and other relevant fields began to come together in groups to debate the latest research and promote high-quality clinical care and teaching in psychological, psychiatric, and social aspects of cancer. Early hospice and palliative care research found a welcome home here, with cancer as the bedrock of much palliative care practice. Soon there were organizations within individual countries across Europe and an international organization—the IPOS—started by Jimmie Holland and others. In 2020, IPOS established a Palliative Care Special Interest Group chaired by Gary Rodin, a journal (*Psycho-Oncology*, edited by Maggie Watson), regular conferences, training courses, and a network to foster the exchange of ideas, all of which continue today.

Despite being an area often overlooked, some international initiatives are developing to promote psychosocial care toward the end of life. An example is the La Caixa Foundation Programme for enhancing comprehensive care for patients with advanced diseases and their families. This social innovation initiative has developed a new model of psychosocial and spiritual care provision that is implemented by 55 psychosocial support teams working alongside palliative care teams across Spain and Portugal. In operation since 2010 in Spain and 2018 in Portugal, the La Caixa Programme supports more than 30,000 patients per year, with benefits in several domains including anxiety and emotional distress for patients and family caregivers and depression and insomnia for family caregivers.[49,50] Concerted and sustained actions such as this have helped trigger societal transformation toward more compassionate and holistic care.

Psychosocial Problems and Concerns in Palliative Care

Palliative care aims to improve the quality of life of patients and their families through assessing and addressing physical, psychological, social, or spiritual problems.[51] Holistic assessment of symptoms and concerns is therefore a critical component of palliative care, one that allows for problems to be identified, treated, and continually monitored over time. The measurement of patient-centered outcomes has been found to improve emotional and psychological symptoms among patients in palliative care settings.[52] The process of completing patient-reported outcome measures encourages patients to reflect on their well-being and allows them to raise issues or concerns with clinicians.[53] Routine holistic assessment of patients is not only advocated within the specialty of palliative care: it can serve to promote a palliative care approach in settings outside of the specialty or may trigger a referral to specialists in palliative care when relevant.[54]

The specialty of palliative care has gained considerable expertise in the area of patient-reported symptom measurement, with a range of measurement tools developed and validated. Given that patients often present with multiple symptoms and concerns at the same time, it is important that assessment tools contain a range of symptoms, covering not only physical domains, but also psychosocial, spiritual, and practical. A widely used patient-centered outcome measure is the Palliative Care Outcome Scale (POS).[55] Although originally developed for a cancer population, the measure has since been updated and adapted to be applicable to both cancer and non-cancer populations as the Integrated Palliative Care Outcome Scale (IPOS).[56] This brief measure is one of the few tools that incorporates the full range of issues and concerns that people with advanced illness deem important, and it has been demonstrated to be valid and reliable.[56] There have also been adaptations made for disease groups with particular issues with communication, such as dementia.[57,58]

Another example of an holistic symptom assessment tool developed for use within palliative care settings is the Edmonton Symptom Assessment System (ESAS).[59] First developed for cancer patients in 1991, ESAS has since been evolved, psychometrically validated, and translated into different languages.[56] A limitation is that there are fewer validations of this measure among patients with non-cancer conditions, which represent most people with serious illness.

Although measurement tools such as IPOS and ESAS have been carefully developed to encompass a range of problems and concerns commonly experienced by people with serious illness, in practice there is variation in how well different domains are assessed and recorded. A descriptive analysis of palliative care consultation documentation in Portugal found that physical symptom items in the ESAS were significantly more likely to be recorded than psychosocial problems such as depression, anxiety, hope, and will to live.[60] This suggests that psychosocial problems are not always considered a critical component of palliative care or not always prioritized when time is limited.

Despite the availability of these patient-centered outcome measures that are brief, valid, and feasible to use in clinical practice, these tools are not yet widely and routinely embedded into clinical practice. Without this standardization of practice, varying degrees of assessment and ongoing monitoring for patients across settings is likely to lead to unwarranted variation in patient outcomes at a population level. There are examples where efforts to embed patient-centered outcome measures in palliative care settings have proved successful. For example, the Palliative Care Outcome Collaborative (PCOC)[61] in Australia maintains a national longitudinal database of palliative care outcome data across care settings. This nationally funded program appears to improve clinical outcomes in palliative care through audit, quality feedback cycles, and benchmarking, and it has led to improvements in clinical outcomes at a service level.[62] Routine assessment of symptoms and concerns using validated patient-centered outcome measures has a multitude of benefits at the level of the individual patient as well as the wider health system.

Barriers to Excellent Care at the End of Life

The WHO considers palliative care an essential service and a basic human right as part of Universal Health Coverage.[51] As discussed, a key part of palliative care is holistic assessment of the physical, psychological, social, and spiritual concerns of the individual and their family. The Academy of Psychosomatic Medicine (APM) has published a position statement on the "Psychiatric Aspects of Excellent Care at the End of Life."[63] It is the APM's position that good end-of-life care requires explicit attention to mental disorders and distress, loss and bereavement, spiritual and religious issues, capacity to make informed decisions, and quality of life. A variety of barriers that interfere with proper recognition and treatment of the full range of problems, including psychiatric and psychological problems, toward the end of life are identified here.

1. *Prognostic uncertainty*, particularly for individuals with less predictable illness trajectories, such as those with chronic disease, multiple coexisting illnesses, and those living with frailty,[64] can create barriers to accessing excellent care at the end of life.[65] Sometimes referred to as *prognostic paralysis*,[66] this phenomenon can mean that the holistic needs of an individual are not considered or discussed with the individual and their family.

2. *Referral to specialist palliative care services early in the progression of an advanced disease* is advocated based on growing evidence that early involvement of specialist palliative care improves patient outcomes in cancer[67] and on emerging evidence within other disease groups.[68] However, it is challenging to implement in practice, in part due to difficulties in prognosis as well as a lack of resources, lack of knowledge of service availability, eligibility restrictions, and patient or family reluctance.[65]

3. *The challenge of diagnosing mental disorders in the setting of serious physical illness.* In the case of even the most common disorders, such as depression, diagnosis is inherently difficult due to the frequent overlap of symptoms (such as fatigue, loss of appetite, or sleep disturbance) that may potentially result from either mental disorder or advanced physical illness.

4. *Confusion about the threshold of clinical significance.* Many believe that symptoms of mental disorder (especially depression) are either so common as to be a normal part of the dying process or are a natural and expected stage in the process of adaptation to impending death. Distinction of clinical syndromes and disorders from transient moods or manifestations of adaptation to change and loss is critical to avoid unnecessary suffering from psychiatric complications of advanced illness.

5. *Prevention, recognition, and management of Alzheimer's disease, other forms of dementia, and cognitive impairment.* As populations age and people die at later ages, cognitive impairment and dementia become more common.

6. *Underemphasis of formal diagnosis (as opposed to symptomatic treatment) in hospice and palliative care.* Any number of problems can mimic, mask, exacerbate, or be attributed to common mental disorders. Especially when treatment considerations include interventions with significant lag time to likely effect (e.g., treatment with standard antidepressants), accuracy in diagnosis is needed to avoid wasting precious time on interventions unlikely to yield much benefit.

7. *Many are unreasonably nihilistic about the potential benefit of treatment of mental disorder and mental distress at the end of life.* This may lead to insufficient vigilance and attention to diagnosis and leave the patient and family to needlessly suffer from treatable problems.

8. *Sadly, mental disorder diagnoses are still associated with stigma.* Patients and families may be embarrassed or ashamed of being diagnosed with a mental disorder or even with making psychological symptoms the focus of treatment. Attribution of such symptoms to moral failings or weakness of character can needlessly complicate the patient and family's suffering.

9. *Members of the palliative care team must guard against countertransference hopelessness (and encourage family members to do so, as well).* Sadness, pessimism, and hopelessness can be contagious to some degree. While it is important to avoid giving false hope or painting too rosy a picture of the patient's situation (in order to avoid a difficult conversation), it is equally important not to collude with hopelessness and pessimism, even inadvertently. A focus on realistic hope and achievable goals is central to good palliative care.

The Interface Between Mind and Body

Psychosomatic medicine, the psychiatric subspecialty dealing with the care of persons with comorbid psychiatric and general medical conditions,[63] shares a common perspective with palliative medicine—a focus on whole-person, integrative care. Parkes[69,70] uses a microscopy metaphor, in which he states that "Much of medicine is high-powered, focused in great detail on one or a few aspects of a person.... Hospice staff, on the other hand, are often low-powered. They are less concerned with the technical aspects of care, and they attempt to take the family (which includes the patient) as the unit of care.... To develop the analogy with microscopy further: Good microscopists know that, to get the best results, they need to rake back and forth between high and low powers. The same applies to the good hospices."

The same also applies to good psychiatric care of patients with serious physical illnesses. Psychosomatic medicine, similar to palliative medicine, requires the physician to be interested and focused on the patient's illness and suffering from both "high-powered" and "low-powered" perspectives. There is a particular skill set and professional temperament needed by those who choose to practice in these fields that bridge disciplines and traditional domains of expertise. They must be able to switch between sophisticated diagnosis and the application of proven and evidence-based therapies to attending to subjective and interpersonal aspects of good care to genuine care and concern for the well-being of patient and family.

The approach illustrated by Parkes's analogy does not imply that holism is an endorsement of any and all unproven or anecdotal treatment (having to "say yes to everything" or what he calls "benevolent amateurism").[69,70] It simply describes the skill and capacity to balance clinical expertise and applied mastery of the knowledge base with a healthy respect for what works, driven by a concern for the suffering and distress of patients and their families.

The intellectual and clinical focus of the psychiatrist in psychosomatic medicine—concerned with how physical illness influences mental illness and distress (and vice versa)—makes the link between psychosomatic medicine and palliative medicine obvious.

An example of this is the management of breathlessness. Breathlessness is a common symptom of advanced disease, found in up to 77% of patients in palliative care and in even more patients with respiratory diseases such as chronic obstructive pulmonary disease and lung cancer.[3] Breathlessness increases with disease progression and often becomes chronic or refractory. The brain (as well as muscle strength and lungs) plays an important part in the generation of breathlessness, leading to an approach to management focused around "breathing, thinking, and functioning."[71,72] Breathlessness-triggered support services that integrate holistic assessment and specialist palliative care input as part of a multiprofessional approach have been developed for this group, offering tailored interventions to support self-management and reduce distress.[73,74] Breathlessness support services involve a combination of holistic assessment, physiotherapy, and palliative care in the management of breathlessness. A novel mantra/poem to help relaxation or other relaxation training during crises is often part of the intervention.[75] Systematic reviews have found holistic breathlessness support services effective in reducing distress and depression and improving quality of life.[73–75]

Future Directions

The holistic practice of hospice and palliative care provides a great and exciting opportunity for the psychiatrist interested in teaching, research, and clinical practice and for all clinicians keen to work on the interface of mind and body. Medical students, residents, and fellows need instruction and supervision in the holistic, psychological, and psychiatric aspects of palliative care. In addition to our non-psychiatric medical colleagues, hospice and palliative care professionals in a variety of other disciplines routinely deal with psychiatric and psychological aspects of care. Opportunities exist to educate patients and families, as well as the public at large, about excellent care at the end of life, especially in holistic care involving psychiatrists, psychologists, and psychosocial professionals.

There are many advances in the development of holistic care. However, there is still much to know about the effects of mental distress and disorder on pain, breathlessness, other symptoms, suffering, and quality of life in advanced disease. There is also much to learn about how these interact with one another and how to develop and apply effective and well-tolerated intervention strategies. Our field must also attend to the need to develop and mentor new investigators in order to maintain this momentum and, indeed, to accelerate the pace of advances in holistic palliative care.

As the field of palliative medicine continues to grow and mature, the clinical and health services evidence base and reimbursement mechanisms must develop apace. It is certain that the demand for excellent palliative care, including attention to holistic (including psychiatric and psychological) aspects of care and specialist-level psychiatric palliative care, will continue to grow. Opportunities for psychiatrists, psychologists, social workers, and psychosocial professionals interested in palliative care abound.

Key Points

- Holistic palliative care provides a unique and exciting opportunity to apply a broad range of skills to the benefit of patients and families.
- The psychiatrist, psychologist, psychosocial professional, or others with the capacity to shift focus from the narrow perspective of symptoms and disorders to the broad view of distress and suffering can provide a uniquely valuable kind of care to those who need it most.
- Routine assessment of symptoms and patient and family concerns using validated outcome measures has a multitude of benefits at the level of the individual patient as well as the wider health system.
- The holistic practice in palliative care, involving a multiprofessional team of nurses; relevant physicians (including palliative specialists and, when appropriate, psychiatrists); social workers; increasingly therapists, such as physiotherapists; and often volunteers provide the opportunity to reconnect with values that give meaning to the practice of medicine and healthcare.

References

1. Solano JP, Gomes B, Higginson IJ. A comparison of symptom prevalence in far advanced cancer, AIDS, heart disease, chronic obstructive pulmonary disease and renal disease. *J Pain Symptom Manage.* 2006;31(1):58–69.

2. Hotopf M, Chidgey J, Addington-Hall J, Ly KL. Depression in advanced disease: A systematic review Part 1. Prevalence and case finding. *Palliat Med.* 2002;16(2):81–97.

3. Moens K, Higginson IJ, Harding R, on behalf of EURO IMPACT. Are there differences in the prevalence of palliative care-related problems in people living with advanced cancer and eight non-cancer conditions? A systematic review. *J Pain Symptom Manag.* 2014;48:660–677.

4. Saunders C. Palliative care for the terminally ill. *Can Med Assoc J.* 1977;117(1):15.

5. National Hospice and Palliative Care Organisation (NHPCO). http://www.nhpco.org.

6. Saunders C. The evolution of palliative care. *J R Soc Med.* 2001;94(9):430–432.

7. Davies E, Higginson IJ. *Palliative Care: The Solid Facts.* Geneva: World Health Organization; 2004.

8. Price A, Hotopf M, Higginson IJ, et al. Psychological services in hospices in the UK and Republic of Ireland. *J R Soc Med.* 2006;99(12):637–639.

9. Saunders C. A personal therapeutic journey. *BMJ.* 1996;313(7072):1599–1601.

10. Kübler-Ross E, Wessler S, Avioli LV. On death and dying. *JAMA.* 1972;221(2):174–179.

11. Tataryn D, Chochinov HM. Predicting the trajectory of will to live in terminally ill patients. *Psychosomatics: Journal of Consultation and Liaison Psychiatry.* 2002;43(5):370–377.

12. Chochinov HM. Dying, dignity, and new horizons in palliative end-of-life care. *CA Cancer J Clin.* 2006;56(2):84–103;quiz 4–5.

13. Chochinov HM. Dignity and the essence of medicine: The A, B, C, and D of dignity conserving care. *BMJ (Clin Res Ed).* 2007;335(7612):184–187.

14. Hinton JM. Problems in the care of the dying. *J Chronic Dis.* 1964;17(3):201–205.

15. Hinton JM. The physical and mental distress of the dying. *Q J Med.* 1963;32:1–21.

16. Cartwright A, Hockey L. *Life Before Death.* London: Routledge & Kegan Paul; 1973.

17. Hinton J. Comparison of places and policies for terminal care *Lancet.* 1979;313(8106):29–32.

18. Hinton J. The progress of awareness and acceptance of dying assessed in cancer patients and their caring relatives. *Palliat Med.* 1999;13(1):19–35.

19. Hinton J. An assessment of open communication between people with terminal cancer, caring relatives, and others during home care. *J Palliat Care.* 1998;14(3):15–23.

20. Hinton J. Sharing or withholding awareness of dying between husband and wife. *J Psychosom Res.* 1981;25(5):337–343.

21. Hinton J. Which patients with terminal cancer are admitted from home care? *Palliat Med.* 1994;8(3):197–210.

22. Hinton J. Can home care maintain an acceptable quality of life for patients with terminal cancer and their relatives? *Palliat Med.* 1994;8(3):183–196.

23. Hinton J. Services given and help perceived during home care for terminal cancer. *Palliat Med.* 1996;10(2):125–134.

24. Parkes CM. Bereavement and mental illness. 2. A classification of bereavement reactions *Br J Med Psychol.* 1965;38:13–26.

25. Parkes CM. Psycho-social transitions: Comparison between reactions to loss of a limb and loss of a spouse. *Br J Psychiatry.* 1975;127:204–210.

26. Parkes CM. Factors determining the persistence of phantom pain in the amputee. *J Psychosom Res.* 1973;17(2):97–108.

27. Williams RM, Parkes CM. Psychosocial effects of disaster: Birth rate in Aberfan. *Br Med J.* 1975;2(5966):303–304.

28. Parkes CM. Determination of outcome of bereavement. *Proc R Soc Med.* 1971;64(3):279.

29. Higginson IJ, Finlay IG, Goodwin DM, et al. Is there evidence that palliative care teams alter end-of-life experiences of patients and their caregivers? *J Pain Symptom Manage.* 2003;25(2):150–168.

30. Parkes CM. Terminal care: Evaluation of in-patient service at St Christopher's Hospice. Part I. Views of surviving spouse on effects of the service on the patient. *Postgrad Med J.* 1979;55(646):517–522.

31. Parkes CM. Terminal care: Evaluation of in-patient service at St Christopher's Hospice. Part II. Self assessments of effects of the service on surviving spouses. *Postgrad Med J.* 1979;55(646):523–527.

32. Parkes CM. Terminal care: Evaluation of an advisory domiciliary service at St Christopher's Hospice. *Postgrad Med J.* 1980;56(660):685–689.

33. Cameron J, Parkes CM. Terminal care: Evaluation of effects on surviving family of care before and after bereavement. *Postgrad Med J.* 1983;59(688):73–78.

34. Gysels M, Richardson A, Higginson IJ. Communication training for health professionals who care for patients with cancer: A systematic review of effectiveness. *Support Care Cancer.* 2004;12(10):692–700.

35. Gysels M, Richardson A, Higginson IJ. Communication training for health professionals who care for patients with cancer: A systematic review of training methods. *Support Care Cancer.* 2005;13(6):356–366.

36. Holland JC. Preliminary guidelines for the treatment of distress. *Oncology (Williston Park).* 1997;11(11a):109–14; discussion 15–17.

37. Holland JC. Improving the human side of cancer care: Psycho-oncology's contribution. *Cancer J.* 2001;7(6):458–471.

38. Holland JC. IPOS Sutherland Memorial Lecture: An international perspective on the development of psychosocial oncology: Overcoming cultural and attitudinal barriers to improve psychosocial care. *Psychooncology.* 2004;13(7):445–459.

39. Holland JC, Morrow GR, Schmale A, et al. A randomized clinical trial of alprazolam versus progressive muscle relaxation in cancer patients with anxiety and depressive symptoms. *J Clin Oncol.* 1991;9(6):1004–1011.

40. Vachon MLS. Grief and bereavement following the death of a spouse. *Can Psychiatr Assoc J.* 1976;21(1):35–44.

41. Vachon ML, Lyall WA, Rogers J, et al. A controlled study of self-help intervention for widows. *Am J Psychiatry.* 1980;137(11):1380–1384.

42. Vachon ML, Rogers J, Lyall WA, et al. Predictors and correlates of adaptation to conjugal bereavement. *Am J Psychiatry.* 1982;139(8):998–1002.

43. Vachon MLS, Stylianos SK. The role of social support in bereavement. *J Soc Issues.* 1988;44(3):175–190.

44. Vachon ML. Staff stress in care of the terminally ill. *QRB Qual Rev Bull.* 1979;5(5):13–17.

45. Vachon ML. Staff stress in hospice/palliative care: A review. *Palliat Med.* 1995;9(2):91–122.

46. Vachon MLS, Kristjanson L, Higginson I. Psychosocial issues in palliative care: The patient, the family, and the process and outcome of care. *J Pain Symptom Manage.* 1995;10(2):142–150.

47. Radbruch L, Payne, S. White paper on standards and norms for hospice and palliative care in Europe: Part 1. *Eur J Palliat Care.* 2009;16(6):278–289.

48. Payne S, Smith P, Dean S. Identifying the concerns of informal carers in palliative care. *Palliat Med.* 1999;13(1):37–44.

49. Gómez-Batiste X, Buisan M, González MP, et al. The "La Caixa" Foundation and WHO Collaborating Center Spanish National Program for enhancing psychosocial and spiritual palliative care for patients with advanced diseases, and their families: Preliminary findings. *Palliat Support Care.* 2011;9(3):239–249.

50. Gómez-Batiste X, Mateo-Ortega D, Lasmarías C, et al. Enhancing psychosocial and spiritual palliative care: Four-year results of the program of comprehensive care for people with advanced illnesses and their families in Spain. *Palliat Support Care.* 2017;15(1):98–109.

51. World Health Organisation. Palliative Care. 2020. https://www.who.int/news-room/fact-sheets/detail/palliative-care.

52. Etkind SN, Daveson BA, Kwok W, et al. Capture, transfer, and feedback of patient-centered outcomes data in palliative care populations: Does it make a difference? A systematic review. *J Pain Symptom Manage.* 2015;49(3):611–624.

53. Greenhalgh J, Gooding K, Gibbons E, et al. How do patient reported outcome measures (PROMs) support clinician-patient communication and patient care? A realist synthesis. *J Patient Rep Outcomes.* 2018;2:42.

54. Lidstone V, Butters E, Seed PT, et al. Symptoms and concerns amongst cancer outpatients: Identifying the need for specialist palliative care. *Palliat Med.* 2003;17(7):588–595.

55. Hearn J, Higginson IJ. Development and validation of a core outcome measure for palliative care: The palliative care outcome scale. *Quality Health Care QHC.* 1999;8(4):219–227.

56. Murtagh FEM, Ramsenthaler C, Firth A, et al. A brief, patient- and proxy-reported outcome measure in advanced illness: Validity, reliability and responsiveness of the Integrated Palliative Care Outcome Scale (IPOS). *Palliat Med.* 2019:0269216319854264.

57. Bone AE, Morgan M, Maddocks M, Sleeman KE, Wright J, Taherzadeh S, et al. Developing a model of short-term integrated palliative and supportive care for frail older people in community settings: Perspectives of older people, carers and other key stakeholders. *Age Ageing.* 2016;45(6):863–873.

58. Ellis-Smith C, Evans CJ, Murtagh FEM, et al. Development of a caregiver-reported measure to support systematic assessment of people with dementia in long-term care: The Integrated Palliative care Outcome Scale for Dementia. *Palliat Med.* 2016;31(7):651–660.

59. Hui D, Bruera E. The Edmonton Symptom Assessment system 25 years later: Past, present, and future developments. *J Pain Symptom Manage.* 2017;53(3):630–643.

60. Julião M, Sobral MA, Calçada P, et al. "Truly holistic?" Differences in documenting physical and psychosocial needs and hope in Portuguese palliative patients. *Palliat Supportive Care.* 2021;19(1):69–74.

61. Palliative Care Outcomes Collaboration. https://www.uow.edu.au/ahsri/pcoc/.

62. Currow DC, Allingham S, Yates P, Johnson C, Clark K, Eagar K. Improving national hospice/palliative care service symptom outcomes systematically through point-of-care data collection, structured feedback and benchmarking. *Supportive Care Cancer.* 2015;23(2):307–315.

63. Academy of Psychosomatic Medicine. Psychiatric aspects of excellent end-of-life care: A position statement of the Academy of Psychosomatic Medicine. *J Palliat Med.* 1998;1(2):113–115.

64. Murray SA, Kendall M, Boyd K, Sheikh A. Illness trajectories and palliative care. *BMJ.* 2005;330(7498):1007–1011.

65. Hawley P. Barriers to access to palliative care. *Palliat Care Res Treatm.* 2017;10:1178224216688887.

66. Epiphaniou E, Shipman C, Harding R, et al. Coordination of end-of-life care for patients with lung cancer and those with advanced COPD: Are there transferable lessons? A longitudinal qualitative study. *Prim Care Respir J.* 2014;23(1):46–51.

67. Haun MW, Estel S, Rücker G, et al. Early palliative care for adults with advanced cancer. *Cochrane Database Syst Rev.* 2017;6(6):Cd011129.

68. Evans CJ, Bone AE, Yi D, et al. Community-based short-term integrated palliative and supportive care reduces symptom distress for older people with chronic noncancer conditions compared with usual care: A randomised controlled single-blind mixed method trial. *Int J Nurs Stud.* 2021;120:103978.

69. Parkes CM. Care of the dying: The role of the psychiatrist. *Br J Hosp Med.* 1986;36(4):250, 2, 4–5.

70. Parkes C. Hospice: A psychiatric perspective. In: Chochinov HM, Breitbart WS, ed. *Handbook of Psychiatry in Palliative Medicine.* New York: Oxford University Press; 2000:3–11.

71. Booth S, Chin C, Spathis A. The brain and breathlessness: Understanding and disseminating a palliative care approach. *Palliat Med.* 2015;29(5):396–398.

72. Spathis A, Booth S, Moffat C, et al. The Breathing, Thinking, Functioning clinical model: A proposal to facilitate evidence-based breathlessness management in chronic respiratory disease. *Primary Care Respirat Med.* 2017;27(1):27.

73. Maddocks M, Brighton LJ, Farquhar M, et al. Holistic services for people with advanced disease and chronic or refractory breathlessness: A mixed-methods evidence synthesis. *NIHR Health Services Delivery Res.* 2019 June, No.7.22.

74. Brighton LJ, Miller S, Farquhar M, et al. Holistic services for people with advanced disease and chronic breathlessness: A systematic review and meta-analysis. *Thorax.* 2019;74(3):270–281.

75. Higginson IJ, Bausewein C, Reilly CC, Gao W, Gysels M, Dzingina M, et al. An integrated palliative and respiratory care service for patients with advanced disease and refractory breathlessness: A randomised controlled trial. *Lancet Respir Med.* 2014;2(12):979–987.

2

Integrating Psychiatry and Palliative Medicine

David W. Kissane

Introduction

Since the early hospices opened over a century ago and modern palliative care was launched by Dame Cicely Saunders in the 1960s, huge growth and development of the discipline has been witnessed across the globe. This is not surprising as projections suggest that 60 million persons will die in 2021, and palliative medicine has become the primary discipline to care for these people. Strong movements have developed to support this growth: the International Association of Hospice and Palliative Care (IAHPC), the European Association for Palliative Care (EAPC), the Asia Pacific Hospice Palliative Care Network (APHPCN), and, as the African Palliative Care Association (APCA) was formed, the World Health Organization (WHO) was brought into strong alignment with these organizations. The provision of essential medicines and the human right to opioid medication for pain relief propelled this development. Policy documents were promoted by these organizations, challenging governments to adopt palliative care as a global initiative.

Psychosocial care is and has always been a key component of what palliative care offers, as psychological, social, existential, and spiritual dimensions contribute to patient distress and suffering. The pursuit of the "good" death has guaranteed the involvement of psychosocial care providers. Yet, while the physician and nurse formed the backbone of any infant palliative care service, resourcing a comprehensive interdisciplinary team with psychiatrists, psychologists, social workers, and chaplains has been challenging in many parts of the world. The rhetoric about including psychosocial and spiritual care has been there, pioneers such as Elizabeth Kubler-Ross, Colin Murray Parkes, and Jimmie Holland have advocated strongly for unmet psychosocial needs to be addressed, yet the financing to support adequate staffing for psychosocial care has not easily followed.

In a less dramatic way, therefore, consultation-liaison psychiatry and psycho-oncology have grown alongside palliative care. Patient advocacy helped as truth-telling movements led by Oken's work in the 1960s advocated for openness about cancer. National and international organizations again formed, from fledgling research efforts like the Psychosocial Collaborative Oncology Group chaired by Arthur Schmale in the United States in the 1970s, to national groups like the British Psycho-Oncology Society (BPOS) and the Academy of Psychosomatic Medicine (APM) in the United States, and to global groups like the International Psycho-Oncology Society and the Federation of Psycho-Social Oncology Societies. Cancer centers became the home of early research endeavors, with the broader focus on cancer control, coping with treatments and survivorship as well as advanced cancer and leading to a stronger research agenda and methodology than developed in the more clinically focused palliative care units. Thus, the early research contribution from psycho-oncology made a major contribution to the development of palliative care.

The Research Agenda of Early Psycho-Oncology Studies

While palliative care focused on the availability of morphine, the behavioral sciences focused initially on tobacco. As awareness of the dangers of smoking grew during the 1960s, behavioral scientists worked on public health campaigns to encourage people to stop smoking. Psychology as a discipline led research groups formed to address the morbidities associated with cancer treatment. In the United States, Cancer and Leukemia Group B started routine quality-of-life (QoL) assessments in every leukemia trial, while Jimmie Coker Holland studied cancer fears caused by the six D's: death, disfigurement, disability, discomfort, dependency and disruption of relationships.[1]

Early attention was directed to the humanistic side of medicine and to understand why patients sought unproved cancer remedies. Studies of communication were launched by Deborah Roter in the 1970s, while Mack Lipkin, a mentee of George Engel's, developed in the 1980s a curriculum for the medical interview and formed a task force that grew into the American Academy on Communication in Healthcare. In the United Kingdom, in parallel during the 1980s, Peter Maguire at the Christie Hospital in Manchester taught communication skills to medical students, demonstrating that empathic behaviors generalized over time and permitted truth-telling in cancer care.

Early observational studies about the impact of cancer and its treatment were led by Arthur Sutherland at Memorial Sloan-Kettering Cancer Center in New York and Avery Weisman at the Massachusetts General Hospital in Boston. Wide publicity given to the work of Elizabeth Kubler Ross about open communication with the dying helped launch a thanatology movement and countered the notion that death was a taboo subject. The growth of consultation-liaison psychiatry since the early 1970s has had a significant impact on patient care.

Measurement development and validation has greatly helped to advance psychosocial research. Measures of anxiety and depression developed by Beck and colleagues, symptom inventories by DeRogatis et al., coping and mental attitudes by Watson in the United Kingdom, and QoL measures refined by the European Organization for Treatment and Research in Cancer ensured good scholarship was conducted in clinical trials. Important measures for palliative medicine included the Edmonton Symptom Assessment Scale by E. Bruera in 1991, the McGill QoL scale by S. R. Cohen and B. Mount in Montreal in 1995, the Schedule of Attitudes toward Hastened Death by B. Rosenfeld and W. Breitbart in 2000, and the Demoralization Scale by D. Kissane and S. Wein in 2004.

Early psychotropic studies assessed the efficacy of antidepressants, anti-anxiety, hypnotic, and neuroleptic medications in palliative medicine. Efficacy studies for the use of tricyclics and selective serotonin reuptake inhibitors (SSRIs) occurred in the 1970–80s, while the benefits of psychostimulants such as methylphenidate were also confirmed in the 1980s. Ultimately, in a meta-analysis in 2010, Rayner and colleagues could demonstrate an odds ratio of 2.25 (95% CI: 1.38–3.67) for the benefit of antidepressants among 12 studies in the palliative care setting.[2] Similarly, the use of neuroleptics to contain agitation in delirium was confirmed,[3] while their antinausea benefits were recognized in opioid toxicity.

The Integrative Model of Consultation-Liaison Psychiatry

The most straightforward role for the psychiatrist working in palliative medicine is as a clinical consultant, offering diagnoses and management guidance, which can be both direct in patient and family care as well as indirect through guiding the actions of other members of the team. Indeed, the liaison role emphasizes the educative and support role played with the multidisciplinary team, countering any compassion fatigue and nihilism that can creep into some palliative care teams.

Many studies have highlighted the ease with which mental disorders can be (1) missed because grief is normalized as commensurate with a dire clinical predicament, (2) undertreated because of failure to adequately titrate dosage or rotate psychotropics when some treatment resistance has emerged, or (3) avoided because of fear of opening a pandora's box of challenges that may be difficult to resolve (see Box 2.1). Lack of screening or inadequate staffing present further difficulties. While some presentations are severe and clear-cut, subsyndromal states are common and raise management uncertainties.

The psychiatrist is well trained in taking a developmental history, understanding transgenerational influences, and making sense of the strengths and vulnerabilities of a person, their coping style, and the family context in which they live. The resulting narrative account of a person's life can enrich understanding for other members of the multidisciplinary team and empower them to better provide person- and family centered care. From time to time, services meet so-called difficult patients whose emotional responsiveness (e.g., anger), personality traits (e.g., narcissism), interpersonal fractures (e.g., splitting of staff into good and bad carers) or eccentric behaviors can make them challenging to look after. The deeper the understanding of the background and dynamics of such a person, the better the resultant care plan can become.

BOX 2.1 Common Reasons Mental Disorders Pass Unrecognized in Palliative Care

1. Grief is normalized and a more detailed assessment is not undertaken.
2. Psychotropic medication titration or rotation is inadequate.
3. There is a fear of opening up issues that need time for assessment and management.
4. Screening tools are not used.
5. Sub-threshold states and existential symptoms not well understood.
6. Skilled staff is lacking to address the psycho-existential needs.

The psychosocial disciplines can offer complementary roles and skills in the overall service of patients, families, and teams. The social worker may have expertise with systems, finances, and family therapy; the psychologist offers mastery of cognitive and behavioral approaches; the music or art therapist delivers a creative skill that will hold appeal to many; the occupational therapist assesses safety, needs to transition home, and activities of daily living; the dietician is responsible for total parenteral nutrition, supplements, and food intake; the physical therapist prescribes rehabilitation exercises; the chaplain or pastoral care worker specializes in spiritual and religious care; and the psychiatrist diagnoses and treats mental illness par excellence. Programs in large institutions can draw diverse contributions from many staff. Small services can struggle to fund a comprehensive program without fostering extensive community linkages; undoubtedly, the quality of care can be deeply enriched when the resources of a full interdisciplinary service are provided.

Screening for Distress

When ships at sea perceive they are in some danger, they put out a distress call to signal their need for help. Distress is seen as a less stigmatized word than depression, making it easier for patients to acknowledge. In distress screening, patients are asked to rate their level of distress on a scale between 0 and 10, where a threshold of 4 or more points indicates some level of clinical need, and a threshold of 7 or more has optimal sensitivity and specificity to detect the presence of clinical depression as measured on the Patient Health Questionnaire-9 (PHQ-9).[4]

Just as hospice associations lobbied successfully to have "pain" assessed as the fifth vital sign after temperature, pulse, blood pressure, and respirations, so, too, did the psycho-oncology societies lobby to have "distress" assessed as the sixth vital sign. The Union for International Cancer Control adopted distress as the Sixth Vital Sign in 2010, and this was followed in 2013 by the World Cancer Declaration setting among its goals that by 2025, Target 08: "effective pain control and distress management services will be universally available."

Although the original Edmonton Symptom Assessment Scale developed by Bruera and colleagues in 1991 included symptoms of anxiety and depression, many services ask only about physical symptoms as they monitor patient well-being. To address this deficit, the Psycho-existential Symptom Assessment Scale (PeSAS) has been introduced to ensure that services do monitor psychological and existential symptoms of importance.[5] See Chapter 26 in this book for more evidence on the demoralization studies involved in the validation of this screening tool to better recognize psycho-existential distress.

The Psycho-Existential Context of Palliative Medicine Today

Human suffering arises from the threat to the wellness and integrity of a person. The biomedical model has its focus on bodily health and function, which can take a disease- or illness-related perspective, most often looking to pharmacological or physical treatments to ameliorate distress from symptoms. The biopsychosocial and spiritual model attends to the needs of the whole person; their emotional and cognitive reaction to illness; the social impact on employment, finances, family, and home life; and any challenges to their spiritual and religious needs. How each individual copes and deals with their illness is central to such a whole person approach.

The existential realm acknowledges challenges that arise from our human nature and that can be universal in that sense, occurring across cultures, creeds, and traditions. Such givens include *mortality*—the finite nature of human life; *freedom*—choice and personal autonomy that we exercise over our lives; *meaning*—whether there is purpose and sense to life; and *aloneness*—our individuality which sits in tension with human relationships. It could be argued that the discipline of psychiatry has brought more study and understanding of these dimensions to palliative care than any other discipline. One of the doyens of psychiatry, Irvin David Yalom, has written an elegant synthesis of the writings of decades of existential philosophers and his text, *Existential Psychotherapy*, is essential reading for all who work in palliative care.[6] Irrespective of such contributions, the psycho-existential realm is vital in understanding and optimally helping the patient and family toward the end-of-life.[7]

These existential realities can act as a catalyst to opportunity and resilience, or a vulnerability that brings suffering to our human experience. Table 2.1 presents the common symptoms that accompany these existential challenges, the adaptive adjustment that is possible, and the maladaptive responses that contribute to clinical issues. The use of a number of psychological therapies supports patients in adopting a resilient posture that helps their overall adaptation.

Over the past decades, psychiatric researchers have built models of therapy which could be understood as responsive to a number of these existential themes. These have made stellar contributions to the discipline of palliative medicine. Each will be presented in some detail in later chapters of this book, but their scholarship is celebrated here as recognition of the contribution of psychiatry to palliative medicine.

TABLE 2.1 Responses to common existential challenges in palliative care[a]

Common symptoms	Nature of existential challenge	Adaptive adjustment	Maladaptive response
Fear of dying; fear of being dead; uncertainty of future	Death anxiety	Courage; open awareness of dying	Panic, dread, angst; anxiety disorders
Waves of tearfulness; sadness; labile emotions	Grief at loss/change	Mourning; continued focus on living	Complicated grief; chronic anger; depressive disorders
Obsessive need for control; fear of dependence; fear of burden	Freedom and autonomy	Treatment adherence; responsibility; acceptance of caregivers	Nonadherence to treatment; fear of being a burden
Shame, embarrassment; body image and identity concerns	Dignity and self-worth	Robust self-esteem; acceptance of frailty; feeling respected	Low self-worth; avoidant, feeling stigmatized; agoraphobic
Loneliness social withdrawal	Fundamental aloneness	Sense of integrity; secure with oneself; connectedness	Feel insecure; Isolated, Alienated
Family conflict relational tension and dysfunction	Human relationships	Well-functioning family; mutual support	Communication breakdown; loss of cohesion and support
Pointlessness, hopelessness, futility, desire to die	Meaning of life	Fulfilled life; accomplishments; Legacy	Demoralization, clinical depression
Guilt; doubt; loss of faith; loss of connection beyond the self	Mystery and the unknowable	Peacefulness; Religious faith; Contentment	Anguish; spiritual doubt; despair

[a] Adapted with permission from Kissane DW. The relief of existential suffering. *Archives of Internal Medicine*, 2012 Oct; *172*(19): 1501–1505, https://doi.org/10.1001/archinternmed.2012.3633

Dignity Therapy

The distinguished Canadian psychiatrist, Harvey M. Chochinov, recognized the concern of palliative care for the dignity of each person, yet the dearth of research examining this important construct. A person preparing for their death deserves to be honored or esteemed because of the intrinsic worth that springs from our common humanity.[8] Developing their sense of dignity is a mark of deep respect for their personhood and an activity which is central to the work of palliative care.

Chochinov and his team in Winnipeg studied dignity, developing an understanding of illness related concerns, dignity-conserving perspectives and practices, together with a social dignity inventory. In Chapter 36 of this book, Chochinov outlines his empirically developed model of therapy and his efficacy trial, confirming its ability to improve quality of life, enhance the patient's sense of dignity and their family's ability to appreciate them more deeply.[9] What a triumph this body of work has been over the past two decades in providing a poignant gift to a dying person and a celebration of their life in a generativity document presented to the patient and their family.

Meaning-Centered Therapy

The internationally renowned American psychiatrist, William Breitbart, recognized the centrality of meaning-based coping to sustain resilience, and achieve fulfilment and joy in life. In his work at Memorial Sloan-Kettering Cancer Center in New York, Breitbart honored the seminal work of Viktor Frankl as a Holocaust survivor and psychiatrist. Frankl emerged from his experiences of intense physical and psychological suffering convinced that man has an inherent drive to connect with something greater than one's own needs and, through this, to find meaning and self-transcendence. In his logotherapy, Frankl made use of a person's freedom to choose what is meaningful in their life and harness what he termed a "will to meaning" to mold their attitude toward suffering, countered by the value and beauty of their life. Breitbart's brilliant work across two decades has adapted these basic tenets to a variety of therapeutic forms, individual[10] or group therapy,[11] delivered not only in the palliative care setting, but also to the caregiver, to the bereaved parent, to people suffering yet striving to celebrate life, its creativity, and its joy.

In Chapter 35 of this book, Breitbart gives an account of how to deliver meaning-centered therapy. This extraordinary body of work exemplifies how well psychiatry has responded to the existential challenges met in palliative medicine. The adaptability of the meaning-centered model is a tremendous strength, as therapists can clearly take it into a variety of clinical settings.

Supportive-Expressive Group Therapy

A third exceptional body of work by another stellar academic psychiatrist is found in the work of David Spiegel from Stanford University, California. Employing a model of emotion-focused, existentially oriented, and relationally nurturing group therapy for patients with advanced breast cancer, Spiegel transformed all that is vital and fundamental in supportive therapy into a well-adapted group format in a palliative care setting. The goals of this therapy are to strengthen relational bonds, express emotions, detoxify death, redefine purpose and meaning, fortify families, enhance doctor–patient relationships, and improve coping.[12]

Spiegel's model is presented in Chapter 40 in this book. One systematic review has confirmed reduced distress and enhanced coping, such as less helplessness and pain from attending group therapy.[13] The existential benefits of this model are undoubted, delivery can utilize the individual or group approach, and, again, a huge body of work was spawned by this psychiatrically led work in the advanced cancer setting.

Integrating Meaning with Good Symptom Management: CALM Therapy

Research in Toronto at the Princess Margaret Cancer Center has integrated Managing Cancer and Living Meaningfully (CALM) for patients with advanced cancer into an approach that combines palliative symptom management with psychological support.[14] Led by the academic psychiatrist, Gary Rodin, and informed by relational, attachment, and existential theories, this model aims to create a reflective space in which to consider symptom management and communication with healthcare providers and changes in self, well-being, relationships, and sense of meaning and purpose, alongside any future-oriented concerns about death and the finitude of life. A detailed account of CALM therapy is provided in Chapter 37 of this book. Trials of CALM Therapy have confirmed reduction in depressive symptoms at 3 months, better end-of-life preparation, and, for patients with moderate death anxiety, improvements in demoralization, anxiety, spiritual well-being, and attachment security.

Family-Centered Therapy

Palliative care has long sought to be family-centered in its orientation. Psychiatric studies have again exemplified a novel model that identifies families that struggle interpersonally toward the end of life yet can be held together by family therapy that begins in palliative care and is extended into bereavement.[15] Kissane has led two randomized controlled trials to show the efficacy of this approach, with prevention of Prolonged Grief Disorder after 13 months of bereavement as a result of these family members being helped to communicate more openly and assist one another more cohesively.[16] The application of this model is explicated in Chapter 17 of this book.

Bereavement Care

Clinical responsibility does not stop with the death of the patient as the multidisciplinary team continues routinely to care for the relatives left bereaved by the loss. Major contributions to studies of grief and bereavement have been led by psychologists and psychiatrists specializing in this domain. The early work of Colin Murray Parkes at St Christopher's Hospice was a sterling contribution focused on *assumptive worlds*, that set of ideas and beliefs about the environment that people carry through transitional experiences in life. Development of acceptance of change was implicit in this work, and Murray Parkes, as a friend of John Bowlby, understood how the nature of attachments impacted upon the work of mourning by a bereaved person.

Holly Prigerson's Inventory of Complicated Grief has been used in a number of studies making sense of chronic grief, which may develop from a very close, interdependent relationship, or in circumstances of trauma, unexpected loss, or where ambivalent attachments have existed. Resultant therapeutic models matured by the psychiatrist, Katherine Shear, involve retelling the story of loss, cognitive restructuring, written exercises to increase exposure, and behavioral activation to resocialize the person.[17] Collaborative endeavor between psychiatry and palliative medicine has been paramount for the field of bereavement care to advance as it has.

When the Psychiatrist Is Needed in Palliative Care

The psychiatrist's contribution to palliative care spans the clinical domain with direct consultations, as well as contributing to education and research.

Clinical Care

While the potential contribution of the psychiatrist is extensive and related to most dimensions of palliative medicine, certain predicaments almost inevitably lead to a referral for psychiatric help. These include patient presentations of severe and treatment-resistant depression, pressing suicidal urges, panic or overwhelming anxiety, agitated and difficult to control delirium, complex pain, steroid-induced hypomania, and concerns about decision-making capacity. In Table 2.2, a summary of these circumstances is presented with reasons that the psychiatrist might be asked to help. The common predicaments are followed by a range of further reasons for the psychiatrist being consulted to assist in diagnosis, in making sense of complex psychodynamics so that a deeper understanding of the patient and family are achieved, and in developing care plans enriched by due attention to relevant psychosocial issues.

Ethical Conundrums

As medical aid in dying (MAID) has expanded internationally over the past decade, as discussed in Chapter 8 of this book, the role of the psychiatrist in the assessment of decision-making capacity is brought into sharper focus. Psychiatry has made its steady contribution here, well exemplified by the research of psychiatrists Appelbaum and Grisso, in validating a structured assessment tool, the MacArthur Competence Assessment Tool-Treatment (MacCAT-T), to assess treatment decisional capacity.[18] This interview assesses the patient's capacity to recall and understand their diagnoses and treatment options, reason about the risks and benefits of these options, appreciate their predicament and the consequences of any decision, and communicate this choice to those involved in their care. One systematic review identified 23 studies of decisional capacity in medical settings, where the weighted average prevalence of incapacity was 34% (95% CI: 25–44%), not statistically different to the prevalence of incapacity of 45% (95% CI: 39–51%) found across 35 studies in psychiatric settings.[19] No formal studies of capacity have been identified in end-of-life care.

In palliative care, where personal autonomy is a primary concern, human agency involves the exercise of freedom in self-governance to achieve competent control and the unencumbered intentionality as people initiate actions in their lives. In the mental state examination, the psychiatrist assesses agency by exploring judgment, insight, and cognition while excluding altered perceptions and delusions that mar reality.[20] Care is taken to understand any systemic influences on human decisions which could act as a tipping point for a patient's judgement. One technique is to make explicit any ambivalent tensions around a judgment and help the patient to work through such ambivalence. In the MacCAT-T studies, this has been described as the "Appreciation test," where an accurate understanding of prognosis alongside perception of the value and worth of future life is teased out and understood. The psychiatrist may play an important clinical role in not only assessing requests for physician aid in dying, but also in treating patients whose judgment is impaired by clinical depression or demoralization.

As the euthanasia debate is played out across countries, the question of the suffering of patients living with chronic mental illness has emerged in the Benelux countries, where

TABLE 2.2 Contributions of the psychiatrist to palliative care

Clinical issue	Presentations	Reasons for referral
COMMON PREDICAMENTS FOR PSYCHIATRIC REFERRAL		
Depression	Severe major depression Treatment-resistance Psychotic features Non-adherence to treatments	Diagnostic dilemmas Psychotropic medication advice Organic etiologies and drug interactions
Suicide	Incipient risk of suicide Suicidal plans Self-harm attempts	Assessment of risk Management advice Assessment of complexity
Panic and anxiety	Panic attacks Overwhelming anxiety Severe insomnia	Diagnostic and management advice
Delirium	Agitated delirium Treatment resistant or prolonged course Cognitive impairment	Diagnostic and management advice Drug interactions and serotonin syndrome
Hypomania	Steroid psychosis Treatment non-adherence	Diagnostic and management advice
Complex pain	Whole body pain Somatizing component to pain Difficult pain syndrome	Diagnostic assessment and understanding of the person Co-analgesic advice
Decision-making capacity	Medical aid in dying requests Treatment refusal Ethical dilemmas	Assessment of agency, judgement, insight, safety Medico-legal support
OCCASIONAL PREDICAMENTS FOR PSYCHIATRIC REFERRAL		
Chronic mental illness	Chronic schizophrenia Bipolar disorder Dementia care Disabled child of dying person	Diagnostic and management advice Medication advice Placement concerns
Substance use/abuse	Alcohol-related syndromes Substance dependence Opioid diversion	Diagnostic and management advice
Complex personalities	Communication difficulties Treatment non-adherence Relationship concerns	Understanding of the person Dealing with anger, conflict Family issues
Child and adolescent concerns	Preparation and talking about death Support needs	Management advice
Marital concerns	Relationship concerns Impact on care	Diagnostic and management advice
Family dysfunction	Communication difficulties Relationship and care concerns	Management advice Difficult family meetings
Ethical dilemmas	Competing care needs Decision-making capacity Domestic violence	Diagnostic and management advice
Complicated grief	Bereavement risk Risk of partner suicide	Management advice and support
Staff support	Burnout and compassion fatigue Debriefing re difficult death Staff conflict	Run staff groups

euthanasia has been granted for treatment-resistant depression, anorexia nervosa, autism, and personality disorder. One survey of Canadian psychiatrists found 71% were not supportive of MAID for mental illness, one telling reason being their prior experience of treating patients who would have qualified for MAID yet recovered fully from this condition.[21] The clinician makes an undeclared commitment to patients to sustain support for them through periods of suffering, thus serving as one source of hope through a time of despair. Such a commitment is invariably altered when physician aid in dying is permitted.

Education

Many opportunities exist for the psychiatrist to contribute educationally, whether through discussion in multidisciplinary team meetings or more formal didactic teaching sessions.

Training of interns, residents and registrars, fellows, and other members of the supportive care team are important to ensure that whole-person and family care can be practiced optimally. The notion of rotations through varied training programs, where the palliative medicine trainee undertakes a 6-month rotation through a psychiatry training post while the consultation-liaison psychiatry trainee spends a complementary 6-month rotation in a palliative medicine role is common in many countries.

Particular thought ought be given to psychotherapy supervision for palliative care clinicians, whether physicians, nurse practitioners or clinical nurse specialists, psychologists, or social workers: building skills in supportive models of counseling, cognitive reframing of negative cognitions, activity scheduling, and use of meaning-centered techniques is critical for anyone aspiring to become a competent clinician. The psychiatrist has a particular skill in providing supervision and technique development and helping supportive care clinicians to better understand these therapies. Training programs need to schedule such practices into the standard working week.

Research

While psycho-oncology research has made a major contribution to the development of the discipline of palliative care, the psychiatrist can also make regular, collaborative contributions to the systematic research conducted in palliative care. Appropriate use needs to be made of QoL, psychosocial, and spiritual measures in assessing outcomes for a range of supportive care studies, whether directed toward pain, nausea, fatigue, insomnia, or the full range of studies undertaken in the palliative medicine discipline.

Future Directions

As the field of palliative medicine continues to grow, with both earlier involvement in the illness trajectory and inclusion of categories of chronic illness alongside cancer, the role of the consultation-liaison psychiatrist remains essential in all these expanding settings. The psychiatrist can bring special expertise to clinical care, education, and research. This chapter has illustrated the extraordinary recent contribution that psychiatry has made to the development of interventions in the palliative setting, work that has expanded exponentially and whose momentum continues. Current research examining psilocybin-assisted therapy, as covered in Chapter 42 in this book, is another illustration of novel developments arising from our richer understanding of the biology of the brain. While research about pain receptors reveals vast complexity, so, too, does research that seeks to understand the human experience of suffering and how to respond psychotherapeutically. The quest to ameliorate human suffering requires an ever deeper understanding of the mind, that seat of consciousness which is quintessentially human and immeasurably complex in its nature.

Key Points

- Psychiatric practice brings many skills that are integral to palliative medicine and whole-person and family-centered care, which lie at the heart of ameliorating human suffering.
- Psychotherapy research has made a gigantic contribution to assuaging suffering through preserving dignity, sustaining meaning, and fostering connections and family support so that improved holistic care can be provided to the patient until death intervenes.
- Palliative medicine clinicians need great skill to guide patients from postures of existential vulnerability and distress to constructive adaptations that empower them to live life out fully.
- Basic aspects of psychiatric practice, such as the effective treatment of depression, anxiety, demoralization, delirium, and suicidal thinking, are critical to the humane conduct of palliative medicine.
- The psychiatrist forms a key and appropriate member of the supportive care team; his absence depletes the quality of care delivery substantially.
- When doubt develops about the value and worth of life, the psychiatrist is best placed to assess, support, and treat patients to sustain their hope and interest in human flourishing.

References

1. Kissane DW. Jimmie C. Holland, MD (1928–2017): A remarkable woman in medicine and cancer care. *Psycho-Oncology*. 2018 May;27(5):1377–1378. https://doi.org/10.1002/pon.4693
2. Rayner L, Price A, Evans A, Valsraj K, Higginson IJ, Hotopf M. Antidepressants for depression in physically ill people. *Cochrane Database Syst Rev*. 2010 Mar;(3):CD007503. https://doi.org/10.1002/14651858. CD007503.pub2
3. Grassi L, Caraceni A, Mitchell AJ, Nanni MG, Berardi MA, Caruso R, et al. Management of delirium in palliative care: A review. *Curr Psychiatry Rep*. 2015 Mar;17(3):550. https://doi.org/10.1007/s11 920-015-0550-8
4. Hegel MT, Collins ED, Kearing S, Gillock KL, Moore CP, Ahles TA. Sensitivity and specificity of the Distress Thermometer for depression in newly diagnosed breast cancer patients. *Psycho-Oncology*. 2008 Jun;17(6):556–560. https://doi.org/10.1002/pon.1289
5. Kissane DW. Education and assessment of psycho-existential symptoms to prevent suicidality in cancer care. *Psycho-Oncology*. 2020 Aug;29(9):1–4. https://doi.org/10.1002/pon.5519
6. Yalom ID. *Existential Psychotherapy*. New York: Basic Books; 1980.
7. Kissane DW. The relief of existential suffering. *Arch Intern Med*. 2012 Oct;172(19):1501–1505. https://doi.org/10.1001/archinternmed.2012.3633

8. Chochinov HM. Dignity-conserving care: A new model for palliative care: Helping the patient feel valued. *JAMA*. 2002;287:2253–2260. https://doi.org/10.1001/jama.287.17.2253

9. Chochinov HM, Kristjanson LJ, Breitbart W, McClement S, Hack TF, Hassard T, et al. The effect of dignity therapy on distress and end-of-life experience in terminally ill patients: A randomised controlled trial. *Lancet Oncol*. 2011 Aug;12(8):753–762. https://doi.org/10.1016/S1470-2045(11)70153-X

10. Breitbart W, Pessin H, Rosenfeld B, Applebaum AJ, Lichtenthal WG, Li Y, et al. Individual Meaning-Centered Psychotherapy for the treatment of psychological and existential distress: A randomized controlled trial in patients with advanced cancer. *Cancer*. 2018 Aug;24(15):3231–3239. https://doi.org/10.1002/cncr.31539

11. Breitbart W, Rosenfeld B, Pessin H, Applebaum A, Kulikowski J, Lichtenthal WG. Meaning-Centered Group Psychotherapy: An effective intervention for improving psychological well-being in patients with advanced cancer. *J Clin Oncol*. 2015 Mar; 33(7):749–754. https://doi.org/10.1200/JCO.2014.57.2198

12. Spiegel D, Classen C. *Group Therapy for Cancer Patients. A Research-Based Handbook of Psychosocial Care*. New York: Basic books, 2000.

13. Beatty L, Kemp E, Butow P, Girgris A, Schofield P, Turner J, et al. A systematic review of psychotherapeutic interventions for women with metastatic breast cancer: context matters. *Psycho-Oncology*. 2018;27:34–42. https://doi.org/10.1002/pon.4445

14. Rodin G, Lo C, Rydall A, et al. Managing Cancer and Living Meaningfully (CALM): A randomized controlled trial of a psychological intervention for patients with advanced cancer. *J Clin Oncol*. 2018 Aug;36(23):2422–2432. https://doi.org/10.1200/JCO.2017.77.1097

15. Kissane DW, McKenzie M, Bloch S, Moskowitz C, McKenzie DP, O'Neill I. Family focused grief therapy: A randomized controlled trial in palliative care and bereavement. *Am J Psychiatry*. 2006 Jul;163(7):1208–1218. https://doi.org/10.1176/appi.ajp.163.7.1208

16. Kissane DW, Zaider TI, Li Y, Hichenberg S, Schuler T, Lederberg M, et al. Randomized controlled trial of family therapy in advanced cancer continued into bereavement. *J Clin Oncol*. 2016 Jun;34:1921–1927. https://doi.org/10.1200/JCO.2015.63.0582

17. Shear K, Wang Y, Skritskaya N, Duan N, Mauro C, Ghesquiere A. Treatment of complicated grief in elderly persons: a randomized clinical trial. *JAMA Psychiatry*. 2014;71(11):1287–1295. https://doi.org/10.1001/jamapsychiatry.2014.1242

18. Grisso T, Appelbaum PS, Hill-Fotouhi C. The MacCAT-T: A clinical tool to assess patients' capacities to make treatment decisions. *Psychiatric Services*. 1997;48(11):1415–1419. https://doi.org/10.1176/ps.48.11.1415

19. Lepping P, Stanly T, Turner J. Systematic review on the prevalence of lack of capacity in medical and psychiatric settings. *Clin Med (Lond)*. 2015 Aug;15(4):337–343. https://doi.org/10.7861/clinmedicine.15-4-337

20. Mendz GL, Kissane DW. Agency, autonomy and euthanasia. *J Law Med Ethics*. 2020 Sep;48(3):555–564. https://doi.org/10.1177/1073110520958881

21. Rousseau S, Turner S, Chochinov HM, Enns MW, Sareen J. A national survey of Canadian psychiatrists' attitudes toward medical assistance in death. *Can J Psychiatry*. 2017 Nov;62(11):787–794. https://doi.org/10.1177/0706743717711174

3

Healing and Whole-Person Care

Tom A. Hutchinson and Nora Hutchinson

Introduction

In 1967, Dr Cicely Saunders opened St. Christopher's Hospice and set the modern model for the care of the dying. Saunders was benefitting from a long history of religious institutions providing care in hospices for dying patients and indeed had worked at St. Joseph's Hospice in London, run by the Irish Sisters of Charity, before she opened St. Christopher's.[1] Her innovation was to combine the excellent spiritual care aimed at healing provided in hospices since medieval times with evidence-based medicine. The combination of modern medicine aimed at cure or control of symptoms and deep personal care aimed at the promotion of healing[2] is whole-person care,[3] the topic of this chapter. Since care as envisaged by Saunders and subsequently developed by Mount and Kearney was the origin of modern whole-person care,[4] it might seem unnecessary to discuss this topic in a book focused on psychiatry in palliative medicine. However, there are both opportunities and challenges created by combining curing and healing that need to be lived out in the day-to-day practice of palliative medicine, which can make a profound difference to the lives of patients with life-threatening illness and have the potential to transform the practice of medicine at all levels of care.[5] We will discuss the topic under the following five headings: the process of healing, curing and healing, institutions and whole-person care, mindful clinical congruence, and the new medical professional and whole-person care.

The Process of Healing

Healing is a move toward a sense of wholeness or integrity that comes from within the patient but can be facilitated by a healthcare practitioner.[2] This sounds like a fairly straightforward linear process that should be relatively easy to observe and support. However, this is not the case because healing is a complex rather than a complicated process and the trajectory is not in one direction (toward integrity and wholeness) but more of a roller coaster ride.[6] In a complicated process we have a detailed plan which we follow step by step to achieve the desired final product or outcome. In a complex process there is no predictable blueprint and it is the moment-to-moment relationships that determine how the process unfolds. The metaphor for the distinction between a complex versus complicated process is the difference between raising a child and sending a rocket to the moon.[7] Healing is more like the complex process of raising a child. This makes most of the usual questions about a process difficult to answer for healing.

For instance, the question "When does healing begin?" is only possible to answer in retrospect, after we have seen the process unfold. This is very important because it means we should treat every moment as the potential start of healing, as in some sense it is or can be. So, when I go to see a patient in a palliative care setting, I should be asking myself what appears to be important to this patient today rather than how can I move this person in a particular direction. The direction and timing of healing comes from the patient. For one person the start of healing might mean refusing to see a family member who has wounded them in the past. For another patient it might mean forgiving and connecting with that family member. And only in retrospect would we be able to see whether the step taken was the beginning of a healing process. This is challenging for healthcare workers who are used to a plan and a defined direction of care. A commitment to healing demands a level of acceptance and openness that is unfamiliar.

The difficulties continue. If we take Joseph Campbells trajectory of the hero's journey as the template for healing,[6] it is actually impossible to know where on that journey the patient is. Campbell outlines various stages: the call, refusal of the call, the descent, the belly of the whale, the ascent, the return. We have described these stages in more detail elsewhere.[6] But those things are also only recognizable in retrospect. The value in the inclusion of healing in the work of palliative care comes from recognizing that there is such a natural process, that this is a process that comes from within the patient, and that the healthcare team's presence and support makes a profound difference in the healing process.

The different stages of the healing journey do provide a context for different understanding and potentially different interventions in the care of palliative patients. For instance, the call and refusal of the call probably describes the very frequent experience with many patients who, on one day, appear to accept that they are dying and need to let go and, on the next day, appear to have an opposite perspective. The descent after acceptance of the call describes many patients' experience that, after being happy with the decision to forego further treatment to control disease and possibly be admitted to a palliative care unit, they now feel overwhelmed and confronted by the full implications of their decision. The "belly of the whale" may describe the lack of meaning that some patients experience in the dying process.[8] The ascent and giving back probably mainly relates to patients' longing for dignity and desire for a legacy.[9] The purpose is not to place patients at a particular stage in the healing journey or push them forward on that journey, but to offer kindness, presence, and support to the patient in what they are experiencing and what appears to be most important to them in this moment, trusting that, regardless of the situation, there is a potential for healing and that we can make a difference in that process. What is required of us in this process is very different from what is needed when our primary focus is to cure or control disease, as will be evident in the section that follows.

Healing and Curing

Curing is a diametrically different process from healing. Curing is an action carried out by a healthcare practitioner to eradicate a disease or correct a problem.[10] It is a simple or complicated process directed by a physician or a healthcare team. The energy for curing comes primarily from outside the patient. Curing often has a clear objective, which can range from controlling symptoms to eradicating disease, and it can often be assessed or measured. It is important to note that curing is usually why patients seek the help of a healthcare practitioner, and this extends to the end of life, where the patient's and the family's main initial concern will often be primarily the control of symptoms.

Table 3.1 outlines the characteristics of curing and healing from different perspectives. At every point, what is required for curing and healing is radically different. For instance,

TABLE 3.1 Curing and healing: Contrasting and synergistic

	Curing	Healing
PATIENT		
Problem	Symptoms or dysfunction	Suffering
Possibility	Control or cure	Healing
Action	Holding on	Letting go
Goal	Survival	Growth
Self-image	At the effect of disease	Responsible for coping
CLINICIAN		
Focus	Disease or symptom	Person with illness
Communication	Content	Relationship
	Digital	Analogue
	Conscious	Unconscious
Power	Power differential	Power sharing
Presence	Competent technician	Wounded healer
Epistemology	Scientific	Artistic
Management	Standardized	Individualized
Process	Simple or complicated	Complex
Reflection	Thinking, Doing, Reflexivity	Being
Framing	Problem to be solved	Mystery to be lived
Wisdom	Practical	Existential
Linear steps	Many[a]	Few[b]

[a]Even when the steps appear few, as in prescribing antibiotics for an infection, there are many preliminary steps leading up to the final decision: steps in the development of the antibiotic, steps in the collection and publishing of evidence for its use, consulting the relevant guidelines, and so on.

[b]Facilitating healing, because it is a complex phenomenon, does not consist of sequential linear steps[7] but the presence necessary to nurture relationship at each stage in the process.[6]

in curing the patient is holding on; in healing the need is to let go. In curing the doctor's main communication is about content; in healing the healthcare worker needs to communicate relationship. And so on for every topic in Table 3.1. Something else is evident from the table. At every point, these diametrically opposed foci are synergistic. If I as a patient perceive that you are expert in the content of my problem, for instance pain control, I will feel more secure in entering into a relationship with you. At the same time, if I perceive you to be an empathic person with whom I want to be in relationship, I will be more likely to listen to you and follow your advice. This means that, as a healthcare practitioner and team, we need to be able to bring these two very different aspects of care to our patient. One might ask whether this is requiring too much. We believe not.

As whole persons we have the capacity to transcend the specifics of the problem that the patient may be experiencing and be present in a way that allows new possibilities to emerge. This means that we need to bring a reflective aspect to our care. Kinsella divides reflection into four kinds[11]: reflective thinking focused on solving problems within a clearly defined framework (as in a homework exercise or an exam question); reflective doing aimed at bringing practical wisdom to a problem in a real-life context (phronesis); reflexivity, the ability to see what lies before us in a wide social context; and reflective being, the ability to bring our full presence as a whole person to our interaction with the whole person of the patient.

An example of a patient with pain may clarify the differences. Reflective thinking is the process that allows us to give a satisfactory answer to the question: "What is the next step in modification of the medication prescription in a patient who is on 5 mg of morphine sc every 4 hours and using 4 breakthrough doses between every regular dose?" It is the kind of problem that could be posed and answered in an exam question to medical students or residents. Reflective doing is adapting this problem-solving skill to the real world. This patient and his family may be scared of morphine and opioids, worry that the patient will become addicted, and resistant to increasing the regular dose. There may also be a strong element of anxiety and total pain that is driving the frequent request for breakthrough doses. Perhaps what is needed at this point is not a new prescription but a more in-depth conversation with the patient and the family about pain control. Reflexivity means putting the problem in a wider context. This patient is part of a religious group which feels that suffering has value and is perhaps a message from God. Strong efforts to control the pain may be seen as going against God's will. And finally, reflective being is the ability to put aside all of our internal reactions and possible prejudices in order to be fully with this patient, to empathize with their perspective—put part of ourselves in their shoes—and be open to what emerges. We need to bring all of these four reflective skills to the bedside. Perhaps the most challenging, and the most important in facilitating the other kinds of reflection, is reflective being. It is easy to see this as a need to listen deeply and be patient for what emerges, but there is also an element of creativity and agency that this form of reflection makes possible.

I was leading a family meeting for a man in his 40s who was dying of colon cancer. The patient was delirious and not part of the meeting. He was an immigrant to Canada, and his family had come from another country to be with their dying son. They were a couple in their 70s who did not speak English. The meeting was conducted with another physician translating. The family were accompanied by some friends from Montreal. Also at the meeting, and one of the main reasons for getting together, was the patient's girlfriend. She was from Montreal and greatly resented by the patient's parents. She was also accompanied by some friends. The two groups were at opposite ends of the room.

There was a serious problem because the patient's parents did not want his girlfriend visiting the patient. She had been very close to the patient and supportive of him during his illness, but the family did not know about her until they came to Montreal. The girlfriend was unhappy, the parents were unhappy, and a conversation about the patient's illness was doing nothing to bring the two sides together.

I realized that nothing I had done so far was working. I needed to step back and see what emerged. I made a speech. I said that we were in the presence of a tragedy. A young man was dying prematurely from cancer with weeks and possibly days to live. But, I said, an even greater tragedy was that the people who were most important to him and loved him most were unable to come together and be at his bedside together in a way that he needed. There was a moment of silence. His girlfriend stood up, walked across the room, and extended her hand to the patient's mother. His mother took the hand, and the group in the room broke into spontaneous applause. It was a pivotal change in their relationship which meant there was no further conflict between the two sides. The parents felt comfortable enough to leave the patient in the care of his girlfriend and returned to their country the following week.

An important point about reflective being and the ways forward it may make possible is that there is no one right approach. For a different person, or at a slightly different time, a completely different approach might have worked as well or better. This is a creative process, no prescription is possible, and yet who we are and who we can bring to the care of the patient is key to the delivery of whole person care. The elements involved in this process are clarified in the last three lines of Table 3.1.

In Table 3.1, the framing of care, the wisdom that is relevant, and the steps involved are given in the last three lines. Framing care as both a problem to be solved and a mystery to be lived combines a practical focus with openness to a much larger context that is particularly relevant to palliative care. On the one hand, this patient has a difficult problem with, for instance, shortness of breath, to which I want to bring all of my medical knowledge and practical wisdom to solve. At the same time, staying aware of the widest possible context, that this patient is dying, that I too will die, opens the mind to the insoluble mystery of life and death and calls on me as a caregiver to be present to this mystery and this person. My experience of this wider awareness is that it has the effect of calmness and moment-to-moment exquisite focus. Everything peripheral drops away and there is nothing but being with this person, right here, right now. In Table 3.1 we have called what becomes available with this wider awareness *existential wisdom*. Jacob Needleman would call it releasing the higher energies of the human mind,[12] which is what is necessary to transcend the polarities of curing and healing in order to provide whole-person care to the patient. The last line of the table points out a final contrast that is of key importance in promoting both curing and healing. Curing is an inherently complicated process that requires multiple steps that need to be followed, usually in a specific order. Knowing such steps and how to complete them is a large part of professional competence. Healing on the other hand is complex, and, surprisingly, this means that the steps required are relatively limited and simple. An example would be the S.T.O.P. technique often promoted in courses on mindfulness. The acronym stands for: Stop, Take a breath, Observe, Proceed. This and other simple slogans and reminders are very helpful to keep us in relationship with ourselves and the patient as the process of healing unfolds.

Institutions and Whole-Person Care

When Saunders combined the focus on healing of traditional hospices with the curative evidence-based approach of modern medicine, she created whole-person care for the dying. To implement her new approach she housed it in a new kind of institution, a modern hospice called St. Christopher's, which became a model for hospices around the world. This brought with it challenges to the healing side of whole-person care. She may have foreseen some of these challenges. She originally envisaged that St. Christopher's would be run by a kind of lay religious ministry, and she planned that the institution would include long-term care patients, avoiding a narrow focus on patients who were actively dying.[13] Both of these ideas fell away in the hospice that she eventually created. The hospice that she founded left unresolved some of the natural tensions between curing and healing and added the pressure for efficiency that most institutions are forced to impose. This was not a bad thing, but maintaining the appropriate balance between efficiency and the requirements for healing care is an ongoing challenge.

When Balfour Mount moved the locus of palliative care from free-standing hospices to units within a general hospital, he widened the availability of care, as he intended[14] and, at the same time, increased further the tension between healing and efficiency. Efficiency is an important objective to be promoted on the curative side of medicine, where measurable outcomes can appropriately be compared with the costs expended to achieve those goals of care. A focus on efficiency works less well on the healing side of medicine, where results are difficult to measure and an emphasis on efficiency can affect the well-being of both patients and staff.

The tensions created by a focus on efficiency play out on a daily basis in the delivery of care in palliative units. With the increasing dominance of top-down management of healthcare in Canada and other countries[15] the balance has shifted heavily toward efficiency. This affects the delivery of whole-person care in multiple ways, but perhaps some simple examples will make the point.

One example is the focus in hospitals generally, including their palliative care units, on length of stay. The average length of stay in the palliative care unit where I worked was 10 to 12 days, which is similar to some other such units in Canada.[16] Patients were admitted to the unit at the very terminal stage in their illness and were expected to die within a week or two. This was not necessarily bad, although it did create a very short time frame to facilitate healing and meant that the care team dealt with recurrent very short-term relationships that may have been taxing over the long term. This was probably part of what Cicely Saunders was originally trying to avoid by including long-stay patients in her hospice. The problem was compounded when patients did not die in the allotted time, as happened relatively frequently. What followed when the patient was still alive after 2 weeks or so was that the team, concerned about efficiency and length of stay, began to explore the transfer of the patient to another institution and had corresponding conversations with the patient and family. As can be imagined, these were not easy conversations. Usually, the patient was very appreciative of the care she was receiving, had adjusted to the unit and the staff, and may even have attributed her continued survival to the excellent care in the palliative care unit. The thought of another transfer in this final phase of her life was very painful and threatening. However sensitively the conversations were conducted, the result was often wounding (a move away from integrity and wholeness) for both patient and caregivers.

The overall concern with efficiency, which focuses primarily on tangible inputs and outputs, values doing over being. This becomes more problematic the more interventions on the curative side of medicine become part of palliative care. For instance, it is now common for some patients to continue to receive "palliative chemotherapy" in palliative care units and intravenous fluids that used to be rare. Other changes that involve additional tasks for palliative care staff and nurses have followed. These are not in themselves bad changes, and they often fit with the wishes of patients and families, but they do create serious challenges for the healthcare team. If the facilitation of healing primarily requires a way of being, which is very difficult to measure, a system focused on efficiency may displace the time and space necessary for whole-person care. This may manifest as a nurse being sure to check the IV when she enters a patient's room but forgetting to touch the patient or sit down by the patient's bedside. To adequately encompass whole-person care and the healing side of medicine will require a profound shift in the overall philosophy of care that we have begun to teach at McGill University.

Mindful Clinical Congruence

Over the past 15 years we have developed and taught an approach to clinical relationships based on the work of John Kabat Zinn[17] on mindfulness and Virginia Satir on congruent relationships.[18] This curricular development began with the vision of Balfour Mount and Michael Kearney who saw that healing, which they recognized was central to the care of very sick and dying patients,[2] was important at all phases of medical care.[4] In order to reincorporate healing into the medical mandate Mount started Programs in Whole-Person Care at McGill in 1999,[19] to reincorporate healing into all aspects of medical care and teach whole-person care to all medical students at McGill.

We have given more detail on the curriculum that we teach elsewhere,[20] but, for our purposes in this chapter, we will outline the main conceptual framework that guides our teaching. When a patient comes to see a doctor or other healthcare professional at any level of care from primary care for a minor illness to palliative care in terminal illness, there is normally one question that is uppermost in the patient's mind: What is the problem? The first step in caring for a patient is usually diagnosing what is wrong and separating the disease or problem from the patient. The diagnosis could be the identification of a disease, like a cancer for instance, or pin-pointing the reason a particular prescription for pain control is not working. The result depicted in the upper left section of Figure 3.1 is a triangle in which the clinician has two therapeutic relationships: her relationship to the disease, where her job is to cure or control, and the relationship to the person of the patient where her job is to facilitate healing.

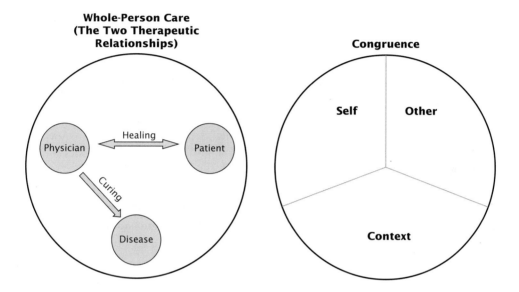

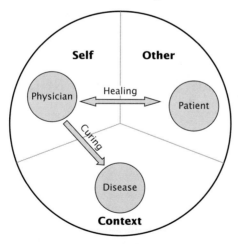

The awareness that arises from paying attention, on purpose and nonjudgmentally, to ourselves, the patient, and the clinical context, in the present moment as it unfolds from moment to moment.

FIGURE 3.1 Whole-person care and mindful clinical congruence.

Mindful clinical congruence allows the healthcare worker to address both curing and healing simultaneously. Congruence, from the work of Virginia Satir,[18] is the ability to remain present to oneself as a person, to the other person as a person, and to the context, shown in the right upper section of Figure 3.1. The context in clinical congruence, shown in the lower section of Figure 3.1, is the particular clinical situation and problem with which we are faced in this interaction. Maintaining clinical congruence is not an easy task, particularly under stress, because, as Satir has pointed out, we automatically adopt limiting communication stances that leave out one or more pieces in the interaction.[21] She described four communication stances: *placating,* in which we leave ourselves out of the relationship; *blaming,* where we leave out the other person; *super-reasonable,* where we leave both ourselves and the other person out as persons and become a pure problem solver; and the *distracting* stance, where we lose touch with ourselves, the other person, and the context. Mindful clinical congruence, shown in the lower section of Figure 3.1, allows us to attend to and become aware of our automatic responses, to notice what we are leaving out, and to make a choice about replacing the missing part with the aim of being clinically congruent. In principle this is a fairly straightforward process, but it requires all of our resources as human beings to enact mindful clinical congruence in stressful clinical situations.

We believe that medicine, particularly in the palliative care context, has an underutilized resource that can make the necessary kind of deep presence to self, other, and clinical context possible. Palliative care, because it deals directly with death and dying, provides a very powerful access to the deepest level of our being. It is not an accident that the recognition of healing as central to healthcare came out of palliative care and that whole-person care originated from the same source. The key element is awareness of death that can either push us into defensive mechanisms if we attempt to deny it or ignore it or open us up to the deepest level of ourselves if we are willing to face and acknowledge death openly.[22] This is the possibility that palliative care opens up, which, we believe, can make it not just another specialty but the seed for the transformation of healthcare.[23]

The New Medical Professional and Whole-Person Care

What will it take to bring mindful clinical congruence and whole-person care to our interactions with patients, not just in palliative medicine but in healthcare across the board? Such a change will require a major shift in how we conceptualize medical care and our work as medical professionals.[24] We need to see healing as the bedrock of our practice. The curing content of our care becomes the important context in which healing takes place. Such a change is already under way with the promotion of relationship-centered care and healing at large medical centers in the United States, including the Cleveland Clinic.[25] Parker Palmer, who has championed a similar reorientation in the context of teaching, has proposed the following: in our interaction with another person what matters most is not only *what* we do, *how* we do it, or *why* we do what we do, but *who* we bring to each interaction.[26] To relate to our patients as whole persons, which we believe is what is required, as medical professionals we will need to learn how to use our full selves in our work.

We realize that such a change will need to occur within a system that continues to value the ability of medicine to fix and cure problems and organizational structures that value efficiency in the delivery of care. These are important objectives but have been pursued to an extent that has affected the balance of medical practice. In another context, that of industrial production, it has been pointed out that a single-minded pursuit of efficiency has a detrimental effect on the resilience of the workforce.[27] We believe that what has been described as an epidemic of burnout in physicians may be evidence of the same effect in healthcare.[28] We are suggesting a new overall framework for healthcare practice that creates space for healing and the one-on-one relationships that allow us to synergize the power of curing and healing for our patients. When we lose the depth and flexibility of those relationships, we damage both ourselves and those who receive care.

I recall a man in his 80s who had been a volunteer in the palliative care unit before he became ill. He had been admitted to the internal medicine service for investigation of progressive weight loss and weakness. After an extensive and exhausting workup that had not yet revealed a diagnosis, he had requested an admission to the palliative care unit to die. His wish was no more tests. When he arrived in palliative care he had lost a lot of weight, was so weak he could barely stand, and did appear to be dying. This was accepted by the doctor who admitted him, and the team began devoting itself to the patient's care and comfort. This changed when the first doctor went on vacation and a new doctor asked "What is the diagnosis?" Since there was no clear answer, he ordered more tests, which the patient at first refused. The team began to doubt how sick the patient really was and whether he really belonged on the palliative care unit. Plans were made to transfer him back to internal medicine, and, under this pressure, the patient did submit to more tests. No definitive diagnosis emerged, but the patient deteriorated and died a little over a week after the new doctor had taken over his care. Neither palliative care nor internal medicine provided the haven that this patient needed.

In this example it is not hard to guess that what that 80-year-old man longed for was probably be to loved, acknowledged, and cared for (possibly in the way that he had provided care for patients as a volunteer) as he entered the last phase of his life. What would have been necessary to provide the kind of care he needed would have been to connect with him at that deep level by using our own longings and yearnings to put part of ourselves in his shoes. That is the level that empathy needs to reach in order to connect us, whole person to whole person. This does not mean that we need to accede to the patient's expectations, agree with his perceptions, share his emotions, or act as he would like us to act, but it does connect us in a way that is deeply nurturing for both of us and makes space for unexpected development.

What we are talking about, however daunting and counter-cultural it may seem, is connecting the soul of the clinician with the soul of the patient. It may be worth remembering that the original meaning of "psychiatry" was "care of the soul." Parker Palmer, who has done so much work to align the souls of individual teachers with their role as guides to the next generation, has pointed out that the soul is like a wild animal: resilient, resourceful, able to survive and thrive in difficult circumstances, and easily startled and frightened off.[29] He points out that if we want to catch a glimpse of a wild animal we do not go crashing through the woods, but must wait patiently and silently. It is that kind of quiet patience and gentleness, combined with clarity and commitment, that we need to bring to our care if we wish to connect at a soul level. It is important to realize that although we are each responsible for making space for our own souls, we need communities to support that space. We believe that it was just such trusting and nurturing environments that the founders of the modern hospice and palliative care movements were committed to creating.[13,30] We need to find more and better ways to create such supportive groups because we believe that the future of healthcare requires the kind of soul-to-soul relationships that heal both patients and those who deliver care.

How will such an approach to healthcare enlarge and prosper? Can the inner lives of clinicians and patients change the outer lives of healthcare institutions? As we have alluded to, there are challenges but also opportunities and openings. In the long run we believe that whole-person care will and must succeed. It is our inner resources as human beings that are the greatest gifts that we can contribute to the ongoing endeavor to provide the best possible care to our patients.

Key Points

The big challenge, in a system which has become increasingly busy and focused on efficiency as judged by measurable outcomes, is to make space and time for healing in all aspects of healthcare, including palliative medicine. We would suggest the following possible approaches:

- Focusing on individual healthcare practitioners, we should develop and teach an approach to care that treats healing as an essential component of healthcare to all clinical workers. We have begun this approach with our teaching of medical students at McGill, but analogous, and possibly different, approaches to meet the same objective need to be taught and promoted more widely in Canada and elsewhere.
- Focusing on the system within which individual healthcare practitioners work, we need a reflective process that openly acknowledges our current difficulties and suggests practical ways to promote a system that gives practitioners the space and time to promote healing. We believe this will both benefit patients and will address the current major problem of clinician burnout.
- One outcome of such a reflective process in Canada would be to have the facilitation of healing included as one of the Royal College of Physicians and Surgeons of Canada Can Meds roles (a set of nationally defined core competencies for Canadian physicians).
- The overall objective would be to start to heal the healthcare system itself, which will require changing the relationships between individuals within the system to create communities of trust that will make space for the whole persons of both patients and healthcare workers.

- A research program must be developed that aims to evaluate some of the above initiatives and uncovers new avenues for the development and dissemination of whole-person care.

References

1. Clark D. Working at St Joseph's Hospice Hackney. In: *Cicely Saunders: Selected Writings 1958–2004.* New York: Oxford University Press; 2006:57–60.
2. Mount B, Kearney M. Healing and palliative care: Charting our way forward. *Palliat Med.* 2003;17:657–658.
3. Hutchinson TA, Hutchinson N, Arnaert A. Whole person care: Encompassing the two faces of medicine. *CMAJ.* 2009;180(8):845–846.
4. Hutchinson TA. Whole person care. In: Hutchinson TA, ed. *Whole Person Care: A New Paradigm for the 21st Century.* New York: Springer Science+Business; 2011:1–8.
5. Hutchinson TA. *Whole Person Care. Transforming Healthcare.* Cham: Springer International; 2017.
6. Hutchinson TA. Healing. In: Hutchinson TA, ed. *Whole Person Care: Transforming Healthcare.* Switzerland: Springer International Publishing; 2017:21–28.
7. Westley F, Zimmerman B, Patton MQ, The first light of evening. In: Zimmerman WF, Westley F, Patton MD, eds. *Getting to Maybe: How the World is Changed.* Toronto: Vintage Canada; 2007:3–26.
8. Kissane DW, Clarke DM, Street AF. Demoralization syndrome: A relevant psychiatric diagnosis for palliative care. *J Palliat Care.* 2001;17:12–21.
9. Chochinov HM, McKeen NA. Dignity therapy. In: Watson M, Kissane D, eds. *Handbook of Psychotherapy in Cancer Care.* Chichester: John Wiley & Sons; 2011:79–88.
10. Cassell EJ. Prologue: a time for healing. In: *The Healer's Art.* Cambridge MA: The MIT Press; 1976:1–8.
11. Kinsella EA. Practitioner reflection and judgment as phronesis: a continuum of reflection and considerations for phronetic judgement. In: Kinsella EA, Pitman A, eds. *Phronesis as Professional Knowledge: Practical Wisdom in the Professions.* Rotterdam: Sense Publishing; 2012:35–52.
12. Needleman J. Attention. In: Needleman J, ed. *The Way of the Physician.* London: Arkana; 1992:38–54.
13. Clark D. St Christopher's Hospice. In: Clark D, ed. *Cicely Saunders. Selected Writings 1958–2004.* New York: Oxford University Press; 2006:115–118.
14. Mount B. The needs of the dying. In: *Ten Thousand Crossroads: The Path as I Remember It.* Montreal and Kingston: McGill-Queen's University Press; 2020:197–223.
15. Laberge M, Gaudreault M. Promoting access to family medicine in Quebec, Canada: analysis of Bill 20, enacted November 2015. *Health Policy.* 2019;123:901–905.
16. Hausner D, Kevork N, Pope A, Hannon B, Bryson J, Lau J, et al. Factors associated with discharge disposition on an acute palliative care unit. *Support Care Cancer.* 2018;26:3951–3958.
17. Kabat-Zinn J. Introduction: stress, pain, and illness: facing the full catastrophe. In: *Full Catastrophe Living: Using the Wisdom of Your Body and Mind to Face Stress, Pain, and Illness.* New York: Delta; 1990:1–14.
18. Satir V, Banmen J, Gerber J, Gomori M. Congruence. In: *The Satir Model: Family Therapy and Beyond.* Palo Alto: Science and Behavior Books; 1991:65–84.
19. Hutchinson TA. A brief recapitulation of medical history in six movements. In: Hutchinson TA, ed. *Whole Person Care: Transforming Healthcare.* Cham: Springer International; 2017:11–20.
20. Hutchinson TA. Whole person care for medical students. In: Hutchinson TA, ed. *Whole Person Care: Transforming Healthcare.* Cham: Springer International; 2017:73–84.
21. Satir V, Banmen J, Gerber J, Gomori M. The survival stances. In: *The Satir Model: Family Therapy and Beyond.* Palo Alto: Science and Behavior Books; 1991:31–64.
22. Solomon S, Lawlor K. Death anxiety: the challenge and the promise of Whole Person Care. In: Hutchinson TA, ed. *Whole Person Care: A New Paradigm for the 21st Century.* New York: Springer; 2011:97–108.
23. Kearney M. Palliative medicine – just another specialty? *Palliat Med.* 1992;6:39–46.

24. Hutchinson TA, Smilovitch M. Experiential learning and reflection to support professionalism and professional identity formation. In: Cruess RL, Cruess SR, Steinert Y, eds. *Teaching Medical Professionalism. Supporting the Development of a Professional Identity.* 2nd ed. New York: Cambridge University Press; 2016:97–112.

25. Cosgrove T. Care should be a healing experience for body and mind. In: *The Cleveland Clinic Way: Lessons in Excellence from One of the World's Leading Healthcare Organizations.* New York: McGraw-Hill Education; 2014:109–131.

26. Palmer PJ. Introduction: teaching from within. In: *The Courage to Teach: Exploring the Inner Landscape of a Teacher's Life.* San Francisco: Jossey-Bass; 2017:1–8.

27. Martin RL. Introduction: a system out of balance. In: *When More Is Not Better: Overcoming America's Obsession with Economic Efficiency.* Boston: Harvard Business School Publishing; 2020:1–17.

28. West CP, Dyrbye LN, Erwin PJ, Shanafelt TD. Interventions to prevent and reduce physician burnout: a systematic review and meta-analysis. *Lancet.* 2016;388:2272–2281.

29. Palmer PJ. Being alone together: a community of solitudes. In: *A Hidden Wholeness: The Journey Toward an Undivided Life: Welcoming the Soul and Weaving Community in a Wounded World.* San Francisco: Jossey-Bass; 2008:51–69.

30. Mount B. First steps. In: *Ten Thousand Crossroads: The Path as I Remember It.* Montreal and Kingston: McGill-Queen's University Press; 2020:256–303.

PART II

Psychiatric Complications of Terminal Illness

4

Diagnosis and Management of Depression in Palliative Care

Nathan Fairman and Scott A. Irwin

Introduction

A commonly held assumption holds that any person with a serious, progressive, life-limiting illness, especially as they near death, must be depressed. This false notion does harm in two ways: first, it obscures the reality that the final period of life may be filled with meaning and purpose, with the possibilities of deepened intimacy in relationships and with transformative personal growth. Second, it draws away attention from the suffering of the *minority* of individuals who *do* experience serious clinical depression as life comes to a close. This chapter focuses on identifying and responding to clinical depression in palliative care settings and near the end of life.

Depression is the leading cause of mental health-related disability worldwide, affecting nearly 300 million people.[1] On a personal level, depression is a profoundly painful experience, with serious physical, emotional, and interpersonal consequences. It robs patients of the ability to experience joy and pleasure; it creates feelings of worthlessness and meaninglessness; it causes profound distress for family and friends; it can worsen physical symptoms and response to disease treatment; and it even has the power to make death itself appealing.

Among patients with serious illness, feelings of depression are common, and they exist on a continuum, ranging from transient feelings of sadness to unrelenting, debilitating impairments in mood, cognition, and judgment that are the hallmarks of a major depressive disorder (MDD; clinical depression). In palliative care settings, the experience of depression is often compounded by burdensome physical symptoms, diminished independence, fear of death, loss of purpose and meaning, anticipatory grief, spiritual crisis, and strained relationships.

While improving, clinicians and caregivers still often overlook the impact of psychological symptoms in patients with serious illness or dismiss them as normal or expected experiences. As with other dimensions of suffering in these individuals, when symptoms of depression are left unaddressed, patients and families may suffer tremendously—through the final stages of life as well as during family bereavement.

Fortunately, many interventions have been shown to alleviate clinical depression in the palliative care setting. As such, prompt identification and effective management of depression is a critical function of the palliative care provider as it can greatly improve outcomes and enhance quality of life for patients and their loved ones.

Epidemiology

Prevalence

Depression is common in palliative care settings. Prevalence estimates range widely, depending on how the condition is defined (e.g., MDD vs. symptoms of depression) and what patient population is studied. In a 2011 meta-analysis of patients in palliative care settings, 14.3% were found to have MDD and 24.6% experienced any form of depressive symptoms and/or disorder.[2]

Reviews consistently indicate that symptoms of depression and depressive disorders occur more often in patients with serious illness than among healthy individuals.[3] For example, while approximately 8.1% of US adults experience major depression,[4] the disorder is believed to be far more prevalent in patients with advanced cancers, with estimates ranging from 14.9% (defined as major depression by the *Diagnostic and Statistical Manual of Mental Disorders* [DSM])[2] to as high as 58% (depression spectrum syndromes).[3] A similar pattern appears to occur in other medical illnesses: elevated rates of depression, as compared to the general population, are seen among those with end-stage heart disease[5] and with advanced kidney disease,[6] for example. Some data also suggest that the incidence of depression may increase as patients become more ill.

Consequences

Left unaddressed, depression results in significant morbidity (physical and psychological) as well as poor caregiver outcomes. Depression can diminish physical health and quality of life, and it can undermine the effectiveness of disease-focused therapy.[7] Depression is a major risk factor for suicide (intentionally taking one's own life driven by psychiatric illness) across all populations. In individuals with an advanced medical disease, it is associated with the desire for hastened death,[8] and it influences the will to live in patients with cancer receiving palliative care.[9] Depression has been correlated with decreased adherence to treatment and increased healthcare utilization. More recent evidence suggests that it may even independently influence mortality in patients with cancer.[10,11] To cite one example, a 2009 meta-analysis found that cancer patients with depressive symptoms experienced a 25% increased mortality rate, and patients with minor or major depression experienced a 39% increased mortality rate.[12]

Differential Diagnosis

Even the most experienced clinicians can have difficulty distinguishing among the various conditions that are marked by depression. Two challenges often arise: first, an advanced disease will frequently produce or mimic symptoms that resemble those seen in states of depression. Somatic symptoms, for example, like poor sleep and weight loss, may be manifestations of medical disease rather than symptoms of a mood disturbance. Second, several discrete mental health conditions share the feature of depressed mood, and effective treatment depends on distinguishing among these conditions. In practice, sorting these findings into discrete etiologic categories, such as "medical" or "psychiatric," is often neither possible nor particularly useful. Nonetheless, accurately characterizing these different entities is important because management strategies will hinge on understanding the etiology of symptoms.

Disease-Related Factors

Many conditions can create or exacerbate symptoms of depression. Some of the possible etiologies of depressive symptoms are presented in Box 4.1. Some medical conditions, such as Huntington's disease, Parkinson's disease, and stroke, appear to play an etiologic role in the development of depression; that is, clinical depression is in some way *caused by* the medical disease, rather than only being a common reaction to the disease.

Similarly, insofar as a serious medical condition involves distressful symptoms or has a serious impact on psychosocial functioning, those conditions often contribute to or amplify existing depressive states. For example, uncontrolled pain, physical exhaustion, insomnia, loss of independence, or concerns about being a burden to others—all common sequelae of a serious medical condition—may contribute to the development of depression or exacerbate an existing depressive state.

Identifying potential medical causes of depression and addressing the factors that can intensify depression are essential first steps in responding to depression in this patient population. Hence, it is important that depression management, like all other components of high-quality palliative care, is rooted in the multidimensional, whole-person approach to care that Cicely Saunders coined as "total pain."[13] Strategies to ameliorate symptoms of depression should occur in the context of broader, interdisciplinary efforts to identify and alleviate all sources of distress.

Mental Health Conditions

In seriously ill patients with symptoms of depression, the second challenging task is to distinguish among the different mental health conditions that share the feature of depressed mood. Table 4.1 describes MDD and the main mental health conditions that are similar.

A severely debilitating episodic disturbance of mood, MDD is characterized by a depressed mood or anhedonia, occurring most days and lasting at least 2 weeks. In addition to these core mood symptoms, cognitive and somatic symptoms also occur in major depression. Poor concentration and indecision are common cognitive symptoms, as are thoughts of worthlessness, hopelessness, guilt, or death. Common somatic symptoms can

BOX 4.1 Etiologies and risk factors for depression

Psychiatric Diseases
- Major Depressive Disorder
- Other mood disorders (e.g., Persistent Depressive Disorder)
- Adjustment Disorder with depressed mood

Risk Factors
- Family history of depression
- History of alcohol use disorder
- Advanced stage of illness
- Diminished functional status
- Left hemispheric strokes
- Pancreatic, breast, and lung cancers
- Younger age with advanced illness
- Spiritual pain
- Poor social support

Psychological, Social, and Spiritual Causes
- Grief
- Existential distress
- Concerns about family
- Overwhelming financial distress
- Hopelessness and meaninglessness
- Guilt
- Sleep deprivation

Medical Causes
- Poorly controlled physical symptoms
- Medications (e.g., opioids, benzodiazepines)
- Tumor involvement of central nervous syste,
- Infections (e.g., Epstein-Barr virus)
- Metabolic disturbances (e.g., abnormal levels of sodium or calcium)
- Nutritional problems (e.g., anemia or deficiencies in vitamin B_{12} or folate)
- Endocrine disorders (e.g., hypothyroidism)
- Neurologic disorders (e.g., Parkinson's disease)

include changes in appetite or weight, changes in sleep, or decreased energy, although, as previously mentioned, these are less helpful in this context. When severe, MDD causes significant functional impairment: major disruptions to relationships, self-care, and key role responsibilities.[14]

As noted above, individuals with serious illness often experience symptoms that overlap with clinical depression: intense sadness, anhedonia, low motivation, and hopelessness, for example. Some may even contemplate death. In isolation, however, none of these phenomena indicates the presence of clinical depression. Similarly, many of the physical symptoms that occur in an advanced medical illness overlap with the somatic dimensions of major depression: for example, changes in sleep, low energy, or changes in weight and appetite. Hence, these are often not reliable indicators of depression in the setting of serious illness. Experts recommend giving greater weight to the emotional and cognitive symptom domains: feelings of sadness, worthlessness, hopelessness, guilt, or thoughts of suicide (intentionally taking one's own life driven by psychiatric illness) point more strongly toward

TABLE 4.1 Differential diagnosis for "depression"

Condition	Characteristics	General treatment approach

Major Depressive Disorder	A. Five or more of the following present, over at least 2 weeks, and at least one of the symptoms is either depressed mood or anhedonia:
	  1. Depressed mood (or, in children/adolescents, irritable mood)
	  2. Anhedonia: markedly reduced interest in most activities
	  3. Changes in weight or appetite
	  4. Insomnia or hypersomnia
	  5. Psychomotor agitation or retardation
	  6. Fatigue or diminished energy
	  7. Feelings of worthlessness or excessive guilt
	  8. Poor concentration, or indecisiveness
	  9. Recurrent thoughts of death, suicidal ideation
	B. Symptoms cause significant distress or functional impairment
	C. Symptoms are not the result of substances or a medical condition
	D. Symptoms are not better explained by a psychotic disorder
	E. The patient has never experienced mania or hypomania
		Medication Therapy
		+
		Psychotherapy

Unspecified Depressive Disorder	Clinically significant distress from depression, accompanied by functional impairment, but which does not meet criteria for any of the more specific depressive illnesses *Note*: This should not be used for patients experiencing normal sadness without clear functional consequences	Continued assessment/ clarification of diagnosis + Psychotherapy
Adjustment Disorder with depressed mood	Depression symptoms that develop within 3 months of a stressor Symptoms are disproportionate to the severity of the stressor *Note*: If criteria are met for Major Depressive Disorder, it should be diagnosed and not Adjustment Disorder.	Problem-solving aimed at resolving/removing stressor Supportive counseling aimed at bolstering resilience and coping skills
Grief	In grief, the predominant emotional state is emptiness and loss; in MDD it is depressed mood and/or inability to experience pleasure. In grief, dysphoria often occurs in waves, generally triggered by thoughts/memories of the deceased; in MDD dysphoria is unrelenting, and cognitions center on worthlessness/hopelessness. In grief, the mood state is reactive; in MDD the mood state can be pervasive or intractable. In grief, self-esteem may be preserved, and feelings of guilt are usually limited to the relationship with the deceased. In grief, thoughts of death often concern "joining" the deceased; in MDD they are aimed at ending one's own life and rooted in feelings of hopelessness and worthlessness. *Note*: Even in the setting of bereavement, if criteria are met for Major Depressive Disorder, MDD should be diagnosed and appropriate treatment initiated.	Supportive counseling/ psychotherapy

(continued)

TABLE 4.1   Continued

Condition	Characteristics	General treatment approach
Demoralization	Marked by subjective incompetence (perceived inability to make progress), hopelessness, despair, loss of meaning/purpose. Often reactivity of mood is preserved. Often develops in serious illness with prolonged hospitalization. Insufficient evidence for Demoralization as its own diagnostic entity.	Supportive counseling/psychotherapy

Notes:
- Descriptions of disorders based on DSM-5.[14]
- Description of demoralization based on Robinson et al.[17]

clinical depression.[15] The presence of true anhedonia (psychological inability to experience joy) also helps to identify major depression. Even when patients are physically unable to engage in previously enjoyable activities, they generally retain the ability to experience joy, for example, in the company of loved ones, unless major depression is present.

As described in Table 4.1, several conditions that are also common in palliative care settings may be mistaken for major depression. *Adjustment disorder*, for example, can produce symptoms of depression (as well as anxiety and behavioral disturbances.) What distinguishes adjustment disorder from clinical depression, however, is that symptoms in adjustment disorder result from an identifiable stressor, and patients do not experience the pattern or severity of associated symptoms consistent with major depression. Nonpharmacologic strategies, which attempt to resolve the stressor or bolster adaptation and coping skills, are the cornerstone of "treatment" for an adjustment disorder, though there may be a role for medications to address specific symptoms, such as insomnia.

Grief is also sometimes mistaken for major depression, since the experience of sadness occurs in both conditions.[16] In grief, however, the fundamental mood experience is one of emptiness, longing, and loss. It often comes in waves that become less intense and less frequent over time. Also, contrary to clinical depression, the mood state in grief is frequently "reactive." That is, grieving individuals can generally experience periods of happiness, laughter, etc., in relation to pleasant or humorous events, while the mood state in clinical depression is generally pervasive or intractable. It is important to note that, if diagnostic criteria are met, major depression should be diagnosed (and treatment should be considered) even in the setting of bereavement.[14] The general approach to addressing grief prioritizes supportive therapeutic interventions rather than drug therapy, though there may be a role for symptom-focused medication trials, as with adjustment disorders.

Demoralization syndrome may also closely mimic clinical depression.[17] The syndrome is not a formal psychiatric diagnosis, but it is often referenced in palliative care. A collection of psychological experiences that frequently occur in patients with advanced disease, demoralization involves feelings of hopelessness, helplessness, meaninglessness, and existential distress. While the core feature of depression is depressed mood or anhedonia, the hallmark of demoralization is "subjective incompetence"—a patient's sense of ineptitude with respect to their internal ability to improve their situation. In major depression, diminished motivation and drive may undermine healing, whereas in demoralization healing is undermined by the patient's feelings of incompetence and hopelessness about the potential for improvement. There is insufficient evidence to establish whether demoralization syndrome can be reliably distinguished from major depression, though many clinicians and patients find it to be a useful construct in helping to characterize and understand a complex set of psychological experiences. Psychotherapy and other nonpharmacologic interventions are generally prioritized when working with a demoralized patient.

Finally, *delirium* and *dementia*, both common in palliative care populations, may also sometimes be mistaken for depression. These two neurocognitive disorders are often marked by social withdrawal, psychomotor retardation, and diminished motivation, which can resemble depression. In delirium and dementia, however, the core symptoms stem from cognitive deficits, whereas in depression, cognitive changes tend to be less prominent and overshadowed by the core symptoms of depressed mood and anhedonia.

Screening Tools and Other Assessment Measures

Major depression is a clinical diagnosis. While some screening tools can be helpful in identifying patients at risk for depression, screening tools themselves do not establish a definitive diagnosis. Instead, diagnosis relies on the patient's subjective history, collateral information, instrument results, and careful clinical assessment/observation with the DSM-5 criteria in mind—informed by knowledge of the different risk factors for and conditions marked by depression.

Choosing an appropriate depression screening tool is a challenge, given the large array of imperfect options in medically ill patients.[18] The most important initial step is to invite discussion about a patient's mood. Simply asking one or two basic questions targeting the core features of depression ("Are you depressed most of the time?" and "Have you lost interest or pleasure?") has documented success in identifying cases of depression, although sensitivities and specificities vary widely (54–100% across reports).[19,20] The best-studied depression screen in palliative care populations remains the Hospital Anxiety and Depression Scale (HADS), though the Edmonton Symptom Assessment Scale (ESAS) and Edinburgh Postnatal Depression Scale (EPDS) are also frequently used in progressive and/or life-threatening illness and cancer.

Management

Depression is a treatable condition, even in patients with serious illness. To dismiss it as "normal" or "expected" in the setting of serious illness likely causes unnecessary suffering for patients and their loved ones. As with other elements of patient care in palliative care, an important first step in addressing depression in seriously ill patients should be to make certain that treatment follows the core tenets of palliative care. These principles are covered thoroughly in other chapters of this book, but in basic terms they include:

- Ensuring that the patient's physical symptoms and other dimensions of distress are assessed and addressed;
- Providing interventions that are concordant with the patient-defined goals of care and medically appropriate given the patient's prognosis;
- Designing time-limited goal-oriented therapeutic trials; and
- Coordinating care with other members of the patient's interdisciplinary team.

In terms of specific treatments for major depression, a multicomponent plan of care could include any of the following but should almost always included nonpharmacological components: interventions to educate and support the patient and family (psychoeducation), supportive psychotherapy, a course of evidence-based psychotherapy, and/or a trial of antidepressant medication. There is now a substantial body of robust evidence demonstrating the effectiveness of this approach using combined modalities, which can be adapted for treating depression in palliative care settings.[21] In addition, some patients may pursue a variety of complementary and alternative medicine (CAM) therapies, as discussed below. An overview of this general approach to managing depression in palliative care settings is presented in Figure 4.1.

Patient and Family Interventions

Psychoeducation involves providing a clear explanation of the diagnostic assessment (and its rationale), addressing any stigma around mental illness, presenting and discussing potential therapies, and addressing any questions or concerns. These first steps are supported by current practice guidelines.[22] Some evidence suggests that psychoeducation interventions may enhance adherence to treatment, improve psychosocial functioning, and even impact prognosis.[23] In some circumstances it may be appropriate to give a firm recommendation for treatment, in particular if patients or family dismiss clinically significant depression that is magnifying the patient's suffering.

Involving loved ones in treatment planning is important, and several studies have examined the interdependent phenomena of depression in patients and their caregivers. There is evidence that depression in caregivers may decrease the likelihood that the patient will respond to both psychiatric and disease-related treatment.[24] In such circumstances, facilitating treatment for both the patient and their depressed caregiver(s) may be valuable.

Psychotherapies

Moderately strong evidence indicates that a variety of psychotherapies can be beneficial for depressed patients with serious illness, although no particular modality has been shown to be superior.[25,26] Hence, it is generally recommended that, where available, formal psychotherapy is offered to patients with significant psychological distress, regardless of etiology or use of medications. Therapy is usually arranged through consultation with psychologists

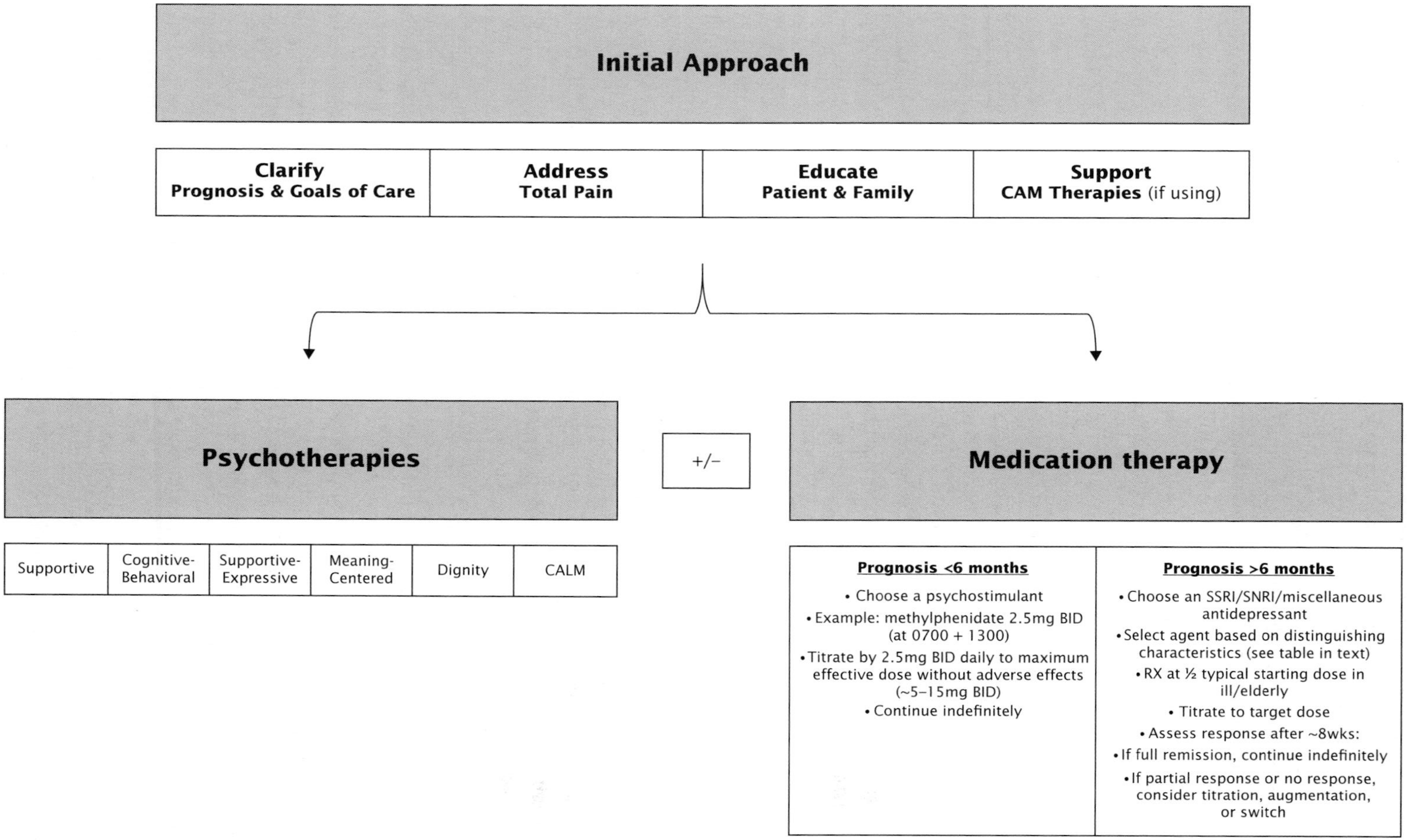

Initial Approach

Clarify Prognosis & Goals of Care	Address Total Pain	Educate Patient & Family	Support CAM Therapies (if using)

+/-

Psychotherapies

Supportive	Cognitive-Behavioral	Supportive-Expressive	Meaning-Centered	Dignity	CALM

Medication therapy

Prognosis <6 months
- Choose a psychostimulant
- Example: methylphenidate 2.5mg BID (at 0700 + 1300)
- Titrate by 2.5mg BID daily to maximum effective dose without adverse effects (~5–15mg BID)
- Continue indefinitely

Prognosis >6 months
- Choose an SSRI/SNRI/miscellaneous antidepressant
- Select agent based on distinguishing characteristics (see table in text)
  - RX at ½ typical starting dose in ill/elderly
  - Titrate to target dose
  - Assess response after ~8wks:
- If full remission, continue indefinitely
- If partial response or no response, consider titration, augmentation, or switch

FIGURE 4.1 Overview of the management of depression in the palliative care setting.

or other licensed therapists. Disease-related factors, such as physical symptom burden and unpredictable disease course, may limit the effectiveness of psychotherapy. Consequently, psychotherapy for depression should be considered as early as possible and aimed at clear goals that can be achieved in a relatively short time frame.

Part VI of this book ("Psychotherapeutic Interventions in Palliative Care") provides a detailed review of evidence-based psychotherapies that may be used in the palliative care setting. Broadly speaking, the following modalities have been developed for and/or tested in populations of seriously ill patients: cognitive-behavioral therapies,[27] supportive-expressive therapy,[28] dignity therapy,[29] meaning-centered psychotherapy,[30] and managing cancer and living meaningfully (CALM).[31]

Complementary and Alternative Therapies

Many patients favor the use of CAM modalities to alleviate depression and other symptoms, either in addition to standard therapies or as stand-alone interventions. A 2010 systematic review examined the efficacy of CAM treatments for symptoms of depression in general populations. Several modalities were found to be modestly helpful, but in general the reviewed studies lacked a robust evidence base. Favorable results were found for omega-3 fatty acids, St. John's Wort, folate, S-adenosyl-L-methionine (SAMe), acupuncture, light therapy, exercise, and mindfulness psychotherapies.[32]

The evidence base is even more sparse for palliative care populations specifically. Some small trials have suggested that music therapy,[33] mindfulness meditation,[34] and massage therapy[35] may alleviate symptoms of depression. Overall, however, trials have generally been of low quality, and the results have been mixed. Hence, there is insufficient evidence to give a strong recommendation for the effectiveness of CAM therapies in alleviating depression in palliative care settings. Nonetheless, many patients report that these interventions are helpful, and they entail few harms save for the potential delay in the use of proven therapies.[32,36] When patients perceive benefit from these interventions, participation should be supported.

Pharmacotherapies

Even in patients with serious illness or approaching the end of life, medication therapy for the treatment of depression has been shown to be efficacious and generally well-tolerated. In a 2011 meta-analysis of patients in palliative care settings, standard antidepressants showed superiority over placebo within 4–5 weeks and increasing in magnitude with time.[37] A more recent meta-analysis, however, found low certainty for the role of antidepressant medications in treating depression in patients with cancer.[38] Nonetheless, expert opinion generally recommends a low threshold to consider a time-limited antidepressant trial since these medications are generally well-tolerated, have few serious side effects, and many have few drug interactions.[7,21,39] Regarding drug selection, in the palliative care setting an important early consideration is the patient's prognosis. As illustrated in Figure 4.1 and discussed below, psychostimulants—not standard antidepressants—are recommended as first-line therapy in patients with a short prognosis since they can be rapidly titrated to effect (or side effect).

Standard Antidepressants

Table 4.2 provides details about the antidepressants commonly used in palliative care settings. *Selective serotonin reuptake inhibitors* (SSRIs) are frequently recommended as an initial option in patients who are naïve to antidepressant therapy. As a class, the SSRIs, such as sertraline or escitalopram, are generally well-tolerated, though they often cause mild, transient gastrointestinal symptoms, headache, and dry mouth. Drugs in this class can also cause significant sexual side effects, which should not be reflexively overlooked or diminished in patients with advanced disease. Therapy with some of the SSRIs (notably, citalopram) should include EKG monitoring, if consistent with the patient's goals, due to a dose-dependent risk of QT_c interval prolongation.

The *serotonin/norepinephrine reuptake inhibitors* (SNRIs) represent a second broad class of first-choice antidepressants. Unlike the SSRIs, SNRIs like venlafaxine and duloxetine also have moderately strong data for efficacy in reducing some forms of neuropathic pain. As a class, the SNRIs have a side-effect profile that generally overlaps with the SSRIs; details are noted in Table 4.2.

A group of *miscellaneous antidepressants* with varied mechanisms of action are also considered first-line antidepressants. Bupropion and mirtazapine are sometimes recommended for patients with serious illness due to some desirable effects. Bupropion inhibits norepinephrine and dopamine, and it often produces a mild stimulant effect that may be desirable in patients whose depression is characterized by significant fatigue, anergia, or lethargy. Mirtazapine has mixed activity on serotonin and norepinephrine receptors, and it is sometimes chosen because it may alleviate insomnia at the lower end of its dose range. It may also positively impact nausea. Newer agents in this group include vilazodone and vortioxetine. In general adult populations, they have been shown to have equivalent efficacy as the other first-choice antidepressants, but there are little data specific to their use in patients with serious illness.

Tricyclic antidepressants (TCAs) are rarely used in palliative care settings, largely because of their anticholinergic effects and the risks of delirium in medically ill patients. However, in patients who are refractory to first-line antidepressants or who have had success in the past with TCAs, these may warrant consideration. TCAs also have good evidence of efficacy in reducing neuropathic pain at lower doses, but, even for this indication, the SNRIs are often preferred due to their more favorable side-effect profile.

Differences in efficacy do not distinguish first-choice antidepressants; none is superior in terms of its likelihood of producing a response or remission or rapidity of effect. As a result, drug selection is guided by familiarity with other features that may be specific to each drug, as shown Table 4.3. A family history, a particular side-effect profile, or unique drug-drug interactions, for example, may be important considerations.

Psychostimulants

Although standard antidepressants are generally first-choice agents for healthy and seriously ill patients alike, they fall short in some circumstances in palliative care. One reason is that they often have a protracted time course to effectiveness: while symptoms may remit quickly for some patients, an adequate trial requires approximately 8 weeks of treatment

TABLE 4.2 Selected drug treatments for depression in palliative care

Drug by class	Suggested dosing/Titration	Notes
SSRIs (Selective Serotonin Reuptake Inhibitors)		Often have sexual side effects Adequate trial requires ~6–8 weeks at therapeutic dose
escitalopram	Start with 5 or 10 mg daily. Increase by 5–10 mg q1–2 weeks to max of 20 mg daily.	Well-tolerated; minimal drug-drug interactions Taper to DC, when possible Available routes: PO (tabs, liq)
sertraline	Start with 25 or 50 mg daily. Increase by 50 mg q1–2 weeks to max of 200 mg daily.	Well-tolerated; few drug-drug interactions Taper to DC, when possible Available routes: PO (tabs, liq)
Other SSRIs: fluoxetine, paroxetine, citalopram		
SNRIs (Serotonin/Norepinephrine Reuptake Inhibitors)		Effective adjuncts for neuropathic pain Often have sexual side effects Adequate trial requires ~6–8 weeks at therapeutic dose
venlafaxine	Start with 37.5 or 75 mg daily. Increase by 75 mg q1–2 weeks to max of 225 mg daily (extended release).	Many common adverse effects (e.g. headache, hypertension) Effective in some types of neuropathic pain Significant discontinuation syndrome; taper to DC; use caution when oral route is unreliable Extended release formulation permits once-daily dosing Available routes: PO (tabs, caps)
duloxetine	Start with 20 or 30 mg daily. Increase by 20–30 mg q1–2 weeks to max of 60–90 mg daily.	Effective in some types of neuropathic pain Significant discontinuation syndrome; taper to DC; use caution when oral route is unreliable Available routes: PO (caps)
Other SNRIs: desvenlafaxine, levomilnacipran		
Miscellaneous Antidepressants		Effective as single agents Also used to augment effectiveness of SSRI/SNRI
bupropion	Start with 150 mg qAM. Increase by 150 mg q1 week to max of 450 mg daily (XL formulation).	Weak norepinephrine and dopamine reuptake inhibitor Contraindicated with seizures or eating disorders Mild stimulant effect; may improve concentration May augment antidepressant effect of SSRIs Multiple formulations available (IR, SR, XL); XL formulation permits once-daily dosing Available routes: PO (tabs, caps)
mirtazapine	Start with 7.5 or 15 mg qHS. Increase by 15 mg q1–2 weeks to max of 45 mg qHS.	Increases central serotonergic and noradrenergic activity At the lower end of the dose range, causes sedation; useful in patients with insomnia Causes orthostatic hypotension Available routes: PO (tabs, ODT)
Other miscellaneous agents: vilazodone, vortioxetine		

TABLE 4.2 Continued

Drug by class	Suggested dosing/Titration	Notes
Psychostimulants		Rapid effect; 1st–choice agents when prognosis is short
methylphenidate	Start with 2.5 or 5 mg qAM. Increase with 2.5 or 5 mg daily, in divided (BID) doses.	May cause/worsen anxiety May cause/worsen insomnia (schedule BID dosing at 0800 + 1400 hrs) Usual effective dose <15 mg BID (doses >30 mg/day usually not necessary) Available routes: PO (tabs, caps, liq)
Novel/experimental "antidepressants"		
ketamine	Recommend reserving for experimental use until stronger data are available	Moderate-strength data in healthy populations using IV route. Intranasal formulation has FDA indication for depression; has specific regulatory administration requirements Limited, low-quality data in palliative care/hospice setting

Note: Dosing guidelines reflect a general, initial strategy, based the clinical experience of the authors and current drug references. Local experts and other resources should be consulted for specific concerns.

at a therapeutic dose in order to determine that an agent is ineffective.[22] Additionally, only about a third of patients respond to initial therapy; many require multiple trials or augmentation in order to achieve remission.[40] Hence, standard antidepressant therapy may be inadequate for patients with a limited life expectancy.

TABLE 4.3 Considerations for antidepressant therapy in the palliative care setting

Factor	Consideration
Prognosis	If prognosis is <6 mos, consider a psychostimulant.
Personal history	If the patient has had a favorable response with a particular agent, consider using the same agent.
Family history	If a first-degree relative has had a favorable response with a particular agent, consider using the same agent.
Common side effects	When possible, choose agents with a side-effect profile that aligns with the patient's symptoms or goals of care. Example: In patients with insomnia, consider mirtazapine. Example: In patients with anergia, consider bupropion.
Presence of neuropathy	Consider SNRIs.
Discontinuation syndromes	If loss of the oral route is anticipated, avoid agents with significant discontinuation syndromes (e.g., paroxetine, venlafaxine); titrate to DC if possible.
Drug-drug interactions	Most antidepressants are P450 substrates, and many also exhibit P450 inhibition. Check interactions with appropriate resource.

Psychostimulants, by contrast, have been associated with rapid reduction in depressive symptoms, and they can be safely titrated over a matter of days—not weeks—in order to assess effectiveness. For these reasons, expert consensus generally supports the use of psychostimulants as first-line agents for treating depression in patients with a short prognosis.[41] Methylphenidate, for example, was shown to produce significant reductions in symptoms of depression in hospice enrollees in a small randomized, double-blind, placebo-controlled trial.[42] Treatment is usually started at a low dose (e.g., methylphenidate 2.5 mg PO BID) and titrated upward daily while assessing for improvement or side effects. Anxiety, restlessness, and insomnia are the common adverse effects, generally occurring in a dose-dependent fashion. Patients with preexisting anxiety may be unable to find a dose that alleviates depression without exacerbating anxiety (unless the anxiety is a symptom of depression rather than a separate etiology). Similarly, in patients with cardiac tachyarrhythmias, psychostimulants may not be appropriate, and the risk/benefit profile should be carefully considered. Experts do not recommend starting a standard antidepressant concurrently to avoid confusing side effects as well as the uncertainty of standard antidepressant therapy as noted above.

Novel Agents for Depression

While antidepressants and psychostimulants play an important role in the treatment of depression in palliative care settings, there remains a need for other medication options that are safe, reliable, and rapidly effective. Recently, ketamine has emerged as a particularly promising candidate. Psychedelic substances have also received attention recently for their potential to alleviate psychological distress near the end of life. (Chapter 42 reviews recent data about psilocybin-assisted therapy and its potential role in palliative care.) Regarding ketamine, a number of well-designed randomized trials have shown rapid antidepressant effects with intravenous administration of sub-anesthetic doses in treatment-resistant depressed, but otherwise healthy, subjects.[43] Ketamine's rapid onset, efficacy in treating pain, and multiple formulations (oral, intranasal, intravenous) offer appealing benefits in the palliative care setting.[44] Indeed, several small pilot studies in the hospice setting have provided hope that there may be a role for oral ketamine in the treatment of depression in hospice patients.[45,46] Furthermore, an intranasal formulation is now approved by the US Food and Drug Administration (FDA) for use in depression, although it has significant barriers to administration due to safety concerns. Larger, multisite randomized trials are needed before ketamine can be recommended for depression in palliative care.

Future Directions

Several important areas of future inquiry and clinician education exist. Further education for palliative care clinicians would improve awareness of the differential diagnosis for symptoms of depression, as reviewed in this chapter. As feelings and states of depression may range widely—including normal sadness, difficulty coping, clinical depression, and other causes (medical and psychiatric)—clinicians will be challenged to distinguish among these states, understand their impact on family systems, and address these various forms of "depression" effectively. Similarly, education and training are needed to help clinicians become more adept at identifying ethically and clinically relevant distinctions among the range of thoughts and behaviors that may influence the timing of death. Specifically, with expanding access to regulated medical aid in dying, clinicians are increasingly called upon to distinguish life-ending acts that are driven by mental illness (like depression) from those that are not (see Chapters 7 and 8). In addition, and notwithstanding the critically important research in this area over the past two decades, substantial opportunities remain to strengthen the evidence base for existing treatments and identify novel, effective interventions for depression in patients with serious illness.

Key Points

- Depression is common among patients with serious illness, and symptoms can range from the normal experience of sadness to clinically significant conditions like major depression.
- Clinical depression is profoundly painful, and, if not correctly identified and effectively addressed, it can cause serious physical, emotional, and interpersonal disability in both patients and their loved ones.
- Since several clinical conditions share the common feature of depressed mood, distinguishing among major depression and its common look-alikes is essential for effective symptom relief.
- Patients with serious illness can often experience relief from depression, even near the very end of life.
- A variety of psycho-therapeutic and alternative modalities have been shown to be effective for treating depression in the palliative care setting, though the quality of evidence is not robust.
- Standard antidepressants are generally appropriate first-line medications in palliative care settings, but psychostimulants are recommended as first-choice medications for patients with a short prognosis.

References

1. Herman H, Kieling C, McGorry P, Horton R, Sargent J, Patel V. Reducing the global burden of depression: A Lancet-World Psychiatric Association Commission. *Lancet.* 2019;393(10189):e42–e43. PMID 30482607.
2. Mitchell AJ, Chan M, Bhatti H, Halton M, Grassi L, Johansen C, et al. Prevalence of depression, anxiety, and adjustment disorder in onological, haematological, and palliative-care settings: A meta-analysis of 94 interview-based studies. *Lancet Oncol.* 2011;12(2):160–74. PMID 21251875.
3. Massie MJ. Prevalence of depression in patients with cancer. *J Natl Cancer Inst Monogr.* 2004;2004(32):57–71. PMID 15263042.
4. Brody DJ, Pratt LA, Hughes JP. *Prevalence of Depression Among Adults Aged 20 and Over: United States, 2013–2016.* NCHS Data Brief, no 303. Hyattsville, MD: National Center for Health Statistics. 2018.
5. Gibbs JS, McCoy AS, Gibbs LM, Rogers AE, Addington-Hall JM. Living with and dying from heart failure: The role of palliative care. *Heart.* 2002;88 Suppl 2:ii36–9. PMID 12213799.
6. Cohen LM, Dobscha SK, Hails KC, Pekow PS, Chochinov HM. Depression and suicidal ideation in patients who discontinue the life-support treatment of dialysis. *Psychosom Med.* 2002;64(6):889–896. PMID 12461194.

7. Wilson KG, Chochinov HM, de Faye BJ, Breitbart W. Diagnosis and management of depression in palliative care. In: Chochinov HM, Breitbart W, eds. *Handbook of Psychiatry in Palliative Medicine*. 2nd ed. New York: Oxford University Press; 2000:25–49.

8. Breitbart W, Rosenfeld B, Pessin H, Kaim M, Funesti-Esch J, Galietta M, et al. Depression, hopelessness, and desire for hastened death in terminally ill patients with cancer. *JAMA*. 2000;284(22):2907–2911. PMID 11147988.

9. Chochinov HM, Tataryn D, Clinch JJ, Dudgeon D. Will to live in the terminally ill. *Lancet*. 1999;354(9181):816–819. PMID 10485723.

10. Spiegel D. Mind matters in cancer survival. *JAMA*. 2011;305(5):502–3. PMID 21285429.

11. Giese-Davis J, Collie K, Rancourt KM, Neri E, Kraemer HC, Spiegel D. Decrease in depression symptoms is associated with longer survival in patients with metastatic breast cancer: A secondary analysis. *J Clin Oncol*. 2011;29(4):413–420. PMID 21149651.

12. Satin JR, Linden W, Phillips MJ. Depression as a predictor of disease progression and mortality in cancer patients: A meta-analysis. *Cancer*. 2009;115(22):5349–5361. PMID 19753617.

13. Clark D. "Total Pain," disciplinary power and the body in the work of Cicely Saunders, 1958–1967. *Soc Sci Med*. 1999;49(6):727–736. PMID 10459885.

14. American Psychiatric Association. *Diagnostic and Statistical Manual of Mental Disorders: DSM-5*. Washington, DC: American Psychiatric Publishing; 2013.

15. Block SD. Perspectives on care at the close of life: Psychological considerations, growth, and transcendence at the end of life: The art of the possible. *JAMA*. 2001;285(22):2898–2905. PMID 11401612.

16. Jacobsen JC, Zhang B, Block SD, Maciejewski PK, Prigerson HG. Distinguishing symptoms of grief and depression in a cohort of advanced cancer patients. *Death Stud*. 2010;34(3):257–273. PMID 20953316.

17. Robinson S, Kissane DW, Brooker J, Burney S. A review of the construct of demoralization: History, definitions, and future directions for palliative care. *Am J Hosp Palliat Care*. 2016;33(1):93–101. PMID 25294224.

18. Wasteson E, Brenne E, Higginson IJ, Hotopf M, Lloyd-Williams M, Kaasa S, et al. Depression assessment and classification in palliative cancer patients: A systematic literature review. *Palliat Med*. 2009;23(8):739–753. PMID 19825894.

19. Mitchell AJ. Are one or two simple questions sufficient to detect depression in cancer and palliative care? A Bayesian meta-analysis. *Br J Cancer*. 2008;98(12):1934–1943. PMID 18506146.

20. Chochinov HM, Wilson KG, Enns M, Lander S. "Are you depressed?" Screening for depression in the terminally ill. *Am J Psychiatry*. 1997;154(5);674–676. PMID 9137124.

21. Block SD. Assessing and managing depression in the terminally ill patient. ACP-ASIM End-of-Life Care Consensus Panel. American College of Physicians – American Society of Internal medicine. *Ann Intern Med*. 2000;132(3):209–18. PMID 10651602.

22. Gelenberg AJ, Freeman MP, Markowitz JC, Rosenbaum JF, Thase ME, Trivedi MH, et al. *Practice Guideline for the Treatment of Patients With Major Depressive Disorder*. 3rd ed. Arlington: American Psychiatric Association; 2010.

23. Tursi MF, Baes CV, Camacho FR, Tofoli SM, Juruena MF. Effectiveness of psychoeducation depression: A systematic review. *Aust N Z J Psychiatry*. 2013;47(11):1019–1031. PMID 23739312.

24. Jacobs JM, Shaffer KM, Nipp RD, Fishbein JN, MacDonald J, El-Jawahri A, et al. Distress is interdependent in patients and caregivers with newly diagnosed incurable cancers. *Ann Behav Med*. 2017;51(4): 519–531. PMID 28097515.

25. Li M, Fitzgerald P, Rodin G. Evidence-based treatment of depression in patients with cancer. *J Clin Oncol*. 2012;30(11):1187–1196. PMID 22412144.

26. Fulton JJ, Newins AR, Porter LS, Ramos K. Psychotherapy targeting depression and anxiety for use in palliative care: A meta-analysis. *J Palliat Med*. 2018;21(7):1024–1037. PMID 29676960.

27. Okuyama T, Akechi T, Mackenzie L, Furukawa TA. Psychotherapy for depression among advanced, incurable cancer patients: A systematic review and meta-analysis. *Cancer Treat Rev*. 2017;56:16–27. PMID 28453966.

28. Kissane DW, Grabsch B, Clarke DM, Smith GC, Love AW, Bloch S, et al. Supportive-expressive group therapy for women with metastatic breast cancer: Survival and psychosocial outcome from a randomized controlled trial. *Psychooncology.* 2007;16(4):277–286. PMID 17385190.

29. Chochinov HM, Kristjanson LJ, Breitbart W, McClement S, Hack TF, Hassard T, et al. Effect of dignity therapy on distress and end-of-life experience in terminally ill patients: A randomised controlled trial. *Lancet Oncol.* 2011;12(8):753–762. PMID 21741309.

30. Breitbart W, Poppito S, Rosenfeld B, Vickers AJ, Li Y, Abbey J, et al. Pilot randomized controlled trial of individual meaning-centered psychotherapy for patients with advanced cancer. *J Clin Oncol.* 2012;30(12):1304–1309. PMID 22370330.

31. Rodin G, Lo C, Rydall A, Shnall J, Malfitano C, Chiu A, et al. Managing cancer and living meaningfully (CALM): A randomized controlled trial of a psychological intervention for patients with advanced cancer. *J Clinical Oncol.* 2018;36(23):2422–2432. PMID 29958037.

32. Freeman MP, Fava M, Lake J, Trivedi MH, Wisner KL, Mischoulon D. Complementary and alternative medicine in major depressive disorder: The American Psychiatric Association Task Force report. *J Clin Psychiatry.* 2010;71(6):669–681. PMID 20573326.

33. Hilliard RE. Music therapy in hospice and palliative care: A review of the empirical data. *Evid Based Complement Alternat Med.* 2005;2(2):173–178. PMID 15937557.

34. Shennan C, Payne S, Fenlon D. What is the evidence for the use of mindfulness-based interventions in cancer care? *Psychooncology.* 2011;20(7):681–697. PMID 20690112.

35. Ernst E. Massage therapy for cancer palliation and supportive care: A systematic review of randomised clinical trials. *Support Care Cancer.* 2009;17(4):333–337. PMID 19148685.

36. Zeng YS, Wang C, Ward KE, Hume AL. Complementary and alternative medicine in hospice and palliative care: A systematic review. *J Pain Symptom Manage.* 2018;56(5):781–794. PMID 30076965

37. Rayner L, Price A, Evans A, Valsraj K, Hotopf M, Higginson IJ. Antidepressants for the treatment of depression in palliative care: Systematic review and meta-analysis. *Palliat Med.* 2011;25(1):36–51. PMID 20935027.

38. Ostuzzi G, Matcham F, Dauchy S, Barbui C, Hotopf M. Antidepressants for the treatment of depession in people with cancer. *Cochrane Database Syst Rev.* 2018 Apr 23;4(4):CD011006. PMID 29683474.

39. Fairman N, Hirst JM, Irwin SA. *Clinical Manual of Palliative Care Psychiatry.* Washington, DC: American Psychiatric Publishing; 2016.

40. Trivedi MH, Rush AJ, Wisniewski SR, Nierenberg AA, Warden D, Ritz L, et al. Evaluation of outcomes with citalopram for depression using measurement-based care in STAR*D: Implications for clinical practice. *Am J Psychiatry.* 2006;163(1):28–40. PMID 16390886.

41. Candy M, Jones L, Williams R, Tookman A, King M. Psychostimulants for depression. *Cochrane Database Syst Rev.* 2008 Apr 16;(2):CD006722. PMID 18425966.

42. Kerr CW, Drake J, Milch RA, Brazeau DA, Skretny JA, Brazeau GA, et al. Effects methylphenidate on fatigue and depression: A randomized double-blind placebo-controlled trial. *J Pain Symptom Manage.* 2012;43(1):68–77. PMID 22208450.

43. Aan Het Rot M, Zarate Jr CA, Charney DS, Mathew SJ. Ketamine for depression: Where do we go from here? *Biol Psychiatry.* 2012;72(7):537–547. PMID 22705040.

44. Goldman N, Frankenthaler M, Klepacz L. The efficacy of ketamine in the palliative care setting: A comprehensive review of the literature. *J Palliat Med.* 2019;22(9):1154–1161. PMID 31090477.

45. Iglewicz A, Morrison K, Nelesen RA, Zhan T, Iglewicz B, Fairman N, et al. Ketamine for the treatment of depression in patients receiving hospice care: A retrospective medical record review of thirty-one cases. *Psychosomatics.* 2015;56(4):329–337. PMID 25616995.

46. Irwin SA, Iglewicz A, Nelesen RA, Lo JY, Carr CH, Romero SD, et al. Daily oral ketamine for the treatment of depression and anxiety in patients receiving hospice care: A 28-day open-label proof-of-concept trial. *J Palliat Med.* 2013;16(8):958–965. PMID 23805864.

47. Micromedex Drugdex [package insert]. Ann Arbor, MI: Truven Health Analytics; 2014. www.micromedexsolutions.com. Accessed on Aug 8, 2021.

5

Anxiety in Palliative Care

Martin S. Chin, Andrew J. Roth, and
Konstantina Matsoukas

Introduction

As patients enter the advanced phases of their illnesses, physical and psychological burdens
change. Anxiety commonly increases as patients become aware of both the relative ineffec-
tiveness of medical treatments in halting the progress of their disease and, consequently, of
approaching death. Fears of death, disability, disfigurement, and dependency loom increasingly large for patients who have been told that medical treatment will not, in all likelihood,
lead to cure but will only be palliative. A 2014 survey on assessment and management of
anxiety in palliative care demonstrated variability in practice suggesting a need for improvement.[1] Awareness of psychological and medical end-of-life issues on the development
and persistence of anxiety allows clinicians to be more effective in helping patients optimize
overall quality of life.

Prevalence of Anxiety in Patients Receiving Palliative Care

Cancer potentially disrupts the roles, interpersonal relationships, quality of life, and the
ways in which patients view their future. Optimal oncology care throughout the disease,
treatment, survivorship, and end-of-life phases requires ongoing attention to palliative and
psycho-oncological needs. Both anxiety and depression are independently associated with
the quality-of-life domains of health status, emotional and cognitive functioning, and fatigue in advanced cancer patients. Anxiety may occur independently or with other psychiatric symptoms. Those with depression and anxiety reported more physical symptoms and

worsened quality of life, and many went untreated.[2] Psychological distress, anxiety, and depression should not be considered normal or expected, in either patients or caregivers.

Distress is associated with greater physical symptom severity, suffering, and mortality, potentially undermining physical and psychosocial quality of life and understanding of test results and prognosis. About a third of patients receiving palliative care in an inpatient cancer setting had significant anxiety,[3] while almost half of all home hospice patients experience moderate to severe depression and anxiety in the last week of life,[4] complicating aspects of existential distress including themes of identity, isolation, responsibility, guilt, death anxiety, deriving meaning, personal growth, spirituality, and religion.

Patients with advanced disease frequently worry that they are losing their race against cancer and that any cessation in chemotherapy or radiation therapy places them closer to the inevitability of death, even though some of those treatments may worsen some aspects of quality of life. Prevalence rates of psychological issues in end-of-life care appear to increase as patients become sicker. Older adults face age-related changes such as frailty, cognitive decline, medical comorbidities, limited mobility, and other issues that warrant attention in assessing anxiety.[5]

Diagnosis of Anxiety

The experience of anxiety is ubiquitous and does not always require diagnosis or intervention beyond reassurance and education. The complete absence of anxiety in all circumstances while maintaining consciousness is unrealistic and unlikely unachievable. Thus the often-heard phrase "Don't worry, everything will be fine" may have a paradoxically chilling effect. Patients may place spiritual, cultural, or religious value on some degree of suffering or mindfulness of its existence. Indeed, the absence of anxiety may produce dysphoria in certain personality types. A clinician must attempt to ascertain the presence and extent of functional impairment and consider the patient's desire for symptom management in determining the need to address anxiety symptoms.

Investigation of anxiety begins with recognition of symptoms. Nonbehavioral health clinicians are important in the identification and initial management of anxiety. Use of assessment instruments may be helpful, but it is important to appreciate that assessment instruments for the measurement of anxiety may be used for the distinct purposes of screening, diagnostic clarification, or monitoring. Care should be exercised to avoid confounding the presence of anxiety symptoms on a screening instrument with the diagnosis or suboptimal management of psychiatric or physical illness. Screening may not identify all patients in need of further attention in regard to anxiety. Demographic factors such as age and gender may affect the sensitivity of instruments. A formalized clinical pathway including routine screening using brief screening tools has been recommended in adult cancer patients by some authors.[6]

Patients with anxiety may report subjective feelings of worry, foreboding, apprehension, or dread, which frequently intensify with worsening illness or when patients perceive that death is imminent. Anxiety symptoms can be classified as either somatic or cognitive.

Somatic symptoms of anxiety are physical in nature and, when prominent, may lead to extensive medical workups seeking an easily treatable or reversible cause. Somatic symptoms often occur in discrete episodes, as in panic attacks. Symptoms of tachycardia, shortness of breath, diaphoresis, gastrointestinal distress, and nausea may also be related to advanced medical illness in the later stages of life, sometimes making diagnosis challenging. Loss of appetite, diminished libido, and insomnia are symptoms associated with both depression and anxiety. Feelings of hyperarousal and irritability are less specific but may also be categorized as somatic. Insomnia may be related to worry or anxiety, often about the future, family, and death. Cognitive symptoms of anxiety in patients with advancing disease include recurrent, unpleasant, or intrusive thoughts about illness, including fears of death, loss of autonomy, loss of dignity, and dependency on others. Overgeneralization, catastrophizing, and dwelling on negative outcomes are not uncommon, and patients view themselves as helpless in a hopeless and inescapable situation.

Though anticipatory nausea and vomiting (ANV) has been associated with anxiety, newer antiemetic regimens have led to decreased nausea with chemotherapy and thus ANV. Patients who do experience nausea with chemotherapy may develop persistent anxiety related to chemotherapy resulting in nausea if chemotherapy is reintroduced with palliative intent. Similarly, patients undergoing palliative radiation therapy may feel apprehensive and anxious. Anxiety associated with radiation therapy may not decline as treatment progresses because of the accumulated side effects and the fear associated with progression of disease.

Suicidal thoughts may present as a manifestation of anxiety in the palliative setting. These thoughts occur on a spectrum from an abstract consideration of the possibility of death to the intention to commit a specific act with the immediate consequence of death. Suicidal ideation is common with uncontrolled pain, thus attempts at pain control should precede a definitive psychiatric diagnosis. Suicidal ideation may represent the patient's desire to express emotion, emphasize distress due to inadequately managed symptoms, feel control rather than a sense of victimhood, or obtain education about hospice options at the end of life. The issue of suicide may arise in the context of a request for physician aid in dying. Suicide and physician aid in dying are addressed in Chapters 7 and 8. Options for management of intractable symptoms exist in all jurisdictions, and palliative sedation is ethically permissible when other interventions prove insufficient to relieve a patient's suffering. The Columbia Suicide Severity Scale[7] may be used in acute care and palliative settings to distinguish passive thoughts of death, wish for hastened death, and active thoughts and plans to hurt oneself.

The *Diagnostic and Statistical Manual of Mental Disorders* (DSM-5) represents a major revision in the organization of anxiety disorder diagnoses from the scheme used in DSM-IV, with removal of obsessive compulsive and trauma-related disorders and inclusion of separation anxiety disorder and selective mutism. The patient who appears anxious may be determined to have "reactive" anxiety or an adjustment disorder (trauma- and stressor-related disorders) or an anxiety disorder (e.g., anxiety that is a manifestation of a preexisting anxiety disorder, anxiety that is secondary to the illness or medication effects, or anxiety that is a manifestation of another psychiatric disorder such as delirium or depression). Increasingly, depression and anxiety are viewed as syndromes existing on a continuum;

there is an overlap in the symptomatology between these two mood states. Depression may be distinguished from anxiety by the presence of psychological symptoms such as hopelessness, anhedonia, worthlessness, and suicidal ideation. Depression and desire for hastened death may become prominent as illness progresses.

Adjustment disorders are diagnosed when the patient's distress is out of proportion to the severity or intensity or the stressor but do not meet criteria for another DSM-5 mental disorder or represent an exacerbation of a preexisting mental disorder.

Anxiety resulting from uncontrolled pain, abnormal metabolic states, pulmonary emboli, and hormone-producing tumors is an *anxiety disorder due to a another medical condition.* Anxiety caused by medication (steroids, psychostimulants, sedatives, hypnotics, anxiolytics, etc.) is called *substance-induced anxiety disorder.*

In the palliative care setting, the presentation of the patient in acute pain is well-known: the patient appears tense and is often restless and perspiring. Undermanaged pain remains a common cause of anxiety, agitation, and diminished quality of life despite the advances of the hospice movement in the understanding and treatment of pain in advanced illness.[8] Understanding the specific nature of a patient's pain phenomenon may be helpful in determining the most appropriate treatment for pain and, consequently, anxiety. Patients with breakthrough pain (episodes of severe or excruciating pain superimposed on relatively stable, well-controlled baseline pain) often report more anxiety and depression than patients who do not report these episodes. Treating a patient's pain with only short-acting opioids, such as oxymorphone, may result in alternation between periods of oversedation and periods of pain. The use of longer-acting or sustained-release opioids dosed around the clock regardless of pain level may provide more consistent pain relief and thus more relief of anxiety. Education that patients need not wait until pain is experienced is essential. Supplemental medication may be dosed in anticipation of pain (e.g., for transportation, manipulation, dressing changes, hygiene, etc.). The patient may achieve more consistent pain control, and the recognition that pain can be controlled may alleviate anxiety. The patient's total pain experience may include components that the clinician might identify as nausea, anxiety, existential distress, or even dyspnea. Careful examination of the possibility that pain is the source of anxiety may reveal that, instead, anxiety is being reported and experienced by the patient as pain.

A change in respiratory or pulmonary status may be heralded by symptoms of anxiety. Suddenly occurring symptoms of anxiety and restlessness with chest pain or respiratory distress may indicate a pulmonary embolus. Patients who are hypoxic often appear anxious and are fearful that they are suffocating or dying. Medications, such as bronchodilators and β-adrenergic receptor stimulants that are commonly used for chronic respiratory conditions, may cause anxiety, irritability, and tremulousness. At the very end of life, respiratory distress or air hunger may be refractory to benzodiazepines. Opiates may be necessary to adequately manage these symptoms.

Delirium, an episode of poor attention, confusion, and impaired sensorium, potentially caused by multiple medical etiologies, may manifest as symptoms of anxiety, restlessness, or agitation. In the palliative setting, the underlying medical issue may not be correctable, thus symptom-directed management may be necessary as delirium may be distressing for both patient and concerned family. Use of behavioral interventions such as reorientation and redirection may be helpful to reduce distress, however pharmacologic interventions including antipsychotics, atypical antipsychotics, benzodiazepines, or opiates may be needed.

A review of medications in the patient with advanced illness is essential to determine potential adverse effects that may present as anxiety. Corticosteroids such as dexamethasone, often used for spinal cord compression or brain metastases, are frequently a cause of motor restlessness and agitation. Anticholinergic medications may also contribute to delirium especially in the context of age, underlying cognitive impairment, or concurrent medical illness. Benzodiazepines, hypnotics, and antiemetics may also be culprits when delirium presents or is exacerbated. Bronchodilators and β-adrenergic stimulants, psychostimulants, and caffeine can cause anxiety, irritability, and tremulousness. Neuroleptic drugs (i.e., metoclopramide, prochlorperazine, chlorpromazine, haloperidol) used to manage nausea or the symptoms of delirium may cause anxiety and restlessness, also known as *akathisia*. Patients may be heard to say, "I feel like I am jumping out of my skin." Fortunately, these symptoms can be controlled by the addition of a benzodiazepine, a β-blocker such as propranolol, or an antiparkinsonian agent such as diphenhydramine.

In addition to the direct effects of medications or substances, withdrawal or discontinuation syndromes of alcohol, antidepressants, stimulants, opioids, benzodiazepines, corticosteroids, anticonvulsants, nicotine, clonidine, and others are often overlooked as causes of anxiety and agitation. The prevalence of alcoholism in studies from different palliative care settings has ranged from 7% to 27% with little data available about the prevalence of other forms of substance abuse.[9] Patients who have been prescribed shorter-acting benzodiazepines for anxiety or nausea may, with frequent use, even within prescribed allowances, experience rebound anxiety between doses, middle of the night awakening insomnia, or withdrawal upon abrupt cessation. These patients may benefit by switching to a longer-acting benzodiazepine such as clonazepam.

It is important to remember that many palliative patients may have preexisting undiagnosed anxiety disorders that may be amenable to treatment. A clinical interview remains the preferred assessment technique for anxiety in the palliative setting; however, diagnosis is often confounded when patients are physically debilitated and/or may have cognitive deficits.

Phobias, panic disorder (PD), posttraumatic stress disorder (PTSD), and generalized anxiety disorder (GAD) may be diagnosed for the first time in the setting of advanced illness, even though the anxiety symptoms may not have come to clinical attention for any number of reasons, including the patient wanting to avoid mental health treatment and stigma, or that the symptoms were managed with mechanisms or tools that are no longer available to the patient., including substances, vigorous exercise, and other hobbies. Advanced illness often brings unwanted changes in physical ability, financial resources, social supports, and cognitive faculties that interfere with a patient's ability to practice hobbies, exercise, meditation, or other adaptive health behaviors. The patient's increasing or decreasing use of alcohol or substances can play a role in the emerging or worsening of anxiety. Earlier, accurate diagnosis and treatment of anxiety disorders may decrease extreme distress and facilitate adequate medical management of the patient.

Patients with advanced cancer may become fearful of falling asleep because they worry that they may not wake up. Common characteristics of all phobias include extreme anxiety on exposure to a feared object or situation and persistent anxiety in anticipation of these situations. Agoraphobia, the most common phobia in the general population, and claustrophobia may appear to present de novo in patients who are confined in a frightening hospital or hospice environment.

Those patients who already have compromised respiratory function may have cyclical exacerbations of their anxiety and breathing problems. Symptoms of a preexisting PD may intensify during the palliative care phase when patients confront increasing physical symptoms and mortality. The persistent or continuous pattern of worry in GAD is distinguished from the situation- or object-defined dread phobias or discrete episodes of PD.

People with advanced cancer may experience the symptoms characteristic of PTSD, similar to those reported by individuals who have been subjected to other types of trauma (e.g., combat, rape, or natural disaster). Alter and colleagues[10] reported that almost half (48%) of a group of cancer survivors reported symptoms related to PTSD, with 4% meeting the criteria for current PTSD diagnosis and 22% meeting the criteria for a lifetime PTSD. Patients with this disorder may repeatedly experience frightening events associated with their cancer diagnosis or treatment in the form of flashbacks, intrusive memories, or nightmares and have chronic, exaggerated startle responses or autonomic hyperactivity. Additionally, patients with PTSD avoid situations, places, people, and other reminders of their trauma. Avoidance behaviors may result in noncompliance with important evaluations or treatments. Intrusive, dehumanizing, or painful medical procedures may be experienced as retraumatizing or triggering in patients with preexisting trauma, leading to exacerbation or relapse of PTSD symptoms. Addressing trauma issues may also be helpful, even toward the end of life.

Treatment of Anxiety

A search of prospective, randomized trials involving the use of pharmacological agents for the treatment of anxiety at the end of life found insufficient data to assess the effectiveness of medications to treat anxiety in palliative care patients.[11] This highlights the important need for prospective randomized controlled trials to establish the benefits and downsides of pharmacological treatment in this area. The most effective management of anxiety is multimodal and usually involves psychotherapy, behavioral therapy, and pharmacological management. Most patients with mild to moderate anxiety can be treated effectively with supportive psychotherapeutic interventions. Emotional support, psychoeducation, and exploration of patients' fears and apprehensions about the progression of disease and psychosocial difficulties, as well as the concerns about suffering during the process of dying and ultimate death, often serve to alleviate a substantial degree of the patient's anxiety. As the patient has the growing realization of the foreshortening of their life, concerns may change or intensify about increased dependence or spirituality, and financial issues may wax or wane.

Psychological Treatment of Anxiety in Palliative Care

Psychotherapy is an effective treatment for anxiety and can be especially beneficial when pharmacologic treatment options are limited by the risks associated with polypharmacy and complex medication interactions. Meta-analysis demonstrates that psychotherapy can be effective in reducing depression and anxiety in a palliative setting.[12] Psychotherapy combined with medication is often more effective than either psychotherapy or medication alone. Commonly used psychosocial interventions in people with advanced cancer fall into four categories: psychoeducational, behavioral, cognitive-behavioral, and group interventions. Additionally, insight-oriented psychodynamic psychotherapy may also be employed.

Although many patients will be quite knowledgeable about the sequelae of particular treatment, providing information about common emotional reactions and palliative therapies may reduce anxiety about the unknown. Providing information to patients' families enables them to cope more effectively, which in turn enhances the patients' sense of support. Educating the patient that "incurable" does not necessarily mean "untreatable" when it comes to evaluating clinical options can be reassuring, hopefully optimizing the patient's ability to function using the psychological resources they already possess.

Behavioral interventions advocating for adaptive behaviors (e.g., writing in a journal, light exercise, meditation, progressive muscle relaxation, guided imagery, desensitization, response prevention, thought stopping, modeling, and distraction) have been demonstrated in a number of studies to be effective in the management of anxiety. In a study comparing the efficacy of relaxation and alprazolam in cancer patients, both treatments were shown to be effective for mild to moderate anxiety, with alprazolam having a slight advantage over relaxation training alone.[13]

Cognitive-behavioral interventions or cognitive-behavioral therapies (CBT) build on behavioral interventions by exploring the links between the patient's thoughts or cognitions and behaviors. Patients are encouraged to identify anxious or maladaptive thoughts, reconsider them more logically, and experiment with alternative viewpoints and behaviors that give them greater control over their situation. Approaching the fear of death, concluding unfinished business, and restructuring one's expectations for life to include finding greater pleasure and purpose in short-term goals rather than in long-term projects are appropriate foci for CBT with terminally ill patients. The structured nature of CBT also allows delivery by mobile device software applications. Greer and colleagues developed a mobile app platform which led to improvements in anxiety, depression, and quality of life.[14]

Insight-oriented psychodynamic psychotherapy seeks to help patients understand the antecedents of their anxiety. This process is often lengthy and thus may be less suited to a patient with a relatively short life expectancy; however, insights gleaned toward the end of life may help a patient place dying in a more meaningful context of their life.

Psychotherapeutic interventions can be provided in individual, family, or group settings. Telephone monitoring has been found to be an effective counseling tool to reduce anxiety and depression in patients too debilitated to come to a therapist's office.[15] Recently, technological solutions have allowed the delivery of these interventions via telemedicine, text messaging, or software applications on mobile devices.

Psychotherapy, in general, has been demonstrated to reduce psychological distress. Individual and group interventions have been used to reduce psychological distress in cancer patients with different stages of cancer. In one study, patients who participated in support groups for at least a year reported less tension than did controls.[16]

Death anxiety, the fear associated with death and dying, is a universal phenomenon. The fear of nonbeing is the ultimate existential concern; however, eliciting the patient's subjective concern is essential. Patients may reveal that they fear the process of dying and symptoms of pain, suffocation, or other distress more than not existing. Some patients may have spiritual belief systems and conviction in the veracity of these systems that allow them to face this transition with diminished anxiety and depression, but it is not uncommon for patients with seemingly well-established spiritual beliefs to decompensate in the face of end-of-life issues. Clergy, chaplains, or other spiritual care professionals can be helpful in exploring the spiritual beliefs of these patients and the role spirituality can play in the terminal phase. Short-duration therapy incorporating spiritual well-being and meaning appear to be beneficial although difficult to examine by rigorous statistical analysis.[17]

In the face of impending death, the goals of psychotherapy are much more finite, and insight is not an essential therapeutic task. Therapy focuses on providing a nurturing, supportive relationship with the dying patient and often with the patient's family. As the patient grapples with the practical fears and anxieties associated with dying (e.g., "How do I want my children reared?," "Who will take care of my autistic sister or my frail father?," "How can I resolve the problems that I am having with my family before I die?"), the therapist may find the need to be active on the patient's behalf by serving as an advocate or ombudsman. Elements not generally present in traditional psychotherapy (e.g., normal conversation) may be present, and defenses such as denial, although acknowledged, may be considered a healthy and adaptive response to impending death and, consequently, may not be challenged.

Ultimately, the goals of therapy with the dying patient are to increase the patient's sense of psychological as well as physical comfort. Research demonstrates that psychotherapeutic interventions can help to achieve these goals.

Frank discussions about the patients' fears and anxieties concerning dying have been shown to be effective in alleviating their anxieties. Patients may find it difficult to raise these issues. Friends and family members may be unwilling or unable to participate in these conversations. They may respond to the patient's overtures with unhelpful advice to avoid thinking about death or empty reassurance that all will be well. Spiegel et al., in their group intervention for women with Stage IV breast cancer, demonstrated that the process of detoxifying and demystifying the experience of death leads to reduced levels of anxiety and psychological distress.[16] Guidance that thoughts of death or the desire to discuss death do not necessarily imply suicidality or will inadvertently bring about death sooner can be provided to family members and allied clinicians. Alternative, complementary, or other symptomatic interventions may be more appropriate, and the patient's preferences and beliefs should be considered.

Relatively short-term psychological interventions may be effective in reducing the distress associated with cancer. The efficacy of psychological treatments without the use of medication depends on the duration and severity of the patient's anxiety. In the case of mild to moderate anxiety, the use of psychological techniques alone may be sufficient to assist patients in managing their anxiety.[18] The presence of functional impairment due to anxiety is often the best indicator that specialist behavioral health evaluation is warranted.

Pharmacological Management of Anxiety

A Cochrane database review found a lack of evidence to draw conclusions about the effectiveness of drug therapy for symptoms of anxiety in adult palliative care patients.[19] Assessing patients' needs regarding anxiety may provide important opportunities where healthcare professionals can make a difference to support anxious patients in their final stage of life and realize tailored palliative care.[20] In deciding whether a pharmacological approach to the management of anxiety may be useful, the severity of the patient's symptoms and the degree to which those symptoms interfere with overall well-being are reliable guides. See Table 5.1 for common medications used to treat anxiety and insomnia in palliative care. Patients with mild "reactive" anxiety that does not respond to either supportive measures or behavioral measures alone may benefit from a brief trial of a benzodiazepine. Given the possibility of decreased hepatic and renal functioning as well as increased sensitivity to pharmacological interventions and multiple medication regimens in patients receiving palliative care, if anxiolytic drugs are to be used, the rubric of starting with lower doses than would be used with physically healthy patients and increasing these doses more cautiously will lead to fewer or more manageable side effects.

For the patient who has felt persistently apprehensive and anxious, the first-line anti-anxiety drugs are the benzodiazepines. In the palliative care setting, however, the excessive use of benzodiazepines may result in mental status changes such as confusion or impaired concentration and memory. These changes are more often seen in elderly patients, those with advanced disease or central nervous system maladies (CNS), those who are taking other CNS depressant medications, or patients with impaired hepatic or renal function. It is important to consider and discuss with patients and caregivers the distinctions between dependence, tolerance, and addiction for all controlled substances, which should be managed with appropriate oversight and monitoring. For patients with compromised hepatic function, the use of shorter-acting benzodiazepines, such as lorazepam, oxazepam for anxiety, or temazepam for insomnia, are preferred, since these drugs are metabolized by conjugation with glucuronic acid and have no active metabolites. Conversely, they should be avoided in those with renal dysfunction. Lorazepam or alprazolam are useful not only for anxiety but also as antiemetic (lorazepam) and anti-panic (alprazolam)

TABLE 5.1 Common medications used to treat anxiety and insomnia in palliative care

Benzodiazepines

- First-line medications for acute worry, phobic situations, panic attacks,, and anxiety related to imaging scans—*scanxiety*—and medical procedures.
- *Can cause drowsiness, unsteadiness, forgetfulness, and lead to falls.*
- If taking for more than 1 month, physical *dependence* can develop, and life-threatening withdrawal is possible if stopped abruptly.
- Physiological *tolerance* (needing higher doses to achieve the same relief) may develop after a few months. This can be mistaken for *addiction.*

	Dose Equiva-lent	Initial Dosage	Absorption/Metabolite	Comments
Alprazolam (Xanax)	0.5	0.25–0.5 mg tid	Intermediate/Yes	Best used *as needed* or for short periods of time at judicious doses. It can have an abrupt end of action experience, leading to *rebound anxiety* at the end of the therapeutic dose. Relieves intermittent panic symptoms quickly. The quick, noticeable onset of action can exacerbate *addictive behaviors*. A long-acting version of alprazolam is available.
Oxazepam (Serax)	10.0	10–15 mg tid	Slow-intermediate/No	Short acting; less hepatotoxic; mostly renal metabolism
Lorazepam (Ativan)	1.0	0.5–2.0 mg tid	Intermediate/No	Moderately long-acting; also used to prevent chemotherapy-induced nausea--may cause amnesia for unpleasant experiences. Good for MRI anxiety. Good for those with liver dysfunction.
Diazepam (Valium)	5	5–10 mg bid	Fast/Yes	Longer acting, with quick, noticeable onset of action. This can provoke *addictive behaviors.*
Clonazepam (Klonopin)	0.25	0.25–1 mg bid	Intermediate/Yes	Longer acting—avoids rebound anxiety, but slower onset of action than alprazolam and diazepam. Good for panic attacks, free-floating anxiety, and inducing and maintaining sleep. Disintegrating wafer available (no swallowing needed).
Temazepam	30.0	15–30 bedtime	Intermediate/No	Used as hypnotic—not anxiolytic.
Antipsychotics	**Initial dosage**		**Comments**	
Haloperidol (Haldol)	0.5–1 mg BID			
Olanzapine (Zyprexa)	2.5–5 mg bedtime			
Quetiapine (Seroquel)	25–50 mg bedtime			

(continued)

TABLE 5.1 Continued

Antidepressants

Selective Serotonin Reuptake Inhibitors (SSRIs) and Serotonin Norepinephrine Inhibitors (SNRIs)

- May treat Panic Disorder and other anxiety syndromes. Need to be taken daily. Beneficial effects take 2–5 weeks or longer at any one dose.
- *Common side effects:* anxiety, restlessness, drowsiness, and gastric upset.
- Antidepressants should be tapered under physician supervision to avoid discontinuation syndrome.
- As with use for depression, treatment lasts 9–12 months.
- Suicidal ideation is rare but should be mentioned to patient and monitored.
- May help with hot flashes for menopause or for those on hormonal treatment.

	Initial dosage	Comments
Sertraline (Zoloft)	12.5–25 mg daily	Wide therapeutic range—up to 200 mg daily. Found to be safe in patients with cardiac disease.
Paroxetine (Paxil)	5–10 mg daily	Shorter acting--May have significant discontinuation syndrome.
Fluoxetine (Prozac)	5–10 mg daily	Longer acting—may alleviate symptoms of discontinuation syndrome; may be energizing and worsen anxiety.
Citalopram (Celexa)	5–10 mg daily	May cause cardiac conduction prolongation at doses above 40 mg daily.
Escitalopram (Lexapro)	5–10 mg daily	May cause cardiac conduction prolongation at doses above 20 mg daily.
Vortioxetine (Trintellix)	5–10 mg daily	May have fewer sexual side effects than other SSRIs.
Other Antidepressants	**Initial dosage**	**Comments**
Venlafaxine (Effexor)	37.5 mg XR daily	Shorter acting—May have significant discontinuation syndrome; extended release less likely to cause increased blood pressure.
Desvenlafaxine (Pristiq)	50 mg daily	Shorter acting—May have significant discontinuation syndrome.
Duloxetine (Cymbalta)	20–30 mg daily	May also treat neuropathic pain syndromes.
Mirtazapine (Remeron)	7.5–15 mg bedtime	Sedating—may help induce sleep; may cause daytime fatigue. May increase appetite. NO gastric side effects.
Trazodone (Desyrel)	25–50 mg bedtime	Sedating—may help induce sleep.
Bupropion (Wellbutrin)	100 mg SR daily	Energizing—may induce anxiety, restlessness or insomnia if taken too late in the day; contraindicated with history of seizures. No sexual side effects. May help with tobacco cessation.

Hypnotics
- Lower risk for tolerance and dependence than benzodiazepines.

	Initial dosage	Comments
Zolpidem (Ambien)	2.5–10 mg bedtime	If sleep does not last long enough through the night, consider Controlled Release formulation.
Zaleplon (Sonata)	5–10 mg bedtime	
Eszopiclone (Lunesta)	1–3 mg bedtime	May cause unwelcome metallic taste.
Ramelteon (Rozerem)	8 mg bedtime	Melatonin receptor Agonist; enhances sleep regulatory mechanisms.
Antihistamines	**Initial dosage**	**Comments**
Hydroxyzine (Vistaril)	As directed	A common ingredient in over-the-counter sleep medications; may cause daytime drowsiness, headache, dry mouth, dizziness, urinary retention, constipation and pounding heartbeat.
Diphenhydramine (Benadryl)		

medications. A longer-acting benzodiazepine such as clonazepam may provide more sustained relief of anxiety symptoms. For insomnia, the benzodiazepine temazepam as well as the nonbenzodiazepine hypnotics zolpidem, zaleplon, eszopiclone, or ramelteon may be effective. In addition, sedating antidepressants such as trazodone or mirtazapine may also help patients with persistent anxiety and insomnia. Duloxetine may be helpful for patients with anxiety and neuropathic pain syndromes. A sedating atypical neuroleptic such as olanzapine or quetiapine may be effective for the patient who is anxious or has trouble sleeping. Antipsychotics may also be useful for the patient whose anxiety is substance-induced (e.g., steroid). Drowsiness and somnolence are the most common adverse effects of benzodiazepines; reductions in dose and the passage of time often mitigate these effects. In anxious patients with severely compromised pulmonary function, the use of benzodiazepines that suppress central respiratory mechanisms may be unsafe. Low doses of atypical antipsychotics such as olanzapine or quetiapine or a low dose of an antihistamine can be useful for these individuals. Structurally, unlike other anxiolytics, buspirone is useful for patients with GAD and for those in whom there is the potential for abuse. Buspirone is not effective on an "as-needed" basis, and, as with antidepressants, its effects are not apparent for 1–2 weeks, which may be problematic in patients who have significant anxiety and who do not have long to live.

For the treatment of PD, the benzodiazepines alprazolam and clonazepam, and antidepressant medications (i.e., serotonin reuptake inhibitors, tricyclic antidepressants, and monoamine oxidase inhibitors) have demonstrated effectiveness. Alprazolam rapidly blocks panic attacks. The tricyclic antidepressant imipramine is effective in the management of PD; its anticholinergic side effects, however, are not well-tolerated by debilitated cancer patients. In the oncology setting, the serotonin reuptake inhibitors (SSRIs) fluoxetine, sertraline, paroxetine, citalopram, escitalopram, and vortioxetine, which have fewer side effects than the tricyclic antidepressants, are effective in the management of depression, generalized anxiety, and PD, but may take 2–4 or more weeks to reach therapeutic levels and therefore may be less useful as patients near the end of life. Serotonin-norepinephrine reuptake inhibitors (SNRIs) such as venlafaxine, desvenlafaxine, and duloxetine are also useful for anxious patients. Mirtazapine is useful for patients who have anxiety as well as difficulty falling asleep and poor appetite or gastric distress. When panic symptoms are caused by air hunger or end-of-life respiratory discomfort, judicious use of opioids may relieve both symptoms.

Provider/Caregiver Anxiety

It is important to recognize that anxiety is often present in families, caregivers, and healthcare providers. Natural, human, empathetic responses to patients experiencing intractable symptoms and existential challenges may result in strong feelings of distress. Caregivers imagine, rightly or wrongly, what the patient feels, and in many cases experience these feelings themselves. Family members may insist that the patient be treated for these imagined symptoms. It is up to the healthcare provider to determine if the patient does indeed experience these symptoms and if these symptoms warrant intervention. Providers may experience distress from pressure to perform interventions for a patient that may be more for the benefit of family. Psychosocial issues for family, caregivers, and healthcare providers are addressed in other chapters of this text.

Future Directions

Development of new and innovative treatments, including randomized control trials for treating anxiety in palliative care, is imperative. New psychotherapies (i.e., meaning-centered psychotherapy, dignity-conserving psychotherapy) for treating anxiety in the field of palliative care have emerged in recent years. Technologies such as mobile software and telehealth hold promise as additional resources in this area. New findings could help develop guidelines for more consistent, appropriate, and timely care for anxiety in palliative care settings as we cannot assume that medications that work in healthy individuals will be as effective or safe in those who are dying. Emerging treatments such as cranial electrotherapy stimulation (CES) have been demonstrated to be safe and effective for anxiety in advanced cancer patients. Use of psychedelics including lysergic acid diethylamide (LSD) and psilocybin for the treatment of anxiety and depression at the end of life is an area of active research. Ketamine has shown benefits in depression, pain management, and sedation without exacerbation of hypotension, thus the sedating effect may have benefits for management of anxiety symptoms in an ICU setting. Use of telehealth, novel mobile software applications, addressing caregiver anxiety, and mitigating provider burnout are other areas in which we hope to see developments in the future. A meditation practice assisted by mobile device software applications may reduce perceived stress in healthcare providers. Use of medication off-label for symptom control has improved quality of life and decreased distress of many patients with advanced disease; this type of innovation must continue within the context of evidence-based medicine through rigorous and disciplined research.

Key Points

- The terminal phase of advanced illness brings challenges in the management of psychological distress in general, and anxiety in particular.
- Clinicians must recognize anxiety through vigilance, screening, and evaluation. The clinician's understanding of the medical and psychological precipitants of anxiety, coupled with an appreciation of available multimodal treatment options, offers patients receiving palliative care the possibility of comprehensive treatment for anxiety.
- Knowledge of standard psychotherapeutic techniques for managing anxiety as well as understanding of patient characteristics can guide the use of various psychotherapy formats (i.e., individual vs. group; insight-oriented vs. interpersonal psychotherapy vs. cognitive behavioral therapy vs. supportive therapy).
- Pharmacologic interventions are effective and safe but must be applied with consideration and care.
- Heightening the attention of and providing education to those who care for patients at the end of life to the existence, multiple causes, management, and sometimes intractable nature of anxiety at the end of life will significantly improve care.

References

1. Atkin N, Vickerstaff V, Candy B. "Worried to death": The assessment and management of anxiety in patients with advanced life-limiting disease, a national survey of palliative medicine physicians. *BMC Palliat Care*. Dec 11 2017;16(1):69.

2. Wilson KG, Chochinov HM, Skirko MG, Allard P, Chary S, Gagnon PR, et al. Depression and anxiety disorders in palliative cancer care. *J Pain Symptom Manage*. Feb 2007;33(2):118–129.

3. Buzgova R, Jarosova D, Hajnova E. Assessing anxiety and depression with respect to the quality of life in cancer inpatients receiving palliative care. *Eur J Oncol Nurs*. 2015;19(6):667–672.

4. Kozlov E, Phongtankuel V, Prigerson H, Adelman R, Shalev A, Czaja S, et al. Prevalence, severity, and correlates of symptoms of anxiety and depression at the very end of life. *J Pain Symptom Manage*. 2019;58(1):80–85.

5. Trevino KM, Saracino RM, Roth AJ. Symptomatology, assessment, and treatment of anxiety in older adults with cancer. *J Geriatr Oncol*. 2021;12(2):316–319.

6. Butow P, Price MA, Shaw JM, Turner J, Clayton JM, Grimison P, et al. Clinical pathway for the screening, assessment and management of anxiety and depression in adult cancer patients: Australian guidelines. *Psycho-oncology*. Sep 2015;24(9):987–1001.

7. Posner K, Brown GK, Stanley B, Brent DA, Yershova KV, Oquendo MA, et al. The Columbia-Suicide Severity Rating Scale: initial validity and internal consistency findings from three multisite studies with adolescents and adults. *Am J Psychiatry*. Dec 2011;168(12):1266–1277.

8. Kolva E, Rosenfeld B, Pessin H, Breitbart W, Brescia R. Anxiety in terminally Ill cancer patients. *J Pain Symptom Manage*. 2011;42(5):691–701.

9. Block SD. Psychological issues in end-of-life care. *J Palliat Med*. Jun 2006;9(3):751–772.

10. Alter CL, Pelcovitz D, Axelrod A, Goldenberg B, Harris H, Meyers B, et al. Identification of PTSD in cancer survivors. *Psychosomatics*. Mar-Apr 1996;37(2):137–143.

11. Jackson KC, Lipman AG. Drug therapy for anxiety in palliative care patients. *Cochrane Database Syst Rev*. 2004;(1):Cd004596.

12. Fulton JJ, Newins AR, Porter LS, Ramos K. Psychotherapy targeting depression and anxiety for use in palliative care: A meta-analysis. *J Palliat Med*. 2018;21(7):1024–1037.

13. Holland JC, Morrow GR, Schmale A, Derogatis L, Stefanek M, Berenson S, et al. A randomized clinical trial of alprazolam versus progressive muscle relaxation in cancer patients with anxiety and depressive symptoms. *J Clin Oncol*. 1991;9(6):1004–1011.

14. Greer JA, Jacobs J, Pensak N, MacDonald JJ, Fuh CX, Perez GK, et al. Randomized trial of a tailored cognitive-behavioral therapy mobile application for anxiety in patients with incurable cancer. *Oncologist*. 2019;24(8):1111–1120.

15. Kornblith AB, Dowell JM, Herndon JE, 2nd, et al. Telephone monitoring of distress in patients aged 65 years or older with advanced stage cancer: A cancer and leukemia group B study. *Cancer*. Dec 1 2006;107(11):2706–2714.

16. Spiegel D, Bloom JR, Yalom I. Group support for patients with metastatic cancer. A randomized outcome study. *Arch Gen Psychiatry*. May 1981;38(5):527–533.

17. Grossman CH, Brooker J, Michael N, Kissane D. Death anxiety interventions in patients with advanced cancer: A systematic review. *Palliat Med*. 2018;32(1):172–184.

18. Maguire P, Faulkner A, Regnard C. Managing the anxious patient with advancing disease–a flow diagram. *Palliat Med*. 1993;7(3):239–244.

19. Salt S, Mulvaney CA, Preston NJ. Drug therapy for symptoms associated with anxiety in adult palliative care patients. *Cochrane Database Syst Rev*. 2017;5(5):CD004596.

20. Zweers D, de Graeff A, Duijn J, de Graaf E, Witteveen PO, Teunissen SCCM. Patients' needs regarding anxiety management in palliative cancer care: A qualitative study in a hospice setting. *Am J Hosp Palliat Care*. 2019;36(11):947–954.

6

Delirium in the Terminally Ill

Christopher Manschreck, Yesne Alici, and
William Breitbart

Introduction

Delirium is a common and often serious neuropsychiatric complication in the management terminally ill patients, characterized by abrupt onset of disturbance in arousal, attention, cognition, and perception that fluctuates over the course of the day. Delirium is a medical emergency that needs to be prevented, identified, and treated vigorously. Delirium is associated with increased morbidity and mortality[1-3] and increased length of hospitalization, causing distress in patients, family members, and staff.[4-6] Delirium is a sign of significant physiologic disturbance, usually involving multiple medical etiologies such as infection, organ failure, and medication adverse effects. Delirium can interfere with the recognition and control of other physical and psychological symptoms, such as pain. Unfortunately, delirium is often underrecognized or misdiagnosed and inappropriately treated or untreated in the medical setting.[7] Clinicians who care for terminally ill patients must be able to diagnose delirium accurately, undertake appropriate assessment of etiologies, and understand the benefits and risks of pharmacologic and non-pharmacologic interventions.

Epidemiology

Delirium is one of the most prevalent neuropsychiatric disorders in inpatient settings, although the reported prevalence and incidence of delirium varies widely in the medical literature. This is due to the diverse and complex nature of delirium and the heterogeneity of sample populations. Many factors, including patient characteristics, setting of care, and the assessment scale used, contribute to disparate estimates of the prevalence and incidence of delirium in the medically ill. The prevalence of delirium at admission to general medical and geriatric wards ranges from 18% to 35%, and the incidence of delirium during such hospitalization ranges from 29% to 64%.[7] Old age is a well-known risk factor for the development of delirium, as is dementia or other cognitive impairment, functional impairment, visual impairment, and a history of alcohol use disorder.[7] Postoperative patients, cancer patients, and acquired immunodeficiency syndrome (AIDS) patients are also at greater risk for delirium.[8] Delirium occurs in up to 51% of postoperative patients.[7] Approximately 25–40% of medically hospitalized cancer patients develop delirium, as do about 85% of terminally ill cancer patients.[8] Severe illness involving multiple organ systems increases the risk of developing delirium. The highest prevalence and incidence of delirium is reported in hospices with terminally ill patients. Prospective studies conducted in inpatient palliative care units have found an occurrence rate of delirium ranging from 13% to 42% on admission and incident delirium developing during admission in 26–62%.[9]

Pathophysiology

As reflected by its diverse symptomatology, delirium is a dysfunction of multiple regions of the brain. A global cerebral dysfunction, delirium arises in the setting of multisystem dysconnectivity and is characterized by concurrent disturbances of level of alertness, awareness, attention, perception, cognition, psychomotor behavior, mood, and sleep-wake cycle.[10] Fluctuations of these symptoms, as well as the abrupt onset of such disturbances, are critical features of delirium.[11] Delirium is conceptualized as a reversible process as opposed to dementia. Reversibility is often possible even in severely ill patients; however, irreversible or persistent delirium has been described in the last days and among elderly patients.[12] If left untreated, however, delirium may irreversibly progress to dementia or exacerbate baseline cognitive dysfunction.[13] The study of the pathophysiology of delirium is vital to our understanding of the phenomenology, prognosis, treatment, and prevention of delirium.

Various hypotheses have been advanced to explain the pathophysiology of delirium, including neuronal aging, neuroinflammatory, oxidative stress, neuroendocrine, circadian rhythm dysregulation, and neurotransmitter hypotheses, among others; none of these is mutually exclusive.[14] In varied measure, each of these hypothesized mechanisms likely plays a part in the development of cognitive and behavioral dysfunctions characteristic of delirium. As detailed in a comprehensive review by Maldonado,[14] delirium is a neurobehavioral syndrome caused by the transient disruption of normal neuronal activity in the setting of multiple systemic disturbances, mediated by failed integration of neuronal networks across domains of integration and processing of sensory information and organization of motor responses. Dysregulation of many neurotransmitter systems, including the serotonin, noradrenaline, endorphin, glutamate, and histamine systems, may be implicated in delirium.[14]

In addition to the prevailing theories focusing on particular neurotransmitter systems or gross cerebral hypoactivity, slowing, and functional dysconnectivity, other pathophysiological mechanisms have been proposed.[14-16] Several studies indicate that neuroinflammatory processes might be central to delirium.[14] Increased cytokine levels have been found in patients with delirium even after controlling for infection, age, and cognitive

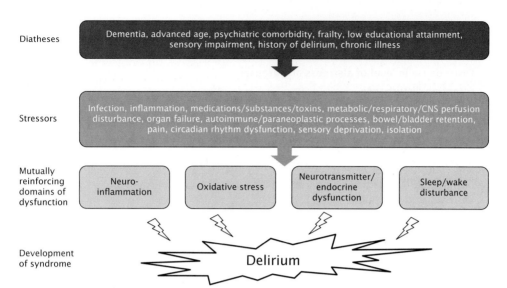

Diatheses	Dementia, advanced age, psychiatric comorbidity, frailty, low educational attainment, sensory impairment, history of delirium, chronic illness

FIGURE 6.1 A schematic representation of aspects of delirium pathophysiology as viewed through the lens of the diathesis-stress model. Risk factors contribute to a *diathesis* for delirium in the context of reversible and irreversible *stressors*. Mutually reinforcing domains of dysfunction are represented by the non-mutually exclusive mechanistic hypotheses which synergistically contribute to the clinical syndrome of delirium. CNS, central nervous system.

impairment. There are also findings suggesting that deficient oxygenation and oxidative stress are key predisposing features in delirium.[15] Another line of work suggests disruption of circadian rhythms is an early disturbance in the cascade of cerebral abnormalities that follows delirium; however, evidence that melatonin[16, 17] and ramelteon[18] is protective against delirium is mixed. The common observation of new or exacerbated delirium following exogenous glucocorticoid administration indicates a potentially powerful role for neuroendocrine dysfunction in delirium. There is likely a heterogenous, overlapping pathophysiological route to the syndrome we observe as delirium. A visual representation of a pathogenesis of delirium as seen through the lens of the diathesis-stress model of illness can be seen in Figure 6.1.

Biomarker research is under way and is of paramount importance since biomarkers may be useful for identifying patients at higher risk for developing delirium and may yield clues to potential underlying pathophysiologic mechanisms.[19] Because delirium can be due to different etiologies, various biomarkers, including inflammatory, neurodegenerative, metabolic, electroneurophysiological (i.e., electroencephalographic), and neurotransmitter-based, have been examined in the last decade.

Clinical Features

The clinical features of delirium are numerous and include a variety of neuropsychiatric symptoms (Box 6.1).[8,11] Main features of delirium include prodromal symptoms (e.g., restlessness, anxiety, sleep disturbances, and irritability), rapidly fluctuating course, abrupt

BOX 6.1 **Common clinical features of delirium**

Disturbance in level of alertness and arousal

Attention disturbance

Rapidly fluctuating course and abrupt onset of symptoms

Increased or decreased psychomotor activity

Disturbance of sleep-wake cycle

Mood symptoms

Perceptual disturbances

Disorganized thinking

Incoherent speech

Disorientation and memory impairment

Other cognitive impairments (e.g., dysgraphia, constructional apraxia, dysnomia)

Asterixis, myoclonus, tremor, frontal release signs

onset of symptoms representing a change from baseline over hours to days, impaired attention (e.g., distractibility), altered awareness of surroundings, altered level of arousal or alertness, increased or decreased psychomotor activity, disturbance of sleep-wake cycle, affective symptoms (e.g., emotional lability, depressed mood, anger, or euphoria), perceptual disturbances (e.g., misperceptions, illusions, and hallucinations), delusions, disorganized thinking and incoherent speech, disorientation, and memory impairment. Language disturbance may be evident as dysnomia (i.e., the impaired ability to name objects) or dysgraphia (i.e., the impaired ability to write). In some cases, the clinician will note poverty of speech/thought, while in others, speech is rambling and irrelevant or pressured and incoherent. Neurologic abnormalities may include motor abnormalities such as tremor, asterixis, myoclonus, frontal release signs, and changes in muscle tone.

Phenomenologic studies have shown cognitive impairment to be common, with disorientation occurring in 78–100%, attention deficits in 62–100%, memory deficits in 62–90%, and diffuse cognitive deficits in 77%; disturbance of consciousness was recorded in 65–100% of patients with delirium; disorganized thinking was found in 95%, language abnormalities in 47–93%, and sleep-wake cycle disturbances in 49–96%.[20] A phenomenologic study by Meagher and colleagues[19] examining 100 palliative care patients showed sleep-wake cycle abnormalities (97%), inattention (97%), long-term memory impairment (89%), reduced visuospatial ability (87%), short-term memory impairment (88%), disorientation (76%), motor agitation (62%), motor retardation (62%), language disturbance (57%), and perceptual abnormalities (50%) to be common features.

There was considerable debate about what changes should be made in the diagnostic criteria in moving from the fourth edition of the *Diagnostic and Statistical Manual of Mental Disorders* to the current DSM-5.[12] In the end, the differences between the two editions are relatively minor with the latest edition focusing on disturbance in awareness and attention rather than in the more nebulous term "consciousness." It is also more explicit in differentiating delirium from coma and makes less of an effort to distinguish it from dementia. According to the DSM-5, the essential features of delirium are disrupted attention (e.g., difficulty directing, focusing, sustaining, or shifting attention) and awareness (i.e., reduced orientation to the environment); a change from baseline that develops over hours to days and fluctuates within a day; additional cognitive problems (e.g., in memory, language, visuospatial ability, or perception); and the condition is not better explained by another neurocognitive disorder and is not associated with a state of severely reduced arousal such as coma; history, physical exam, or lab findings suggest the patient's mental state is a direct physiological result of another medical condition, substance intoxication or withdrawal, exposure to a toxin, or multiple etiological factors. Abrupt onset and fluctuation of the signs and symptoms are necessary diagnostic criteria. DSM-5, similar to the previous edition of the manual, does not place diagnostic emphasis on disturbance of sleep-wake cycle or disturbances in psychomotor activity.

On the basis of psychomotor behavior and arousal levels three subtypes of delirium are described. The subtypes include the hyperactive (or agitated, or hyperalert) and the hypoactive (or lethargic, hypoalert, or hypoaroused). A mixed subtype is the third, with alternating features of hypo- and hyperactive delirium.[21] The hypoactive subtype is characterized by psychomotor retardation, lethargy, sedation, and reduced awareness of surroundings. Hypoactive delirium is often mistaken for depression and is difficult to differentiate from sedation due to opioids or obtundation in the last days of life.[22] The hyperactive subtype is commonly characterized by restlessness, agitation, hypervigilance, hallucinations, and delusions. The hyperactive delirium is more easily recognized by clinicians and is more likely to be referred to psychiatrists compared to patients with other subtypes of delirium.

A meta-analysis of delirium subtypes suggests that the mean prevalence of the hypoactive subtype is 48% (ranging between 15% and 80%) of those diagnosed with delirium.[22] The prevalence of hyperactive delirium ranges from 13% to 46%.[22] The mixed subtype has a prevalence ranging from 17% to 55%. The mixed subtype may be less frequently identified and may be more likely to be classified as hypoactive delirium.[22] In the palliative care setting, hypoactive delirium is most common.[23]

Both hypoactive and hyperactive subtypes of delirium have been shown to cause distress in patients, family members, clinicians, and staff.[24, 25] In a study of 101 terminally ill cancer patients, Breitbart et al.[6] found that 54% of patients recalled their delirium experience after recovering from the episode. Patients with hypoactive delirium (i.e., with few outward manifestations of discomfort or distress) were just as distressed as patients with hyperactive delirium.

There is evidence suggesting that the subtypes of delirium may be related to different causes and may have different treatment responses.[8] Hypoactive delirium has generally been found to occur due to hypoxia, hepatic encephalopathies, and other metabolic disturbances.[22] Hyperactive delirium is correlated with alcohol and drug withdrawal, drug intoxication, or medication adverse effects. A randomized controlled trial of haloperidol and chlorpromazine found that both medications were equally effective in hypoactive and hyperactive subtypes of delirium.[26] The hypoactive subtype of delirium is also associated with higher risk of mortality.[27]

Etiologies and Reversibility of Delirium

Delirium can have multiple etiologies. In the terminally ill, delirium can result either from the direct effects of the primary illness on the central nervous system (CNS), secondary illnesses arising independently, or from the indirect CNS effects of diseases or treatments (e.g., medications, electrolyte imbalance, dehydration, major organ failure, infection, vascular complications, autoimmune/paraneoplastic encephalitides). For a summary of potentially reversible contributors to delirium see Box 6.2.

The diagnostic workup of delirium should include an assessment of potentially reversible causes. The clinician should obtain a detailed history from family, caregivers, and staff of the patient's baseline mental status to determine whether an abrupt change in mental status or fluctuating mental status is present. It is important to inquire about alcohol or other substance use disorders in hospitalized patients to be able to recognize and treat alcohol or other substance withdrawal or intoxication delirium appropriately. A full physical examination and laboratory studies should assess for evidence of sepsis, dehydration, or major organ failure (renal, hepatic, pulmonary). Medications that could contribute to

---

BOX 6.2 Potentially reversible factors contributing to delirium

Medication/substance use
Medication/substance withdrawal
Medication/substance interaction
Electrolyte and metabolic disturbance
Poisons and environmental toxins
Nutritional deficiency
Dehydration
Hypoxia
Hypercapnia
Reduced cerebral perfusion
Major organ failure
Infection
Systemic inflammation
Vascular insult
Autoimmune/paraneoplastic encephalitides
Bowel/bladder obstruction/retention
Pain
Sleep/circadian rhythm disturbance
Sensory deprivation/impairment
Loss of familiar orientation cues
Prolonged isolation

delirium should be reviewed, and possible medication interactions should be carefully considered. Opioid analgesics, benzodiazepines, and anticholinergic drugs are common causes of delirium, particularly in the elderly and the terminally ill. The challenge of assessing the relative contribution of medications to an episode of delirium is often compounded by the presence of many other potential contributors to cognitive changes, such as infection, metabolic disturbance, dehydration, pain, or medication withdrawal.

A screen of laboratory parameters will allow assessment of the possible role of metabolic abnormalities, such as hypercalcemia or thiamine deficiency, hypoxia, or disseminated intravascular coagulation, for example. In some instances, an EEG (to rule out seizures), brain imaging studies (to rule out brain metastases, intracranial bleeding, or ischemia), D-dimer or computed tomography (CT) angiogram of chest (to rule out pulmonary embolism), and lumbar puncture (to rule out leptomeningeal carcinomatosis, subarachnoid hemorrhage, or meningitis) may be appropriate. There are select times when more specialized laboratory workup is indicated, such as when anti-NMDA (N-methyl-D-aspartic acid) receptor encephalitis or another autoimmune encephalitis or paraneoplastic syndrome is suspected.

In terminally ill patients, the extent of diagnostic workup and treatment of reversible causes of delirium is intrinsically linked to goals of care. When assessing etiologies of delirium, an important challenge is the differentiation of delirium as either a reversible complication or an integral element of the dying process in terminally ill patients. When diagnostic information points to a likely etiology, specific therapy may be able to reverse delirium; however, the set of reversible etiologies of delirium may be limited by overall prognosis and goals of care. There is an ongoing debate about the appropriate extent of diagnostic evaluation that should be pursued in a terminally ill patient with delirium. When confronted with delirium in terminally ill patients, the clinician must take an individualized and judicious approach, consistent with the goals of care. Care must be taken to select only diagnostic studies which do not incur excessive discomfort and those for which the results may be actionable by employing treatments consistent with the goals of care. In an otherwise healthy patient, for illustration, endocarditis, requiring several weeks of antibiotics, may be reversible, whereas in another patient with hours to days to live, such an etiology may be, for practical purposes, irreversible. On the other hand, in the same two patients, hypomagnesemia requiring simple repletion may be practicably reversible.

An etiology is discovered in about 40% of terminally ill patients with delirium, and about one-third to half of the patients with delirium improve with treatment of the specific etiologies.[28] Reversibility of delirium is most commonly associated with opioids, other psychoactive medications, and dehydration. Irreversibility of delirium is associated with hypoxic encephalopathy and metabolic factors related to major organ failure, including hepatic and renal insufficiency and refractory hypercalcemia.

In light of the several studies on reversibility of delirium, the prognosis of patients who develop delirium is defined by the interaction of the patient's baseline physiologic susceptibility to delirium (e.g., predisposing factors), the precipitating etiologies, and any response to treatment. If a patient's susceptibility or resilience is modifiable, then targeted interventions may reduce the risk of delirium upon exposure to a precipitant and enhance the capacity to respond to treatment. Conversely, if a patient's vulnerability is high and resistant to modification, then exposure to precipitants enhances the likelihood of developing delirium and may diminish the probability of a complete restoration of cognitive function. A good example of an irreversible risk factor that may contribute to such a situation is the recent finding by Root et al.[29] of an association between preoperative white matter pathology seen on magnetic resonance imaging (MRI) and postoperative delirium in non-small cell lung cancer patients.

The Contribution of Delirium to Prognosis

Delirium in terminally ill cancer patients is a relatively reliable predictor of approaching death in the coming days to weeks. The death rates among hospitalized elderly patients with delirium over the 3-month post-discharge period range from 22% to 76%.[7] In the palliative care setting, several studies support delirium reliably predicting impending death in patients with advanced cancer. Several prognostic tools for predicting survival in terminally ill cancer patients include delirium as a variable. Recognizing an episode of delirium in the late phases of palliative care is critically important in treatment planning and in advising family members on what to expect. Observational data show that delirium is associated with an OR 11.9 ([95% CI: 7.29–19.6]; p < 0.001) of developing dementia[30] and with an increased risk of developing depression and anxiety symptoms.[31] Although the associations are concerning, the long-term sequelae may be less clinically significant in presumed terminal delirium, and there is inadequate evidence to show that aggressive treatment of delirium symptoms can modify outcomes.

Assessment of Delirium

Clinically, the diagnostic gold standard for delirium is the clinician's assessment utilizing the DSM-5 criteria.[32] Several delirium screening and evaluation tools have been developed to maximize diagnostic precision for clinical and research purposes and to assess delirium severity.[33] Examples of delirium assessment tools used in cancer patients and in palliative care settings include the Memorial Delirium Assessment Scale (MDAS),[34] the Delirium-Rating Scale-Revised 98 (DRS-R-98),[35] the 4 A's Test for Delirium (4AT),[36] and the Confusion Assessment Method (CAM).[37] Each of these scales has good reliability and validity. Ely and colleagues have also extended use of the CAM to mechanically ventilated patients in intensive care units (ICUs) with the creation of the CAM-ICU.[38]

Differential Diagnosis

Many of the clinical features of delirium can also be associated with other psychiatric disorders, such as depression, mania, psychosis, and dementia, making diagnosis more challenging. Because of delirium's fluctuating course, there may be disagreement between clinicians evaluating the patient at different times of day about whether there is any abnormality at all. Assessments that differ widely between time points within the same day are suggestive of delirium. When delirium presents with mood symptoms such as depression, apathy, euphoria, or irritability, these symptoms are not uncommonly attributed to depression or mania, especially in patients with a past psychiatric or family history of these conditions. This is particularly concerning as attribution of delirium symptoms to comorbid psychiatric disorders may delay recognition and treatment of a reversible etiology of the delirium. The hypoactive subtype of delirium is commonly misdiagnosed as depression. Symptoms of major depression, including decreased psychomotor activity, insomnia, reduced ability to concentrate, depressed mood, and even suicidal ideation, can overlap with symptoms of delirium. In distinguishing delirium from depression, particularly in the context of advanced cancer, an evaluation of the onset and temporal sequencing of depressive and cognitive symptoms is particularly helpful. It is important to note that the degree of cognitive impairment is much more pronounced in delirium than in depression, and delirium has a more abrupt onset. Also, in delirium, the characteristic disturbance in level of alertness is present, while it is not usually a feature of depression. Similarly, a manic episode may share some features with delirium, particularly the hyperactive or mixed subtypes, but it is not common for mania to feature disturbances in awareness of surroundings. Symptoms such as severe anxiety and autonomic hyperactivity can lead the clinician to an erroneous diagnosis of a panic attack. Again, time course is crucial; a panic attack reaches its peak and remits within minutes, while delirium fluctuates throughout the day. Delirium causing vivid hallucinations and delusions must be distinguished from schizophrenia spectrum disorders. Delusions in delirium tend to be poorly organized and of abrupt onset, while hallucinations are predominantly visual or tactile rather than auditory, as is typical of schizophrenia. Acute onset, fluctuating course, disturbances of cognition, and reduced awareness of surroundings, all in the presence of one or more etiologic causes, are helpful in differentiating delirium from other psychiatric disorders.

The most challenging differential diagnostic issue is whether the patient has delirium, dementia, or a delirium superimposed on a preexisting dementia. Both delirium and dementia are disorders of cognition and share common clinical features, such as disorientation, memory impairment, aphasia, apraxia, agnosia, and executive dysfunction. Impairments in judgment, abstract thinking, and disturbances in thought process are seen in both disorders. Furthermore, delusions and hallucinations can be central features of certain types of dementia (e.g., Lewy body dementia). Collateral informants who can attest to the patient's baseline cognitive function are indispensable in differentiating the delirium from dementia. Abrupt onset (precipitated by a known or as yet unknown medical cause), fluctuating course, and disturbance of arousal differentiate delirium from dementia. The temporal onset of symptoms in dementia is more insidious (or, in the case of vascular dementia, acute and stepwise in onset) and the course is more chronically progressive. In delirium superimposed on a premorbid dementia, differential diagnosis becomes even more challenging. Signs of dementia that might otherwise be obvious tend to be eclipsed by the more acute signs of delirium. Again, resolving the diagnosis may hinge on reliable collateral information regarding the recent baseline cognitive function of the patient. Delirium, unlike dementia, is often reversible, although in terminally ill patients, as noted previously, it may not be.

Management of Delirium in the Terminally Ill

The standard approach to managing delirium in in the terminally ill, even in those with advanced disease, includes a search for underlying causes, correction of those factors, and management of the symptoms of delirium. Treatment of the symptoms of delirium should be initiated before or concurrent with a diagnostic assessment of the etiologies to minimize distress to patients, staff, and family members. The desired and often achievable outcome is a patient who is awake, alert, calm, comfortable, cognitively intact, and communicating coherently with family and staff.

Since publication of the American Psychiatric Association (APA) guidelines for treatment of delirium in 1999,[10] a number of systematic reviews and guidelines have been released based on evidence-based management of delirium. In 2014, the American Geriatrics Society and the American College of Surgeons jointly released clinical practice guidelines for the prevention and treatment of postoperative delirium in older adults.[1] The guidelines highlight the importance of multicomponent nonpharmacologic prevention strategies, education of healthcare professionals, medical evaluation of delirium etiology, optimizing pain management with nonopioids, and avoiding high-risk medications. The guidelines included avoidance of drug treatment for hypoactive delirium and avoidance of benzodiazepines for treatment of delirium except in cases of alcohol or benzodiazepine withdrawal.

In the terminally ill patient who develops delirium during the last days of life, the management of delirium is unique, presenting a number of dilemmas, and the desired clinical outcome may be significantly altered by the dying process.[9] The goals of care in the terminally ill may shift to providing comfort through the judicious use of sedatives, even at the expense of alertness.

Nonpharmacological Interventions

Promising studies,[39] a strong evidence base supporting a multicomponent nonpharmacological intervention to prevent delirium, and the low-risk nature of a subset of these interventions lead the authors to recommend their use for treatment as well as prevention of delirium (see details in "Prevention" section, below). It should be noted, however, that the available body of evidence remains insufficient to support nonpharmacologic interventions for treatment (as opposed to prevention, which is well supported) of delirium. Those nonpharmacological interventions most appropriate for treatment of delirium involve greater attention to supportive management, gentle reorientation, attention to sleep-wake cycle, and the presence of familiar objects and people, whereas those interventions requiring significant patient participation, such as early mobilization or cognitive remediation, may indeed prove counterproductive.[40] A prospective risk model validation study showed that nonpharmacologically reversible risk factors (i.e., those risk factors that can be modified without the use of medications) predict delirium at hospital discharge,[41] and a predominantly nonpharmacological multicomponent delirium intervention in elderly patients (mean age 83 years) in general hospital wards showed more rapid remission of delirium and improved cognition at 6-month follow-up, although there was no mortality or institutionalization benefit.[42] To date, most nonpharmacological delirium treatment research has occurred outside of a palliative care setting.[43]

Pharmacological Interventions

Very often, nonpharmacologic interventions and supportive measures alone are often not effective in controlling the symptoms of delirium in terminal illness. Symptomatic treatment with psychotropic medications is often essential to control the symptoms of delirium, although there are no US Food and Drug Administration (FDA)-approved medications for treatment of delirium.

Antipsychotic Medications

The APA provided guidance for the use of antipsychotics in the treatment of delirium[11] in 1999. Antipsychotic use has been studied in many settings and patient populations in the two decades since.[44–50]

Treatment with antipsychotic agents has been the norm in the everyday management of delirium across settings and different patient populations for more than two decades.[49] The past decade has seen a surge in treatment trials in delirium. Several recent studies did not show benefit of antipsychotics in decreasing the duration or severity of delirium; however, a 2016 systematic review examined antipsychotic drugs including oral risperidone, oral olanzapine, oral quetiapine, intramuscular ziprasidone, and oral, intravenous, and intramuscular haloperidol[46] and concluded that the current evidence does not support the use of antipsychotics for treatment (or prevention) of delirium in hospitalized older adults. There was no significant decrease in delirium incidence among 19 studies and no change in delirium duration, severity, hospital or intensive care length of stay, or reduction in mortality. Potential harm was demonstrated in two studies, in which more patients required institutionalization after treatment with antipsychotics.

A subsequent high-quality randomized controlled trial (RCT) showed no effect of ziprasidone versus haloperidol versus placebo on delirium-free days in delirious ICU patients.[51] In a more recent systematic review of antipsychotics in treatment of delirium, among 16 RCTs and 10 observational studies, there was no difference in sedation status, delirium duration, hospital length of stay, or mortality between haloperidol and atypical antipsychotics versus placebo.[45] There was no difference in delirium severity and cognitive functioning for haloperidol versus second-generation antipsychotics. The authors noted that heterogeneity was present among the studies in terms of dose, administration route of antipsychotics, outcomes, and measurement instruments. There was insufficient or no evidence regarding multiple clinically important outcomes.

In an RCT[47] of atypical and conventional antipsychotic drugs in palliative care settings, participants receiving oral risperidone or haloperidol had higher delirium symptom scores and were more likely to require breakthrough treatment compared with participants receiving placebo. This study was largely publicized due to the finding that participants in the placebo group had better overall survival compared to those in the haloperidol group. An important point to make here is that the survival was not one of the primary study outcomes, and the patients in the haloperidol arm were medically sicker with greater opioid use and more severe delirium.

A 2020 Cochrane review on drug therapy for delirium in the terminally ill[44] concluded that there was no high-quality evidence to support or refute the use of drug therapy for delirium symptoms in terminally ill adults. As noted eloquently in a debate article by Meagher et al.,[40] evidence-based concerns must be applied to all interventions, both pharmacological and nonpharmacological, with equal vigilance.

Management of delirium in terminally ill is nuanced, and goals of care must be central to pharmacological decision making. Short term use of low-dose antipsychotics continues to be the mainstay of treatment for symptoms of delirium (e.g., severe agitation, delusions and hallucinations interfering with care) with the understanding that antipsychotics are not expected to cure the underlying etiologies or prolong survival, but to allow for patients to safely and successfully be managed and to ameliorate patient, staff and caregiver distress, especially during the dying process. In the light of the recent research on use of antipsychotics, it is important to emphasize that in hypoactive delirium lacking symptoms interfering with management, or delirium of all subtypes that is of mild to moderate severity, antipsychotics are best avoided or only used if the benefits of medications clearly outweigh the risks associated with their use (see Table 6.1).

Haloperidol (a "typical" antipsychotic) remains the gold standard medication for treatment of symptoms of delirium among cancer patients due to its efficacy in managing symptoms of delirium and its safety. Haloperidol has few anticholinergic effects, lacks active metabolites, and is formulated for several routes of administration.[49] Haloperidol, used at dosages lower than those commonly used in medically healthy adults (1–3 mg/day), is usually effective in targeting agitation and psychotic symptoms.[49] In general medical and psychiatric settings, doses of haloperidol need not exceed 20 mg in a 24-hour period; however, some clinicians advocate higher doses in selected cases.[49] In severe agitation related to delirium and in terminal delirium, clinicians may add lorazepam to haloperidol. This combination may be more effective in rapidly sedating patients and may help minimize any extrapyramidal adverse effects of haloperidol.[49] There is evidence benzodiazepines can worsen delirium;[26] however, a trial by Hui and colleagues of haloperidol alone versus haloperidol plus lorazepam for agitation in delirium in a palliative care population found that the combination resulted in greater reduction in agitation.[52] Where there is concern that lorazepam is worsening symptoms of delirium, switching to monotherapy with a more sedating antipsychotic, such as olanzapine or chlorpromazine, is an option. The FDA has issued a warning about the risk of QTc prolongation and torsades de pointes with intravenous haloperidol,[53] thus monitoring QTc intervals daily among medically ill patients receiving intravenous haloperidol has become the standard clinical practice.

Oral or intravenous chlorpromazine is considered to be an effective alternative to haloperidol (with or without lorazepam) when increased sedation is required, especially in the ICU setting, where close blood pressure monitoring is feasible, and for severe agitation in terminally ill patients to decrease distress for the patient, family, and staff. It is important to monitor chlorpromazine's anticholinergic and hypotensive side effects, particularly in elderly patients.[49]

TABLE 6.1 Antipsychotic medications in the treatment of delirium

Medication	Initial dose range in terminally ill	Routes of administration	Side effects	Comments
TYPICAL ANTIPSYCHOTICS				
Haloperidol	0.25–2 mg every 2–12 hr	PO, IV, IM, SC	Extrapyramidal adverse effects can occur at higher doses Monitor QT interval on EKG	Remains the gold-standard therapy for delirium May add lorazepam (0.5–1 mg every 2–4 hr) for agitated patients
Chlorpromazine	12.5–50 mg every 4–6 hr	PO, IV, IM, SC, PR	More sedating and anticholinergic compared with haloperidol Monitor blood pressure for hypotension	May be preferred in agitated patients due to its sedative effect
ATYPICAL ANTIPSYCHOTICS				
Olanzapine	1.25–5 mg every 12–24 hr	PO[a] IM	Sedation is the main dose-limiting adverse effect in short-term use	Older age, preexisting dementia, and hypoactive subtype of delirium have been associated with poor response
Risperidone	0.125–1 mg every12–24 hr	PO[a]	Extrapyramidal adverse effects can occur with doses >2 mg/day Orthostatic hypotension	Clinical experience suggests better results in patients with hypoactive delirium
Quetiapine	12.5–50 mg every 12–24 hr	PO	Sedation, orthostatic hypotension	Sedating effects may be helpful in patients with sleep-wake cycle disturbance
Ziprasidone	10–20 mg every 12–24 hr	PO, IM	Monitor QT interval on EKG	Has not been found to be effective in controlling symptoms of delirium in ICU settings.
Aripiprazole	2–5 mg every 24 hr	PO,[a] IM	Monitor for akathisia	Evidence is limited to case reports, case series, and open label trials. Clinical experience suggests better results with hypoactive delirium.
Asenapine	2.5-10mg every 24 hr	SL, TD	Sedation, insomnia	While SL may be favorable in some cases (e.g., dysphagia, gastric tube use), compliance with SL administration instructions may be limited in delirium and oral bioavailbility is low. Evidence limited to single case report of SL use in end-stage cancer delirium with aphagia.

[a]Risperidone, olanzapine, and aripiprazole are available in orally disintegrating tablets.

EKG, electrocardiogram; IM, intramuscular; IV, intravenous; PO, per oral; PR, per rectum; SC, subcutaneous; SL, sublingual; TD, transdermal.

"Atypical" antipsychotic agents (i.e., risperidone, olanzapine, quetiapine, ziprasidone, and aripiprazole) are increasingly used in the treatment of delirium due to decreased risk of extrapyramidal adverse symptoms (EPS). In the light of existing literature, risperidone may be used in the treatment of delirium, starting at doses ranging from 0.125 to 1 mg and titrated up as necessary, with particular attention to the risks of EPS, QTc prolongation, orthostatic hypotension, and sedation at higher doses. Olanzapine can be started between 1.25 and 5 mg nightly and titrated up, with sedation being the major limiting factor, although this may be favorable in the treatment of hyperactive delirium, where twice-daily divided dosing may be used. The current literature on the use of quetiapine suggests a starting dose of 12.5–50 mg and a titration up to 100–200 mg/day (usually at twice-daily divided doses). Sedation and orthostatic hypotension are the main dose-limiting factors. Limited evidence supports the use of aripiprazole, especially in hypoactive delirium.[54] Findings to date and our clinical experience suggest a starting dose of 2–5 mg daily for aripiprazole, with a maximum dose of 15 mg daily. There is a promising case report supporting the tolerability and efficacy of asenapine at doses from 2.5 to 10 mg daily in antipsychotic-resistant delirium in terminal cancer;[55] this is notable because asenapine is available in sublingual and transdermal formulations.

Important considerations in starting treatment with any antipsychotic for delirium include EPS risk; sedation; anticholinergic side effects; cardiac arrhythmias, particularly prolonged QTc interval; and drug-drug interactions. Importantly, the FDA has issued a "black box" warning of increased risk of death associated with the use of typical and atypical antipsychotics in elderly patients with dementia-related psychoses.[56]

Mood Stabilizers

Valproic acid and its oral counterpart divalproex have been suggested as a potentially useful alternative or adjunct to antipsychotic medications due to their multiple hypothesized deliriolytic mechanisms of action.[57] While clinical case series have shown these agents apparently successful at reducing agitation in refractory delirium, RCTs to test the effectiveness of valproic acid in delirium have not been undertaken.

Psychostimulants

Some clinicians have suggested that the hypoactive subtype of delirium may respond to psychostimulants, such as methylphenidate and amphetamine, or to combinations of antipsychotics and psychostimulants or antipsychotics and wakefulness agents such as modafinil.[41] However, studies with psychostimulants in treating delirium remain limited to case reports and open-label studies.[49] The risks of precipitation or exacerbation of agitation or psychotic symptoms should be carefully evaluated when psychostimulants are considered in the treatment of delirium.

Cholinesterase Inhibitors

Impaired cholinergic function has been implicated in the neuropathogenesis of delirium. Despite case reports of beneficial effects of donepezil and rivastigmine, current evidence does not support use of cholinesterase inhibitors in the treatment of delirium.[49]

α-2 Agonists

Dexmedetomidine, an α-2 agonist mostly studied for use postoperatively and in critical care settings, has been compared to standard sedatives such as midazolam and propofol, to opioids and to placebo in randomized controlled trials. A systematic review and meta-analysis with incidence and duration of delirium as the primary outcomes showed that the administration of dexmedetomidine was associated with significantly lower overall incidence and duration of delirium when compared to placebo, propofol, midazolam, and opioids. The main side effects were increased risk of bradycardia and hypotension.[58] It is important to emphasize that dexmedetomidine is used intravenously in postsurgical and critical care settings and primarily for mechanically ventilated patients. Evidence for its use in palliative care settings remains limited; however, a 2021 open-label trial supports further study of dexmedetomidine for hyperactive delirium in a palliative care setting by a continuous subcutaneous infusion route.[59]

Prevention of Delirium

To date, the majority of delirium prevention has focused on secondary prevention via early detection with risk models to predict those patients at risk for developing delirium and pharmacological and nonpharmacological interventions to minimize risk of development of delirium symptoms. Primary prevention efforts have focused on educating clinicians about deliriogenic drugs, such as in the American Geriatrics Society 2019 Updated AGS Beers Criteria.[60]

Research into prevention of delirium in the ICU setting has identified sedative and analgesic use, age, educational attainment, hypertension history, alcohol use disorder history, and elevation of Acute Physiology, Age, Chronic Health Evaluation II (APACHE-II) scores as risk factors for delirium.[61] Use of physical restraints has also been identified as an independent risk factor for delirium persistence at the time of hospital discharge.[41] Physical restraints should be avoided in all patients with delirium or at risk for delirium. To date, several risk models have been proposed for predicting those at risk for delirium in the ICU setting,[61] however whether they may have any value within a palliative care setting is not yet known.

Researchers have studied both pharmacologic and nonpharmacologic interventions in the prevention of delirium among older patient populations, particularly in surgical settings. The applicability of these interventions to the prevention of delirium in palliative care settings has not been widely studied.[62] A 2016 Cochrane review examined prophylactic antipsychotics for preventing delirium in hospitalized non-ICU medical and surgical patients 16 years or older and found no clear evidence of an effect of antipsychotics on incidence of delirium.[63]

Prevention of delirium with multicomponent nonpharmacologic approaches has been shown to be effective and has gained widespread acceptance as the most effective strategy for delirium prevention.[63] Multicomponent nonpharmacological approaches studied include individualized care, use of checklists/protocols, education/training, reorientation, attention to sensory deprivation, nutrition/hydration, electrolytes, oxygenation, identification of infection, mobilization, sleep hygiene, multidisciplinary team-based care, pain control, familiar objects, cognitive stimulation, medication review, mood assessment for anxiety/depression, bowel/bladder care, and management of postoperative complications. In a meta-analysis of 14 interventional studies based on the American Geriatrics Association Hospital Elder Life Program, multicomponent approaches significantly reduced the risk of incident delirium by 53%, and the risk of falls by 62%, among hospitalized, non-ICU patients 65 years and older.[62] In the terminally ill, the effect of these interventions on delirium incidence has been more limited. In a study of 1,516 patients with terminal cancer, Gagnon et al.[43] were not able to reduce incidence of delirium with a multicomponent intervention including early assessment of patient risk factors, active engagement of physicians in planning for delirium, and education of family members. We advocate for a common-sense approach to implementing multicomponent nonpharmacological interventions in the setting of terminal illness, one guided by goals of care and with recognition that many of these interventions are low risk and are likely to have benefits well beyond the endpoint of incidence of delirium.

Special Considerations

Delirium and Pain

It is well recognized that success in the treatment of pain is highly dependent on proper assessment. However, the assessment of pain intensity becomes very difficult in patients with delirium. Delirium can interfere dramatically with the recognition and control of pain and other physical and psychological symptoms in advanced cancer patients, particularly in the terminally ill. Patients with severe pain are particularly at risk of delirium due to their high opioid requirements.[64] Where there is reversal of sleep-wake cycle, patients with delirium use a significantly greater number of "breakthrough" doses of opioids at night compared to patients without delirium. In turn, agitation may be misinterpreted as uncontrolled pain, resulting in inappropriate escalation of opioids, potentially exacerbating delirium. Accurate pain reporting depends on the ability to perceive the pain normally and to communicate the experience appropriately. Delirium may impair the ability to both perceive and report pain. Patients' ability to manage their own pain through patient-controlled analgesia should be considered carefully where applicable. Efforts have been made to improve assessment of pain in nonverbal palliative care patients, and some pain management strategies show promise of reducing pain without increasing risk of delirium. Reducing the dose of opioids or switching to another opioid has been demonstrated to reverse delirium due to opioids. Rotation to methadone from other opioids has potential to attenuate pain while also improving mental status in inpatients and outpatients.[65] A study by Arai et al.[66] demonstrating reduced pain and reduced incidence of terminal delirium with neurolytic celiac plexus block in patients with pancreatic cancer is a good example of non-opioid pain management strategies that reduce risk for delirium.

Caregiver and Family Distress

Both hypoactive and hyperactive subtypes of delirium have been shown to cause distress in family members, clinicians, and staff. Studies suggest the experience of caring for a delirious family member or patient is perhaps more distressing than the experience of the patient,[21,22] may induce symptoms of anxiety and depression,[67] and may persist for at least 12 months following the delirious episode.[68] In a study of delirium-related caregiver distress, Breitbart et al.[6] found that caregivers including spouses, family members, and staff experienced significant levels of distress. Predictors of spouse distress included the patients' Karnofsky Performance Status, as well as the presence of hyperactive delirium and delirium related to brain metastases.[6] Predictors of staff distress included delirium severity, the presence of perceptual disturbances, paranoid delusions, and sleep-wake cycle disturbance. A study by Bruera et al.[5] replicated the finding of even greater distress in family caregivers compared to patients, but, in contrast to the earlier study, found quite low levels of delirium-related distress in nurses and palliative care specialists. A review by Finucane et al. found that, specifically within palliative care settings, delirium may trigger acute distress in caregivers related to the uncertainty of being able to reestablish the relationship between the caregiver and patient before the patient dies. Clinicians may mitigate this distress by facilitating communication and emphasizing aspects of the caregiver relationship that remain intact, in addition to managing symptoms of delirium.[69]

Controversies in the Management of Terminal Delirium

As noted above, the use of antipsychotics and other pharmacologic agents in the management of delirium in the dying patient remains controversial. Some researchers have argued that pharmacologic interventions are inappropriate in the dying patient. Delirium is viewed by some as a natural part of the dying process that should not be altered. Clearly, there are many patients who experience hallucinations and delusions during delirium that are pleasant and in fact comforting, and many clinicians may justifiably question the appropriateness of intervening pharmacologically in such instances. Another concern is that these patients are so close to death that aggressive treatment is unnecessary, and antipsychotics or sedatives may be inappropriately avoided because of exaggerated fears that they might hasten death through hypotension or respiratory depression.

Clinical experience in managing delirium in dying patients suggests that the use of antipsychotics in the management of agitation, paranoia, hallucinations, and altered sensorium is safe, effective, and often quite appropriate. Management of delirium on a case-by-case basis is most prudent. The agitated, delirious dying patient should probably be given antipsychotics to help restore calm. A "wait-and-see" approach may be appropriate with some patients who have a lethargic or somnolent presentation of delirium or who are having frankly pleasant or comforting hallucinations. Such a wait-and-see approach must, however, be tempered by the knowledge that a lethargic or hypoactive delirium may very quickly and unexpectedly become an agitated or hyperactive delirium that can threaten the serenity and safety of the patient, family, and staff. It is important to remember that, by their nature, the symptoms of delirium are unstable and fluctuate over time.

Perhaps the most challenging clinical problem is the management of the dying patient with a terminal delirium that is unresponsive to standard pharmacologic interventions. Approximately 30% of dying patients with delirium do not have their symptoms adequately controlled by antipsychotic medications. Addition of benzodiazepines to haloperidol appears to control agitation better in the setting of terminal delirium than haloperidol alone.[52] Palliative sedation may be performed in terminally ill patients to manage one or more refractory symptoms. About a quarter to a third of all terminally ill patients undergo palliative sedation. The most frequent refractory adverse effects are delirium and dyspnea. And yet in studies on the use of palliative sedation for symptom control, delirium was identified as the target symptom in up to 40% of cases.[70] The most widely used drugs for palliative sedation are midazolam and haloperidol for refractory delirium, but chlorpromazine and other neuroleptics are also effective. When patients experience refractory symptoms during the last hours or days of life, palliative sedation is a medical intervention aimed at managing the suffering.[70] Clinicians are sometimes concerned that the use of sedating medications may hasten death via respiratory depression, hypotension, or even starvation. However, studies have found that the use of opioids and psychotropic agents in hospice and palliative care settings is associated with longer rather than shorter survival.[71] A national multicenter study on palliative sedation in terminal cancer patients showed the feasibility of it in both home and inpatient hospice settings.[72]

The clinician must always keep in mind the goals of care and communicate these goals with staff, patients, and family members when treating delirium in the terminally ill. The clinician must weigh competing clinical imperatives when deciding how to best manage the dying patient with delirium in a manner that preserves and respects the dignity and values of the patient and family.

Future Directions

Delirium is a frequently encountered complication of underlying disease and symptom management treatments in the terminally ill. In the past decade, there has been an exponential increase in the number of studies for delirium across all settings and age groups. Advances in screening methods, biomarker and risk modeling studies to identify high risk patients, and pathophysiologically targeted interventions to prevent and treat delirium and its long-term cognitive outcomes will continue to move the field forward. Proper assessment, diagnosis, and management of delirium are essential to minimizing the impact on patients, family and caregivers for the terminally ill.

Key Points

- Delirium is a common and often serious neuropsychiatric complication in the management terminally ill patients, characterized by abrupt onset of disturbance in awareness, attention, cognition, and perception that fluctuates over the course of the day.

- Delirium is a medical emergency that needs to be prevented, promptly identified, and treated vigorously.
- Optimal treatment of delirium in terminally ill patients should be individualized, symptom-directed, and informed by goals of care.
- Delirium is a major source of patient, caregiver, and family distress.

References

1. American Geriatrics Society Expert Panel on Postoperative Delirium in Older A. American Geriatrics Society abstracted clinical practice guideline for postoperative delirium in older adults. *J Am Geriatr Soc.* 2015;63(1):142–150. doi:10.1111/jgs.13281
2. Leslie DL, Zhang Y, Holford TR, Bogardus ST, Leo-Summers LS, Inouye SK. Premature death associated with delirium at 1-year follow-up. *Arch Intern Med.* July 2005;165(14):1657. doi:10.1001/archinte.165.14.1657
3. Markar SR, Smith IA, Karthikesalingam A, Low DE. The clinical and economic costs of delirium after surgical resection for esophageal malignancy. *Ann Surg.* July 2013;258(1):77–81. doi:10.1097/sla.0b013e31828545c1
4. Cohen MZ, Pace EA, Kaur G, Bruera E. Delirium in advanced cancer leading to distress in patients and family caregivers. *J Palliat Care.* September 2009;25(3):164–171. doi:10.1177/082585970902500303
5. Bruera E, Bush SH, Willey J, et al. Impact of delirium and recall on the level of distress in patients with advanced cancer and their family caregivers. *Cancer.* 2009;115(9):2004–2012. doi:10.1002/cncr.24215
6. Breitbart W, Gibson C, Tremblay A. The delirium experience: Delirium recall and delirium-related distress in hospitalized patients with cancer, their spouses/caregivers, and their nurses. *Psychosomatics.* May 2002;43(3):183–194. doi:10.1176/appi.psy.43.3.183
7. Inouye SK, Westendorp RGJ, Saczynski JS. Delirium in elderly people. *Lancet (London, England).* 2014;383(9920):911–922. doi:10.1016/S0140-6736(13)60688-1
8. Breitbart W, Alici Y. Agitation and delirium at the end of life. *JAMA.* December 2008;300(24):2898–2910. doi:10.1001/jama.2008.885
9. Hosie A, Davidson PM, Agar M, Sanderson CR, Phillips J. Delirium prevalence, incidence, and implications for screening in specialist palliative care inpatient settings: A systematic review. *Palliative Medicine.* September 2012;27(6):486–498. doi:10.1177/0269216312457214
10. Practice guideline for the treatment of patients with delirium. American Psychiatric Association. *Am J Psychiatry.* May 1999;156(5 Suppl):1–20.
11. American Psychiatric Association. *Diagnostic and Statistical Manual of Mental Disorders (DSM-IV).* New York: Springer-Verlag; 1994.
12. Leonard M, Raju B, Conroy M, et al. Reversibility of delirium in terminally ill patients and predictors of mortality. *Palliative Medicine.* August 2008;22(7):848–854. doi:10.1177/0269216308094520
13. Davis DH, Muniz Terrera G, Keage H, et al. Delirium is a strong risk factor for dementia in the oldest-old: A population-based cohort study. *Brain.* Sep 2012;135(Pt 9):2809–2816. doi:10.1093/brain/aws190
14. Maldonado JR. Delirium pathophysiology: An updated hypothesis of the etiology of acute brain failure. *Int J Geriatr Psychiatry.* December 2017;33(11):1428–1457. doi:10.1002/gps.4823
15. Maldonado JR. Acute brain failure: Pathophysiology, diagnosis, management, and sequelae of delirium. *Crit Care Clin.* Jul 2017;33(3):461–519. doi:10.1016/j.ccc.2017.03.013
16. Al-Aama T, Brymer C, Gutmanis I, Woolmore-Goodwin SM, Esbaugh J, Dasgupta M. Melatonin decreases delirium in elderly patients: A randomized, placebo-controlled trial. *Int J Geriatr Psychiatry.* 2010/09/15 2010;26(7):687–694. doi:10.1002/gps.2582
17. Jaiswal SJ, McCarthy TJ, Wineinger NE, et al. Melatonin and sleep in preventing hospitalized delirium: A randomized clinical trial. *Am J Med.* 2018;131(9):1110–1117.e4. doi:10.1016/j.amjmed.2018.04.009

18. Hatta K, Kishi Y, Wada K, et al. Preventive effects of Ramelteon on delirium. *JAMA Psychiatry*. April 2014;71(4):397. doi:10.1001/jamapsychiatry.2013.3320

19. Hall RJ, Watne LO, Cunningham E, et al. CSF biomarkers in delirium: A systematic review. *Int J Geriatr Psychiatry*. Nov 2018;33(11):1479–1500. doi:10.1002/gps.4720

20. Meagher DJ, Trzepacz PT. Delirium phenomenology illuminates pathophysiology, management, and course. *J Geriatr Psychiatry Neurol*. Fall 1998;11(3):150–156; discussion 157–8. doi:10.1177/089198879801100306

21. Association AP. *Practice Guideline for the Treatment of Patients With Delirium*. Washington, DC: American Psychiatric Association; 1999.

22. Stagno D, Gibson C, Breitbart W. The delirium subtypes: A review of prevalence, phenomenology, pathophysiology, and treatment response. *Palliat Support Care*. June 2004;2(2):171–179. doi:10.1017/s1478951504040234

23. Hosie A, Davidson PM, Agar M, Sanderson CR, Phillips J. Delirium prevalence, incidence, and implications for screening in specialist palliative care inpatient settings: A systematic review. *Palliat Med*. Jun 2013;27(6):486–498. doi:10.1177/0269216312457214

24. DiMartini A, Amanda Dew M, Kormos R, McCurry K, Fontes P. Posttraumatic stress disorder caused by hallucinations and delusions experienced in delirium. *Psychosomatics*. September 2007;48(5):436–439. doi:10.1176/appi.psy.48.5.436

25. Buss MK, Vanderwerker LC, Inouye SK, Zhang B, Block SD, Prigerson HG. Associations between caregiver-perceived delirium in patients with cancer and generalized anxiety in their caregivers. *J Palliat Med*. October 2007;10(5):1083–1092. doi:10.1089/jpm.2006.0253

26. Breitbart W, Marotta R, Platt MM, et al. A double-blind trial of haloperidol, chlorpromazine, and lorazepam in the treatment of delirium in hospitalized AIDS patients. *Am J Psychiatry*. February 1996;153(2):231–237. doi:10.1176/ajp.153.2.231

27. Fang CK, Chen HW, Liu SI, Lin CJ, Tsai LY, Lai YL. Prevalence, detection and treatment of delirium in terminal cancer inpatients: A prospective survey. *Jpn J Clin Oncol*. Jan 2008;38(1):56–63. doi:10.1093/jjco/hym155

28. Bruera E, Miller L, McCallion J, Macmillan K, Krefting L, Hanson J. Cognitive failure in patients with terminal cancer: A prospective study. *J Pain Symptom Manage*. May 1992;7(4):192–195. doi:10.1016/0885-3924(92)90074-r

29. Root JC, Pryor KO, Downey R, et al. Association of pre-operative brain pathology with post-operative delirium in a cohort of non-small cell lung cancer patients undergoing surgical resection. *Psychooncology*. 2013;22(9):2087–2094. doi:10.1002/pon.3262

30. Pereira JV, Aung Thein MZ, Nitchingham A, Caplan GA. Delirium in older adults is associated with development of new dementia: A systematic review and meta-analysis. *Int J Geriatr Psychiatry*. July 2021;36(7):993–1003. doi:10.1002/gps.5508

31. Davydow DS. Symptoms of depression and anxiety after delirium. *Psychosomatics*. July 2009;50(4):309–316. doi:https://doi.org/10.1176/appi.psy.50.4.309

32. American Psychiatric Association. *Diagnostic and Statistical Manual of Mental Disorders: DSM*-5. 5th ed. Arlington: American Psychiatric Association; 2013.

33. Oh ES, Fong TG, Hshieh TT, Inouye SK. Delirium in older persons: Advances in diagnosis and treatment. *JAMA*. 2017;318(12):1161–1174. doi:10.1001/jama.2017.12067

34. Breitbart W, Rosenfeld B, Roth A, Smith MJ, Cohen K, Passik S. The memorial delirium assessment scale. *J Pain Symptom Manage*. March 1997;13(3):128–137. doi:10.1016/s0885-3924(96)00316-8

35. Trzepacz PT, Mittal D, Torres R, Kanary K, Norton J, Jimerson N. Validation of the Delirium Rating Scale-Revised-98. *J Neuropsychiatry Clin Neurosci*. May 2001;13(2):229–242. doi:10.1176/jnp.13.2.229

36. Bellelli G, Morandi A, Davis DHJ, et al. Validation of the 4AT, a new instrument for rapid delirium screening: A study in 234 hospitalised older people. *Age Ageing*. 2014;43(4):496–502. doi:10.1093/ageing/afu021

37. Inouye SK, van Dyck CH, Alessi CA, Balkin S, Siegal AP, Horwitz RI. Clarifying confusion: The confusion assessment method. A new method for detection of delirium. *Ann Intern Med*. Dec 1990;113(12):941–948. doi:10.7326/0003-4819-113-12-941

38. Ely EW, Inouye SK, Bernard GR, et al. Delirium in mechanically ventilated patients: Validity and reliability of the Confusion Assessment Method for the Intensive Care Unit (CAM-ICU). *JAMA.* 2001;286(21):2703–2710. doi:10.1001/jama.286.21.2703

39. Waszynski CM, Milner KA, Staff I, Molony SL. Using simulated family presence to decrease agitation in older hospitalized delirious patients: A randomized controlled trial. *Int J Nurs Stud.* Jan 2018;77:154–161. doi:10.1016/j.ijnurstu.2017.09.018

40. Meagher D, Agar MR, Teodorczuk A. Debate article: Antipsychotic medications are clinically useful for the treatment of delirium. *Int J Geriatr Psychiatry.* July 2017;33(11):1420–1427. doi:10.1002/gps.4759

41. Inouye SK, Zhang Y, Jones RN, Kiely DK, Yang F, Marcantonio ER. Risk factors for delirium at discharge. *Arch Intern Med.* July 2007;167(13):1406. doi:10.1001/archinte.167.13.1406

42. Pitkälä KH, Laurila JV, Strandberg TE, Tilvis RS. Multicomponent geriatric intervention for elderly inpatients with delirium: A randomized, controlled trial. *J Gerontol A Biol Sci Med Sci.* Feb 2006;61(2):176–181. doi:10.1093/gerona/61.2.176

43. Gagnon P, Allard P, Gagnon B, Mérette C, Tardif F. Delirium prevention in terminal cancer: Assessment of a multicomponent intervention. *Psychooncology.* December 2010;21(2):187–194. doi:10.1002/pon.1881

44. Finucane AM, Jones L, Leurent B, et al. Drug therapy for delirium in terminally ill adults. *Cochrane Database Syst Rev.* 2020;(1)doi:10.1002/14651858.CD004770.pub3

45. Nikooie R, Neufeld KJ, Oh ES, et al. Antipsychotics for treating delirium in hospitalized adults. *Ann Intern Med.* September 2019;171(7):485. doi:10.7326/m19-1860

46. Neufeld KJ, Yue J, Robinson TN, Inouye SK, Needham DM. Antipsychotic medication for prevention and treatment of delirium in hospitalized adults: A systematic review and meta-analysis. *J Am Geriatr Soc.* 2016;64(4):705–714. doi:10.1111/jgs.14076

47. Agar MR, Lawlor PG, Quinn S, et al. Efficacy of oral risperidone, haloperidol, or placebo for symptoms of delirium among patients in palliative care: A randomized clinical trial. *JAMA Intern Med.* Jan 1 2017;177(1):34–42. doi:10.1001/jamainternmed.2016.7491

48. Patel AK, Bell MJ, Traube C. Delirium in pediatric critical care. *Pediatr Clin North Am.* October 2017;64(5):1117–1132. doi:10.1016/j.pcl.2017.06.009

49. Breitbart W, Alici Y. Evidence-based treatment of delirium in patients with cancer. *J Clin Oncol.* 2012;30(11):1206–1214. doi:10.1200/JCO.2011.39.8784

50. Burry L, Mehta S, Perreault MM, et al. Antipsychotics for treatment of delirium in hospitalised non-ICU patients. *Cochrane Database Syst Rev.* 2018;(6)doi:10.1002/14651858.CD005594.pub3

51. Girard TD, Exline MC, Carson SS, et al. Haloperidol and ziprasidone for treatment of delirium in critical illness. *N Engl J Med.* December 2018;379(26):2506–2516. doi:10.1056/NEJMoa1808217

52. Hui D, Frisbee-Hume S, Wilson A, et al. Effect of lorazepam with haloperidol vs haloperidol alone on agitated delirium in patients with advanced cancer receiving palliative care: A randomized clinical trial. *JAMA.* 2017;318(11):1047–1056. doi:10.1001/jama.2017.11468

53. Haloperidol Tablet FDA Label. FDA.gov. https://www.accessdata.fda.gov/spl/data/9d955576-92e6-471f-a42b-14bd224c942a/9d955576-92e6-471f-a42b-14bd224c942a.xml, 2010.

54. Boettger S, Breitbart W. An open trial of aripiprazole for the treatment of delirium in hospitalized cancer patients. *Palliat Support Care.* 2011;9(4):351–357. doi:10.1017/S1478951511000368

55. Osawa K, Ukai S, Kuriyama T. A case report of the efficacy and usefulness of asenapine in the treatment of a cancer patient with delirium and aphagia. *Palliat Support Care.* Aug 2019;17(4):488–491. doi:10.1017/s1478951518000962

56. Yan J. FDA extends black-box warning to all antipsychotics. American Psychiatric Association. July 18, 2008. Accessed September 6, 2021. https://psychnews.psychiatryonline.org/doi/full/10.1176/pn.43.14.0001

57. Sher Y, Miller Cramer AC, Ament A, Lolak S, Maldonado JR. Valproic acid for treatment of hyperactive or mixed delirium: Rationale and literature review. *Psychosomatics.* Nov-Dec 2015;56(6):615–625. doi:10.1016/j.psym.2015.09.008

58. Flükiger J, Hollinger A, Speich B, et al. Dexmedetomidine in prevention and treatment of postoperative and intensive care unit delirium: A systematic review and meta-analysis. *Ann Intensive Care.* 2018;8(1):92. doi:10.1186/s13613-018-0437-z

59. Thomas B, Lo WA, Nangati Z, Barclay G. Dexmedetomidine for hyperactive delirium at the end of life: An open-label single arm pilot study with dose escalation in adult patients admitted to an inpatient palliative care unit. *Palliat Med*. Apr 2021;35(4):729–737. doi:10.1177/0269216321994440

60. American Geriatrics Society 2019 Updated AGS Beers Criteria for potentially inappropriate medication use in older adults. *J Am Geriatr Soc*. Apr 2019;67(4):674–694. doi:10.1111/jgs.15767

61. Ruppert MM, Lipori J, Patel S, et al. ICU delirium-prediction models: A systematic review. *Crit Care Explor*. Dec 2020;2(12):e0296. doi:10.1097/cce.0000000000000296

62. Martinez F, Tobar C, Hill N. Preventing delirium: Should non-pharmacological, multicomponent interventions be used? A systematic review and meta-analysis of the literature. *Age Ageing*. November 2014;44(2):196–204. doi:10.1093/ageing/afu173

63. Siddiqi N, Harrison JK, Clegg A, et al. Interventions for preventing delirium in hospitalised non-ICU patients. *Cochrane Database Syst Rev*. March 2016;doi:10.1002/14651858.cd005563.pub3

64. Oosten AW, Oldenmenger WH, van Zuylen C, et al. Higher doses of opioids in patients who need palliative sedation prior to death: Cause or consequence? *Eur J Cancer*. October 2011;47(15):2341–2346. doi:10.1016/j.ejca.2011.06.057

65. Parsons HA, de la Cruz M, El Osta B, et al. Methadone initiation and rotation in the outpatient setting for patients with cancer pain. *Cancer*. 2010;116(2):520–528. doi:10.1002/cncr.24754

66. Arai Y-CP, Nishihara M, Kobayashi K, et al. Neurolytic celiac plexus block reduces occurrence and duration of terminal delirium in patients with pancreatic cancer. *J Anesth*. September 2012;27(1):88–92. doi:10.1007/s00540-012-1486-3

67. Rosgen BK, Krewulak KD, Davidson JE, Ely EW, Stelfox HT, Fiest KM. Associations between caregiver-detected delirium and symptoms of depression and anxiety in family caregivers of critically ill patients: A cross-sectional study. *BMC Psychiatry*. Apr 2021;21(1):187. doi:10.1186/s12888-021-03200-7

68. Partridge JSL, Crichton S, Biswell E, Harari D, Martin FC, Dhesi JK. Measuring the distress related to delirium in older surgical patients and their relatives. *Int J Geriatr Psychiatry*. Jul 2019;34(7):1070–1077. doi:10.1002/gps.5110

69. Finucane AM, Lugton J, Kennedy C, Spiller JA. The experiences of caregivers of patients with delirium, and their role in its management in palliative care settings: An integrative literature review. *Psychooncology*. Mar 2017;26(3):291–300. doi:10.1002/pon.4140

70. Garetto F, Cancelli F, Rossi R, Maltoni M. Palliative sedation for the terminally ill patient. *CNS Drugs*. 2018/09/27 2018;32(10):951–961. doi:10.1007/s40263-018-0576-7

71. Lo B, Rubenfeld G. Palliative sedation in dying patients. *JAMA*. 2005;294(14):1810–1816. doi:10.1001/jama.294.14.1810

72. Caraceni A, Speranza R, Spoldi E, et al. Palliative sedation in terminal cancer patients admitted to hospice or home care programs. Does the setting matter? Results from a national multicenter observational study. *J Pain Symptom Manage*. July 2018;56(1):33–43. doi:10.1016/j.jpainsymman.2018.03.008

7

Suicide and Desire for Hastened Death in the Terminally Ill

Leah E. Walsh, Laura C. Polacek, Marjorie Heule, and Barry Rosenfeld

Introduction

Patients with advanced illness are often faced with the potential that the disease may result in deteriorating health or even death. Especially in the context of palliative care, where symptom management is prioritized over curative treatments, the idea of death is often in the forefront of patient's minds. The shift from curative to palliative treatment can signify to the patient that recovery from the illness is no longer possible and the most that medical care can offer is physical comfort. Unfortunately, many patients respond to worsening medical illness by wishing to expedite death, as evidenced by the elevated rates of suicide in medically ill populations and growing political movements to legalize medically hastened death. However, understanding and responding to a severely ill patient's expression of the wish to end their life has become more complicated over the past decades.

The wish to end one's life in the context of medical illness is typically conceptualized as two related constructs: suicide (or suicidal ideation, SI) and the desire for hastened death (DHD). While the constructs of SI and suicide are applicable to both physically healthy and medically ill individuals, DHD is specific to those with advanced illness because it refers to wanting to quicken the dying process. Thus, DHD can include thoughts of suicide, but also encompasses requests for physician-assisted suicide, and more indirect means of hastening death (e.g., rejecting potentially life-sustaining interventions). An extensive research literature exists examining the correlates of or reasons for SI and attempted or completed suicide, but studies focusing squarely on suicide in patients with advanced or terminal medical illness are less common.

Research on DHD (and the term itself) first emerged in the 1990s, but the lack of a formal definition of what this term means, and how it is distinguished from suicide more generally, has hindered research into these related fields. In 2016, Balaguer and colleagues published a consensus definition of DHD and related terminology in patients with advanced illness.[1] After reviewing the existing literature, an international group of experts used the Delphi process to develop a consensus definition of the desire or wish for hastened death: "a reaction to suffering, in the context of a life-threatening condition, from which the patient can see no way out other than to accelerate his or her death."[1] Importantly, this definition distinguished DHD from an acceptance of one's impending death, or even wishing to die soon but without any intention to hasten death. They concluded that DHD can be driven by present or anticipated physical symptoms, psychological distress, existential suffering, or social stressors (e.g., feeling like a burden to family or friends). This definition provides a framework for researchers to use when studying DHD across different illnesses and settings, and it can help clinicians identify the basis for these thoughts and wishes in their patients who express similar ideas. Notably, DHD is not rare, with studies of terminally ill patients identifying an elevated desire to die in 8–45% of the samples studied.[2,3] In palliative care settings, clinicians often encounter patients who articulate thoughts of death and may even express a wish to speed up the disease process, making this construct an important topic for any professional working in the palliative care setting.

This chapter aims to provide a broad overview of the reasons for, assessment of, and possible responses to suicidality and DHD in those with advanced medical illness. Much of this research is drawn from the field of psycho-oncology, though research has focused on a range of life-limiting medical illnesses and is therefore applicable to most palliative care settings. This chapter will occasionally use the terms "suicide" and "DHD" interchangeably but will distinguish the two constructs when it is important to contextualize the research literature more clearly. The first part of this chapter details risk factors for suicide and DHD. Subsequently, the available tools to assess for suicidality and DHD are presented, focusing on both research and clinical applications, as well as potential interventions in the medical context. Finally, we discuss the role of culture on SI in palliative care, as well as legal and ethical issues regarding physician-assisted suicide and euthanasia. We conclude with future directions and suggestions for ways to conceptualize and provide care for those who may be suicidal or wish to hasten their death in the context of palliative care.

Risk Factors for Suicide and DHD

It is crucial for researchers and clinicians working in palliative care settings to understand the risk factors for SI and DHD as many patients may express thoughts about death and dying even when they are not considering hastening their death. A systematic review of SI and its associated risk factors in patients with cancer determined that many of the risk factors that are relevant to suicide in the general population also apply to those with a

TABLE 7.1 Risk factors for suicidal ideation, desire for hastened death, and completed suicide

SUICIDAL IDEATION	Desire for hastened death	Completed suicide
DEMOGRAPHIC AND SITUATIONAL FACTORS		
Male gender		Male gender
Single/not partnered		Single/not partnered
		Young age or older age*
		Non-Hispanic ethnicity
		Racial minority
		Low socioeconomic status
Access to life-threatening means		Access to life-threatening means
Substance abuse		Substance abuse
PHYSICAL AND DISEASE-RELATED FACTORS		
Diagnosis of head and neck, gastric, lung, or pancreatic cancers	Symptom distress	Recent diagnosis of terminal illness
Very advanced disease stage		
Pain		
Fatigue		
PSYCHOLOGICAL AND DISTRESS-RELATED FACTORS		
Depression	Depression	Poor quality of life
Hopelessness	Hopelessness	
History of psychiatric illness	Feeling like a burden	

* Younger and older palliative care patients are both at elevated risk for completed suicide.

life-threatening medical illness.[4] However, other risk factors appear to be unique to the context of medical illness (see Table 7.1). For example, male gender and individuals who are single, depressed, and those with a history of psychiatric illness are risk factors that are typical of the general public but also put individuals in palliative care settings at higher risk for suicide. Likewise, controlled substance misuse and access to life-threatening means also suggest a more serious risk for suicide in both the general public as well as palliative care patients.

A population-based study of suicide in US cancer patients examined records from more than 3 million individuals diagnosed with cancer between 2000 and 2010.[5] Mortality ratios identified several socioeconomic variables that increased the risk of death by suicide based on the ratio between the observed number of completed suicides in the sample versus completed suicides in a demographically similar non-cancer cohort of individuals in the United States during the same time period. Some of the risk factors identified in this study mirror those found in the general population, such as older age and male gender. Racial minorities (Asian/Pacific Islander, African American, Indigenous American) also showed a higher risk of completing suicide, although Hispanic individuals were at lower risk. Individuals who reported being divorced had twice the risk of completed suicide compared to those who were not divorced. Other demographic characteristics associated with increased risk of suicide in patients with cancer included being from a region of the country with low levels of education, high levels of unemployment, counties where a majority of residents fell below the poverty line, and regions with less urban development. Of course, many of these risk factors can co-occur, and individuals who exhibited both demographic and socioeconomic risk factors (e.g., males living in a county with significant poverty) showed an even greater likelihood of suicide. These results highlight the importance of considering an individual's demographic background when assessing considering suicide risk, as well as the environment in which they reside.

Research has also identified a number of disease-specific factors that increase a patient's risk for SI or completed suicide. The highest risk for completing suicide is during the first year after diagnosis, with the first week being a particularly sensitive timeframe.[4] While suicide risk in patients with cancer does decrease over time, it still remains elevated during the first 5 years of the illness when compared to the general population. Of particular importance in palliative care settings, advanced cancer stage (i.e., stage III and IV) is also associated with an increased risk of suicide, likely corresponding to the lower likelihood of cure or remission.[2,4] Some medical interventions are also associated with a higher risk of suicide, such as cancer patients who undergo surgery, perhaps due to concerns about disfigurement or the pain and stress surrounding recovery from surgery. Additionally, certain types of cancers, such as head and neck, gastric, lung, and pancreatic, have been associated with elevated rates of suicide.[4] Relatedly, greater physical symptom distress has also been correlated with SI in cancer patients (particularly those patients endorsing pain or fatigue).[4] Patients who are relatively young at time of an initial cancer diagnosis also display some of the highest rates of both SI and completed suicide, with rates that exceed those of older cancer patients.[4] However, research on age and suicide (and SI) has generated mixed results, suggesting that cancer patients at either end of the age spectrum (younger and much older) are at elevated risk for suicidality.

Multiple psychological constructs, most of which have also been linked to suicide and SI in physically healthy adults, have also been linked to SI in the palliative care setting.[4] Not surprisingly, one widely researched risk factor for SI in patients with cancer is the presence of depressive symptoms and/or clinically diagnosed depression; both have been strongly linked to SI in patients with cancer. Furthermore, studies that assessed for demoralization, hopelessness, existential distress, and anxiety have typically found strong relationships with SI. Perhaps the most important of these risk factors is hopelessness, which was originally conceptualized as a symptom of depression but has increasingly been recognized as a related but independent construct.[6] Characterized by the loss of future goals or plans, hopelessness is strongly associated with an increased likelihood of SI for those with advanced illness.

Research focused on patients suffering from the neurodegenerative disorder Huntington's disease also demonstrates the link between mental health symptoms and SI.[7] In a sample of nearly 2,000 patients with Huntington's disease, depression/anxiety and aggression/irritability were associated with greater likelihood of SI. Moreover, within the group of individuals who endorsed the highest level of SI, alcohol abuse was also a significant predictor of SI, in addition to psychological distress. Thus, while the cognitive and motor sequelae of Huntington's disease often receive the most attention, these findings suggest that the psychiatric symptoms are crucial to assess for when considering SI in patients with Huntington's disease.

In addition to the extensive literature on suicide and SI in patients with a life-limiting medical illness, a substantial body of research has focused on DHD, almost exclusively studying patients in palliative care settings. One distinction in the research literature examining DHD is the stronger emphasis on physical symptom distress. Both physical symptom distress and the perception of oneself as a burden to others were associated with DHD in patients with advanced HIV/AIDS who were living in a skilled nursing facility.[2] Overall quality of life (QoL) is another important risk factor for both suicide and DHD as the loss of physical functioning abilities or loss of meaning in life has been linked to an increased desire to die. While symptoms such as pain have not been strongly linked to DHD, this is likely due to adequate management of symptoms by the palliative care services where much of the published research has taken place. Of course, pain and symptom management should always be prioritized, as expressions of DHD may reflect an indirect way for a patient to communicate physical symptom distress.[8] The relationship between physical functioning and DHD also highlights the important role of palliative care in addressing risk for suicide and SI, as symptom burden can often be treated effectively with palliative care services, which may reduce thoughts or feelings about wanting to die.

Not all patient expressions of DHD are driven by physical symptoms, as depression and hopelessness also impact DHD. Breitbart and colleagues, in their study of 92 patients with terminal cancer found that both hopelessness and depression independently contributed to DHD, with the combination of high levels of hopelessness and severe depression being linked to particularly high levels of DHD.[2] In their analyses, perceived social support and physical functioning also contributed to predicting DHD, albeit more modestly, highlighting the additive effect of these risk factors (i.e., more risk factors correspond to a greater level of DHD or risk of suicide). Clearly, psychological distress impacts how patients feel about their future and can fuel thoughts of suicide or DHD. Importantly, psychological distress often responds to mental health interventions, which will be discussed later in this chapter. Moreover, while highlighting risk factors for SI and DHD is critical to patient care, reinforcing protective factors can also help patients who are struggling. Protective factors are attributes of a person, their social context, or their community that help buffer against risk, in this case for SI or DHD. A first defense is high-quality palliative care for the entire patient—not only the physical disease, but also for the patient's psychological need through evidence-based psychotherapy or other forms of emotional support. Feeling connected to others can provide patients with reasons to live, even in the context of physical or existential suffering. Hence, reinforcing connections between patients and their family and community support, as well as to other sources of meaning in their lives, can be critically important. Additionally, cultural and religious beliefs may discourage suicide and/or help patients find adaptive ways to cope with their physical limitations as well as providing additional sources of support for patients who are suffering.[3] Self-efficacy has also been found to protect against SI in patients with advanced cancer who have less than 6 months to live.[9]

These are just a few of the protective factors that patients may respond to and can be used to combat the distress and hopelessness that may lead to SI.

Assessment of Suicide Risk and DHD

Assessment of suicide risk varies across studies, and no gold standard approach currently exists for palliative care or even general medical settings. Measurement approaches used in published research vary and include clinical interviews, single items drawn from established measures of depression and symptom burden (e.g., one item from the Patient Health Questionnaire asks specifically about SI), and measures specifically developed to quantify severity of SI, intent and/or actions (e.g., the Beck Scale for Suicidal Ideation).[4] One measure that has been widely used in research and clinical settings and that has been recommended by the US Food and Drug Administration for community settings is the Columbia Suicide Severity Rating Scale (CSSRS).[10] The CSSRS measures intensity and severity of SI, as well as suicide attempts and self-injurious behavior without suicidal intent. While the CSSRS and other measures of SI can be quite useful among the general population, unique challenges arise when these measures are used in the context of terminal illness. For example, thinking about whether one would be better off dead is less pathological in a palliative care sample than in the general population. As such, risk assessment approaches that are more sensitive to the mortality concerns of those with terminal illness are necessary.

Given the challenges posed by existing measures of suicide risk, many palliative care researchers have focused on the assessment of DHD. Initial research attempted to identify DHD as a construct distinct from both suicidality and requests for physician-assisted suicide (PAS) by focusing on understanding the meaning of and motivations for DHD.[11] In other words, they aimed to differentiate between a wish to die, a wish to die *soon*, and a request for medical assistance to expedite the dying process. To accomplish this, researchers have developed quantitative measures of DHD that have helped better define the construct and pinpoint its clinical relevance.

Chochinov and colleagues published the first quantitative measure of DHD, which they termed the Desire for Death Rating Scale (DDRS).[3] They administered semi-structured interviews to 200 terminally ill cancer inpatients, beginning with the question "Do you ever wish that your illness would progress more quickly so that your suffering could be over sooner?" If the patient responded affirmatively to this question, follow-up questions were asked to determine the extent and frequency of those feelings. Clinicians then assigned a score ranging from 0 (no desire for death) to 6 (extreme desire for death), with scores of 4 or greater considered to be indicative of clinically significant DHD. Chochinov and colleagues classified 8.5% of the patients in their sample as having clinically significant DHD, 59% of whom were also diagnosed with a depressive disorder. Although the DDRS has been used to measure DHD in a number of subsequent studies, its utility is limited because it relies on structured interviews and clinician ratings, which hinders application in many clinical and research settings.

To address these limitations, Rosenfeld and colleagues developed a self-report measure called the Schedule of Attitudes Toward Hastened Death (SAHD).[8] The scale was originally developed in a sample of 195 patients with HIV/AIDS but has subsequently been applied to patients with a range of terminal illnesses (cancer, Parkinson's disease) and has been translated into multiple languages (e.g., Spanish, Greek, German, Korean). The SAHD includes 20 true/false questions, and a score of 10 or greater typically indicates clinically significant DHD. In multiple studies, the SAHD has demonstrated strong internal consistency and significant correlations with measures of depression, hopelessness, spiritual well-being, and QoL. The SAHD differs from the DDRS in that it captures *patient-reported* levels of DHD, rather than requiring a clinician's assessment of patient DHD. As a result, it is easy to use, quick, and reliable. Furthermore, the availability of the SAHD in multiple languages and abbreviated (7-item) versions make it an accessible and useful tool to assess DHD in both clinical and research settings. However, it is unclear how often measures like the DDRS or SAHD are used in routine clinical care, given that many clinicians are reticent to raise issues (like SI or DHD) that they are uncomfortable discussing or feel ill-equipped to address. Hence, the importance of clinical interventions for patients at risk for suicide or expressing clinically significant DHD is clear.

Interventions for Patients with Elevated Risk of Suicide or DHD

Given that depression and hopelessness play a significant role in suicide and DHD, the treatment of depression, whether psychopharmacological or psychological (or both), has been a primary starting point for many mental health professionals working in palliative care and psycho-oncology. In fact, purely pharmacological interventions have shown some success in reducing both SI and DHD among individuals with terminal illnesses. For example, Breitbart and colleagues examined the use of selective serotonin reuptake inhibitors to treat depression among individuals with advanced AIDS.[12] They observed significant and substantial declines in DHD among those participants who experienced improvement in depressive symptoms. Fan and colleagues have also found that a single dose of ketamine was effective in treating SI among patients with cancer, with results lasting for 3 days following administration.[4]

Psychotherapeutic approaches have also shown effectiveness in reducing depression and DHD in terminally ill cancer patients. Although cognitive behavioral therapy (CBT) is the most well-established and widely used psychological treatment for depression in physically healthy individuals, many of the negative thoughts that are typically addressed through a CBT approach are realistic and rational in the context of terminal illness. Therefore, other psychological treatment approaches may be more useful when working with palliative care or terminally ill patients. In fact, preliminary research has supported the use of behavioral activation, problem-solving interventions, spiritual care, and nurse-administered psychoeducation to reduce SI among patients with cancer.[4] Even stronger support exists for psychological interventions that focus on existential distress by enhancing the patient's sense of meaning and dignity and thereby reducing DHD and other aspects of psychological distress. There are several treatment approaches that show promise in addressing the existential distress that often underlies SI and DHD, such as dignity therapy and meaning-centered psychotherapy (MCP).

Dignity therapy was developed by Chochinov and colleagues,[13] based on the hypothesis that a loss of dignity is an integral component of the existential distress often experienced by individuals with terminal illness. This brief intervention focuses on questions around the patient's sense of self, dignity, and values that are discussed with a mental health professional. Sessions are recorded, transcribed, and arranged chronologically to generate a cohesive narrative that the mental health provider reads back to the patient and then provides a copy for the patient to share with loved ones. Although their randomized clinical trial (RCT) of 441 palliative care patients from the United States, Australia and Canada indicated little benefit from this intervention on systematic measures of DHD, feelings of hopelessness, or perceived burden, patients reported significantly better quality of life, and the intervention was perceived as more helpful than other interventions by both patients and their family members. Moreover, the widespread dissemination of this intervention highlights the intuitive appeal for clinicians worldwide.

Another promising intervention to address DHD is MCP, which was developed specifically for patients with advanced and terminal cancer.[14] This intervention can be delivered in a group or individual format, typically over 7 or 8 weekly sessions. Rooted in the work of existential philosophers and psychologists like Frankl and Nietzsche, MCP aims to enhance a sense of meaning in the face of severe suffering through manualized sessions that incorporate psychoeducation, question prompts, and homework. Each session focuses on a particular topic, including an introduction to the concept of meaning; the patient's cancer history; historical, attitudinal, creative, and experiential sources of meaning; and transitions or plans for the patient's future. Patients are also encouraged to complete a "legacy project," which can range from completing a lifelong goal (e.g., writing a song or poem) to mending strained relationships. Multiple RCTs have shown consistently strong benefits for MCP, with significantly greater reductions in DHD and hopelessness and improved QoL compared to patients receiving supportive psychotherapy in both group and individual formats.[15] Considering these promising results, researchers have adapted MCP for use with other populations, cultures, and settings.

Although not an exhaustive summary of the available psychotherapeutic interventions, dignity therapy and MCP are two of the most widely used interventions for patients with advanced and terminal illness and highlight the importance of addressing existential distress rather than focusing exclusively on symptoms such as anxiety and depression.[16] As an understanding of DHD continues to grow, including its etiology, pathogenesis, and methods of treatment, it is also important to consider the high rates of comorbidity with other forms of psychological and existential distress. It is also imperative that palliative care interventions extend past the medical or physical symptoms so that physicians are better able to assess (and when appropriate, treat) DHD among their patients, with the aim of reducing stigma and maximizing access to appropriate psychological care.

Physician Hastened Death

Complicating the understanding of, and response to expressions of suicide and DHD is the growing acceptance of PAS. PAS involves *patient administration* of physician-prescribed lethal drugs with the intention of ending life.[17] This practice is distinct from euthanasia (which is legal in a handful of countries, but not the United States), which involves *physician administration* of a lethal medication. Legalization of PAS and euthanasia, often referred to as physician hastened death (PHD), has steadily increased worldwide over the past two decades. In fact, while only three countries in Europe and three US states had legalized PHD in 2010, just a decade later that number had more than doubled, with PHD legal in seven countries and nine US states and the District of Columbia.

Many safeguards exist before a PHD request is granted, and these have important implications for broader questions about how to respond to patient expressions of SI or DHD more generally. Most legislation requires the patient to consent and then reiterate that consent at a later date (e.g., a minimum of 48 hours later) as well as obtain verification from two physicians of the patient's mental competence and the irreversibility and unbearable degree of patient suffering.[18] However, the clinical conditions that would make a patient eligible for PHD differ across jurisdictions. For example, in some countries, PHD is available to minors whereas most countries prohibit this practice. Likewise, the Netherlands and Belgium permit PHD on the grounds of psychological suffering in addition to physical suffering, whereas most countries require a diagnosis of terminal illness and preclude psychological suffering as a sole basis for PHD.[18] Despite these and other policy differences across jurisdictions, the common emphasis is a requirement that the patient be capable of competent decision-making.

Factors influencing decision-making among patients are variable. In a report of 56 individuals who requested PHD, the most common reason for the request was to foster a sense of increased autonomy over the circumstances of death. Other important reasons cited included a wish to avoid a loss of independence and concerns about future pain, poor QoL, and loss of dignity.[19] Interestingly, inadequate social support and depressed mood were not cited as important reasons for requesting PHD. However, the fact that patients did not report depression as an important reason for requesting PHD does not mean that depression or distress were not influential, as depression is often observed among patients who request PHD. For example, in an analysis of 66 PHD cases in the Netherlands between 2011 and 2014, 49 individuals had either a primary or secondary diagnosis of depression.[20] Another study estimated that 25–50% of patients expressing interest in PHD present with significant depressive symptoms and that 2–10% of patients who followed through with PHD were considered clinically depressed.[21] Thus, the extent to which depression or distress compromises decision-making competence requires careful attention by clinicians faced with a patient request for PHD. Indeed, research has suggested that depressed individuals often have difficulty appreciating the potential benefits from available interventions and may perceive PHD as the only option to avoid eventual suffering.[22] Hence, attention to subtle but potentially important influences on patient decision-making when PHD is raised highlights the need for careful consideration in how to respond. This response to PHD differs from patients who express SI and/or DHD, which more often reflect a "cry for help," particularly when PHD is not a legally sanctioned option.

Moreover, while the decisional impairments observed in depressed, terminally ill patients may not rise to the level of incompetence, the intervention research described previously highlights the potential for change in an individual's interest in PHD or suicide. This possibility is evident in the finding that many individuals who request PHD never follow through with the procedure. In one study of 100 patients requesting assisted suicide, 38 withdrew their requests before a decision was made by physicians, and, of the 48 patients who were provided with a prescription that could be used to end life, 11 postponed or never followed through with the suicide.[23] In fact, some commentators have suggested that merely knowing that the option of PAS exists can help alleviate the anxiety and distress associated with terminal illness.[24]

Of course, depression is not the only mental health condition that might impact requests for PHD, as neurological disorders and dementia have also been observed in patients requesting PHD, albeit less frequently. Understanding when or if psychological symptoms are driving a request for PHD (or SI more generally) is crucial to determining the appropriate response. However, evaluating depression in the palliative care setting also poses unique challenges, especially among older adults. Many of the diagnostic criteria for depression, such as sleep and appetite disturbance, fatigue, and psychomotor retardation, may reflect normative aging or can be symptoms of disease progression. Saracino and colleagues recommended alternative criteria, such as feeling a loss of meaning and purpose in life, feelings of boredom ("having nothing to do"), and social withdrawal as useful in helping identify depression in older, medically ill adults.[25] Coupled with careful attention to the patient's decision-making capacity, these criteria can help clinicians differentiate between "rational" requests for PHD and those that might respond to intervention. This is not to suggest that a competent request for PHD requires the absence of depressive symptoms or perfect ability to articulate the basis for one's decision, but differentiating a "cry for help" from a well-thought out decision can help patients, their family members, and treatment providers have confidence that the decision is consistent with the patient's values and beliefs. While PHD can provide comfort and protect patient autonomy, careful assessment of requests for PAS is no less important than other expressions of SI or DHD.

Future Directions

The loss of a patient or family member to an unanticipated suicide can be traumatic for family members as well as for the patient's healthcare providers. Understanding the risk factors for suicide and DHD can help the palliative care clinician navigate these challenging situations by identifying and responding to patient expressions of SI or DHD—regardless of whether PHD is a legally sanctioned option. Although tools are available to help clinicians screen for SI and DHD, they are infrequently used in routine clinical practice. Instead, clinicians typically rely on their judgement, hopefully guided by existing research. While a substantial area of research has focused on evaluating SI and DHD in the palliative care context, more research is needed on the effect of psychotherapy or psychopharmacotherapy on SI and DHD. As detailed in this chapter, several psychotherapeutic interventions have been shown to help alleviate SI and DHD in the palliative care context. However, there is limited research on how or if pharmacotherapy may be useful in reducing wishes to hasten death. When an elevated risk of suicide or DHD is identified, the clinician will need to determine what, if any, intervention is warranted, ranging from more aggressive pain and symptom management to psychotherapeutic interventions (e.g., antidepressant medication, existential psychotherapy). Critical to any clinical decision-making is vigilance to the parallel goals of optimizing the patient's mental and physical health while still respecting their autonomy to determine how to spend their remaining days, weeks, or months.

Key Points

- Demographic and disease-specific factors put patients with advanced illness at heightened risk for suicidal ideation, desire for hastened death, and completed suicide.
- Multiple measures exist to assess for depression, suicidal ideation, and desire for hastened death in the palliative care community and can provide critical information for clinicians on the safety and wishes of the patient.
- Interventions, such as MCP and dignity therapy, are efficacious treatment options to decrease existential distress, hopelessness, and perceived burden in patients with advanced illness, which in turn may impact levels of suicidality or DHD.
- PAS, the administration of physician-prescribed lethal drugs by the patient intended to end life, and euthanasia, which involves physician-administered lethal medication, are often referred together as "physician-hastened death" and are becoming more available across the United States and globally.

References

1. Balaguer A, Monforte-Royo C, Porta-Sales J, Alonso-Babarro A, Altisent R, Aradilla-Herrero A, et al. An international consensus definition of the wish to hasten death and its related factors. *PLoS One.* 2016;11(1):e0146184.
2. Breitbart W, Rosenfeld B, Pessin H, Kaim M, Funesti-Esch J, Galietta M, et al. Depression, hopelessness, and desire for hastened death in terminally ill patients with cancer. *JAMA.* 2000;284(22):2907–2911.
3. Chochinov HM, ilson KG, Enns M, Mowchun N, Lander S, Levitt M, et al. Desire for death in the terminally ill. *The Am J Psychiatry.* 1995;152(8):1185–1191.
4. Kolva E, Hoffecker L, Cox-Martin E. Suicidal ideation in patients with cancer: A systematic review of prevalence, risk factors, intervention and assessment. *Palliat Support Care.* 2020;18(2):206–219.
5. Abdel-Rahman O. Socioeconomic predictors of suicide risk among cancer patients in the United States: A population-based study. *Cancer Epidemiol.* 2019;63:101601.
6. Rosenfeld B, Pessin H, Lewis C, Abbey J, Olden M, Sachs E, et al. Assessing hopelessness in terminally ill cancer patients: Development of the Hopelessness Assessment in Illness Questionnaire. *Psychol Assess.* Jun 2011;23(2):325–336. doi:10.1037/a0021767
7. Wetzel HH, Gehl CR, Dellefave–Castillo L, Schiffman JF, Shannon KM, Paulsen JS, et al. Suicidal ideation in Huntington disease: The role of comorbidity. *Psychiatry Res.* 2011;188(3):372–376.

8. Rosenfeld B, Breitbart W, Stein K, Funesti-Esch J, Kaim M, Krivo S, et al. Measuring desire for death among patients with HIV/AIDS: The schedule of attitudes toward hastened death. *Am J Psychiatry.* 1999;156(1):94–100.

9. Trevino KM, Balboni M, Zollfrank A, Balboni T, Prigerson HG. Negative religious coping as a correlate of suicidal ideation in patients with advanced cancer. *Psycho-Oncology.* 2014;23(8):936–945.

10. Posner K, Brent D, Lucas C, Gould M, Stanley B, Brown G, et al. *Columbia-Suicide Severity Rating Scale (C-SSRS).* New York: Columbia University Medical Center. 2008;10.

11. Monforte-Royo C, Villavicencio-Chávez C, Tomás-Sábado J, Mahtani-Chugani V, Balaguer A. What lies behind the wish to hasten death? A systematic review and meta-ethnography from the perspective of patients. *PLoS One.* 2012;7(5):e37117.

12. Breitbart W, Rosenfeld B, Gibson C, Kramer M, Li Y, Tomarken A, et al. Impact of treatment for depression on desire for hastened death in patients with advanced AIDS. *Psychosomatics.* 2010;51(2):98–105.

13. Chochinov HM, Hack T, Hassard T, Kristjanson LJ, McClement S, Harlos M. Dignity therapy: A novel psychotherapeutic intervention for patients near the end of life. *J Clin Oncol.* 2005;23(24):5520–5525.

14. Breitbart W. Spirituality and meaning in supportive care: Spirituality-and meaning-centered group psychotherapy interventions in advanced cancer. *Support Care Cancer.* 2002;10(4):272–280.

15. Breitbart W, Breitbart W, Pessin H, Rosenfeld B, Applebaum AJ, Lichtenthal WG, Li Y, et al. Individual meaning-centered psychotherapy for the treatment of psychological and existential distress: A randomized controlled trial in patients with advanced cancer. *Cancer.* 2018;124(15):3231–3239.

16. Kredentser MS, Chochinov HM. Psychotherapeutic considerations for patients with terminal illness. *Am J Psychotherapy.* 2020;73(4):137–143.

17. Booker R, Bruce A. Palliative sedation and medical assistance in dying: Distinctly different or simply semantics? *Nurs Inq.* 2020;27(1):e12321.

18. Vergallo G, Gulino M, Bersani G, Rinaldi R. Euthanasia and Physician-Assisted Suicide for Patients With Depression: Thought-Provoking Remarks. *Riv Psichiatr.* 2020;55(2):119–128.

19. Ganzini L, Goy ER, Dobscha SK. Oregonians' reasons for requesting physician aid in dying. *Arch Intern Med.* Mar 9 2009;169(5):489–492. doi:10.1001/archinternmed.2008.579

20. Kim SY, De Vries RG, Peteet JR. Euthanasia and assisted suicide of patients with psychiatric disorders in the Netherlands 2011 to 2014. *JAMA Psychiatry.* 2016;73(4):362–368.

21. Levene I, Parker M. Prevalence of depression in granted and refused requests for euthanasia and assisted suicide: A systematic review. *J Med Ethics.* 2011;37(4):205–211.

22. Hindmarch T, Hotopf M, Owen GS. Depression and decision-making capacity for treatment or research: A systematic review. *BMC Med Ethics.* 2013;14(1):54.

23. Thienpont L, Verhofstadt M, Van Loon T, Distelmans W, Audenaert K, De Deyn PP. Euthanasia requests, procedures and outcomes for 100 Belgian patients suffering from psychiatric disorders: A retrospective, descriptive study. *BMJ Open.* 2015;5(7):e007454.

24. Rosenfeld B. *Assisted Suicide and the Right to Die: The Interface of Social Science, Public Policy, and Medical Ethics.* American Psychological Association; 2004.

25. Saracino RM, Nelson CJ. Identification and treatment of depressive disorders in older adults with cancer. *J Geriatr Oncol.* 2019;10(5):680–684.

8

Medical Assistance in Dying

Aliza A. Panjwani, Gary Rodin, and Madeline Li

I should only make myself ridiculous in my own eyes if I clung to life and
hugged it when it had no more to offer.
—Socrates

Introduction

Dr. A is an 82-year-old philosophy professor approaching the end of life with advanced
ovarian cancer. She is single, has no children, and had been living alone until admission to
hospice. Recognizing the inevitable continued loss of daily function, she described her experience as "every morning, little increments of my person are gone." She requested assisted
dying primarily so that "I can leave with my cognitive faculties."

Few topics in medicine are as polarizing as assisted dying. For this and other reasons, there
is considerable variability in assisted dying terminology. The definitions and terms commonly used to refer to assisted dying are listed in Table 8.1. Terms such as "euthanasia" are
not used in some regions due to connotations of eugenics. Moreover, the designation of an
assisted death as a "suicide" has largely been eliminated because of the stigma associated
with suicide. The phrases "physician-assisted dying/death" or "medical assistance in dying"
(MAiD) are preferred by some because of the legitimacy and support associated with a
medical act. Others argue that this association may heighten misperceptions that palliative
care will shorten life. In the absence of international consensus regarding terminology, we
use "MAiD" to include both clinician administration of a lethal substance at a patient's request (euthanasia) and prescription of a lethal substance to a patient for self-administration
(assisted suicide) in this chapter.

TABLE 8.1 Terms and definitions

Term(s)	Definitions
Euthanasia, Voluntary (active) euthanasia	The intentional ending of the life of a mentally competent patient by a physician via the administration of lethal substance, based on the explicit request of the patient
Assisted suicide, Physician-assisted suicide (PAS), Physician aid in/assisted dying (PAD), Voluntary assisted dying (VAD)	The provision of medication or a prescription to a patient at his or her explicit request with the understanding that the patent intends to self-administer the medication to end his or her life
Assisted dying/death, Medical assistance in dying (MAiD)	Either clinician administration of a lethal substance at a patient's request or prescription of a lethal substance to a patient for self-administration

In countries and jurisdictions where it is legal, MAiD accounts for less than 5% of deaths.[1] This is a substantial number, although the vast majority of individuals at the end of life do not request this intervention even in jurisdictions where it is legal. With or without an accompanying request for MAiD, assessment of the desire for death is an integral part of palliative psychiatry. Dr. A did not evidence a clinical disorder, such as depression (Chapter 4), demoralization (Chapter 26), or other psychosocial vulnerability, that led her to impulsively decide to end her life. She reflected on MAiD over a long period of time and ultimately sought it so that she could reach the end of life with her cognitive functioning intact. In the case of Dr. A and others like her, it is often unclear if a psychosocial intervention is clinically indicated or desired by the patient, or if it would even alter the core desire to control circumstances of death.

Astute clinical judgment is required to ensure access to MAiD when clinically appropriate and to identify psychiatric disorders or social circumstances that may limit the capacity for informed consent or benefits from other interventions. At minimum, distinguishing MAiD as a rational and capable choice from a decision to die that is heavily influenced by depression or social isolation is paramount. Nevertheless, whether MAiD should be associated with palliative care remains a highly controversial topic.

This chapter provides an overview of the historical and global context of MAiD, the role of palliative care and psychiatry, practice points with case illustrations, and the impacts of MAiD on patients and family, the practice of medicine, and on healthcare providers.

Historical Evolution

Etymologically, "euthanasia" is derived from the early 17th-century Greek *eu* "well" + *thanatos* "death," meaning a "good death." For some philosophers, a central consideration in care for the dying was prioritizing quality rather than quantity of life. Voluntary and involuntary "mercy killings" were therefore accepted in ancient Greece and Rome, especially when the alternative was prolonged agony. Some have suggested that the presumed forbidding of euthanasia in the Hippocratic Oath—"I will not give a lethal drug to anyone if

I am asked"—may actually have been intended to prohibit collaboration in political murder, which was common in Ancient Greece and for which physicians were sought due to their expertise in poisons.

The arrival of Christianity in the 12–15th centuries reinforced the view that human life is a trusted gift from God. During this time, the presence of a physician in the final hours of life was actively discouraged, and the notion that medicine is powerless against incurable illness was fortified. To call for a physician while on one's deathbed was considered a sign of weakness and a spurning of spiritual deliverance. With the evolution of scientific knowledge, technological and economic advancement, and industrialization in the 19th century, the physician's role at the dying patient's bedside became central, not to shorten life but to ensure provision of adequate care. Not until the 20th century were open discussions about death and dying and the limiting of futile, burdensome medical interventions deemed acceptable in some settings.

Attempts to legalize MAiD in Britain and the United States in the first half of the 20th century were unsuccessful, and caution about MAiD was heightened by the Nazi use of involuntary euthanasia. Proponents continued to argue that *voluntary* euthanasia be allowed for competent, terminally ill patients to preserve their dignity, a view that became more accepted in the 1960s and 1970s with the rising interest in individual rights and freedoms in the Western and European world. The Harvard Medical School's definition of irreversible coma as a new criterion for death in 1968 and the 1976 US Supreme Court ruling that a respirator may be removed from a patient in a permanent neurovegetative state further affirmed the human right to death when meaningful life is no longer possible. In 1990, the US Congress passed the Self-Determination Act, which required hospitals receiving national funds to inform patients of their right to refuse treatment. However, the greatest impetus for the growing legalization of MAiD in the Western world came not from medicine but from the convergence of social factors, including an increasing emphasis on individual autonomy and secular values, the movement of consumerism and patient empowerment, and the aging population.

International MAiD Legislation

In 1942, Switzerland became the first country to decriminalize physician-assisted suicide. Oregon became the first jurisdiction to permit assisted suicide in 1997, and Netherlands the first country to legalize MAiD (both assisted suicide and euthanasia) in 2001. To date, 8 countries (Switzerland, Netherlands, Belgium, Luxembourg, Columbia, Canada, New Zealand, Spain), 11 American states (Oregon, Montana, Washington, Vermont, Maine, California, District of Columbia, Colorado, Hawaii, New Mexico, and New Jersey), and 5 Australian jurisdictions (Victoria, Tasmania, Western Australia, South Australia, and Queensland) have legalized euthanasia, assisted suicide, or both. The adoption of MAiD has expanded, with several countries recently passing court rulings but awaiting legislation for implementation (Germany, Austria, Portugal). Legalization of MAiD is also being considered in Italy, the United Kingdom, France, and South Africa.

There is variability in MAiD laws and eligibility criteria across jurisdictions (see Table 8.2). The Benelux countries generally have the most permissive laws, allowing for both euthanasia and assisted dying in the absence of terminal illness, as well as permitting MAiD for children, individuals with mental illness, and as advance requests. The American states are at the other end of the spectrum, where assisted suicide is restricted to capable adults with terminal illness, and euthanasia is not permitted. Countries with permissive MAiD laws have seen a continual increase in deaths due to MAiD over time, while its prevalence has largely remained stable in countries with more restrictive legislation.[1]

MAiD and Palliative Care

The role of palliative care in MAiD remains controversial. Virtually all palliative care professional societies or organizations have taken the position that MAiD should be separate from palliative care practice. Individual practitioners involved in MAiD may experience tension or conflict with the positions of their professional bodies. Although some have argued that the implementation of MAiD will limit access to palliative care, research on MAiD in North America and Europe indicates that 70–87% of those who request assisted dying also receive palliative care services.[2,3] Among the minority of individuals who receive MAiD but not palliative care, the primary reasons for not accessing palliative care were that their palliative and support needs were sufficiently addressed or they did not desire a referral.[2] These findings provide strong support for the notion that MAiD requests are not typically driven by lack of access or referral to palliative services. However, more research is needed on the type, extent, and comprehensiveness of palliative care services provided to those who request and receive MAiD.

Studies of the perspectives of palliative care physicians and nurses have generated contrasting views and identified several practical challenges in MAiD. One of these is the need to balance the dosage of sedating medications to manage symptoms while maintaining the capacity of the patient for informed consent at the time of assisted death. Palliative care physicians may then face the paradoxical scenario of employing strategies such as the use of opioid antagonists or antipsychotics to achieve lucidity in patients with terminal delirium so that MAiD can then be provided.

Palliative care associations have accepted *palliative sedation*, or the administration of sedative drugs to decrease consciousness of a terminally ill patient in order to relieve intractable symptoms, as an intervention within their purview. Alongside symptom relief, death may be an unintended consequence of palliative sedation, a concept referred to as "double effect." MAiD is heavily publicized in the media, whereas palliative sedation is often not known to patients. Advocates of palliative sedation suggest that more patients would opt for sedation if they were made as aware of its availability as they are for MAiD.[4] Variations in both guidelines and practice have been observed across countries, particularly regarding existential distress as an indication for palliative sedation. Table 8.3 outlines features that are generally common to palliative sedation, contrasting them to MAiD.

TABLE 8.2 Summary of assisted dying laws globally

	Switzerland (1942)	Oregon, United states (1997)[a]	Netherlands (2001)	Belgium (2002)	Luxembourg (2009)
Assisted suicide	✓Article 115, Swiss Penal Cade: Legal if offered without selfish motive, Additional guidelines and criteria put forth by individual right-to-die organizations (RDOs)	✓Death with Dignity Act	✓Termination of Life on Request and Assisted Suicide Act	✓Not explicitly mentioned in Belgian law but accepted as form of euthanasia by Federal Control and Evaluation Committee on Euthanasia	✓Law Euthanasia and Assisted Suicide
Euthanasia	✗	✗	✓	✓Belgian Act on Euthanasia	✓
			SUBSTANTIVE SAFEGUARDS[B]		
Non-terminal illness	✓	✗Terminal illness, death<6 months	✓	✓	✓
Mental illness as sole condition	✓	✗	✓Determined that there is no reasonable alternative	✓Only for adults; in minors, mental illness and intellectual disabilities excluded; determined that there is no reasonable alternative	✓
Children	✓Age unspecified in law	✗	✓16 to 17 years: Require parentalinvolvement; 12 to 15 years: Require parental consent; 1–12 years: Plans approved to extend law	✓Minor <18 years; Require parental consent, except emancipated minors deemed to have capacity; unbearable, unrelievable, and incurable physical suffering due to medical condition; death expected in short-term	✗
Advance requests	✗	✗	✓	✓Patients with serious incurable disorder, no longer conscious, and both unconsciousness and underlying condition are irreversible	✓Patients with serious incurable illness who are no longer conscious, and situation is irreversible

(continued)

TABLE 8.2 Continued

	Switzerland (1942)	Oregon, United states (1997)[a]	Netherlands (2001)	Belgium (2002)	Luxembourg (2009)
PROCEDURAL SAFEGUARDS					
	✗ Physician assesses person's decisional capacity & prescribes medication; additional guidelines by RDOs	✓Attending and consulting physician	✓Attending and consulting physician; multidisciplinary committee to verify service provided in accordance with law	✓Attending and consulting physician; third expert physician in patient's condition consulted if death not foreseeable or I request by minor	✓Attending and consulting physician
Written request	Guidelines determined by RDOs	✓Two oral and one written requests	✗	✓Two written requests	✓One written request
Waiting period	Guidelines determined by RDOs	✓15 days between oral requests; 48 hours between written request and filling prescription; waived if patients expected to die within waiting periods	✗	✓One month waiting period required between second request and administering of euthanasia when death is not foreseeable	✗
	Colombia (2015)	Canada (2016)	Victoria, Australia (2017)[c]	New Zealand (2019)	Spain (2021)
Assisted suicide	✗Assisted suicide remains illegal	✓Model Assistance in Dying (MAiD) Law	✓Voluntary Assisted Dying {VAD} Act: Passed in 2017, enacted in 2019	✓End of Life Choice Act: Passed in 2019, enacted in 2021	✓Organic Law for regulation of Euthanasia
Euthanasia	✓Court ruling legalizing euthanasia in 1997. No regulated guidelines developed until 2015	✓	✓Only if physically incapable of taking medication themselves	✓	✓
SUBSTANTIVE SAFEGUARDS					
Non-terminal illness	✗	✓	✗Terminal illness, death <6 months; neurodegenerative disease, death <12 months	✗Terminal illness, death <6 months; mental illness or disorder, including dementia, excluded	✓
Mental illness as sole condition	✗	✗Will be permitted as of March 2023	✗	✗	✓

TABLE 8.2 **Continued**

	Switzerland (1942)	Oregon, United states (1997)[a]	Netherlands (2001)	Belgium (2002)	Luxembourg (2009)
Children	✓Minor ≥15 years: do not need parental consent; 7–14: consent from both parents; 12–14: if discrepancy between parents, child's will prevails	✗	✗	✗	✗
Advance requests	✓	✗	✗	✗	✓
PROCEDURAL SAFEGUARDS					
Attending and consulting physician and/or committee	✓Attending physician and interdisciplinary committee of physician (specialist in medical condition), lawyer, psychiatrist or clinical psychologist)	✓Two independent physicians, and, in some provinces, nurse practitioners	✓Attending and consulting physician	✓Attending and consulting physician	✓Attending and consulting physician; multidisciplinary committee to verify service provided in accordance with law
Written request	✓Written or oral request	✓One written request	✓Two oral and one written requests	✓Oral request, later reconfirmed in writing	✓Two written requests
Waiting period	✓15 days between committee approval and receipt of MAiD	✓90-day assessment period only for non-terminal illness, no waiting period for terminal illness	✓Minimum 10 days between first request and permit to receive MAiD; waived if person expected to die within this period	✓	✓15 days between written requests, unless patient at risk of losing capacity; ~40 days between first request and approval for MAiD

Note: This table depicts MAiD criteria across jurisdiction where legislation is available or accessible.

[a]The following US jurisdictions also allow assisted suicide: Washington (2008), Montana (2009), Vermont (2013), California (2015), Colorado (2016), Washington, D.C. (2017), Hawaii (2019), New Jersey (2019), Maine (2019), New Mexico (2021).

[b]Jurisdictions specify the following in some form: voluntary well-informed request made by capable persons; suffering must be intolerable, with no prospect for improvement.

[c]In addition to Victoria, Western Australia has also passed legislation on MAiD in 2019, and the law is currently in effect. Tasmania, South Australia, and Queensland passed legislation in 2021 that is expected to go into effect in 2022–2023.

TABLE 8.3 Differences between MAiD and palliative sedation

	Medical assistance in dying	Palliative sedation
Goal	Reduce suffering	Reduce suffering
Intent	To end patient's life, at patient's request	To reduce consciousness
Cause of death	Respiratory followed by cardiac arrest due to administered medication	Natural progression of illness
Indication	Subjective physical or psychological suffering, intolerable to the patient	Intractable symptom (e.g., dyspnea, pain, nausea and vomiting, existential distress)
Who drives the process	Requested by the patient (personal autonomy)	Offered by the palliative care physician as a treatment of last resort
Consent	Capacity and consent by patient	Consent by patient and/or substitute decision maker
Availability	Often weeks to arrange assessments and pass any required reflection periods	Available urgently for symptom crisis
Control	Patient can stay conscious to the last moment and is able to choreograph their death	Patient is unconscious before death
Duration	Immediate	Hours to short weeks to death
Process	Burdensome evaluation and legal forms required by patient	Usually documented as routine clinical care by physician

MAiD and Psychiatry

Research from North American countries shows that up to 72% of psychiatrists support MAiD for advanced and incurable illness, and approximately 30% are in favor of permitting it for the relief of suffering due to mental illness.[5] Surveys from the Benelux countries suggest that up to 75% of psychiatrists may support MAiD for suffering due to psychiatric conditions.[6] Notably, MAiD for psychiatric disorders remains rare even in jurisdictions where it is permitted. In 2019, only 1% of all MAiD cases in the Netherlands were for suffering related to psychiatric disorders alone.[7]

Concerns about MAiD for psychiatric disorders include the risk of psychosocial vulnerability driving MAiD requests in this population, the difficulty distinguishing suicidality as a rational choice from a symptom of mental illness, and the interpersonal and multiple meanings of such requests, particularly in patients with personality disorders. Determining what is "irremediable" in mental illness is also unclear, although there is an emerging acceptance of the treatment of severe and treatment-resistant mental illness as palliative care (Chapter 9). Whether and how MAID should be incorporated into such an approach has not yet been clarified.

Psychiatric comorbidity has been found in up to 40% of individuals who request MAiD for medical conditions, with depression being the most identified psychiatric disorder.[8] In such research, it is often unclear to what extent the low mood or degree of impairment associated with the medical condition contributes to the MAiD request, or even whether the reported diagnosis of depression was historical or current. Often, distinctions between depression as a clinical disorder and nonpathological forms of existential distress are not made or recorded.

Depression (Chapter 4), demoralization (Chapter 26), and death anxiety (Chapter 5) have been previously defined as distinct forms of existential distress. Death anxiety and demoralization may predict the desire to hasten death in advanced cancer (Chapter 7). Social and spiritual distress may also drive requests for MAiD in patients with advanced disease (Chapters 25 and 27). Although determination of capacity is often the reason for psychiatric consultation in MAiD, the role of psychiatry extends far beyond capacity determination. Psychiatrists also bring key expertise in the diagnostic assessment of mood or other psychiatric disorders, elucidation of psychosocial factors that may contribute to a MAiD request, and consideration of interventions to relieve psychological suffering due to disease burden and end-of-life distress.

Several existential or meaning-based supportive interventions have been shown to reduce demoralization, death anxiety, and desire to hasten death. These psychotherapeutic interventions include meaning-centered psychotherapy (Chapter 35), dignity therapy (Chapter 36), and managing cancer and living meaningfully (CALM) therapy (Chapter 37). More recently, psychedelics are being investigated as rapidly acting interventions for psychological distress in palliative care (Chapter 42). There is hope by some that such rapidly acting interventions may clarify the underlying motivation for MAiD in patients with comorbid depression or high existential distress at end of life, a significant clinical challenge faced by palliative psychiatrists.[9]

MAiD Practice Points

Enduring psychological distress is included as an eligibility criterion in most MAiD legislation, and a proportion of patients experiencing existential distress will go on to request MAiD. Psychiatrists working in palliative care have traditionally regarded existential distress as a target for psychological intervention, but most MAiD laws do not require patients who request MAiD to have had a trial of treatment for suffering of this kind. The frequency, acceptability, or efficacy of psychological interventions for patients who request MAiD is not known, although the unwillingness of such individuals or their providers to consider them can be a source of moral distress for palliative psychiatrists. Two concrete and practical entry points will be used to illustrate this dilemma.

This case illustrates that urgent requests for MAiD may be problematic when there is insufficient time to ensure sustained intent. Mr. B's case also illustrates the important role of the healthcare provider in helping patients to reflect on the decision to pursue MAiD. This discussion can include asking patients to imagine swallowing or holding their arm out for lethal medications to ensure that it is a moment that they can face. Providers may also discuss with patients what their natural deaths might look like. The intent of such conversations is not to dissuade patients from pursuing MAiD but to allow reflection and ensure fully informed consent.

Urgent Requests for MAiD

Mr. B was a 58-year-old journalist with widely metastatic melanoma. He had recently stopped an immunotherapy trial due to disease progression, and his expected survival was only a few weeks. He was highly anxious about death, not wanting to know his prognosis, engage in psychotherapy, or discuss his cancer. Mr. B was admitted to the ICU for respiratory distress. He refused do-not-resuscitate (DNR) status and was still interested in pursuing a phase 1 immunotherapy trial if he could regain enough strength to qualify. He had also requested MAiD, wanting to secure this option in case it was needed in future.

Mr. B had enjoyed a successful career and felt well-supported by his wife, children, and a large network of friends. He was not depressed, nor was he taking psychotropic medication. He met all eligibility criteria, including the capacity to consent, and was provisionally approved for MAiD pending his decision to select a date to proceed. After an acute aspiration event, he urgently asked for MAiD and arrangements were made to provide MAiD the next day. His family and friends held a special gathering to say good-bye the night before, and he prepared for this by refusing pain or sedating medications to avoid cognitive impairment the next morning. Unexpectedly, at the moment of final confirmation, Mr. B changed his mind about proceeding with MAiD for reasons that were not known, and the procedure was aborted. Support was then provided to the patient, family, and healthcare team, who were all distressed by the sudden turn of events. The following morning, Mr. B again refused his pain medications to prepare for receiving MAiD that day, evidently having no memory of changing his mind about MAiD the day prior.

Once patients are approved for MAiD, providers often withdraw from further discussions about it to avoid unduly influencing their patients' decisions. However, patients may actually benefit from ongoing discussions about MAiD along the course of their disease; their views may even change with the unpredictable and sometimes precipitous nature of decline as death nears. Individuals who want to die by MAiD should understand that they may miss the window of opportunity to receive it by losing the capacity to consent. Palliative psychiatrists can play an important role in helping patients and clinical teams navigate these complex discussions and decisions. Mr. B was advised that MAiD is not optimal as an emergency intervention, and he was supportively engaged in a detailed discussion about his care at end of life. For example, his anxiety about suffering that might occur if he lost the ability to swallow pills was diminished when he learned that pain medications could be delivered subcutaneously. He was also enormously relieved to understand that palliative sedation could be made urgently available for an intractable symptom crisis and that his natural death would likely take place over days, not months in a lingering unconscious state as he had initially feared. Mr. B died a peaceful natural death with comfort measures.

Ms. C's case illustrates the well-known clinical challenge of diagnosing depression in the context of terminal illness (Chapter 4) and determining whether depressive symptoms impair capacity to consent to MAiD. The accepted standard for medical decision-making capacity is the ability to understand, appreciate, reason, and communicate the relevant information needed to inform treatment choices. Some have argued for higher thresholds and stringency for irreversible life-and-death decisions that comprehensively assess rationality of emotional decision-making.[10] This recommendation has been made because depressive

---

Capacity Assessment

Ms. C was a 67-year-old married woman with an unresectable pancreatic cancer. She had recently retired as head of social work at a major urban hospital. Her first cycle of chemotherapy was poorly tolerated, and, in follow-up with her oncologist, she stated, "I've had enough. I can no longer go to the cottage, travel, or do anything. I can't enjoy my retirement. I hate every day that I am alive." After discussing the remaining treatment options, namely dose-reduced chemotherapy or best supportive care, she stated "What do I need to do—go into the woods with a rope and noose?" Ms. C's oncologist determined that she was not at imminent risk of attempting suicide and referred her for MAiD assessment.

Ms. C had a preexisting history of mild persistent depressive disorder for which she had sought help but never found the right fit with a psychotherapist. Her MAiD assessors were divided on whether she now met diagnostic criteria for a major depressive episode. She was very knowledgeable about the symptoms of depression, attributing her sadness to her medical condition and denying anhedonia. Ms. C had stopped all of her usual pleasurable activities, such as playing computer games or seeing friends, stating that fatigue from cancer treatment prevented her from engaging in valued activities. She was also experiencing intense restless agitation in the evenings, causing severe insomnia. When interviewed during the day, she was composed and clear-minded, able to smile and reflect on her life with satisfaction. Despite mild psychomotor slowing, she scored perfectly on cognitive testing. However, she had been uncharacteristically indecisive and lacking her usual confidence, frequently turning to her husband to confirm answers to questions and deferring all daily decisions to him. They both noted an emotional lability that was atypical for her, in which she would suddenly become a "blubbering idiot" when reflecting on her past.

Ms. C stated that she was requesting MAiD because she had observed the course of pancreatic cancer with many of her former patients. She believed that it was senseless to prolong an inevitable death, that she would only become weaker and more bedridden, and that her days were already endlessly "dragging on." She stated that her request for MAiD was in no way related to depression but rather to her poor quality of life.

hopelessness and anhedonia may influence the ability to appreciate that the quality of life might improve or be preserved in the face of terminal illness in patients who meet formal criteria for informed consent. Table 8.4 presents suggested question prompts that may be helpful in assessing the capacity for MAiD, as well as clinical red flags for when to question it.

Ms. C refused psychological counseling but agreed to a trial of ketamine at the urging of her husband who was hoping for more time with her. She experienced a marked improvement in mood after the first dose, with resolution of anhedonia, agitation, and insomnia. She resumed playing online solitaire and enjoying dinner outings with her family. Ms. C was no longer bothered by crying and was able to enjoy her days without the previous impatience for death. Her desire for MAiD, though, did not waiver. She discontinued chemotherapy and enjoyed a good quality of life while receiving palliative care. Several months later, she hosted her own "living wake" with friends and former colleagues before receiving MAiD.

TABLE 8.4 Questions and red flags related to capacity and voluntariness

Questions to assess capacity	Questions to assess voluntariness	When to question capacity or voluntariness (red flags)
1. What is your understanding of your condition?	1. Why do you want MAiD?	1. Psychological suffering unrelated to medical condition
2. What is your understanding of MAiD?	2. Is there a wish, real or imagined, that would change your mind about MAiD?	2. Irrational pessimism about alternatives
3. Aside from MAiD, what else can we do to help you?	3. When did you first start thinking about MAiD?	3. Disproportionate guilt/self-perceived burden.
4. What do you think will happen if you are able to receive MAiD?	4. Is anyone encouraging you to ask or not ask for MAiD?	4. Severe anhedonia impairing quality of life
5. What would happen if you do not receive MAiD?	5. How do the opinions and feelings of your family influence you?	5. Sense of urgency or impulsivity
6. What makes you believe that MAiD is the best option for you?	6. What supports do you have personally and socially?	6. Ambivalence
7. How sure are you about dying through MAiD?	7. Are there pressures from society at large (i.e., ableism, ageism, racism, sexism) influencing your decision-making?	7. Requests during acute symptom crisis
8. Are you afraid of dying?	8. Do you feel financial or other sorts of pressures to ask for MAiD?	
9. [If primarily psychological suffering] Do you think supportive counseling would help?	9. Have you felt so depressed that you've thought about taking your own life?	
10. Could you help me understand why you refused _____?		

Ms. C's case demonstrates that both rational and irrational thinking can influence the desire for MAiD in patients with depression. Recognition of depression requires a higher index of suspicion in such high-functioning patients who are often overrepresented among those who request MAID. Ms. C held the irrational belief that her anhedonia and agitated insomnia were unrelated to her depression and therefore could not be improved. This view coexisted with her rational desire to control the circumstances of her death. The clinical task in such cases is to offer therapeutic interventions to address irrational assumptions, even when they do not indicate ineligibility for MAiD.

Patient Factors and Family Impacts of MAiD

Individuals who request MAiD are more likely to be non-Hispanic White, well-educated, and to have higher income than their counterparts.[11] Whereas suicide is more common in older men than women of the same age, consistent gender differences have generally not been found in MAiD requests or completions.[11] Cancer is the most common medical condition underlying requests for MAiD, accounting for more than 70% of cases in most jurisdictions, followed by neurological and respiratory illnesses.

Consistent findings regarding psychological factors motivating MAiD requests and completions include a loss of autonomy, dignity, and ability to enjoy valued activities.[11] Select studies also demonstrate greater mastery, attachment avoidance, and fear of the unknown and future suffering as well as less religiosity in patients who pursue MAiD.[11,12] Although hopelessness, loneliness, thoughts of being a burden, and depressive symptoms are related to pursuit of MAiD, these same factors may also result in refusal of MAiD requests.[13]

MAiD requests that do not result in provision may be due to multiple factors. For example, patients who are depressed are less likely to be approved for MAiD.[13] MAiD may not be delivered when death occurs naturally, before MAiD can be provided, or when the patient subsequently becomes ineligible or withdraws the request. Factors associated with withdrawals of MAiD requests include having fewer general health problems, alternative treatment options, less unbearable or pointless suffering, and fewer concerns about loss of dignity.[14]

Studies have shown comparable or better family bereavement outcomes with MAiD deaths than with deaths due to other causes.[15,16] Several reviews suggest that, compared to bereaved caregivers of patients who died of other causes, bereaved caregivers of those who received MAiD were more reconciled to the patient's death, had less complicated grief, found that MAiD preserved patient dignity and alleviated suffering, and viewed MAiD as compassionate and humane. Caregivers of patients who received MAiD have reported less physical exhaustion, caregiving burden, and regret about the death and dying process.[16,17] These outcomes may be partly due to the comfort family members find in having honored the patient's wishes, being more prepared for death, and having more opportunities to say goodbye.[17] However, further research is warranted as family members' adjustment may also depend on factors such as the nature of MAiD delivery, extent of family involvement in and agreement with MAiD decisions, nature of caregiving, and level of support from the medical team.

Impacts of MAiD on Medicine

There has been a profound shift in the roles of patients and physicians in medical decision-making during the age of MAiD. Patients now have the right to not only refuse treatments clinically recommended by their physicians but also request alternative interventions. The emergence of patient empowerment in medical care has many advantages, although it may have consequences that are unintended by the patient. As with Mr. B, the increasing proximity to death may heighten the desire for MAiD in some patients. Additionally, the pursuit of MAiD at the very end of life can result in suboptimal symptom control in order to maintain capacity to provide informed consent. The logistical requirements of the MAiD process can also take precious time away from engagement in other meaningful activities of patients and families. These outcomes might be viewed as iatrogenic consequences of the availability of MAiD.

Many providers report a hesitation to discuss MAiD if it is not first raised by the patient, for fear of upsetting the patient or damaging the patient–physician relationship.[18] However, research has found that more than 90% of patients with advanced cancer do not find discussion of the wish to hasten death to be upsetting, and almost 80% prefer the physician to be proactive in assessing and discussing the desire to hasten death.[19] Nevertheless, raising the question of MAiD during goals of care discussions with patients and family members requires careful consideration regarding clinical timing and the presentation of the full range of appropriate, available treatment options. The skills employed in end-of-life discussions (Chapter 12) can be leveraged in clinical decisions about whether, when, and how to initiate discussions of MAiD.

A patient's spontaneous statement regarding the wish to hasten death does not necessarily require a referral for consideration of MAiD. It does, however, present an opportunity to start a discussion of the patients' values, beliefs, and wishes regarding their care and the adequacy of current symptom management. An initial request for MAiD should be regarded as an opportunity to explore motivations and feelings about MAiD *before* being viewed as a request for action. As with discussion of other goals of care, such conversations can be ongoing and evolving. Some distress may be relieved by existential and supportive psychotherapies and pharmacotherapy among a subset of patients who pursue MAiD (Part VI of this volume), although the approval for MAiD may itself restore a sense of control and dignity and promote quality of death and dying.

Impact of MAiD on Healthcare Providers

Concerns about burden and distress among healthcare providers engaged in MAiD are common, although the impact of MAiD on clinicians varies based on their personal opinions and feelings about the intervention as well as their professional and clinical affiliations. Individual factors include previous personal and professional experiences, religious or spiritual beliefs, comfort with death and dying as well as attitudes about care at end of life, and the impact of these attitudes on providing MAiD. Professional factors that affect MAiD providers include the organizations within which they work, perceived impact of their participation in MAiD on their relationships with colleagues and patients, and extent to which MAID is perceived to fit within the policy or model of care in the program or clinical setting in which they work.

Conscientious objection of physicians ranges from an unwillingness to discuss MAiD with patients, refer patients for MAiD assessment, or participate in the assessment or delivery of MAiD. These positions are supported to a greater or lesser extent in different jurisdictions and clinical settings, and distress is common in providers when they feel pressured to participate in activities that they find morally unacceptable. Even among providers who are accepting of MAiD, requests for this intervention by patients may be experienced as undermining their sense of competence and professional identity, which is typically based on the medical mandate to treat suffering and preserve life.

Future Directions

The introduction of palliative care and MAiD into medical practice has served to normalize the discussion and acceptance of dying and death. Much is now known about the motivations for MAiD and its impact on patients, families, and healthcare providers as well as optimal means of delivering this intervention. However, controversy and knowledge gaps remain in the optimal criteria for eligibility, factors that result in refusal or prevent the delivery of MAiD to those who have been approved, and considerations that could or should determine the delivery of MAID versus palliative sedation. Furthermore, a careful delineation of the different forms of the desire for death, ranging from a passive wish to hasten death to active suicide attempts, is needed to guide appropriate safeguarding of MAiD practice.

The initial feared "slippery slope" that the elderly, socioeconomically disadvantaged, or disabled would disproportionately receive MAiD or receive it against their will has not materialized in jurisdictions where MAiD has been legal for decades.[20] There are, however, concerns about another slippery slope, which includes expanding the indications for MAiD, including for mature minors, for suffering associated with psychiatric disorders, as an advance directive, and for relatively healthy but elderly patients who feel they have "completed life." Expansion of MAiD to these areas may result in increased utilization of MAiD. As such, each of these scenarios requires thorough examination to balance access to MAiD with its imposition on individuals who may lack sufficient knowledge, mental capacity, or resources to utilize reasonable alternatives. In this regard, palliative psychiatry can offer valuable perspectives in the development of frameworks with carefully considered safeguards and rigorous assessment protocols.

Key Points

- An initial request for MAiD should be viewed as an opportunity for exploration of the desire for death *before* a request for action.
- The role of palliative psychiatry in MAiD extends beyond capacity assessment to include identification and management of psychological suffering at end of life.
- Caution should be exercised in clinical situations where the availability of MAiD at the end of life can have iatrogenic adverse effects on the quality of death and dying.
- Although psychosocial vulnerabilities are observed in a significant proportion of individuals who request MAiD, approval and receipt of MAiD is typically not driven by the presence of a psychiatric disorder.
- The majority of patients who receive MAiD have also received palliative services. However, the nature and type, extent, and comprehensiveness of these services are unknown.
- For a small minority of patients with advanced disease, approval for MAiD may restore a sense of control and dignity, promote quality of death and dying, and relieve psychological distress.

References

1. Borasio GD, Jox RJ, Gamondi C. Regulation of assisted suicide limits the number of assisted deaths. *Lancet*. 2019;393(10175):982–983. doi:10.1016/S0140-6736(18)32554-6
2. Dierickx S, Deliens L, Cohen J, Chambaere K. Involvement of palliative care in euthanasia practice in a context of legalized euthanasia: A population-based mortality follow-back study. *Palliat Med*. 2018;32(1):114–122. doi:10.1177/0269216317727158
3. Emanuel EJ, Onwuteaka-Philipsen BD, Urwin JW, Cohen J. Attitudes and practices of euthanasia and physician-assisted suicide in the United States, Canada, and Europe. *JAMA*. 2016;316(1):79–90. doi:10.1001/jama.2016.8499
4. Koksvik GH, Richards N, Gerson SM, Materstvedt LJ, Clark D. Medicalisation, suffering and control at the end of life: The interplay of deep continuous palliative sedation and assisted dying. *Health*. 2020:1363459320976746. doi:10.1177/1363459320976746
5. Rousseau S, Turner S, Chochinov HM, Enns MW, Sareen J. A national survey of Canadian psychiatrists' attitudes toward medical assistance in death. *Can J Psychiatry*. 2017;62(11):787–794. doi:10.1177/0706743717711174
6. Verhofstadt M, Audenaert K, Van den Broeck K, Deliens L, Mortier F, Titeca K, et al. Belgian psychiatrists' attitudes towards, and readiness to engage in, euthanasia assessment procedures with adults with psychiatric conditions: A survey. *BMC Psychiatry*. 2020;20(1):374. doi:10.1186/s12888-020-02775-x
7. Regional Euthanasia Review Committees. *Annual Report 2019*. Netherlands; 2019. https://english.euth anasiecommissie.nl/the-committees/documents/publications/annual-reports/2002/annual-reports/ annual-reports
8. Isenberg-Grzeda E, Nolen A, Selby D, Bean S. High rates of psychiatric comorbidity among requesters of medical assistance in dying: Results of a Canadian prevalence study. *Gen Hosp Psychiatry*. 2021;69:7–11. doi:10.1016/j.genhosppsych.2020.12.017
9. Rosenblat JD, Li M. Is ketamine a litmus test for capacity in assisted dying with depression? *Psychooncology*. 2021;30(3):417–420. doi:10.1002/pon.5586
10. Charland L, Lemmens T, Wada K. Decision-making capacity to consent to medical assistance in dying for persons with mental disorders. *JEMH*. 2016:1–14.

11. Castelli Dransart DA, Lapierre S, Erlangsen A, Canetto SS, Heisel M, Draper B, et al. A systematic review of older adults' request for or attitude toward euthanasia or assisted-suicide. *Aging Ment Health*. 2021;25(3):420–430. doi:10.1080/13607863.2019.1697201

12. Smith KA, Harvath TA, Goy ER, Ganzini L. Predictors of pursuit of physician-assisted death. *J Pain Symptom Manage*. 2015;49(3):555–561. doi:10.1016/j.jpainsymman.2014.06.010

13. Lewis P, Black I. Adherence to the request criterion in jurisdictions where assisted dying is lawful? A review of the criteria and evidence in the Netherlands, Belgium, Oregon, and Switzerland. *J Law Med Ethics*. 2013;41(4):885–898. doi:10.1111/jlme.12098

14. Marcoux I, Onwuteaka-Philipsen BD, Jansen-van der Weide MC, van der Wal G. Withdrawing an explicit request for euthanasia or physician-assisted suicide: A retrospective study on the influence of mental health status and other patient characteristics. *Psychol Med*. 2005;35(9):1265–1274. doi:10.1017/S0033291705005465

15. Ganzini L, Goy ER, Dobscha SK, Prigerson H. Mental health outcomes of family members of Oregonians who request physician aid in dying. *J Pain Symptom Manage* 2009;38(6):807–815. doi:10.1016/j.jpainsymman.2009.04.026

16. Lowers J, Scardaville M, Hughes S, Preston NJ. Comparison of the experience of caregiving at end of life or in hastened death: A narrative synthesis review. *BMC Palliat Care*. 2020;19(1):154. doi:10.1186/s12904-020-00660-8

17. Goldberg R, Nissim R, An E, Hales S. Impact of medical assistance in dying (MAiD) on family caregivers. *BMJ Support Palliat Care*. 2021;11(1):107–114. doi:10.1136/bmjspcare-2018-001686

18. Ho A, Norman JS, Joolaee S, Serota K, Twells L, William L. How does Medical Assistance in Dying affect end-of-life care planning discussions? Experiences of Canadian multidisciplinary palliative care providers. *Palliat Care Soc Pract*. 2021;15:26323524211045996. doi:10.1177/26323524211045996

19. Porta-Sales J, Crespo I, Monforte-Royo C, Marin M, Abenia-Chavarria S, Balaguer A. The clinical evaluation of the wish to hasten death is not upsetting for advanced cancer patients: A cross-sectional study. *Palliat Med*. 2019;33(6):570–577. doi:10.1177/0269216318824526

20. Reggler J. The slippery slope argument and medical assistance in dying. *CMAJ*. 2017;189(12):E471. doi:10.1503/cmaj.732886

9

Palliative Care for People Who Experience Severe Persistent Mental Illness

Alan Bates, John-Jose Nunez, Alexandra Farag,
David Fudge, Timothy O'Shea,
Kathleen Baba Willison, and Anne Woods

Introduction

Two systematic reviews on palliative care for people who experience SPMI[1, 2] identified almost identical themes. Each discussed difficulties with regard to (1) capacity, autonomy, and their roles in decision-making and care planning; (2) access to care; (3) complexity of care provision; and (4) vulnerability.

The two reviews also made similar recommendations: (1) to recognize heterogeneity and "seek diversity when investigating the experiences of people with SPMI"[2]; (2) to include the voices of people who experience SPMI in both research and care; (3) to address institutional and system issues; and (4) for mental health and palliative care to work together.

Since the second review in 2019, literature in this area has burgeoned, with a focus on commonalities between palliative care and psychiatry—their shared goals of reducing suffering and improving quality of care; their patient-centered focus that tries to honor autonomy; and their skill in communication. Lines between the two disciplines blur further when SPMIs are conceptualized as life-limiting illnesses and key questions emerge. How do we ensure maximal appropriate, curative, and recovery-focused care without being overly aggressive and harming the person or their identity? How do we attend to the person's desires, abilities, and personhood when these seem to be in conflict with treatment?

These questions are not different from those in diseases like cancer or heart disease, but the balance between life-prolonging treatment, bodily and personal integrity, and comfort can be significantly more complex. The intent of this chapter is to take a step toward addressing some of the recommendations above by (1) describing the population of people with SPMI in terms of diagnoses in order to identify issues and questions specific to each diagnosis, and (2) discussing how mental health and palliative care might work together. This chapter does not, however, contain patient voices. While recent literature reflects the increased experience and reflection of healthcare providers, with the exception of Foti's[3,4] early work, the voices of patients remain absent.

SPMI Diversity and Mimics

SPMI is a collection of multiple diverse syndromes or diagnoses that are chronic and disabling and cause serious functional impairment. Depending on the syndrome, the degree of impairment may be primarily related to emotion, behaviors, perception, cognition, or some combination of those and other variables. While common in some SPMIs, phenomena such as psychosis or irritability with decreased need for sleep are not always the product of long-standing psychiatric illness in people with SPMI. Distinguishing psychosis in delirium from long-standing psychotic illness is important as it signals an underlying change in non-psychiatric illness that might be reversible. Fluctuating course within 24 hours and new disturbances in sleep, awareness, orientation, and attention are indicators of overlying delirium. Psychosis or mania-like symptoms can also be medication-induced, with steroids such as prednisone or dexamethasone being common culprits. Steroid dose adjustments or addition or increase of an antipsychotic such as olanzapine should be considered to reduce steroid-induced changes in mental status.

Schizophrenia

Schizophrenia

Bill had lived quietly in the community for years, coming to hospital when his neighbors became worried about odd behavior. He had developed a large tumor on his face and didn't look well. The tumor was resected in a surgery that required the removal of one of his eyes, as well as a skin graft. He survived this and was moved out of hospital, but developed COVID, from which he also recovered. Then he had a recurrence of his cancer. He stayed in the hospital, rarely saying anything, curling up in bed when he was tired, and walking the halls when awake. As he became sicker, he slept more. He didn't complain of pain and rarely took analgesics. His swallowing became difficult and speech and language pathology recommended a pureed diet and thickened fluids. Bill would be found in the bathroom drinking from the tap. Gradually he was unable to take oral medications including his neuroleptics. He became agitated only when he developed pneumonia, a high fever, and shortness of breath. Escalating doses of parenteral medications were required—well beyond normal doses.

Schizophrenia occurs in 0.5–1% of the population and is characterized by "positive symptoms" including hallucinations and delusions; "negative symptoms" such as social withdrawal, flat affect, or amotivation; and disorganized speech and behavior. Positive symptoms tend to respond better to antipsychotics, while negative symptoms tend to be more intractable, and a portion of patients do not see significant benefit from medications.

Mean onset of psychotic symptoms is late 20s in men and early 30s in women with a course that tends to be chronic, resulting in major impact on social, educational, and vocational functioning.

Poverty, homelessness, and related issues such as substance abuse and a history of interactions with law enforcement may be present. However, though psychosis is a risk factor for unpredictable behavior, people with schizophrenia are much more likely to be victims of violence than violent themselves, and a patient's history can be used to predict risk.

Although the 10- to 20-year reduced life expectancy of people with schizophrenia is partially explained by premature death by suicide or injury, the majority of the increased mortality risk is related to natural causes including cardiovascular and respiratory illness. Part of that risk, including increased rates of lung cancer, is explained by a much higher rate of smoking. Other factors such as poor diet, lack of exercise, and metabolic side effects of antipsychotic medications also contribute. People with schizophrenia who die from cancer are likely to present with more advanced illness, die at a younger age (mean of 8 years earlier in a French study), and die sooner after diagnosis.[5] Despite the well-known risk of premature death in schizophrenia, a Canadian study found the median age of death to be 77.[6]

People with history of psychosis are less likely to have formulated advance directives.[7] However, this does not appear to be because they are not capable of it. Foti and colleagues[3] have demonstrated effective use of the Health Care Preferences Questionnaire in eliciting desire for a substitute decision-maker and concerns related to pain, family, finances, spiritual distress, and funeral arrangements. Compared to the general population, people with serious mental illness are less likely to want a substitute decision-maker,[3] an end to life support if they were in an irreversible coma,[4] or medical assistance in dying.[8] Unfortunately, people with schizophrenia are sometimes not provided full opportunity in informed healthcare decision-making at end of life because of stigma, incorrect assumptions about their ability to make decisions about their non-psychiatric care, and/or unfair assumptions about their quality of life.

Care planning is not a single event and often requires multiple conversations over time as both understanding and health change. People with schizophrenia are likely to have a long-standing connection to a mental health clinic, and efforts should be made to keep a community psychiatrist, social worker, or case manager engaged as they may have good rapport with the patient and can provide invaluable collateral information. Family caregivers should be similarly integrated into care as appropriate, and family meetings may be needed to optimize planning and communication. However, people with schizophrenia are more likely to have lost connections to friends and family who might otherwise be advocates or caregivers. As a result, it may also be difficult to find an appropriate substitute decision-maker when one is needed, and a public guardian, or equivalent, may have to be involved.

Without the luxury of collateral, capacity assessments may be challenging when a patient's wishes differ greatly from what most reasonable people would want but seem aligned with long-standing values or choices. Interventions should not be ruled out just because they're more challenging than usual to implement, but providing medical interventions against a patient's will is always problematic and is less likely to be justifiable at end of life where focus is on quality of life rather than treating a reversible condition in order to extend life significantly.

In a large Canadian study, Chochinov et al.[9] found that, at end of life, people with schizophrenia spend more time in nursing homes, receive less hospital care or home care, see fewer specialists other than psychiatrists (with even the frequency of psychiatry visits declining), and are less likely to receive opioid analgesia or formal palliative care. The finding of less provision of analgesics may be related to physician concern about history of comorbid substance abuse, concern about worsening cognitive state, thought disorder preventing patients from clearly describing their pain, and/or to people with schizophrenia possibly being less sensitive to pain. While care in a nursing home may be appropriate, there is need for greater will and creativity in adapting home hospice to settings like social housing, perhaps through dedicated beds or units that serve particular group homes or shelters, including appropriate staffing. For outpatient palliative care services, treating patients closer to where they live also eliminates possible barriers related to transportation.

Changes in antipsychotic dosing may be required at end of life as a result of liver dysfunction, medication interactions, the addition of medications for symptom management, delirium, or change of environment (e.g., if a smoker is moved to a facility where smoking is not permitted, it is important to consider dose reductions of medications whose metabolism is accelerated by smoking via CYP1A2 induction, with clozapine and olanzapine being prime examples). Virtually all antipsychotics can impact QT interval or lower seizure threshold.

Mood Disorders

Bipolar Disorders

Bipolar disorders (BDs) are mood disorders affecting 2–3% of the population and defined by patterns of manic, hypomanic, and major depressive episodes, with bipolar I disorder (BD1) being characterized by history of mania and bipolar II disorder (BD2) being characterized by history of depressive and hypomanic episodes. Many people return to functional baseline between episodes, but a significant number face prolonged challenges with social, educational, and occupational activities. However, some people achieve remarkable things during hypomanic episodes, which can feature increased productivity and creativity.

People with BD have increased all-cause mortality including a significantly increased risk of suicide, as well as an increased risk of dying sooner from natural causes such as respiratory and cardiovascular disease. According to a large epidemiological study in France,[10] people who experience BD and cancer die younger (mean of 66 vs. 72 years old), have increased occurrence of some cancers, and have less metastatic disease, with the differences unexplained by cancer screening, which is less common in individuals with SPMI.

There is sparse literature about end-of-life decision-making and advance care planning, but manic episodes can impair decision-making capacity, and the increased prevalence of substance use disorders can also pose challenges. A large epidemiological study found cancer patients with BD access more palliative care.[10] They found evidence of "better" end-of-life care including less chemotherapy, surgery, imaging, and admissions to acute care in their last 31 days of life.

People with BD may have difficulty with impulsivity and emotion regulation as well as with accurate emotion recognition (e.g., a tendency to overly interpret the actions of others as hostile). This may impact treatment adherence[10] and lead to strained relationships with healthcare providers. In addition, patients with BD1 may have increased or atypical reactions to pain[11] that could be difficult to interpret. Managing mania is challenging, and recommendations include clear limit-setting, avoiding excessive enforcement of rules, finding common ground for collaboration, and providing day/night structure, as well as medication changes if needed.

Particularly as patients get closer to end of life, mood stabilizing medications are often reduced or discontinued as a result of organ failure, other medications being used for palliative symptom management, or mood symptoms no longer being a prime focus of care. When continued, it is important to maintain monitoring, such as lithium levels. Lithium excretion is 95% renal, and levels can by impacted by fluid intake, perspiration, diuretics, and nonsteroidal anti-inflammatory drugs (NSAIDs). Valproic acid elimination is varied, but largely depends on initial liver metabolism. Serum levels can change significantly with body weight, as can serum protein levels, and it can also increase serum levels of other medications including some antidepressants, antipsychotics, and benzodiazepines. Serum level monitoring is less common for other mood stabilizers, but toxicity can still develop. Rare, potentially fatal skin disorders can occur with both lamotrigine and carbamazepine, though this usually occurs in the weeks following initiation. When possible, mood stabilizers should be discontinued gradually to minimize risk of seizures. Antipsychotics are commonly used in BD and may be safer alternatives, though they can prolong QT and lower seizure threshold. Though rare, there is risk of serotonin syndrome from interactions between serotonergic antidepressants and medications commonly used at end of life, including antiemetics and synthetic opioids.

Long-Standing Depressive Disorders

Major depressive episodes are characterized by low mood or anhedonia for most of the day for days on end, as well as symptoms such as hopelessness, changes in sleep or appetite, and decreased energy or concentration. Suicidal ideation may also be present. Criteria for persistent depressive disorder include depression lasting at least 2 years, without a 2-month or longer reprieve. The condition is associated with anxiety, personality and somatic disorders, more severe health outcomes, impairment in social and occupational function, and lower income. Lifetime prevalence of chronic major depressive disorder and dysthymia are estimated at 1–6%. Women are affected 2:1 compared with men.

While there is a literature on depression in the context of life-limiting illness (Chapter 4), there is little written about palliative and end-of-life care for people who have depressive disorders that are severe and persistent. A large French epidemiological study examined cancer patients with a "severe lifetime/chronic recurrent form of depression."[12] Compared to other cancer patients, they had more medical comorbidities, higher rates of certain cancers, and fewer metastases. This group also died an average of 3 years earlier. Curative and palliative care utilization at end of life varied in this group, with more artificial nutrition, specialized cancer center care, and acute care unit admissions, as well as a longer length of palliative care and fewer interventions. In this study, unlike others, patients were less likely to live in socially deprived areas.

Considering how often depression is a factor considered in capacity assessments, there is little literature on how long-standing depressive disorders affect decision-making capacity at the end of life. Depression and hopelessness are both medically addressable variables known to be associated with desire for hastened death.[13]

Treatment for long-standing depressive disorders requires a combined approach using medication and psychotherapy, focusing on quality of life and addressing demoralization and hopelessness. Antidepressant medications are used, sometimes with adjuvant medications from different classes. Tricyclic antidepressants and monoamine-oxidase inhibitors require significant caution in acute medical environments. Citalopram, escitalopram, and antipsychotics can affect QT interval (though aripiprazole has minimal effect on QT). The risk of serotonin syndrome should be considered whenever multiple medications could contribute. Mirtazapine is a common choice in the medically frail as it increases appetite, reduces nausea, and helps with sleep, while activating antidepressants such as venlafaxine or even stimulants like methylphenidate may be used for mental energy. Medication dosing may need to be lowered in renal and hepatic impairment.

Anxiety Disorders

Similar to long-standing depression, it is common for people to arrive at end of life with a long-standing anxiety disorder. Prior history, diagnoses, experiences, triggers, and interventions (successful or unsuccessful) related to anxiety should be explored early. The focus of anxiety may become fear of death or dying, or fear of failures in the medical system that might lead to increased suffering or a missed opportunity for further treatment. Clinicians sometimes feel unprepared to assist with existential distress, but specific interventions are described in earlier chapters and treating anxiety as one would in other settings may improve the overlying existential distress as well. As with depressive disorders, selective serotonin reuptake inhibitors (SSRIs) are the most common medications used and teams should be aware of risk for QT prolongation (citalopram, escitalopram) and serotonin syndrome. Benzodiazepines present a number of challenges in the setting of comorbid serious non-psychiatric illness, including risk of respiratory depression (particularly in combination with opioids), contribution to delirium, and risk of dangerous withdrawal if discontinued abruptly.

Personality Disorders

Personality traits are conceptualized as enduring patterns of the ways in which people relate to others and the world that are repeatedly demonstrated in several contexts. An individual with a personality disorder (PD) consistently demonstrates inflexible and maladaptive patterns of relating to and perceiving themselves and others. At end of life, clinicians encounter a variety of PDs, including those less common in other medical settings. People with PDs can be challenging to care for due to the presence of distressing physical symptoms and loss of control which can amplify underlying maladaptive coping mechanisms. Serious illness may be an unacceptable "failure" in an otherwise flawless self-image of someone oblivious to their narcissistic PD, and team members may struggle to establish trust with someone with antisocial PD or set appropriate limits with someone with histrionic PD. People with schizoid and avoidant PD may be experienced as cold or unfriendly by team members, and clinicians may struggle to avoid making decisions for people with dependent PD. People with schizotypal PD may be difficult to collaborate with due to odd decisions or behavior, and people with obsessive-compulsive PD may have unrealistic expectations of the care team, while people with paranoid PD may make accusations related to perceived intentional deficiencies in care.

Borderline personality disorder (BPD) is the best-studied personality disorder due to being a relatively common and frequent presentation to healthcare facilities, given the propensity for emotional and behavioral dysregulation and suicidal behaviors. BPD develops in adolescence, has an incidence of between 1% and 2%, and is twice as common in women as in men. Worsening of signs and symptoms can occur during times of increased psychosocial or physical distress and may include immature, overaggressive defense mechanisms including splitting, idealization, denial, and projective identification. Individuals may experience dissociation and pseudo-psychosis and alternate from being acutely dysregulated and agitated to being withdrawn and dysphoric. The combination of primitive defense mechanisms and a wildly fluctuating mental status can bewilder and engender a sense of chaos among treating teams. A focused, evidence-based, coherent treatment plan to address issues can lead to improved care for the patient and also decreased distress for the care team.

There is no medication specifically indicated for BPD, but several may help with associated symptoms. Low-dose antipsychotics may reduce impulsivity, hostility, affective instability, and pseudo-psychosis and help with delirium, nausea, and loss of appetite (e.g., olanzapine). Antidepressants may assist with depression, worsening dysregulation, and anger. Valproic acid may also be helpful in the treatment of emotional dysregulation, impulsivity, and anger. Benzodiazepines may cause disinhibition and should be avoided outside times of extreme agitation or anxiety. As with mood and anxiety disorders, medication interactions and possible adverse effects must be considered with all medication options.

The fundamental treatment for BPD is psychotherapeutic interventions such as dialectical behavioral therapy (DBT). In the context of a severe life-limiting illness, most people are not able to attend the relatively rigorous commitment of formal DBT, but the team may still employ aspects of it. For example, distress tolerance skills can be taught to both the patient and the team, and the patient may benefit from learning a mindfulness meditation exercise. Consultation with psychiatry, when available, and involvement of the patient in establishing a behavioral plan, including mutually agreed-upon expectations of the patient and the team, is suggested. Psychoeducation for the treating team is important to discuss regression, splitting, and the importance of firm boundaries. The treating team should also receive emotional support as the behaviors that are characteristic for BPD can cause distress and burnout to healthcare providers.

Anorexia Nervosa

Onset of anorexia nervosa (AN) is often early in life (rarely after the age of 40), has a 12-month prevalence of about 0.5% in young females, and females are affected 10 times more often than males. Although most people who develop AN experience remission within 5 years, fewer than 50% recover, and 20% progress to a severe and enduring form of the illness. The mortality rate is about 5% per decade of illness, making AN the psychiatric illness with the highest mortality rate,[14] with death most often a result of suicide or medical complications of nutritional deficits.

Where there is sustained treatment failure, a stepwise approach from active treatment to harm reduction to palliative care is suggested. Active treatment, including involuntary admission and forced/enforced feeding, has as its goals cure, remission, and weight gain/maintenance. When this is not possible, the focus of harm reduction moves to what is reasonable, acceptable, and can be maintained rather than what is ideal. People for whom palliative care is adopted are those for whom active treatment is unlikely to help and who are unable to make the agreements necessary to participate in harm reduction.[14]

There is debate about when transition to palliative care may be appropriate. Some argue that active, possibly forced, treatment is always appropriate as life must be preserved if at all possible. Others may point to objective evidence of need for a transition to a palliative focus such as[15] multiple treatment failures, lack of sustained response to a wide range of evidence-based treatment provided by competent providers, longer periods of failed treatment, continued physical and physiological decline, poor prognosis or the appearance of inexorable and terminal course, judgment that real treatment options do not exist, and a sustained desire to stop treatment by someone with greater age/lived experience.

Capacity is often questioned in severe AN, but even if a person is found to lack capacity to make a particular decision, success of treatment tends to ultimately rely on the person's willingness to collaborate with long-term change in behavior, and there is little anyone can do to "force" that. Focus often shifts to vigilance for moments when the person is ready to initiate positive change themself. Unfortunately, cognitive distortions related to body image and weight are often a core feature, and cognition, particularly executive function, is impaired by poor nutrition, sometimes leading to increasingly worse decision-making capacity as the illness progresses. Often, family, healthcare providers, ethics committees, and/or courts become involved in decision-making.

Even with diminished capacity, a person "is still likely capable of appraising his or her own suffering,"[14] and combining this with knowledge held and shared by others, not only of who the person is but who they were and who they hoped to be—a form of relational autonomy—may be appropriately used to create collaborative supported decision-making, rather than substitute decision-making.[16]

Posttraumatic Stress Disorder

Approximately 75% of Canadian adults report some form of trauma exposure in their lifetime, but less than 10% ever meet criteria for posttraumatic stress disorder (PTSD). People who are structurally vulnerable and/or experience racism, sexism, or income inequality are disproportionately impacted by trauma.

About a third of people with PTSD recover within 1 year, but a small proportion continue to have symptoms for several years, even decades. People with PTSD are more likely to develop chronic illnesses such as cardiovascular disease, arthritis, asthma, chronic pain, and gastrointestinal disorders,[17] and are at 2–3 times higher risk of attempting suicide.

PTSD can first present or worsen as patients become seriously ill, complicating their end-of-life care. Life-limiting illnesses such as cancer increase risk for PTSD. Pain, anxiety, and thoughts about impending mortality may trigger reminders of traumatic experiences and memories and precipitate PTSD symptoms. These symptoms can present as increased pain, agitation, irritability, and nightmares. Studies with veteran populations have shown higher healthcare utilization and antipsychotic use in patients with PTSD at the end of life, suggesting that patients with PTSD may be at a higher risk of terminal delirium.[18] People with PTSD may have difficulty trusting authority figures, which can manifest as "difficult" interactions with care providers. Being aware of the impacts of trauma can help providers contextualize these difficult symptoms.

There is significant debate about screening patients for trauma experiences and PTSD. Several tools to screen for PTSD have been described, but universal screening is not recommended as discussing trauma histories can be triggering or retraumatizing for patients. Universal trauma precautions, such as allowing for choice and collaboration and focusing on patient strengths and skills, should be applied to the care of all patients facing serious illnesses.

Symptom management of PTSD at end of life can be difficult. People approaching end of life may not have the time or mental or physical stamina for therapies such as cognitive behavioral therapy (CBT) or eye movement desensitization and reprocessing (EMDR). Medications with sedative properties, such as benzodiazepines, can be disinhibitory and precipitate intrusive symptoms. First-line pharmacological treatment includes SSRIs and serotonin/norepinephrine reuptake inhibitors (SNRIs). Mirtazapine is a second-line option but may be useful given its side effects of sedation and appetite stimulation. Atypical antipsychotics can also be used as alternative agents and are particularly beneficial for intrusive symptoms (e.g., distressing dreams and flashbacks). Prazosin can also be used for nightmares and has demonstrated significant improvements in sleep quality in people with

PTSD. As with the diagnoses above, possible medication interactions and adverse effects must be considered.

Substance Use Disorders

Substance use disorders (SUDs) have an estimated lifetime prevalence of around 10%, with significant comorbidity with other psychiatric diagnoses and with the highest rates in men, White or Indigenous individuals, and those with lower education and income (see Chapter 10).

SUDs are associated with a number of behavioral and cognitive patterns, such as impairments in impulse control, abstract reasoning, attention, executive functioning, and memory. States of intoxication or withdrawal can be particularly challenging. For example, intoxication with stimulants can lead to agitation, euphoria, disordered thinking, and paranoia, and use of sedating substances can lead to poor attention, decreased level of consciousness, and apathy. Individuals who lack safe and reliable access to their substance of choice may spend a great deal of time and energy focused on obtaining it, even in acute medical settings.

Individuals with SUD have reduced overall health and decreased life expectancy related to increased risks, including intentional and unintentional injuries; liver disease and cirrhosis from alcohol; infections such as osteomyelitis, endocarditis, hepatitis, or HIV from injection drug use; chronic cardiac and/or pulmonary disease related to stimulant abuse; and deaths directly attributable to substances.

Individuals with a history of SUD often report experiencing stigma in their interactions with the healthcare system and may find it difficult to trust healthcare providers. Each patient should be approached with a plan to establish trust while incorporating trauma-informed care. Inadequate pain control in patients with substance use is an issue that extends into many areas of healthcare and one that has been well documented. The reasons for this are many and include beliefs and attitudes of the treating team, as well as a poor understanding of tolerance, especially for patients with preexisting opioid use disorder. Incorporating individuals with expertise in the management of SUDs, including peer support workers, into palliative care teams may help.

Vulnerability

People with SPMI often experience deficits in the social determinants of health, such as poverty, insecure housing, or racism. This "structural vulnerability" is further compounded by the diagnosis of other life-limiting illnesses that impair ability to maintain autonomy, independence, and self-determination. People who are structurally vulnerable may experience fewer social supports, lack financial resources, and typically die alone, in either an acute care setting or in shelters or transitional housing while being cared for by workers who have limited palliative care training. They often experience significant stigma and discrimination when interacting with the medical system, which leads to lack of trust and difficulty accessing palliative care services. Ideally, palliative care services for structurally vulnerable populations meet people where they are (whether in hospital, shelters, or on the street) and include cultural safety training for providers, a focus on building trust, a flexible approach, and harm-reduction strategies.

Psychiatry and Palliative Care: Similarities, Integration and Cross-Training

Prior to the discovery of chlorpromazine, much of psychiatry for people with severe and persistent psychotic illness was essentially a form of palliative care. It is only in relatively modern times that psychiatry has tended to aim for a "cure" or near-complete symptom resolution in many SPMIs through use of medications to complement psychotherapy. Even today, antipsychotics are relatively ineffective in up to a quarter of people with schizophrenia, and psychiatrists often speak of walking alongside people with SPMIs over the course of their illness, not always being able to provide symptomatic relief, but at least being an empathic witness. This is not unlike aspects of palliative care, where clinicians also use medications to their very limits in resolving or minimizing pain, nausea, shortness of breath, and other symptoms but are, nonetheless, ultimately forced to be empathic guides to inexorable courses of progressive terminal illness. Palliative care has long grappled with supporting people through illness that threatens life and therefore personhood, while psychiatry often grapples with loss of reality-based personhood that can become an early threat to life. The commonalities in the disciplines have led to approaches such as "palliative psychiatry" that addresses physical, mental, social, and spiritual needs and focuses on harm reduction and avoidance of interventions with questionable impact.[19]

A number of models—consultative, co-consultative, collaborative, shared or integrated care—have been developed in which psychiatry and palliative care work together, along with other disciplines including family medicine. However, multidisciplinary teams are still often born out of necessity or fortunate availability rather than created by design. Ideally, mental health clinicians would have training in palliative care and vice versa, but cross-training has yet to become a reality in most centers despite being described by Foti[20] almost 20 years ago. Suggestions for training psychiatrists have included an elective or mandatory clinical rotation in palliative care.[19] More in-depth experiences, within both palliative care and psychiatry fellowships are needed, particularly longitudinal experiences.

Future Directions

Much of the available research on palliative care for people with SPMI focuses on schizophrenia, and greater focus on other syndromes is needed. There has also been very little work examining ideal locations and models of care. The feasibility and effectiveness of hospice facilities within social housing or shelters, for example, requires more analysis. Ideal composition of multidisciplinary teams is also poorly defined at this time. Clearly, there should be more patient-oriented or patient-informed research, and some advances are likely to be in ethical standards or frameworks rather than somewhat simpler clinical variables such as mood or pain.

Events such as the COVID-19 pandemic reveal the importance of being members of communities of belonging, meaning, and security. System gaps and inequities have had disproportionate and terrible impacts on vulnerable populations. Addressing these gaps in care will require new ways of thinking and a willingness to embrace new models. We can advance equity by creating compassionate communities, taking a public health approach to SPMIs and palliative care, and by integrating new models of care into existing structures and financing of health services. In all of these endeavors, the experiences and opinions of people with SPMI and their families are critical.

Key Points

- Thoughtful capacity assessment, trauma-informed care, and coordinated team-based care are key to caring for people with SMPI at end of life.
- Interactions between psychiatric and non-psychiatric medications need to be carefully considered in end-of-life care for people with SPMI.
- There are many similarities between psychiatry and palliative care, with management of severe anorexia nervosa demonstrating a clear example of overlap.
- There is need for more cross-training in mental health and palliative care, as well as care models designed for people with SPMI that can be applied in non-traditional settings.

References

1. Woods A, Willison K, Kington C, Gavin A. Palliative care for people with severe persistent mental illness: A review of the literature. *Can J Psychiatry Rev Can Psychiatr*. 2008;53(11):725–736. doi:10.1177/070674370805301104

2. Donald EE, Stajduhar KI. A scoping review of palliative care for persons with severe persistent mental illness. *Palliat Support Care*. 2019;17(4):479–487. doi:10.1017/S1478951519000087

3. Foti ME, Bartels SJ, Merriman MP, Fletcher KE, Van Citters AD. Medical advance care planning for persons with serious mental illness. *Psychiatr Serv Wash DC*. 2005;56(5):576–584. doi:10.1176/appi.ps.56.5.576

4. Foti ME, Bartels SJ, Van Citters AD, Merriman MP, Fletcher KE. End-of-life treatment preferences of persons with serious mental illness. *Psychiatr Serv Wash DC*. 2005;56(5):585–591. doi:10.1176/appi.ps.56.5.585

5. Fond G, Salas S, Pauly V, Baumstarck K, Bernard C, Orleans V, et al. End-of-life care among patients with schizophrenia and cancer: A population-based cohort study from the French national hospital database. *Lancet Public Health*. 2019;4(11):e583–e591. doi:10.1016/S2468-2667(19)30187-2

6. Martens PJ, Chochinov HM, Prior HJ. Where and how people with schizophrenia die: A population-based, matched cohort study in Manitoba, Canada. *J Clin Psychiatry*. 2013;74(6):e551–e557. doi:10.4088/JCP.12m08234

7. Cai X, Cram P, Li Y. Origination of medical advance directives among nursing home residents with and without serious mental illness. *Psychiatr Serv Wash DC*. 2011;62(1):61–66. doi:10.1176/ps.62.1.pss6201_0061

8. Elie D, Marino A, Torres-Platas SG, Noohi S, Semeniuk T, Segal M, et al. End-of-life care preferences in patients with severe and persistent mental illness and chronic medical conditions: A comparative cross-sectional study. *Am J Geriatr Psychiatry.* 2018;26(1):89–97. doi:10.1016/j.jagp.2017.09.018

9. Chochinov HM, Martens PJ, Prior HJ, Kredentser MS. Comparative health care use patterns of people with schizophrenia near the end of life: A population-based study in Manitoba, Canada. *Schizophr Res.* 2012;141(2-3):241–246. doi:10.1016/j.schres.2012.07.028

10. Fond G, Baumstarck K, Auquier P, Pauly V, Bernard C, Orleans V, et al. End-of-life care among patients with bipolar disorder and cancer: A nationwide cohort study. *Psychosom Med.* 2020;82(7):722–732. doi:10.1097/PSY.0000000000000839

11. Minichino A, Delle Chiaie R, Cruccu G, Piroso S, Di Stefano G, Francesconi M, et al. Pain-processing abnormalities in bipolar I disorder, bipolar II disorder, and schizophrenia: A novel trait marker for psychosis proneness and functional outcome? *Bipolar Disord.* 2016;18(7):591–601. doi:10.1111/bdi.12439

12. Fond G, Baumstarck K, Auquier P, Fernandes S, Pauly V, Bernard C, et al. Recurrent major depressive disorder's impact on end-of-life care of cancer: A nationwide study. *J Affect Disord.* 2020;263:326–335. doi:10.1016/j.jad.2019.12.003

13. Breitbart W, Rosenfeld B, Pessin H, Kaim M, Funesti-Esch J, Galietta M, et al. Depression, hopelessness, and desire for hastened death in terminally ill patients with cancer. *JAMA.* 2000;284(22):2907–2911. doi:10.1001/jama.284.22.2907

14. Westmoreland P, Mehler PS. Caring for patients with severe and enduring eating disorders (SEED): Certification, harm reduction, palliative care, and the question of futility. *J Psychiatr Pract.* 2016;22(4):313–320. doi:10.1097/PRA.0000000000000160

15. Geppert CMA. Futility in chronic anorexia nervosa: A concept whose time has not yet come. *Am J Bioeth AJOB.* 2015;15(7):34–43. doi:10.1080/15265161.2015.1039720

16. Stienstra D, Chochinov HM, 2006.Vulnerability, disability, and palliative end-of-life care. Accessed September 6, 2021. https://journals.sagepub.com/doi/10.1177/082585970602200307

17. Pacella ML, Hruska B, Delahanty DL. The physical health consequences of PTSD and PTSD symptoms: A meta-analytic review. *J Anxiety Disord.* 2013;27(1):33–46. doi:10.1016/j.janxdis.2012.08.004

18. Bickel KE, Kennedy R, Levy C, Burgio KL, Bailey FA. The relationship of post-traumatic stress disorder to end-of-life care received by dying veterans: A secondary data analysis. *J Gen Intern Med.* 2020;35(2):505–513. doi:10.1007/s11606-019-05538-x

19. Trachsel M, Irwin SA, Biller-Andorno N, Hoff P, Riese F. Palliative psychiatry for severe persistent mental illness as a new approach to psychiatry? Definition, scope, benefits, and risks. *BMC Psychiatry.* 2016;16(1):260. doi:10.1186/s12888-016-0970-y

20. Foti ME. "Do it your way": A demonstration project on end-of-life care for persons with serious mental illness. *J Palliat Med.* 2003;6(4):661–669. doi:10.1089/109662103768253830

10

Palliative Care in the Patient with Substance Use Disorder

Jaya S. Amaram-Davila and Joseph A. Arthur

Introduction

Substance use disorders (SUDs) are a recurrent problem in the United States. In 2015, 19 million people aged 12 or older reported using prescription medications that were not prescribed to them, and the majority of these were prescription pain relievers.[1,2] In a survey, 57.4% of adolescents and young adults reported buying these drugs or taking them from friends and relatives.[1] The opioid crisis has been associated with a growth in opioid-related overdoses. In 2019, the United States had nearly 71,000 deaths from drug overdose. Seventy percent of these involved opioids, and, of these, 73% were from synthetic opioids.[3]

SUDs can have consequences on multiple stages of life, resulting in homelessness, financial losses, loneliness, relationship problems, inability to fulfill obligations, and unemployment.[4] Adolescents with SUDs may face all the above issues along with academic struggles and risky behaviors. Furthermore, people with SUDs eventually develop chronic conditions such as diabetes, hypertension, cancer, growing resistance to illicit drugs, withdrawal symptoms, and overdose leading to premature death.[4] In 2016, the National Survey on Drug Use and Health (NSDUH) reported only 10% of the 19.9 million affected adults 18 or older received treatments for SUD.[2]

Considering the widespread nature of the phenomenon in the general population, medically ill patients with co-occurring substance abuse problems are being encountered more frequently.[4,5] Substance abuse issues are among the most serious and complicated challenges faced by clinicians in the palliative care setting.[5] The presence of a substance abuse problem in terminally ill patients can be extremely problematic, creating additional obstacles throughout treatment and pain management.[6]

Even though national guidelines exist for the treatment of pain in medically ill populations such as the cancer patients, pain continues to be undertreated even at the end of life.[6] Reports have indicated that the prevalence of moderate to severe pain is as high as 75% among those with advanced disease for whom curative therapy was no longer feasible. A systematic review of the literature also found that the prevalence of cancer pain was 39% after curative treatment, 55% during anticancer treatment, and increased to 66% for patients with metastatic disease.[7] Since the undertreatment of pain is already a significant problem in the palliative care setting, particular attention to substance abuse among these patients is critical for the proper management and treatment of their pain.[7]

Substance Use Issues in Palliative Care

Initial studies that evaluated the epidemiology of SUD in patients with advanced illness indicated that SUDs appeared to be relatively rare within the tertiary care population with cancer and other advanced diseases.[8] Findings from a review of consultations performed by the Psychiatry Services at Memorial Sloan-Kettering Cancer Center (MSKCC) revealed that requests for management of issues related to substance abuse comprised only 3% of consultations.[5] However, recent evidence shows that substance abuse issues among palliative care patients is more common than previously thought. Some studies have suggested that at least one in five cancer patients might be at risk of inappropriate use of opioids.[9] In a prognostic study of patients receiving opioids for cancer pain, 19% of patients developed nonmedical opioid use behavior within a median duration of 8 weeks after an initial supportive care clinic consultation.[10]

Terminology

When caring for a person with SUD, it is essential to understand the medical language and the various terminologies used to describe the conditions related to the use of opioids (Table 10.1).[11] It has been reported that some of these words might be perceived as stigmatizing and pejorative and could potentially affect their ability to receive appropriate care. There have therefore been proposals to use alternative terms that are neutral, respectful, precise, and nonjudgmental.[12] For example, the term "nonmedical opioid use" (NMOU) is a proposed alternative to terms such as "opioid abuse" or "opioid misuse." "Substance use disorder" is suggested instead of "substance abuse" or "addiction." Providers must maintain a nonjudgmental language while addressing their patients if they are to build trust and increase adherence with treatment. The neutral language will remind the clinician, patients, and families that patients are humans first who are secondarily diagnosed with a disease.[12,13]

When an opioid is prescribed for medical purposes, it is necessary to consider NMOU behaviors along a continuum. The spectrum may range from relatively lower risk conditions such as hoarding of medication and unauthorized dose escalation, to more severe conditions such prescription forgery and selling prescription drugs, which usually result in hazardous use.[12] According to the *Diagnostic and Statistical Manual of Mental Disorders*

TABLE 10.1 Common terms related to opioids and their definitions

Common term	Definition
Aberrant drug-related behavior	Any behavior outside the boundaries of the agreed- treatment plan, which is established as early as possible in the doctor-patient relationship
Abuse	The intentional self- administration of a medication for a nonmedical purpose, such as altering one's state of consciousness, or the use of any illegal drug
Addiction	A primary, chronic, neurobiological disease that occurs due to genetic, psychosocial, and environmental factors. Characterized by one or more of the following features: • Impaired control, • Overuse, compulsive use • Continued use despite harm • Craving
Binge	Heavy drinking episodes or other substance use, like cocaine or Marijuana
Chemical coping	A term used to describe an inappropriate and excessive use of opioids to cope with the various stressful events associated with the diagnosis and management of cancer
Diversion	The intentional transfer of a controlled substance from legitimate distribution and dispensing channels
Medical marijuana	Cannabis prescribed by a licensed medical provider
Meth	Used as an abbreviation for multiple products and medications. Methadone, Methamphetamine, Methylphenidate
Misuse	The use of a medication for purpose other than directed or indicated, either intentionally or unintentionally. It does not refer to use for the mind- altering purposes.
Nonmedical opioid use	Use of opioids without a prescription, use with a prescription but not as prescribed or use simply for the experience or feeling caused by the opioids
Physical dependence	A physiological adaptation characterized by the onset of withdrawal symptoms after sudden opioid cessation, rapid dose reduction, reduction in blood drug levels and/or administration of an opioid antagonist
Pseudo- addiction	The clinician misinterprets a syndrome of abnormal behavior resulting from undertreatment of pain as inappropriate drug-seeking behavior. This behavior resolves once the pain is adequately managed.
Relapse	Use, return to use, or disorder vs. remission specifiers (early or sustained) as defined by DSM-5
Substance use disorder	A pattern of symptoms due to recurrent use of the substance despite considerable clinical and functional impairments as a result. It is defined using 11 diagnostic criteria based on evidence of impaired control, social impairment, risky use, and pharmacological criteria. It is classified: • Mild (2–3 criteria), • Moderate (4–5 criteria) • Severe (≥6 criteria)
Tolerance	A physiological adaptation characterized by the need to use increasing opioid doses to maintain the same effects. Persistent exposure to the opioid results in a decrease in one or more opioid effects over time

TABLE 10.2 Four Main domains and 11 criteria of DMS-5 definition for substance use disorder[14]

IMPAIRED CONTROL	
Criterion 1	Large amount or for prolonged period
Criterion 2	Persistent desire to reduce, regulate and multiple failed attempts
Criterion 3	Spending time on obtaining, using and recovering from the side effects of the substance
Criterion 4	Craving, intense desire or urge for the substance
SOCIAL IMPAIRMENT	
Criterion 5	Missing or failure to meet obligations at work, school or home
Criterion 6	Straining interpersonal relationships
Criterion 7	Withdrawing from social connections and activities. Development of isolation
RISKY USE	
Criterion 8	Use of substance in physically hazardous situations
Criterion 9	Continued use, despite of knowing they have a persistent or recurrent psychosocial or physical problem
PHARMACOLOGICAL CRITERIA	
Criterion 10	Tolerance: requiring an increased dose to achieve the desired effect or having reduced effect with usual dose
Criterion 11	Withdrawal: cluster of symptoms or syndrome due to reduced concentration of substance in the blood or tissue.
DIAGNOSTIC CRITERIA FOR SUBSTANCE USE DISORDER	

- Mild: 2–3 criteria
- Moderate: 4–5 criteria
- Severe: ≥6 criteria

(DSM-5), SUD may be classified as mild (2–3 criteria), moderate (4–5 criteria), or severe (≥6 criteria) depending on the number of items from the 11 diagnostic criteria (Table 10.2) which are grouped into four main domains: (1) evidence of impaired control, (2) social impairment, (3) risky use, and (4) pharmacological criteria.[14]

Approach to Care for Patients with SUD or NMOU

Initial Patient Evaluation

During the early patient encounters, it is essential to screen all patients to identify any current or previous history of SUD, risk stratify them, and tailor the care accordingly (Figure 10.1). Following a general set of guidelines can be helpful for the proper management of opioid therapy.[11] Studies have shown that male gender, younger age (<45 years), family or personal history of mental health disorder or SUD, alcohol, or tobacco use are considered

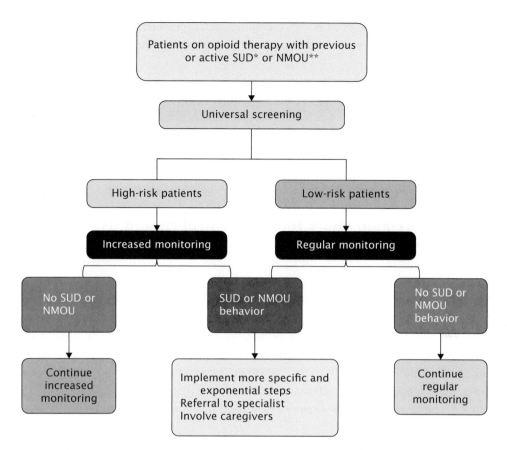

*SUD: Substance use disorder; **NMOU: Non-medical Opioid Use

FIGURE 10.1 Approach to patients on long-term opioid therapy.

some of the risk factors of developing NMOU.[15] Unfortunately, no single risk factor or set of risk factors has shown to have higher predictability over the others. For that reason, we must combine the clinical history and the screening tools to identify the patients who are at risk of NMOU.[13]

Comprehensive History and Physical Examination

All clinicians should consider universal screening for all their patients by obtaining a comprehensive clinical history, psychosocial and family histories, and substance abuse history.

In many instances, clinicians are uncomfortable and knowingly avoid asking patients about drug abuse.[11,16] However, we must obtain history on the duration, frequency, desired drugs, and time they last used. Using open-ended questions in a nonjudgmental approach with empathy and compassion will promote trust and help obtain reliable history.[16] It is equally vital to document patient history with neutral terms to avoid any prejudice from other professionals. While interviewing, it is essential to note that the patient might misinterpret the questions for many reasons: fear of judgment, mistrust, legal problems, concern, or fear of undertreatment of pain.[7,11,16] Therefore, clinical providers must be open and explain the need for accurate drug dosage use to prevent withdrawal, interactions, or even overdose.

The clinician should carefully structure the interview, start with a broad spectrum of questions, and narrow the discussion to closing the problems. They may start with general inquiries about the use of caffeine or tobacco smoking and gradually proceed to more specific questions related to illicit drugs.[11,16] This approach helps understand the other comorbidities such as psychosocial issues, family history of SUD, and any coexisting mental health issues that can play a role in NMOU.[4] Moreover, this style of interview develops trust and helps formulate treatment strategies with safety and decreased potential for relapse.[11,16]

Risk Assessment Tools for Nonmedical Opioid Use

Several screening tools are available to identify SUD or NMOU among patients receiving long-term opioid therapy (Table 10.3). The Cut down, Annoyed, Guilty, and Eye-opener (CAGE) questionnaire is a popular tool exclusively used for screening alcohol use, which is a known risk factor for NMOU. It is either administered by the clinician or self-administered by the patient. It consists of the following four questions: (1) Have you ever felt you should cut down on your drinking? (2) Have people annoyed you by criticizing your drinking? (3) Have you ever felt bad or guilty about your drinking? (4) Have you ever had a drink first thing in the morning to steady your nerves or get rid of a hangover (eye-opener)? A total score of 2 or more indicates problematic alcohol use and therefore a high risk for NMOU.[15] The CAGE-Adapted to Include Drugs (CAGE AID) questionnaire substitutes "drink" with "drink or drugs."[15]

The Screener and Opioids Assessment for Patients with Pain (SOAPP) form helps identify patients who might be at risk of developing NMOU with long-term opioid therapy. It consists of questions related to the patient's history of substance use, medication-related behaviors, and psychiatric and neurobiological need for medicine. There are three different versions available: SOAPP-Original, SOAPP-Revised, and SOAPP-Short Form, each consisting of 14, 24, and 5 question items, respectively, with cutoff scores of ≥ 7, ≥ 18, and ≥ 4, respectively. It is a clinician or patient self-administered tool.[15]

The Opioid Risk Tool (ORT) is a patient self-administered questionnaire consists of 10 questions that evaluates the risk factors in five categories: (1) family history of substance abuse, (2) personal history of substance abuse, (3) age 16 to 45 years, (4) history of preadolescent sexual abuse, and (5) psychological disease. The scoring ranges from 0 to 26: patients with a score of 0–3 are at low risk, 4–7 are at moderate risk, and greater than or equal to 8 are at high risk.[15]

The Diagnosis, Intractability, Risk and Efficacy Inventory (DIRE) is a clinician-administered screening tool. This questionnaire helps determine patient compliance with long-term opioid therapy and the efficacy of analgesia. This questionnaire consists of risk factors in four categories. The total score ranges from 7 to 21, with lower scores indicating higher risk, and a cutoff score of 13 carries a sensitivity and specificity of 94% and 87%, respectively. Other tools, such as the Current Opioid Misuse Measure (COMM) and the

TABLE 10.3 Screening tools for substance use disorder[15]

Administered by	Tool	Remarks	Number of questions	Score range	Cut-off score for increased risk of SUD
Clinician or Patient	CAGE[a]	Assessment of risk of alcohol use or other SUD[c], including patients for LOT[d]; not specific to only patients with pain or alcohol dependency	4	0–4	≥2
	CAGE-AID[b]	A version of CAGE for the assessment of both alcohol and illicit drug use	4	0–4	≥2
Clinician	DIRE inventory[e]	Assessment of risk of NMOU in patients considered for LOT; helps with proper estimation of patients who will benefit and have effective analgesia and be compliant with opioid therapy	7	7–21	≤13
	ABC[f]	Identification of SUD, or NMOU[g] in patients who are on LOT by tracking their behaviors	20	0–20	≥3
Patient	SOAPP V.1[h]	Assessment of risk of NMOU in patients considered for LOT	14	0–56	≥7
	SOAPP-Revised	Revised version of SOAPP V.1	24	0–96	≥18
	SOAPP-Short Form	An abbreviated version of SOAPP V.1	5	0–20	≥7
	ORT[i]	Assessment of risk of NMOU in patients considered for LOT	10	0–26	• Low 0–3 • Moderate 4–7 • High ≥8
	PMQ[j]	Identification of NMOU in patients who are on LOT	26	0–104	≥30
	COMM[k]	Identification of NMOU in patients who are on LOT and need monitoring	17	0–68	≥9

[a]CAGE: Cut down, Annoyed, Guilty and Eye-opener.

[b]CAGE-AID: CAGE Adapted to Include Drugs.

[c]SUD: Substance use disorder.

[d]LOT: Long-term opioid therapy.

[e]DIRE: Diagnosis, Intractability, Risk and Efficacy.

[f]ABC: Addiction Behavior Checklist.

[g]NMOU: Nonmedical opioid use.

[h]SOAPP: Screener and Opioid Assessment for Patients with Pain.

[i]ORT: Opioid Risk Tool.

[j]PMQ: Pain Medication Questionnaire.

[k]COMM: Current Opioid Misuse Measure.

Addiction Behavior Checklist (ABC), are used for patients who are on long-term opioids and need continued monitoring.[15]

Subsequent Patient Care

Patients on long-term opioid therapy require a close and periodic evaluation after the initial risk assessment. The treatment plan may subsequently be revised based on patients' response to the ongoing treatment, adherence to the opioid therapy, adverse effects, and other clinical findings.[8,17] Before initiating opioids, providers must explain to patients about initial dosing, subsequent titration, selection of the opioids, and rotation of opioids if necessary based on the patient's ongoing clinical condition and symptoms.[17] The doses may need to be adjusted based on hepatic and renal function. In addition, clinicians should be proactive and discuss the clear plan of weaning off the opioids if the pain etiology is transient, such as self-limiting postsurgical pain or after receiving radiation for head and neck cancers. At every visit, clinicians should be able to identify any behavior suggestive of NMOU, otherwise known as "red flags" (Box 10.1), whenever present and utilize the prescription drug monitoring program (PDMP) and urine drug test (UDT) when necessary.[9]

BOX 10.1 Behaviors related to nonmedical opioid use

- Frequent unscheduled appointments or telephone calls for early opioid refills
- Self-escalation or request for excessive increase in the opioid dosage not consistent with the patient's pain syndrome
- Reports of lost or stolen opioid prescriptions or medication
- Frequent emergency room visits for opioids
- Seeking opioids from multiple providers ("doctor shopping")
- Requests for a specific opioid
- Resistance to changes in the opioid regimen even when clinically indicated
- Use of non-prescribed restricted medications or illicit drugs
- Requesting opioids for their euphoric effect or for symptoms such as anxiety or insomnia
- Reports of impaired functioning in daily activities owing to opioid use
- Family members and/or caregivers expressing concern over patient's use of opioids
- Reports of hoarding drugs
- Obtaining opioids from nonmedical sources
- Reports of stealing, tampering, or forging opioid prescriptions
- Discrepancy in pill counts without good explanation

Adapted with permission from ref.[15] **Nature** Reviews.

Behaviors Suggestive of Nonmedical Opioid Use

According to the literature, there are certain behaviors that patients on opioid therapy may display that are suggestive of NMOU. Examples of such behaviors are shown in (Box 10.1). Different behaviors may represent different levels of concern. Certain behaviors such as "injection drug use" are more indicative of NMOU than "requesting dose escalation for uncontrolled pain." In a longitudinal study conducted among cancer patients receiving opioids at an outpatient setting, "requests for early refills" were the most commonly observed behaviors.[13] Deviation from opioid adherence to NMOU might be very subtle and easily missed. Clinicians should always be vigilant in monitoring their patient's behavior related to opioid therapy and combine that information with other aspects of patients' care in making the ultimate therapeutic decision.

For patients displaying NMOU behavior who are closer to the end of life, therapy goals should focus on optimization of symptom burden and emotional support. Complete behavior transformation in a short life span may not be achievable. On the other hand, patients with curable disease exhibiting NMOU behaviors need closer attention, more aggressive strategies, and, if warrantied, SUD specialist involvement.

Prescription Drug Monitoring Program

PDMPs are state-run programs which manage secure electronic databases with prescriber and pharmacy dispensing information on controlled substances. The data are available to authorized users, including regulatory boards, law enforcement agencies, and prescribes. PDMPs help identify those patients who obtain prescriptions from multiple providers (doctor shopping) and/or fill their prescriptions from various pharmacies (pharmacy shopping).[18] PDMPs are available in North America, Australia, and some parts of Europe. In the United States, all the states have some form of PDMPs in place. Twenty-four states in the United States showed a reduction of greater than 30% in the rate of prescribing scheduled II opioid prescriptions over 10 years with the implementation of PDMP. This rate of decline was sustainable for the subsequent 2 years. PDMPs help providers identify patients with NMOU, support clinical decision-making, and guide clinicians during opioid therapy.[18]

Urine Drug Testing

UDT is an effective test utilized in the course of managing patients receiving chronic opioid therapy. The two commonly used UDTs in the clinical practice include screening tests or immunoassays and confirmatory tests or laboratory-based specific drug identification tests, such as gas chromatography-mass spectrometry and liquid chromatography-mass spectrometry.[17] UDTs provide data on opioids and their metabolites and can direct opioid therapy by showing treatment adherence. It also helps identify NMOU by detecting the presence of undisclosed medications, the use of illicit drugs, and the absence of prescribed medications. Although UDTs may be helpful, they also have certain limitations. A normal result does not always indicate normal drug-taking behavior because a patient may have a normal UDT but might be using opioids in an excessive or maladaptive manner as a way of coping with stressful situations such as cancer diagnosis or progression. Similarly, an abnormal result may not always indicate NMOU and sometimes require that other potential causes be carefully explored. UDT interpretation can be challenging considering the complex metabolic pathway of opioids.[17] Wrong interpretation of UDT results can have negative outcomes for the patient, such as deterioration of physician–patient relationship, unfair loss of opioid privileges, and potential inability to receive appropriate therapy from other physicians.[9]

Management of Nonmedical Opioid Use

Once patients demonstrate NMOU behavior, clinicians should initiate an open and candid conversation. This discussion should focus on the concerns about the patient's safety and well-being. Some rudimentary measures that can be implemented to ensure adherence to safe opioid use include intensifying patient and caregiver education on safe opioid use, storage, and disposal; decreasing the time interval between follow-ups for refills;[17] augmenting patient monitoring with relatively more frequent UDT;[17] providing smaller quantities and lower doses of opioids refills at a time; weaning off opioids when possible; and referring to a specialist in pain medicine, palliative care, mental health, or drug addiction for co-management where necessary.[8,13]

Additional strategies that might be considered when managing patients with NMOU are described below with some supporting evidence.

Opioid Characteristic

Certain characteristics of opioids, such as the opioid agent, formulation, route of administration, dosing, and timing of opioid intake can determine the risk of NMOU and opioid overdose.

> *Opioid agent*: The abuse liability potential is universal for all opioids, although a few studies have shown relatively higher abuse potential with oxycodone and relatively lower potential with buprenorphine and tapentadol.[19] Clinicians should be aware of this when selecting opioids for pain management in patients with SUD.
>
> *Opioid dose*: The abuse liability effect of opioids generally increases with increasing opioid dose. Clinicians should titrate the dose to a minimum effective dose to achieve desired pain control. Guidelines by the US Centers for Disease Control and Prevention (CDC) for noncancer pain recommended caution for opioid titration above 90 mg of daily morphine milligram equivalent.[8,13] Some states in the United States have legislation prescribing opioids for noncancer pain for no more than 7 days for acute pain and a 30-day supply for chronic pain. However, applying the dose- and time-related limitations for terminally ill patients and cancer-related pain is challenging. Patients with cancer-related pain usually require higher strength and prolonged courses of opioids.[15]
>
> *Opioid formulation*: Immediate-release formulations are more preferred among patients with SUD. The rapid onset and short-term effect of the immediate-release

opioids is associated with high reward potential and can be a high risk for NMOU compared to extended-release opioids. Immediate-release opioids penetrate the limbic system faster than extended-release formulations and provide higher levels of reward. On the contrary, extended-release opioids have an increased risk of fatal and nonfatal overdose in the initial 2 weeks of therapy than immediate-release.[16,19] Opioid dosing should be personalized to each individual and their medical condition. Consider extended-release opioids for patients with cancer-related pain and NMOU.[8,16,20] Agents such as buprenorphine and methadone are highly effective for the management of cancer-related pain and SUD, but prescribers need to be cautious with prescribing methadone as it is related to many fatal overdoses.[8]

Abuse-deterrent opioid formulations (ADFs) have properties that reduce the potential for NMOU when injected or snorted, making the product less rewarding. Unfortunately, the high cost of ADFs has made it challenging to access among terminally ill and cancer patients. On the other hand, ADFs can increase relapses in NMOU patients to heroin use and injection-related complications due to the dangerous methods patient invent to overcome the tamper-deterring properties.[15]

Route of administration: Faster administration of intravenous opioids is associated with increased patient-reported abuse liability effects compared with slower infusion. This has immediate implications for opioid administration in the inpatient setting where intravenous opioids are frequently administered to achieve a rapid onset of pain relief.[15,16,20]

Timing of opioid intake: Patients with a history of NMOU and SUD are highly vulnerable to overdose after a period of abstinence through detoxification or incarceration.[15] Although they might continue to desire opioids, they have lost the tolerance to them. The opioid dose they have used before the abstinence could therefore cause overdose, leading to respiratory depression and sedation. Loss of tolerance occurs within days of opioid discontinuation. On the contrary, the craving and desire to use opioids in patients with NMOU and SUD remains for many years. [8]

Benzodiazepines and Adjuvant Analgesics

Benzodiazepines and opioids can work synergistically to cause increased sedation and respiratory depression. Concurrent use of these medications is associated with increased opioid-related deaths and contributes to one-third of opioid overdoses in the United States.[8] Similarly, the concurrent use of gabapentin and opioids is also associated with dose-dependent opioid-related deaths compared to opioids alone.[8,13,15]

Terminally ill patients and cancer patients usually receive benzodiazepines to help with anxiety and gabapentinoids for neuropathic pain. In these situations, efforts to reduce the dose or replace the medications with alternatives are crucial. Olanzapine for anxiety and duloxetine for neuropathic pain are appropriate alternatives.[8,15] So far, these medications have not shown to be associated with opioid-related deaths when combined. Opioid-sparing agents and adjuvant analgesics should always be considered wherever possible in treating cancer-related pain.[8,13,15]

Naloxone Co-Prescription

Naloxone, a short-acting opioid antagonist that can reverse an opioid overdose in less than 5 minutes, can be beneficial in patients at risk of NMOU.[17] CDC guidelines on pain recommend prescription of naloxone to the patient on opioids with high-risk factors such as the previous history of overdose, history of SUD, or a median morphine equivalent dose (MMED) of greater than 50 mg/day. Other considerations for naloxone co-prescription include patients on methadone; history of chronic renal, pulmonary, or hepatic disease; and recent history of incarceration.[8,15,17]

Interdisciplinary Team Approach

The care of patients who display NMOU behavior can be complex due to multiple underlying biomedical, psychosocial, and financial factors. Utilizing a treatment plan that involves a team approach that recognizes and responds to these complex needs is the most efficient way to treat such patients in the palliative care setting. Interdisciplinary teams consisting of diverse clinician experts may be better equipped to manage these patients and are more likely to adopt more structured, rigorous risk evaluation strategies and established risk mitigation measures to care for such patients.[5,9] A specialized opioid stewardship program was developed to care for patients receiving opioids in the supportive care clinic of a tertiary cancer center.[13] It was modeled after concepts from well-established behavioral therapies such as screening, brief intervention, referral and treatment, and motivational interviewing techniques. The care is delivered by a team consisting of a physician, a registered nurse, and one or more of other team members, including a pharmacist, psychologist, counselor, social worker, and patient advocate. A preliminary study to evaluate the efficacy of this intervention found that the intervention was associated with a significant reduction in the frequency of NMOU-related behaviors from a median of 3 per month before the intervention to 0.4 postintervention ($P < 0.0001$).[15,17] The daily morphine equivalent dose went down from a median of 165 mg/day at the initial intervention visit to 112 mg/day at the last follow-up visit ($P = 0.02$) with no significant change in their pain intensity. Such efforts have proved effective in managing opioid therapy for patients with cancer pain and NMOU.[13] During the COVID-19 pandemic, the intervention was modified to adapt to the changing healthcare environment due to unintended disruptions in patient care as a result of the pandemic.[17]

Comorbid Psychologic Conditions

Mental health disorders are common among patients with a history of SUD or NMOU. Early evaluation and treatment of any underlying psychiatric condition enhances the chances of recovery from SUD and minimizes the risk of relapses. American Society of Clinical Oncology guidelines on cancer pain suggest including adjuvant therapies when appropriate. Psychological interventions, such as cognitive-behavioral therapy, relaxation techniques, biofeedback, distraction techniques, problem-solving techniques, and other coping strategies are some of the beneficial adjuvant therapies that may be utilized when caring for patients with NMOU.[8,17]

Family Sessions and Meetings

To increase and strengthen a patient's support system, the clinician should involve family members and friends in the treatment plan. These family meetings serve many purposes. One is to familiarize the clinician with the patient's support system; this may help the clinician better understand a patient's history of aberrant drug-taking behaviors. These meetings may also help to identify any family members who are using illicit drugs so that further help can be offered.[20] Clinical experience has shown that encouraging family members to make changes in deference to the patient and to support them with specific referrals can be useful.[5] Special attention is needed when a family member or friend has an SUD, either active or in remission. The patient should be made aware of the possibility that family members or friends may attempt to buy or sell the patient's medications and should be counseled not to encourage such activity. Family members of palliative care patients are particularly vulnerable because of their increased involvement in the patients' care, which usually results in increased access and excessive exposure to the patients' medications. This eventually creates a perfect arena for opioid diversion or development of NMOU. Studies have shown that more than 45.5% of those who engage in NMOU obtained prescription opioids from a friend or relative for free, and 5.4% bought opioids from a friend or relative.[1] The meetings can also help identify very reliable individuals who can serve as an integral source of strength and support for the patient during treatment.[20]

Referral to Specialized Programs for Co-Management

Clinicians taking care of patients with NMOU or SUD should utilize the services of specialized programs and experts such as psychiatrists and addiction medicine specialists whenever possible. The care of these patients has multiple layers such as biomedical, psychosocial, legal, and financial domains, and involvement of these supporting services will likely increase the rate of successful patient outcomes. Within the context of outpatient management, a clinician may choose to refer patients to a 12-step program. This referral must stipulate that documented attendance is a condition for ongoing drug prescriptions. Clinical providers may consider communicating with the sponsor beforehand regarding the patient's illness and the reason for prescribing opioids. Establishing this contact will also limit any ostracism the patient may experience because of perceptions of not being compliant with the ideals of the 12-step program.[20] A 12-step program can be confusing in this patient population because the patient's condition might warrant them using opioids while making efforts to remain sober. The programs may not support the liberal use of opioids despite the patient's terminal status and may also misunderstand the side effects of the opioids.[16]

Patient-Physician Communication Surrounding NMOU

Patients may misrepresent their drug use for a variety of logical reasons, such as stigmatization, mistrust of the clinician, or concerns regarding fears of undertreatment. Thus, clinicians need to employ the right techniques and communication skills in order to navigate these conversations.[16,20] A practical way to approach this is to start with a broad spectrum of topics and gradually narrow the interview as it proceeds. More specifically, this approach would begin with general inquiries regarding the role of drugs, such as caffeine and nicotine, in the patient's life and gradually proceed to more specific questions regarding illicit drugs. An advantage of employing this interview style is that it may distinguish any coexisting psychiatric disorders, many of which can significantly contribute to NMOU behavior. Identifying these comorbidities and further treating them can aid in developing management strategies and minimize the risk of relapse.[16,20]

One approach to navigate these conversations describes five key communication strategies in a way that maintains the therapeutic alliance between provider and patient while decreasing the stigma surrounding discussions about substance use. These include (1) exploring and validating the patient's pain and experience of suffering in an empathic manner, (2) directly inquiring about nonmedical use and SUDs in a neutral and non-judgmental manner rather than circumventing the issue, (3) expressing to the patient the clinician's concerns for harms associated with NMOU, (4) setting clear limits and boundaries including re-outlining the necessary steps to be taken with repeated medication non-compliance, and (5) voicing a commitment to ongoing treatment and assuring the patient of non-abandonment as much as possible.[11]

Conclusion

Evidence supports the use of opioid analgesics for cancer-related pain and in terminally ill patients. Ensuring safe opioid use among patients with NMOU can be challenging, especially with the increasing opioid crisis in the United States and worldwide. Through a stepwise approach with ongoing monitoring; timely identification; extensive education; utilization of resources such as PMPD, UDT, and interdisciplinary care, healthcare providers can optimize prescribing opioids for symptom management while minimizing NMOU. Further research is needed in finding safer and novel pharmacological options with minimum risk of NMOU and better symptom control.

Future Directions

More evidence-based recommendations on managing palliative care patients with cancer pain and NMOU are needed. Timely implementation of educational resources for palliative medicine trainees and healthcare providers in caring for patients with SUD should be considered.

Key Points

- Opioids remain the gold standard for treating cancer-related pain and among patients under palliative care.

- Those patients who receive opioids for cancer pain are at risk for NMOU, diversion, chemical coping, opioids-related side effects, accidental overdose, and even death.
- Increasing data suggest that NMOU is more prevalent among cancer patients than previously thought.
- It is essential to obtain a consistent patient history, including prior SUD or NMOU behavior; screen all patients with validated risk assessment tools; and provide proper education on safe opioid use and storage.
- Utilize PDMPs and UDTs to help monitor adherence to the prescribed opioids, detect any NMOU behavior, and make well-informed therapeutic plans.
- Avoid prescribing high doses of gabapentin, pregabalin, and benzodiazepines for patients on opioids.
- Consider prescribing naloxone nasal spray for all patients who are at risk for opioid overdose.

References

1. Lipari HA. How people obtain the prescription pain relievers they misuse. The CBHSQ Report: January 12, 2017. Center for Behavioral Health Statistics and Quality, Substance Abuse and Mental Health Services Administration, Rockville, MD. https://www.samhsa.gov/data/sites/default/files/report_2686/ShortReport-2686.html. Published 2018. Accessed May 12, 2018.
2. Park-Lee E, Lipari RN, Hedden SL, Kroutil LA, Porter JD. Receipt of services for substance use and mental health issues among adults: Results from the 2016 National Survey on Drug Use and Health. In: *CBHSQ Data Review*. Rockville, MD: Substance Abuse and Mental Health Services Administration; 2012:1–35.
3. Centers for Disease Control and Prevention. Opioid overdose. 2020. Centers for Disease control and Prevention. https://www.cdc.gov/drugoverdose/epidemic/index.html. Updated March 19, 2020. Accessed March 19, 2020.
4. Ebenau A, Dijkstra B, Ter Huurne C, Hasselaar J, Vissers K, Groot M. Palliative care for people with substance use disorder and multiple problems: A qualitative study on experiences of patients and proxies. *BMC Palliat Care.* 2019;18(1):56.
5. Kirsh KL, Passik SD. Palliative care of the terminally ill drug addict. *Cancer Invest.* 2006;24(4):425–431.
6. Ward SE, Goldberg N, Miller-McCauley V, Mueller C, Nolan A, Pawlik-Plank D, et al. Patient-related barriers to management of cancer pain. *Pain.* 1993;52(3):319–324.
7. van den Beuken-van Everdingen MH, Hochstenbach LM, Joosten EA, Tjan-Heijnen VC, Janssen DJ. Update on prevalence of pain in patients with cancer: Systematic review and meta-analysis. *J Pain Symptom Manage.* 2016;51(6):1070–1090 e1079.
8. Arthur J, Hui D. Safe opioid use: Management of opioid-related adverse effects and aberrant behaviors. *Hematol Oncol Clin North Am.* 2018;32(3):387–403.
9. Meghani SH, Wiedemer NL, Becker WC, Gracely EJ, Gallagher RM. Predictors of resolution of aberrant drug behavior in chronic pain patients treated in a structured opioid risk management program. *Pain Med.* 2009;10(5):858–865.
10. Yennurajalingam S, Arthur J, Reddy S, Edwards T, Lu Z, De Moraes AR et al. Frequency of and factors associated with nonmedical opioid use behavior among patients with cancer receiving opioids for cancer pain. *JAMA Oncol.* 2021;7(3):404–411.
11. Sager Z, Childers J. Navigating challenging conversations about nonmedical opioid use in the context of oncology. *Oncologist.* 2019;24(10):1299–1304.

12. Saitz R. Recommended use of terminology in addiction medicine. In: Herron, Abigail J., ed. *The ASAM Essentials of Addiction Medicine.* 3rd ed. Philadelphia: Wolters Kluwer; 2020:7–10.

13. Arthur J, Edwards T, Reddy S, Nguyen K, Hui D, Yennu S, et al. Outcomes of a specialized interdisciplinary approach for patients with cancer with aberrant opioid-related behavior. *Oncologist.* 2018;23(2):263–270.

14. Association AP. *Diagnostic and Statistical Manual of Mental Disorders (DSM-5)* 5th ed. Washington, DC: American Psychiatric Association Publishing; 2013:10.

15. Arthur J, Bruera E. Balancing opioid analgesia with the risk of nonmedical opioid use in patients with cancer. *Nat Rev Clin Oncol.* 2019;16(4):213–226.

16. Passik SD, Portenoy RK, Ricketts PL. Substance abuse issues in cancer patients. Part 2: Evaluation and treatment. *Oncology (Williston Park).* 1998;12(5):729–734; discussion 736, 741–742.

17. Amaram-Davila JS, Arthur J, Reddy A, Bruera E. Managing nonmedical opioid use among patients with cancer pain during the COVID-19 pandemic using the CHAT model and telehealth. *J Pain Symptom Manage.* 2021;62(1):192–196.

18. Bao Y, Wen K, Johnson P, Jeng PJ, Meisel ZF, Schackman BR. Assessing the impact of state policies for prescription drug monitoring programs on high-risk opioid prescriptions. *Health Aff (Millwood).* 2018;37(10):1596–1604.

19. Comer SD, Sullivan MA, Whittington RA, Vosburg SK, Kowalczyk WJ. Abuse liability of prescription opioids compared to heroin in morphine-maintained heroin abusers. *Neuropsychopharmacology.* 2008;33(5):1179–1191.

20. Kirsh KL, Rzetelny A, Passik SD. Substance use disorders. In: Holland JC, Breitbart WS, Jacobsen PB, et al, eds. *Psycho-Oncology.* New York: Oxford University Press; 1998:317–322.

11

Difficult Personality Traits and Disorders in Palliative Care

John Wynn

I do not like that man. I must get to know him better.
—Abraham Lincoln

Introduction

Terminal illness is a crisis. Patients and families coping with terminal illness experience extremes of emotional, cognitive, social, and spiritual strain. Many, perhaps most, cope effectively within their premorbid repertoire of responses, experiencing only transient dysfunction. They compensate effectively with the disruptions of their bodily functions, self-image, work, and relationships. They can accommodate the life changes without overwhelming strain. They have a flexible self-concept and supportive, understanding people to help them.

Less fortunate patients, however, are not so resilient. Their established ways of coping do not meet the challenge, and they respond to crisis with self-defeating, isolating, alienating strategies that stymie the most well-intentioned and sophisticated clinicians. They may be experienced by staff as aggravating, aggrandizing, chaotic, dramatic, or odd, and their dysfunctional responses may appear as attempts to foil treatment or monopolize resources.

Staff may experience feelings of anger, disinterest, neglect, and guilt, or even extreme feelings such as hatred. Despite their attempts to cope with such strong and "unprofessional" feelings, clinicians may view the patient as unreachable, uncooperative, bizarre, dramatic, or demanding; in other words, "impossible."

The question that should arise in such instances is "Why, in a setting of care and attention, when most patients are so collaborative, would this person behave so badly? Furthermore, how could caring, thoughtful, hardworking clinicians be so angry, impatient, frustrated, or dismissive of a patient's suffering?"

Answering these questions requires that we (1) identify dysfunctional working relationships between patients, family, and staff, and (2) facilitate quality care for all patients. This is an especially challenging task when working with the patients discussed in this chapter.

Defining Difficult Personality Traits and Disorders in Palliative Care Settings
Elements of Personality Functioning

Section III of the *Diagnostic and Statistical Manual of Mental Disorders* (DSM-5) presents a conceptual model of personality that incorporates disorders of self and interpersonal functioning.[1] "Self" comprises identity and self-direction, referring to the long-term stability and integrity of one's self-image and orientation relative to internal standards and goals. "Interpersonal functioning" is expressed in one's capacity for empathy and intimacy, how we understand others' feelings and our impact on them as well as our ability to connect with them at various levels of intimacy. Deficits in any of these areas limits coping. This may be through misperception of oneself and others, an inability to organize behavior around internal and interpersonal demands and expectations, a lack of strategies for integrating those demands, or a failure to develop social ties in times of need. The misperceptions and limited repertoire are expressed in character rigidity.

Character Rigidity

All patients long to trust someone who will understand their predicament and respond compassionately to their needs. Clinicians easily overlook how terribly stressful routine medical care can be for anxious, insecure patients. Close contact activates feelings of fear and at times desperate maneuvers to avoid emotional vulnerability and pain. Feelings of shame and guilt may interfere with expressing these needs, leading to fears of being forgotten, abandoned, or rejected. Interpersonal difficulties are caused by idiosyncratic perceptions, distorted cognitions, unstable or confusing affects, and troublesome behaviors. *Labeling patients and their distortions is of little value.* Identifying and addressing their fears with care and reassurance, however, will go a long way to resolving conflict and supporting patients, families, and staff.

Character rigidity is the essential presenting feature of a personality disorder: a limited ability to think about oneself and others in varied or new ways, combined with a limited repertoire of behaviors in challenging circumstances. Distorted cognitions—"ways of perceiving and interpreting self, others, and events"—surface as differences with staff, conflicts with family, or preoccupation with specialness, suspicions, guilty rumination, or self-criticism.[1]

By definition, the personality disorders of the DSM-5 are comprised of stable and enduring patterns of thinking, feeling, and behaving. In fact, however, personality features and disorders are not stable over time.[2-7] In longitudinal studies, many patients are later found to meet other personality disorder diagnostic criteria or to have no diagnosis at all. In one study of college students, "change was typically and uniformly in the direction of decreasing personality disorder features over time."[5]

Clinicians must use caution assessing troubling behaviors in difficult circumstances. Responses to crisis may be mistaken for longstanding patterns of behavior.[3,5] Maladaptive responses may only represent an initial stumble in a steady march from diagnosis and treatment until death. The inpatient Ms. North, admitted in October, may be very different from the Ms. North we met last May.

Clinicians often underestimate patients' potential for improvement over time.[8] Properly addressed, troubling behaviors often lead to maturation and emotional growth.[9] A personality disorder diagnosis may be wrong and yet indelibly, authoritatively inscribed in the patient's chart, only to mislead subsequent clinicians.

DSM-5

DSM classifies personality disorders into three categories, or clusters, of disorders: A. *odd or eccentric*; B. *dramatic, emotional, or erratic*; and C. *anxious or fearful*. These are listed in Table 11.1.

Personality establishes the context in which mood, anxiety, and other mental disorders take place: schizoid and schizotypal patients are more vulnerable to psychosis; borderline and narcissistic patients are prone to depression, irritability, and egotism; and cluster C patients often develop anxiety disorders.[11-14] Personality disorders increase exposure and vulnerability, perhaps through a distortion of social perception and alienating interpersonal styles.[15-17] Distorted perceptions isolate patients, leaving them without social buffers against adverse life events. Solitary coping is less effective and reinforces aberrant patterns of thinking, feeling, and relating.

Alternatively, other disorders may be precursors to personality disorder.[18,19] Chronic mood, anxiety, or substance disorders may restrict social interactions and obscure opportunities to learn social coping strategies. This restricted repertoire of interpersonal interactions constitutes the character rigidity that defines personality disorders.

In one large study, patients with schizotypal and borderline personality disorders were found to have significantly more impairment at work, in social relationships, and at leisure than patients with major depressive disorder.[20] Patients with co-occurring personality and mood disorders fare even worse than those with mood disorder alone: spontaneous remission rates and treatment responses are worse when disorders co-occur.[15,17,18,21-28] In this light, personality disorder might be seen as a severity marker for other major mental disorders. Perhaps personality disorders are neither cause nor consequence of other mental illness, but merely occur beside the others, with overlapping symptoms or diatheses.[16] This comorbidity alone may suffice to worsen patient outcomes.

TABLE 11.1 Personality disorders: Diagnostic features and typical interactions with clinical staff

Diagnosis	Dominant features	Typical caregiver interactions	Helpful interventions	Diagnostic confounds, Rx options
Cluster A: Paranoid	Difficulties understanding others' actions, especially distrust and suspiciousness; others' motives are interpreted as malevolent. Deteriorate under stress.	Patient may make angry accusations, withdraw from staff. Staff has difficulty engaging and may feel misunderstood and wrongly accused.	Take extra time to explain and clarify problems and procedures, expect need for repetition and reassurance. Seek out patient's understanding of problems and procedures.	Consider schizophrenia, psychotic depression and mixed mania Autism spectrum disorders, limbic encephalitis, frontal abulia, steroid psychosis, or aphasia may be mistaken for the detachment and eccentricities seen in cluster A patients.
Schizoid and Schizotypal	Social detachment, restricted range of emotional expression masks shame and feelings of inadequacy. Acute discomfort in close relationships, cognitive or perceptual distortions, and eccentricities of behavior.	Patient perceived as odd, even frightening by staff who thus misinterpret patient's intent and needs and do not perceive intense anxiety and suffering. (Note absence of delusions and hallucinations seen in other conditions, including delirium, schizophreniform and bipolar disorders.)	Recognize diminished needs for interpersonal connection and lesser skills in relating to others. Explain restricted range to staff and reassure regarding unusual behaviors, especially "unfriendliness." Encourage simple, straightforward social interactions without humor, irony, or sarcasm. Beware of interpersonal over-stimulation.	Schizoid/schizotypal symptoms respond only weakly to neuroleptic treatment, but trial of an antidepressant or atypical neuroleptic may reduce comorbid depression and anxiety. Nonpsychotic patients may be more sensitive to neuroleptic side effects; *start low and go slow.*
Cluster B: Antisocial	Disregard for and violations of the rights of others.	Staff split between feeling special and rejected; patient has angry outbursts that exacerbate staff splits; staff feel seduced, deceived, loved, manipulated. Patient responds to confrontation with glib explanations of outrageous behavior or sham contrition.	Anticipate, educate, and address splitting. Encourage staff to discuss various impressions and to share information with one another. Reinforce what is to be done and who will do it, address needs for consistent, coherent responses to complaints, demands and threats.	All Cluster B: Mood disorders, especially bipolar II (hypomania). Depressive disorders are common complications, especially with threats of surgical disfigurement, diminished autonomy, and increased need to trust others.

TABLE 11.1 Continued

Diagnosis	Dominant features	Typical caregiver interactions	Helpful interventions	Diagnostic confounds, Rx options
Borderline	Unstable relationships, self-image, and affects, with marked impulsivity. Intense sensitivity to threats of rejection or abandonment.	Patient is panicky and needy, stimulating staff fantasies of specialness and rescuing the patient (e.g., from other staff). Staff reactions range from deep attachment to hatred and aggressive fantasies.	Clarify dysfunctional help-seeking style and disentangle (un)realistic expectations without blame. Be alert to bargaining, seduction, and manipulation. Reassure patient and facilitate staff alignment with role and task clarity. Help staff appreciate and discuss their own emotional responses, especially anger, neediness, and low self-worth.	Frontal disinhibition syndromes due to brain tumor, corticosteroids, drug abuse (intoxication), or delirium may cause marked impulsivity and socially inappropriate behavior.
Histrionic	Excessive emotionality and attention seeking.	Staff repelled by dramatic attention seeking, but may experience sexual attraction and arousal; splitting.		Reduce polypharmacy when possible; consider episodic use of antidepressant, antipsychotic, and anxiolytic medication.
Narcissistic	Grandiosity, need for admiration, and lack of empathy.	Angry outbursts, pitiful apologies, dramatic withdrawal. Staff feel special or worthless; patient "demanding & unreasonable" or "misunderstood & special."		
Cluster C: Avoidant	Social inhibition, feelings of inadequacy, and hypersensitivity to negative evaluation.	Patient seems fearful or uninterested, staff feel clumsy, intrusive, or unjustly accused of same.	Explain patient vulnerability and aversions to staff. Attend to dependency needs to the extent that they do not compromise staff or disrupt patient care.	Depression, social anxiety disorder and obsessive-compulsive disorder are obvious overlap syndromes.

(continued)

TABLE 11.1   Continued

Diagnosis	Dominant features	Typical caregiver interactions	Helpful interventions	Diagnostic confounds, Rx options
Dependent	Submissive, clinging behavior from excessive need to be taken care of, and terrible fear of being alone. Helpless, guilty, and indecisive.	Patient needy, demanding, childlike, and vulnerable. Staff feel protective or repelled by excessive demands for care and attention.	Describe and explain problems and procedures; give patient options and clear role in decision making as tolerated. Return locus of control to patient whenever possible.	Depression is common, as are generalized, phobic and obsessive-compulsive anxiety disorders. Mood, neurovegetative and disruptive anxiety symptoms strongly urge an
Obsessive-Compulsive	Preoccupation with orderliness, perfectionism, and control.	Patient may seem the ideal patient or staff may feel their performance is being monitored and harshly judged.	Encourage staff discussion of their own sensitivities, dependency needs, and meticulousness.	antidepressant trial that may efface dependent or avoidant behavior.[2]
Diagnosis	Dominant features	Typical caregiver interactions	Helpful interventions	Diagnostic confounds, Rx options

OT, occupational therapy; PT, physical therapy.

From Shedler J, Westen D. Refining personality disorder diagnosis: integrating science and practice. *Am /Psychiatry.* Aug 2004;161(8):1350–1365; American Psychiatric Association[1]; and Fava et al.[18]

The DSM-5 Personality Disorders

Clinical characteristics of patients with personality disorders are listed in Table 11.1. The DSM-5 diagnostic categories represent extremes that are rarely encountered,[29] and "the typical patient meeting criteria for a specific personality disorder frequently also meets criteria for other personality disorders."[1 (p. 761)] *Note especially that the vast majority of uncooperative patients do not have a personality disorder.* Nevertheless, the DSM categories provide us with clear examples of personality dysfunction that strongly correlate with functional impairment and human suffering.[17,20,30–33] Understanding these types sensitizes us to their manifold presentations and strengthens our treatment strategies.

Cluster A. The odd or eccentric patients of cluster A all struggle with some degree of social discomfort. Interpersonal closeness may be unpleasant or simply of no interest, leading to avoidant and frankly odd behaviors.[34] Getting to know cluster A patients may be not only difficult, but also actually alienating or frightening for the patient.

> Like many patients, this 37-year-old woman brought her favorite pillow and stuffed animal into the hospital with her. After several days staff became aware that she "consulted" her teddy bear regarding difficult treatment decisions and urged her husband to bring several other trusted plush toy "counselors" from home. She arranged the dolls at her bedside and grew angry if they were disturbed around bedtime.

Social alienation can be increased by cluster A patients' unusual beliefs. Magical thinking and paranoid ideas may be alarming to staff (but note the absence of delusions and hallucinations seen in psychotic disorders). Patients may experience others' judgments with blithe indifference, total ignorance, or dramatic secrecy breached only with selected staff. At times patients' unusual beliefs get in the way of proper care. Standard procedures are experienced as menacing, routine questions feel like threatening interrogation, and innocent jokes are deeply offensive. Uncovering these treatment-foiling beliefs or attitudes can be quite difficult, often requiring collateral interviews with family, friends, or trusted staff.

Cluster B. Cluster B patients may also be particularly vulnerable in medical settings, especially when circumstances demand high levels of stress tolerance, decision-making, and shifting relationships. Uncomfortable with the passive role that many patients readily adopt, they need frequent reassurance that they are valued and safe. The subgroups—antisocial, borderline, narcissistic, and histrionic—are distinguished by their reactions to interpersonal ambiguity or strain.

Antisocial patients are often extraverted (socially outgoing) and manipulative: their focus is on interpersonal advantage. When secure they may be pleasantly thoughtful and ingratiating, even charming. They engage others not so much for security or affection, however, but for leverage and dominance: all relations are ultimately seen as instrumental; that is, as means to particular ends. Rageful, even violent reactions, may occur when they feel disadvantaged or threatened. The change of attitude may be shocking (and frightening) to staff unaccustomed to the sudden appearance of rude, demanding, demeaning, or threatening behavior. Threats—even escalating to physical violence—may dissipate as soon as the desired result is obtained; the patient will then express surprise at others' angry, distancing reactions, as if their distressing behavior were well within acceptable norms. Nonchalance in violating accepted norms is the hallmark of the disorder.

Borderline patients may exhibit many of the same behaviors but tend to be less organized and less in control. They are more likely to be self-destructive than threatening to others and pursue relationship attachments for their own sake rather than interpersonal advantage per se. Under duress their perception of others is distorted by black-and-white thinking that sees only enemies and allies without nuance. They respond to distress with impulsive desperation that may include sexual adventurism, substance abuse, and self-mutilation. Offers of nurturance may be surprisingly sexualized, for example, a nurse's eagerness to provide physical comfort may be experienced as seductive or a physician's concern may be seen as an offer of lifelong affection.

> Margaret is an attractive 42-year-old twice-divorced attorney with widely metastatic lung cancer. Hours after a difficult meeting with her oncologist, she has paged the palliative care physician on call to ask more questions about her symptoms and prognosis. After a few minutes of conversation with the empathic doctor Margaret begins to cry and asks, "Can you meet me somewhere? I really need to talk this over."
>
> The doctor, a bit taken aback, replies, "I know you are worried about all of this, but I think you should talk things over with your oncologist."

"You seem so much more compassionate," she explains. "I feel like you really understand what I'm going through. Your office is right next to my doctor's, isn't it? I saw you earlier today. You have such a warm smile, such a kind way with everyone around you. Are you married?"

Borderline and antisocial patients' dramatic behavior may be seen as goal-oriented and manipulative, but for the borderline patient it is more often simply an insecure, impulsive way of coping with extreme distress. It is striking to see the disparate responses of involved clinicians to these behaviors: some will be angry and alienated, while others are moved to tears and rescue efforts. Staff conflict may ensue. This staff splitting is commonplace in work with borderline patients: *multiple clinicians working on the same team experience the patient very differently.* Productively responding to the patient can tax even the most experienced clinicians.

Histrionic and narcissistic patients are far more predictable and less threatening. Like the borderline, they are motivated by a need for love and security rather than interpersonal advantage. But while the borderline patient is often eager to be whatever the person in front of her demands, histrionic and narcissistic patients have a much more solidly established personality and sense of self. Histrionic patients are pervasively insecure and attention seeking: it is their dominant mode of relating to others whether or not they are in distress. Rather than feeling manipulated, staff tend to feel entertained, exhausted or, eventually, bored and annoyed. Histrionic patients may elaborate dramatic stories, offer fantastic rewards, and look for special treatment. Both borderline and histrionic patients may be highly intolerant of being alone; the former needs to be reassured that she is loved, the latter to be reminded that she is still alive.

The narcissistic patient is the least likely of the cluster B patients to elicit psychiatric consultation. The medical care setting, directed toward the patient's comfort and well-being, may be experienced as supremely reassuring. But the narcissist responds to interpersonal threat by highlighting deficits in others. The feelings that narcissistic patients arouse in staff—including guilt, shame, and inadequacy—are often very hard for staff to identify as emanating from the patient rather than originating in their own high professional standards.

Although instrumentally oriented like the antisocial patient, seeing others as means to their own esteem and gratification, the narcissist feels and often gets others to feel that he deserves whatever he wants. When ill, he is whiney and demanding, even infantile and petulant. Mature nursing staff will quickly identify the narcissist and simply become more efficient in meeting his needs while dismissing unreasonable behaviors and demands. Other clinicians, however, may find themselves mired in the low self-esteem, guilt, and self-doubt that reside at the core of the narcissistic personality.[35]

Cluster C. Avoidant patients experience extremes of social inhibition that may extend to all interpersonal relations. Some will avoid all human touch whenever possible, making physical care extremely difficult: the patient may freeze, panic, or dissociate. Puzzled staff responses may reveal their own elevated sensitivity to negative evaluation, manifest as withdrawal, depression, or overt anger in response to the patient's indifference, aversion, and avoidance.

Dependent patients tend to be extremely compliant and submissive and are thus less likely to alienate clinicians. Their high degree of deference, clinging behavior, and intense need for direct care may overtax clinicians, especially nurses running interference for physicians. In extremis these patients demonstrate regressive, childlike neediness that may intensely engage or repel staff.

Obsessive-compulsive personality disorder (OCPD) must be distinguished from *obsessive-compulsive disorder* (OCD). OCD manifests with ritualized thoughts and behaviors that interfere with daily activities. The personality disorder presents as a preoccupation with orderliness, perfectionism, and control that clinicians may find endearing, inspiring, or maddening. For the most part these patients are not clinically problematic; they are more likely to be seen as ideally organized, adherent, and predictable. This need for order may be challenged by the unpredictability and messiness of terminal illness, arousing intense anxiety and agitation when things cannot be "just so."

Etiology

The personality disorders encompass very heterogeneous groups of people with wide varieties of family makeup, developmental history, traits, and disease course. No single cause will suffice to create adult traits or disorder. Genetic endowment, parental influences, social learning, and trauma are well-established contributors.[36,37] The cluster B disorders, for example, may be seen as resulting from an amalgam of genetic predisposition, childhood neglect, and lack of developmental resources.[38]

Genetic influences may impact regulation of affects, impulse/action patterns, cognitive organization, and anxiety/inhibition.[14,39,40] Heritable traits may include deficits "in recruitment of brain mechanisms of emotion regulation, and this process may be potentiated by . . . particularly stressful or negative contexts."[41] Compelling epigenetic studies link genetic endowment and early life experience to phenotypic expression in adrenal reactivity, stress tolerance, and other personality traits, perhaps even suicidality.[35,38,42] This may explain the stymied maturation of brain mechanisms regulating impulse control and identity formation.

These mechanisms may be impacted more acutely as well. Orbitofrontal insult from trauma or surgery may be associated with new onset of personality disorder features,[43] reflecting, for example, regional dysfunction in antisocial and borderline disorders.[14,41,44,45]

Diagnostic Challenges

The distinction between normality, major mental disorder, and personality disorder has vexed clinicians for more than a century.[37] Kraepelin observed that "wherever we try to mark out the frontier between mental health and disease, we find a neutral territory, in which the imperceptible change from the realm of normal life to that of obvious derangement takes place."[51 (p. 295)] This is especially true of personality disorders, which present on a continuum with normal adaptive behavior and yet often overlap genetically and phenomenologically with other mental disorders.[36,37,52–57]

Establishing a personality disorder diagnosis presents multiple challenges. Rapport with such patients is by definition difficult, and is often the reason for consultation. Much time may be required to avoid premature diagnostic closure, to sort through the range of traits, assess their stability over time, and link them to significant dysfunction. The presence of longstanding dysfunction is clearly not enough: concomitant mood, anxiety or psychotic disorder, substance abuse, and circumstantial chaos may be more causative than the patient's personality per se. The traits must be the cause of "significant functional impairment or subjective distress."[1] There is no substitute for a detailed history, sensitively elicited and supplemented by collateral sources.

Cultural determinants of coping behavior must also be addressed, including beliefs that might be mistaken for magical thinking, fastidiousness misconstrued as compulsive neatness, or dramatic self-expression confused with histrionics.[58]

Hazards and Value of Diagnostic Labeling in End-of-Life Settings

It is not surprising that some patients are hard to engage in frightening circumstances. But clinicians' fear, ignorance, and frustration may lead to pejorative labeling and a downward spiral of clinician frustration, mutual avoidance, and patient deterioration. A personality diagnosis may be less a guide to diagnosis and treatment than dismissive shorthand applied to a difficult patient.

Skillfully used, however, the diagnosis can help staff recognize patients' morbidity and suffering. A named disorder with established treatments can demystify and destigmatize the patient, and reduce staff helplessness, frustration, and anger.[59] Diagnostic clarity often gives staff permission to express confusion, frustration, anger, or guilt over their own feelings and behaviors. Awareness of avoidant, paranoid, shame-prone, or rejection-sensitive vulnerabilities allows staff to address their own feelings of rejection, guilt, or sadism that challenging patients may engender, and it promotes multidisciplinary collaboration around shared understandings and goals.[60,61]

Management of Patients with Difficult Personality Traits and Disorders

Diagnostic assessment of disruptive behavior should be approached with an emphasis on interactions between patients and staff. Most difficult patient encounters may be organized into a small number of such interactions.

General Principles in Working with Personality Disorder Patients

Cluster A: Patients Who Are Odd or Eccentric

- Seek out the patient's understanding of what is happening.
- Take extra time to clarify problems and procedures, expect need for repetition and reassurance. When possible, engage familiar, trusted friends or family members to support, encourage and reassure patient.

- Recognize diminished needs for interpersonal connection and limited skills relating to others. Beware of interpersonal overstimulation.
- Explain restricted range to staff and reassure regarding unusual behaviors, especially "unfriendliness."
- Encourage simple, straightforward social interactions without humor, irony, or sarcasm.

Cluster B: Patients Who Are Dramatic, Emotional, or Erratic

- Anticipate, educate, and address staff about splitting.
- Encourage staff to share information and discuss differing impressions with one another.
- Engage familiar, trusted friends or family members to support, encourage, and reassure patient.
- Reinforce clear staff and patient roles and responsibilities, especially the need for consistent, coherent responses to complaints, demands, and threats. Clarify dysfunctional help-seeking style and disentangle (un)realistic expectations without blame.
- Be alert to bargaining, seduction, and manipulation.
- Help staff appreciate and discuss their own emotional responses, especially anger, neediness, and low self-worth.

Cluster C: Patients Who Are Anxious or Fearful

- Describe and explain problems and procedures; give patient options and clear role in decision making as tolerated.
- Return locus of control to patient whenever possible. Engage familiar, trusted friends or family members to support, encourage, and reassure patient.
- Explain patient vulnerability and aversions to staff.
- Attend to dependency needs to the extent that they do not compromise staff or disrupt patient care.
- Encourage staff discussion of their own sensitivities, dependency needs, and meticulousness.

Problematic Patient Encounters

Regardless of the DSM diagnosis, clinical personnel find patients to be

- *Lost*, overwhelmed, and chaotic;
- *Seeking*, thoughtful, misguided, and uncooperative;
- *Smiling*, superficially agreeable but foiling care;
- *Limitless*, needy, or overentitled;
- *Baffling*, perplexing, frightening, or repellent;
- *Anomalous*, odd, confusing, or daunting.

Lost. Some patients may disagree with the care plan because they do not understand explanations of the disease or the treatments or because the information is so overwhelming they cannot collaborate effectively with the care team. We may see them as overwhelmed and chaotic

> Roberta was 29 years old when her suspicious mammogram led to an abnormal biopsy and, the day after her son's first birthday, a diagnosis of cancer. The oncologist explained to this intelligent, thoughtful, bewildered woman that her ductal carcinoma *in situ* would require lumpectomy and a brief course of radiation therapy. An excellent outcome was all but assured.
>
> Roberta's response was to sit down and make a list of women for her husband to date after her death. She became irritable, tearful, and angry. She consulted megavitamin gurus and researched alternative treatments on the web. She refused to return to the oncologist's office. Anguished and desperately suicidal, she drafted a farewell letter to each of her family members, including one to be read to her son on his thirteenth birthday. Despite her minimal disease and excellent prognosis, no matter who tried to reassure her, all she could hear was the first thing her oncologist had told her: you have cancer.

Roberta demonstrates extreme narcissistic vulnerability and fears of abandonment, along with unstable identity, mood, and impulse control. These borderline traits are dramatically expressed, leaving those around her as bewildered as she is. But Roberta's frantic behavior diminished as she gradually yielded to the pleas of her family and friends to again review her diagnosis and treatment plan. The oncologist patiently re-explained what to expect, she discussed her fears of disfigurement and death with a psychiatrist, and an oncology social worker helped Roberta meet other patients who demonstrated better coping strategies.

Overwhelmed and confused patients like Roberta are *Lost*: they foil care because they cannot take in the information and work with the team. They experience the diagnosis and plan as "too much, too fast," and they panic. We err by using jargon or otherwise missing the level at which a particular patient should be approached. Or we may simply misread a superficially agreeable, compliant patient.

The clinician may take time to carefully and thoroughly present information, leaving ample room for questions, only to find that the patient adamantly refuses to cooperate. These patients are hard to read, because they appear calmer than they feel, they have difficulty relating to authority figures, or they simply fear or detest the patient role. They demand our best clinical communication skills. We have to repeatedly back up and make sure we understand what they heard us say, not just the factual details, but especially the meanings and consequences. Eye contact, body language, and patience are essential.[62] And check at each step for signs of miscommunication and mistrust.

Seeking. Terminally ill patients and their families are increasingly educated by an infinite array of information sources. Disagreements with the care plan may stem from differences in "expert opinion" or from the intrusion of unproved (or disproved) therapies. The patients feel they have valuable information that contradicts what the care team is offering.

They rationally disagree with the care plan, demand care the team feels is not indicated, or refuse treatments considered essential. Clinical staff may see them as thoughtful and misguided or odd and irksome. Such patients may prefer complementary or alternative treatments with clinicians they find less threatening or more reassuring.

Sometimes we are arguing with folk beliefs that have great currency in certain ethnic groups. For example, "you should never have surgery for cancer, because when the air hits the tumor it spreads everywhere."[63,64]

Such "uncooperative patients" are often thoughtful, rational, and misinformed. Their ignorance is sometimes misread as a refusal to cooperate with care when in fact it is precisely the opposite: by *Seeking* they are trying to join the treatment team and collaborate. When treated with consideration and respect they routinely come around—or get the medical team to reconsider their recommendations.

Smiling. Patients may agree with the care plan but not behave the way staff expect: they may miss scheduled appointments, lab draws, examinations, and consultations. They don't stick to the treatment plan, even after they appear to understand and agree. The cues we expect when people disagree never appear. Everything looks fine until they have to follow through.

Overwhelmed by the facts, these *Smiling* but mistrustful, fearful, or anxious patients may anticipate disapproval or punishing responses to their questions or problems. Lengthy, detailed conversations may be entirely forgotten because anxiety prevents them from taking in the information. And the odd patient, preoccupied with unusual beliefs and fears, just has a different, often unpredictable way of hearing and responding that the clinician may not fully appreciate.

The "perfect patient" is an interesting variant. Passively cooperative, they never complain or object. Uncertain of how staff will react to their disagreement, they smile and go their own way—or obey with mounting anxiety. These ideal patients often deteriorate as effective treatments are exhausted, when the reward for their obedience is painfully absent.

Again, we may be misreading their understanding of the facts and consequences of care, or we may be underappreciating how much their emotional responses are interfering with their ability to act on the information. These patients should be carefully questioned about the treatment plan, with special attention paid to their reluctance to disclose unspoken fears: the emphasis must be on shared understanding, rather than the shared commitment that will hopefully follow.

Limitless. Some patients understand, agree, participate with care-as-planned, and drive the staff batty: they talk at great length, call frequently, and ask infinite questions—or the same questions over and over. Others do everything as clinically expected, but the rest of their life takes over and complicates the clinician–patient relationship beyond recognition. Clinicians find these patients needy and demanding, clinging, or overentitled.

Such patients run the gamut from the anxious-but-endearing elderly woman to the obsessive-compulsive young man who always has just one more question. They may be anxious worriers or odd ducks with magical thinking, but often, with time and familiarity, what emerges is that they are terribly lonely and scared.

The treatment team is their newfound and only social outlet, and they have a difficult time managing the attachments. Every test, drug, side effect, risk-benefit ratio, or research controversy is another opportunity to engage and not let go.

These patients cry out for reassurance and constancy: they need to know that the team will stand by them. Every superfluous question is another plea for a reliable caretaker; any rebuff is an affirmation of their worst fears: namely, that you will not be there when they really need you. Such patients generally respond well to clear, compassionate boundaries, as long as they are accompanied by calm, reassuring office visits. They are brilliant readers of body language, so the clinician's words and actions must be consistent. Remember to use lots of eye contact (they're used to being avoided), and keep your hand off the doorknob until the visit is officially (and explicitly) over.

Alternatively, it may be the patients' advocates—family members, well-intentioned friends, or clergy—who frustrate clinical staff. The patient may express helpless frustration or passive acquiescence, but however they handle things the family is now your problem.

The patient is not actually *Limitless*, and neither are you. Presence, clarity and consistency, reassurance, and clear boundaries—when you are available, what you can offer, and what you cannot—will go a long way to engaging without overengaging or alienating these patients and caregivers.

Baffling. Some patients do everything we require of them, but they do other things that perplex, frighten, or repel. They may threaten, alienate, or seduce us, leaving the clinician feeling like the vulnerable person in need of specialized care. These patients, because of their dramatic presentations and emotionally challenging engagements, can bring out the worst in us. We feel a need to fight or flee, to put them in their place or take them home with us, to kick them out or kick ourselves. We may label them out of frustration or anger: crock, kook, borderline, crazy.

The seductive patient presents a more sophisticated version of the limitless, clinging group. Rather than clinging with infinite questions or requests, such patients invite us into their life's drama. They convince you that you are very special, that you are the only one who understands their dilemmas, and that only your powers will suffice. Of course, once you sit down with your team you realize that everyone gets that message from the patient: *only you can help me!* We feel drawn in and may not realize how involved we are until we wake up in the middle of the night, wondering how to extricate ourselves without giving up our values of gracious, compassionate care. Recall the story of Margaret's after-hours phone call, above.

Margaret is obviously frightened and in need; she is asking for comfort and reassurance; you dole out comfort and reassurance all day. You're still at the office, you haven't had dinner yet, she is only a short drive away . . . what could it hurt?

The answer is to be mindful of your position and your limitations. Consider the role(s) you have taken on, the tasks you perform, and the constraints of time and place that define your roles and responsibilities. Are you responding to requests beyond these roles, tasks, and situations? Are you the only one who can fulfill these requests? *Generally speaking, the more unique you feel the more the patient needs a team approach.* If you find yourself increasingly drawn to special care arrangements with the patient, consider transferring care to a colleague. Your worst fantasies about the patient's reaction to your rejection are still better than the path to increasing entanglement, confusion, and catastrophe. At the very least, if you are uncomfortable or preoccupied with a clinical relationship, discuss it with a colleague who can help you think it through.

Threats and instances of self-harm should be seen as "a means of managing emotional pain and not as a deliberate attempt to control others"[59] Staff focused on patient care may feel betrayed by such behavior, and it is important to distinguish among dramatic help-seeking, despondent suicidality, and rational euthanasia.[65,66] Confusion in such situations should prompt psychiatric or clinical ethics consultation.

Anomalous. While not exactly uncooperative, some patients still do not meet staff demands or expectations. They may appear "distant" or "needy" in ways that are oddly unresponsive, incurious, or passive. This inert, unreactive style sometimes alternates with prolonged, disproportionate distress that demands additional time from nursing and physicians. The staff winds up feeling confused, disoriented, and guilty, incapable of connecting through collaboration or consolation.

Clinicians often overread such odd patients. Their distance may be interpreted as a retreat or withdrawal while in fact they are just most comfortable staying apart. Their emotional storms are confusing, overvalued, or underappreciated. They don't know how to use the interpersonal supports offered by staff; *their habit and skills are in righting their own ships without ballast or direction from others.* Only patience and trial and error can reveal and repair the mismatches of expectations and understanding.

The Consultant's Role: Enhancing Resilience of Patients with Difficult Personality Traits

As with all patients, the consultant must use and provide a biopsychosocial perspective (see Box 11.1).

- *Identify destabilizing biological influences*: Medication, tumor effect, infection, sleep deprivation, malnutrition, and physical deconditioning;
- *Clarify psychological dysfunction*: Depression, hopelessness, psychosis, emotional lability, cognitive distortions, irritability, impulsivity, and passive resistance;
- *Address social complications*: Legal or financial problems, family chaos, staff conflicts, and distortions of social perception; and
- *Give voice to spiritual needs*: Loss of faith, despair, preoccupations with persecution abandonment.

Personality disorders are treatable conditions. Multiple treatment modalities can reduce symptoms of depression and anxiety, enhance global functioning, and improve social adjustment.[8,9,26,67–69] Even with adequate skills, however, treatment can be challenging, frustrating, and prolonged.[20,70]

Proper care of patients with difficult personality traits demands patience and creativity. Regardless of the patient's diagnosis, interpersonal problems are generally most prominent at the time of consultation. An empathic, supportive approach demands attention to

---

BOX 11.1 Biopsychosocial dimensions of clinical care

Destabilizing biological influences

Infection (CNS or systemic)

    Malnutrition (global or nutrient deficiency)

    Medication

    Physical deconditioning

    Sleep disruption

    Tumor effect (direct or paraneoplastic)

Psychological vulnerabilities

    Anxiety

    Cognitive distortions

    Depression

    Emotional lability

    Hopelessness

    Impulsivity, irritability, aggression

Social complexity

    Distortions of social perception

    Isolation (chronic or recent onset)

    Family challenge, criticism, chaos

    Staff conflicts

Spiritual crisis

    Existential guilt or despair

    Loss of faith

    Persecutory or grandiose preoccupations

---

the stage of treatment and essential areas in which the patient needs immediate assistance. This will often require attention to biological, psychological, and social dimensions, any of which may be threatened throughout the course of care.[71]

Psychotherapy and medication strategies developed to prevent or diminish trauma-related symptoms may be helpful in terminal illness, particularly hyperarousal and dysphoric mood.[72–74] Medication benefits in cluster B personality disorder may be limited, although antidepressants do have some supporting evidence.[75] Meditation, including imagery, relaxation, and mindfulness strategies, are helpful for many patients alone or in conjunction with structured psychotherapy.[68,76]

Psychotherapy should be problem-focused and activate psychosocial strengths (see Chapters 33, 35, 36, 37, 38, 39, 40, 42). Social complications, including family conflict and financial and legal concerns, must be addressed as precipitants of distress and disruptive behavior. Individual, family, and group therapies may powerfully assist with relating to caregivers, strengthening outside sources of nurturance, and self-esteem.[8,26,77–79] (See Part VI: "Psychotherapeutic Interventions in Palliative Care.")

Beyond the problem focus that consultation initially demands, we must anticipate pitfalls, bolster mature defenses, and encourage productive coping. Diagnostic assessment that clarifies the patient's personality features will facilitate predicting the patient's reactions to each stage of care. An appreciation of the patient's strengths and limitations will help build rapport and support dignity and remoralization.[80]

The same may be said of clinicians working with these patients; they need clarity and encouragement for such challenging work. We can greatly enhance patients' resilience by supporting the staff and families that care for them.

Future Directions

Progress in helping populations with challenging personality traits and disorders requires research that clarifies the processes of human development and socialization, as well as clinical interventions to address the inevitable mismatches between patients, families, and clinical staff. Enhanced training of clinical staff must anticipate and appreciate the diversity of our patients and their families: how they cope, and how we can flexibly adapt to meet their needs.

Key Points

- A small fraction of terminally ill patients will puzzle and stymie clinical staff with self-defeating, alienating behavior.
- Proper care of patients with difficult personality traits demands patience and creativity.
- Diagnosis can help staff recognize patients' morbidity and suffering.
- Consultation should clarify the patient's self-image and interpersonal functioning, to help staff anticipate pitfalls, bolster mature defenses, and encourage productive coping.
- Identifying personality features will facilitate predicting patient and staff reactions at each stage of care. Heading off stigmatization and dysfunctional relations between staff and patient will benefit everyone.
- An appreciation of the patient's strengths and limitations will help build rapport, support dignity, and promote remoralization.

References

1. American Psychiatric Association. DSM-5 Task Force. *Diagnostic and Statistical Manual of Mental Disorders: DSM-5*. 5th ed. Washington, DC: American Psychiatric Association; 2013.
2. Drake RE, Vaillant GE. A validity study of axis II of DSM-III. *Am J Psychiatry*. 1985 May; 142(5):553–558.
3. Ferro T, Klein DN, Schwartz JE, Kasch KL, Leader JB. 30-month stability of personality disorder diagnoses in depressed outpatients. *Am J Psychiatry*. 1998 May;155(5):653–659.
4. Johnson JG, Williams JB, Goetz RR, Rabkin JG, Lipsitz JD, Remien RH. Stability and change in personality disorder symptomatology: Findings from a longitudinal study of HIV+ and HIV- men. *J Abnorm Psychol*. 1997 Feb;106(1):154–158.
5. Lenzenweger MF, Johnson MD, Willett JB. Individual growth curve analysis illuminates stability and change in personality disorder features: The longitudinal study of personality disorders. *Arch Gen Psychiatry*. 2004 Oct;61(10):1015–1024.

6. Loranger AW, Lenzenweger MF, Gartner AF, Susman VL, Herzig J, Zammit GK, et al. Trait-state arti-facts and the diagnosis of personality disorders. *Arch Gen Psychiatry.* 1991 Aug;48(8):720–728.

7. Jorm AF, Duncan-Jones P, Scott R. An analysis of the re-test artefact in longitudinal studies of psychi-atric symptoms and personality. *Psychol Med.* 1989 May;19(2):487–493.

8. Zanarini MC, Frankenburg FR, Hennen J, Silk KR. The longitudinal course of borderline psychopa-thology: 6-year prospective follow-up of the phenomenology of borderline personality disorder. *Am J Psychiatry.* 2003 Feb;160(2):274–283.

9. Perry J, Banon E, Ianni F. Effectiveness of psychotherapy for personality disorders. *Am J Psychiatry.* 1999;156:1312–1321.

10. American Psychiatric Association. *Diagnostic and Statistical Manual of Mental Disorders: DSM-III.* 3rd ed. Washington, DC: American Psychiatric Association; 1980:23.

11. Akiskal HS. Demystifying borderline personality: Critique of the concept and unorthodox reflections on its natural kinship with the bipolar spectrum. *Acta Psychiatr Scand.* 2004 Dec;110(6):401–407.

12. Orstavik RE, Kendler KS, Czajkowski N, Tambs K, Reichborn-Kjennerud T. The relationship between depressive personality disorder and major depressive disorder: A population-based twin study. *Am J Psychiatry.* 2007 Dec 1;164(12):1866–1872.

13. Ramklint M, Ekselius L. Personality traits and personality disorders in early onset versus late onset major depression. *J Affect Disord.* 2003 Jun;75(1):35–42.

14. Skodol AE, Siever LJ, Livesley WJ, Gunderson JG, Pfohl B, Widiger TA. The borderline diagnosis II: Biology, genetics, and clinical course. *Biol Psychiatry.* 2002 Jun 15;51(12):951–963.

15. Viinamaki H, Tanskanen A, Koivumaa-Honkanen H, Haatainen K. Cluster C personality disorder and recovery from major depression: 24-month prospective follow-up. *J Personal Disord.* 2003 Aug;17(4):341–350.

16. Gamez W, Watson D, Doebbeling BN. Abnormal personality and the mood and anxiety dis-orders: Implications for structural models of anxiety and depression. *J Anxiety Disord.* 2007;21(4):526–539.

17. Morse JQ, Pilkonis PA, Houck PR, Frank E, Reynolds CF, IIIrd. Impact of cluster C personality dis-orders on outcomes of acute and maintenance treatment in late-life depression. *Am J Geriatr Psychiatry.* 2005 Sep;13(9):808–814.

18. Fava M, Farabaugh AH, Sickinger AH, Wright E, Alpert JE, Sonawalla S, et al. Personality disorders and depression. *Psychol Med.* 2002 Aug;32(6):1049–1057.

19. Kasen S, Cohen P, Skodol AE, Johnson JG, Smailes E, Brook JS. Childhood depression and adult per-sonality disorder: Alternative pathways of continuity. *Arch Gen Psychiatry.* 2001 Mar;58(3):231–236.

20. Skodol AE, Gunderson JG, McGlashan TH, Dyck IR, Stout RL, Bender DS, et al. Functional impair-ment in patients with schizotypal, borderline, avoidant, or obsessive-compulsive personality disorder. *Am J Psychiatry.* 2002 Feb;159(2):276–283.

21. Brieger P, Ehrt U, Bloeink R, Marneros A. Consequences of comor-bid personality disorders in major depression. *J Nerv Ment Dis.* 2002 May;190(5):304–309.

22. Fournier JC, Derubeis RJ, Shelton RC, Gallop R, Amsterdam JD, Hollon SD. Antidepressant medica-tions v. cognitive therapy in people with depression with or without personality disorder. *Br J Psychiatry.* 2008 Feb;192:124–129.

23. Grilo CM, Sanislow CA, Shea MT, Skodol AE, Stout RL, Gunderson JG, et al. Two-year prospective naturalistic study of remission from major depressive disorder as a function of personality disorder comorbidity. *J Consult Clin Psychol.* 2005 Feb;73(1):78–85.

24. Hirschfeld RM. Personality disorders and depression: Comorbidity. *Depress Anxiety.* 1999;10(4):142–146.

25. Iacovides A, Fountoulakis KN, Fotiou F, Fokas K, Nimatoudis I, Kaprinis G. Relation of personality dis-orders to subtypes of major depression according both to DSM-IV and ICD-10. *Can J Psychiatry.* 2002 Mar;47(2):196–197.

26. Joyce PR, McKenzie JM, Carter JD, Rae AM, Luty SE, Frampton CM, et al. Temperament, character and personality disorders as predictors of response to interpersonal psychotherapy and cognitive-behavioural therapy for depression. *Br J Psychiatry.* 2007 Jun;190:503–508.

27. Kool S, Dekker J, Duijsens IJ, de Jonghe F. Major depression, double depression and personality dis-orders. *J Personal Disord.* 2000 Fall;14(3):274–281.

28. Shea MT, Pilkonis PA, Beckham E, Collins JF, Elkin I, Sotsky SM, et al. Personality disorders and treatment outcome in the NIMH Treatment of Depression Collaborative Research Program. *Am J Psychiatry.* 1990 Jun;147(6):711–718.

29. Coid J, Yang M, Tyrer P, Roberts A, Ullrich S. Prevalence and correlates of personality disorder in Great Britain. *Br J Psychiatry.* 2006 May;188:423–431.

30. Ansell EB, Sanislow CA, McGlashan TH, Grilo CM. Psychosocial impairment and treatment utilization by patients with borderline personality disorder, other personality disorders, mood and anxiety disorders, and a healthy comparison group. *Compr Psychiatry.* 2007 Jul-Aug;48(4):329–336.

31. Kunkel EJ, Woods CM, Rodgers C, Myers RE. Consultations for 'maladaptive denial of illness' in patients with cancer: Psychiatric disorders that result in noncompliance. *Psychooncology.* 1997;6(2):139–149.

32. Skodol AE, Gunderson JG, Pfohl B, Widiger TA, Livesley WJ, Siever LJ. The borderline diagnosis I: Psychopathology, comorbidity, and personality structure. *Biol Psychiatry.* 2002 Jun 15;51(12):936–950.

33. Skodol AE, Oldham JM, Bender DS, Dyck IR, Stout RL, Morey LC, et al. Dimensional representations of DSM-IV personality disorders: Relationships to functional impairment. *Am J Psychiatry.* 2005 Oct;162(10):1919–1925.

34. Spitzer RL, Endicott J, Robins E. Research diagnostic criteria: Rationale and reliability. *Arch Gen Psychiatry.* 1978 Jun;35(6):773–782.

35. Kraus G, Reynolds DJ. The "A-B-C's" of the cluster B's: Identifying, understanding, and treating cluster B personality disorders. *Clin Psychol Rev.* 2001 Apr;21(3):345–373.

36. Reichborn-Kjennerud T, Czajkowski N, Torgersen S, Neale MC, Ørstavik RE, Tambs K, et al. The relationship between avoidant personality disorder and social phobia: A population-based twin study. *Am J Psychiatry.* 2007 Nov 1;164(11):1722–1728.

37. Sass H, Junemann K. Affective disorders, personality and personality disorders. *Acta Psychiatr Scand Suppl.* 2003(418):34–40.

38. Caspi A, McClay J, Moffitt TE, Mill J, Martin J, Craig IW, et al. Role of genotype in the cycle of violence in maltreated children. *Science.* 2002 Aug 2;297(5582):851–854.

39. Coccaro EF, Bergeman CS, McClearn GE. Heritability of irritable impulsiveness: A study of twins reared together and apart. *Psychiatry Res.* 1993 Sep;48(3):229–242.

40. Goldsmith H, Buss K, KS L. Toddler and childhood temperament: Expanded content, stronger genetic evidence, new evidence of the importance of environment. *Dev Psychobiol.* 1997;33:891–905.

41. Siegle GJ. Brain mechanisms of borderline personality disorder at the intersection of cognition, emotion, and the clinic. *Am J Psychiatry.* 2007;164(12):1776–1779.

42. McGowan PO. Epigenetic regulation of the glucocorticoid receptor in human brain associates with childhood abuse. *Nature Neuroscience.* 2009;12:342–348.

43. Witt J-A. The impact of lesions and epilepsy on personality and mood in patients with symptomatic epilepsy: A pre- to postoperative follow-up study. *Epilepsy Research.* 2008;82:139–146.

44. Damasio H, Grabowski T, Frank R, Galaburda AM, Damasio AR. The return of Phineas Gage: Clues about the brain from the skull of a famous patient. *Science.* 1994 May 20;264(5162):1102–1105.

45. Silbersweig D, Clarkin JF, Goldstein M, Kernberg OF, Tuescher O, Levy KN, et al. Failure of frontolimbic inhibitory function in the context of negative emotion in borderline personality disorder. *Am J Psychiatry.* 2007 Dec;164(12):1832–1841.

46. Casey PR, Dillon S, Tyrer PJ. The diagnostic status of patients with conspicuous psychiatric morbidity in primary care. *Psychol Med.* 1984 Aug;14(3):673–681.

47. Casey PR, Tyrer PJ, Platt S. The relationship between social functioning and psychiatric symptomatology in primary care. *Soc Psychiatry.* 1985;20(1):5–9.

48. Reich J, Boerstler H, Yates W, Nduaguba M. Utilization of medical resources in persons with DSM-III personality disorders in a community sample. *Int J Psychiatry Med.* 1989;19(1):1–9.

49. Lyons MJ, Jerskey BA. Personality disorders: Epidemiological findings, methods and concepts. In: Tsuang MT, Tohen M, eds. *Textbook in Psychiatric Epidemiology.* 2nd ed. New York: Wiley-Liss; 2002:563–599.

50. Grant BF, Hasin DS, Chou SP, Stinson FS, Dawson DA. Nicotine dependence and psychiatric disorders in the United States: Results from the national epidemiologic survey on alcohol and related conditions. *Arch Gen Psychiatry.* 2004 Nov;61(11):1107–1115.

51. Kraepelin E. *Lectures on Clinical Psychiatry*. 3rd ed. New York: William Wood; 1917.

52. Maser JD, Patterson T. Spectrum and nosology: Implications for DSM-V. *Psychiatr Clin North Am*. 2002 Dec;25(4):855–885.

53. Tyrer P. Personality diatheses: A superior explanation than disorder. *Psychol Med*. 2007 Nov;37(11):1521–1525.

54. Lenzenweger MF. Schizotaxia, schizotypy, and schizophrenia: Paul E. Meehl's blueprint for the experimental psychopathology and genetics of schizophrenia. *J Abnorm Psychol*. 2006 May;115(2):195–200.

55. Tsuang MT, Stone WS, Gamma F, Faraone SV. Schizotaxia: Current status and future directions. *Curr Psychiatry Rep*. 2003 Jun;5(2):128–134.

56. Gunderson JG, Weinberg I, Daversa MT, Kueppenbender KD, Zanarini MC, Shea MT, et al. Descriptive and longitudinal observations on the relationship of borderline personality disorder and bipolar disorder. *Am J Psychiatry*. 2006 Jul;163(7):1173–1178.

57. Zimmerman M, Ruggero CJ, Chelminski I, Young D. Is bipolar disorder overdiagnosed? *J Clin Psychiatry*. 2008;6:e1–e6.

58. Bhugra D, Bhui K. *Textbook of Cultural Psychiatry*. Cambridge; New York: Cambridge University Press; 2007.

59. Nadine N. Borderline personality disorder: The voice of patients. *Res Nurs Health*. 1999;22(4):285–293.

60. Schwartz H. A person is a person and a shpos is not. *Man Med*. 1980;5(3):226–228.

61. Strauss A. "Shpos". *South Med J*. 1983 Aug;76(8):981–984.

62. Lee SJ, Back AL, Block SD, Stewart SK. Enhancing physician-patient communication. *Hematology Am Soc Hematol Educ Program*. 2002:464–483.

63. Kaptchuk TJ, Eisenberg DM. Varieties of healing. 2: A taxonomy of unconventional healing practices. *Ann Intern Med*. 2001 Aug 7;135(3):196–204.

64. Kaptchuk TJ, Eisenberg DM. Varieties of healing. 1: Medical pluralism in the United States. *Ann Intern Med*. 2001 Aug 7;135(3):189–195.

65. Chochinov HM, Wilson KG, Enns M, Lander S. Depression, hopelessness, and suicidal ideation in the terminally ill. *Psychosomatics*. 1998;39(4): 366–370.

66. Breitbart W, Rosenfeld B, Pessin H, Kaim M, Funesti-Esch J, Galietta M, et al. Depression, hopelessness, and desire for hastened death in terminally ill patients with cancer. *JAMA*. 2000 Dec 13;284(22):2907–2911.

67. Clarkin JF, Levy KN, Lenzenweger MF, Kernberg OF. Evaluating three treatments for borderline personality disorder: A multiwave study. *Am J Psychiatry*. 2007 Jun;164(6):922–928.

68. Bartak A, Andrea H, Spreeuwenberg MD, Ziegler UM, Dekker J, Rossum BV, et al. Effectiveness of outpatient, day hospital, and inpatient psychotherapeutic treatment for patients with cluster B personality disorders. *Psychother Psychosom*. 2011;80:28–38.

69. Storebø OJ, Stoffers-Winterling JM, Völlm BA, Kongerslev MT, Mattivi JT, Jørgensen MS, et al. Psychological therapies for people with borderline personality disorder. *Cochrane Database Syst Rev*. 2020;5:CD012955. doi:10.1002/14651858.CD012955.pub2.

70. Bender DS, Dolan RT, Skodol AE, Sanislow CA, Dyck IR, McGlashan TH, et al. Treatment utilization by patients with personality disorders. *Am J Psychiatry*. 2001 Feb;158(2):295–302.

71. Holland JC. Improving the human side of cancer care: Psycho-oncology's contribution. *Cancer J*. 2001 Nov-Dec;7(6):458–471.

72. Bennett WRM, Zatzick D, Roy-Byrne P. Can medications prevent PTSD in trauma victims? *Curr Psychiatry Online*. 2007;6(9):47–55.

73. Davidson JR, Payne VM, Connor KM, Foa EB, Rothbaum BO, Hertzberg M, et al. Trauma, resilience and saliostasis: Effects of treatment in post-traumatic stress disorder. *Int Clin Psychopharmacol*. 2005 Jan;20(1):43–48.

74. Yen S, Shea MT, Battle CL, Johnson DM, Zlotnick C, Dolan-Sewell R, et al. Traumatic exposure and posttraumatic stress disorder in borderline, schizotypal, avoidant, and obsessive-compulsive personality disorders: Findings from the collaborative longitudinal personality disorders study. *J Nerv Ment Dis*. 2002 Aug;190(8):510–518.

75. Stoffers J, Völlm BA, Rücker G, Timmer A, Huband N, Lieb K. Pharmacological interventions for borderline personality disorder. *Cochrane Database Syst Rev*. 2010;6:CD005653. doi:10.1002/14651858. CD005653.pub2.

76. McMain S. Dialectic behaviour therapy reduces suicide attempts compared with non-behavioural psychotherapy in women with borderline personality disorder. *Evid Based Ment Health*. Feb 2007;10(1):18.

77. de Figueiredo JM. Demoralization and psychotherapy: A tribute to Jerome D. Frank, MD, PhD (1909–2005). *Psychother Psychosom*. 2007;76(3): 129–133.

78. Dimeff L, Koerner K. Overview of dialectical behavior therapy. In: Dimeff L, Koerner K, eds. *Dialectical Behavior Therapy in Clinical Practice: Applications Across Disorders and Settings*. New York: Guilford Press; 2007:1–18.

79. Lacy TJ, Higgins MJ. Integrated medical-psychiatric care of a dying borderline patient: A case of dynamically informed "practical psychotherapy." *J Am Acad Psychoanal Dyn Psychiatry*. 2005 Winter;33(4):619–636.

80. Slavney PR. Diagnosing demoralization in consultation psychiatry. *Psychosomatics*. 1999 Jul-Aug;40(4):325–329.

PART III

Psychosocial Issues in Palliative Care

12

Screening for Psychological Distress in the Palliative Care Setting

Bryan Gascon, Gary Rodin, Camilla Zimmermann, and Madeline Li

Introduction

Optimal psychosocial care for patients with terminal illness requires that clinicians routinely identify psychological distress. This is particularly important in palliative care, where psychological distress is highly prevalent but often undetected for variety of reasons. Patients in this setting may be too unwell to reflect on or communicate their emotional state, clinicians may be more focused on physical than psychological symptoms, and both may mistakenly regard emotional distress as understandable and therefore irremediable.[1] The routine identification of psychological distress in palliative care can be enhanced with the systematic use of patient-reported outcome measures (PROMs). A patient-reported outcome (PRO) is a self-report on the status of health conditions that matter to the patient, with psychological distress commonly identified as an important PRO. PROMs are psychometrically validated PRO measurement tools. Such tools can be used to screen for a broad range of psychological disturbances, including those that meet criteria for a psychiatric disorder, to implement appropriate therapeutic interventions and to facilitate rigorous research.

A growing body of research in oncology has demonstrated that the use of PROMs to inform symptom management improves patient–provider communication and quality of life of patients, reduces emergency department visits, and increases survival.[2,3] Implementation science research supports the inclusion of PROMs to screen for psychological distress, many of which are now commonly used in clinical care and research in diverse clinical populations. Validated screening tools can range in length from a brief single-item screen that takes only a few seconds to complete to more comprehensive PROMs with well over 30 items that take several minutes for patients or clinicians to complete. Administration of such measures typically constitutes the first of several steps in psychological distress management, in which positive screening results signal the need for a more comprehensive assessment by the oncology clinicians and/or by psychosocial care professionals. PROMs also have value in palliative care in monitoring symptom course, measuring treatment response, and in facilitating research.

The term "distress" is used to refer to a broad construct, first introduced in cancer care and defined as "the multifactorial unpleasant emotional experience of a psychological, social, and/or spiritual nature, ranging from normal feelings of vulnerability, sadness, and fears to problems that can become disabling, such as depression, anxiety, panic, social isolation, and existential and spiritual crisis" (National Comprehensive Cancer Network).[4] This definition captures the wide continuum of distress that may be identified in palliative care settings, ranging from nonpathological symptoms of depression, anxiety, or demoralization to full-syndrome psychiatric disorders. Interventions to alleviate both full-syndrome and subthreshold disorders have the potential to increase psychological well-being, improve quality of life and quality of dying and death, and prevent progression of psychological distress.

Patients near the end of life may experience existential or spiritual distress concerns, which may be detected by distress screening. While there is a lack of consensus on a precise definition, existential distress has been operationalized in the context of advanced disease in constructs such as death anxiety, demoralization, hopelessness, dignity-related distress, spiritual distress, and the wish to hasten death (WTHD) (Section IV). Spiritual distress can be considered a subset of existential distress that relates to a crisis in religious or spiritual concerns within oneself or to connection to a higher being (Chapter 27).

This chapter provides an overview of considerations for optimal emotional distress screening and clinical response mechanisms in the palliative care setting. The utility of specific screening tools to identify psychological distress most relevant to patients receiving palliative care will be highlighted. While the identification of psychological distress among family caregivers of patients in palliative care is equally important, this is beyond the scope of this chapter. From the plethora of available PROMs, we have highlighted tools that are brief enough to have practical utility for screening purposes and that have been validated in palliative populations. We also suggest future directions for research in palliative care utilizing validating screening tools.

Screening Implementation

Improving health outcomes in palliative care by screening for psychological distress requires careful attention to when, where, and how to screen, as well ensuring that clinicians to respond to psychological distress using best practice care pathways.[5] These core principle of screening for distress to achieve these goals include the following:

1. Screening should be performed for all patients at the initial assessment, and periodically thereafter, particularly during points of potential vulnerability. These include the initiation of a new medical treatment, enrolment in a clinical trial, disease progression, or transition to end-of-life care. Screening for psychological distress at these times may provide valuable information regarding the psychological wellbeing of patients at these times and a baseline to allow assessment of change over time.

2. Screening tools may be completed online before a clinic visit, in the clinic waiting room by patients themselves or with the aid of caregivers or clinic volunteers, or with clinicians during the clinical encounter. Verbal administration of the screening tool by clinicians may be helpful for patients who are too ill to self-report or who are otherwise reluctant to disclose distress. However, completion of screening measures by caregivers or clinicians on behalf of patients is not recommended as symptom severity tends to be overestimated by caregivers and underestimated by clinicians.

3. Brief validated screening tools should be used to capture psychological distress, physical symptoms, and practical needs. Electronic screening requires information technology investment but allows for more items to be administered in the same time period and more reliable data capture.

4. Training for clinicians is necessary to ensure that they review the distress screening results, conduct an appropriate secondary assessment, and implement a clinical response triaged to the level of psychological distress. As with any screening test, a positive primary screen only identifies distress. A secondary assessment is necessary to determine the need for an intervention and its nature.

5. The secondary assessment should be followed by the implementation of a stepped level of care. Patients with mild distress should be provided with clinic-based emotional support and validation of distress and with self-management resources, such as psychoeducation and connection to peer support groups. Persistent distress not responding to these initial interventions or moderate to severe initial distress may warrant referral for specialized psychosocial care.

6. Documentation of distress screening results and the clinical response, with repeat screening to monitor treatment delivery and changes in distress, is necessary to ensure optimal outcomes. This is best facilitated when electronic screening results can be directly linked to the patient's electronic medical record, where the clinical response can then also be documented.

The successful institutional implementation and sustainability of screening for psychological distress requires attention to change management principles to guide the process. Their application to systematic distress screening has included obtaining top-down leadership support, engaging clinical teams in the initiative using a bottom-up approach, establishing a joint partnership with clinical champions from the psychosocial and palliative care teams, and using quality improvements strategies such as regular team feedback and iterative Plan-Do-Study-Act (PDSA) cycles.[6] PDSA cycles are a process of cycling through Planning (e.g., planning for when, where, and how to screen and identifying screening rate goals), Doing (e.g., observing and noting any issues during screening, such as clinical backlog, patient feedback, etc.), Studying (e.g., determining whether screening rates were met), and Acting (e.g., identifying barriers to successful screening and planning for improvements for the next PDSA cycle).

The greatest challenge, by far, in implementing screening for distress is engagement of the front-line clinical teams in responding to positive screening results. The bottom-up approach to ensure this includes efforts to make mental health be understood by clinicians as an important and meaningful outcome, engaging teams in developing clinical workflow processes following distress screening, providing regular distress screening data feedback to clinicians on their patient population, and establishing brief and efficient review and response pathways following distress screening.[6]

Psychometrics of Measures

The selection of a particular screening tool in a clinical setting is based on its relevance in that setting, the feasibility of its application, and the evidence for its psychometric properties. The latter refers to the validity and reliability of a screening tool in the population, language, and culture in which it is used and the demonstration of clinically relevant cutoff points. The most common types of validity that are assessed for screening tools are content/face, concurrent, and predictive validity. *Content* or *face validity* refers to whether a screening tool measures what it is intended to measure and is typically assessed through expert and nonexpert evaluation of the individual items included in the measure, often using confirmatory factor analysis. *Concurrent validity* refers to the performance of a screening tool against a gold standard test for the same condition at the same time. This is assessed in terms of sensitivity (i.e., ability of a positive screen to correctly detect the presence of the condition) and specificity (i.e., ability of a negative screen to correctly identify those without the condition). *Predictive validity* refers to the degree to which the screening cut-score predicts a related health outcome, measured against a criterion standard at a future time. The reliability of a measurement tool refers to its consistency over time (test-retest reliability), across items (internal consistency), and across different researchers (inter-rater reliability).

The psychometric properties of a screening tool are specific to the patient population, setting, and language in which the screening tool was developed or evaluated. Therefore, the use of a screening tool in a setting other than the one it was developed or evaluated in requires repeat assessment of its validity. Translation and back-translation and assessment of the cultural relevance and equivalence of constructs in other languages ensures retention of meaning and allows for greater comparability of findings across regions and settings.

The length of a screening tool often determines its utility in screening, assessment, or research. PROMs can be categorized as ultrashort (i.e., 1–4 items), short (i.e., 5–20 items), and long (i.e., >20 items). Ultrashort tools have limited specificity but are most useful to employ in routine screening efforts when results are followed-up by secondary clinical assessment. Short and long tools have better specificity than ultrashort tools. Long tools having the greatest utility and clinical relevance when used for assessment, case-finding, and research.

Longer screening tools have greater sensitivity and specificity but impose more burden on patients for their completion. Therefore a two-step screening approach is increasingly being adopted in distress screening programs as an efficient compromise between brevity, sensitivity, and specificity. This may be used when a highly sensitive ultrashort tool is administered and then sequentially followed by a longer tool with greater specificity administered to those who screen positive. Such an approach can be facilitated by computer adaptive testing (CAT), in which this process is automated electronically on a tablet or desktop computer. The Patient-Reported Outcomes Measurement Information System (PROMIS, https://www.promishealth.org/) utilizes a CAT approach based on item-response theory and is gaining uptake for distress screening in institutions where established electronic health records systems are available.

Screening Tools

A myriad of screening tools for psychological distress have been developed, studied, and employed in routine practice and research. Most validation studies in palliative care populations have been conducted in patients with advanced cancer, with fewer in non-cancer palliative care patients. The following sections discuss several commonly used screening tools for psychological distress, with attention to briefer screening tools that are practical to utilize during clinical encounters. They will be discussed in terms of the constructs they were designed to measure, their psychometrics, and their utility in routine screening. These screening tools are presented in Table 12.1.

Several cancer care agencies and national palliative care distress management guidelines recommend screening for distress comprehensively, covering psychological, physical, social, and practical patient concerns.[7,4] One of the most widely studied and implemented ultrashort distress screening measures is the Distress Thermometer (DT). The DT is a visual, single-item, 11-point rating scale for generalized distress over the past week. Developed by the National Comprehensive Cancer Network (NCCN), the DT is implemented in many cancer centers internationally. While its use has been recommended for use in all phases of cancer care, several studies have examined its validity in diverse palliative care setting. Meta-analytic subanalyses of DT data in patients with cancer near the end of life have led to recommendations to use a cutoff of $\geq$4–6 on the DT, providing adequate sensitivity but limited specificity (ranging from 0.52 to 0.73).[8,9] For this reason, secondary assessment by clinicians for threshold distress reported on the DT is recommended.

To identify the nature of patient-reported distress identified by the DT, the NCCN Problem List is often administered concurrently. This 39-item checklist asks patients to identify problems they have experienced in the past week related to the domains of practical, emotional, physical, spiritual, and familial matters.[1] Combining both tools identifies both the severity and potential cause of heighted distress (i.e., DT $\geq$4), which may inform the selection of the most appropriate treatment pathways (e.g., psychiatry, psychology,

TABLE 12.1 Selected screening tools for psychological distress in palliative care

Measures	Scoring	Description
PSYCHOLOGICAL DISTRESS SCREENING TOOLS		
DT (Distress Thermometer) and Problems Checklist[9,39]	▪ Cut scores ranging from ≥4–6 (cut score of ≥5 recommended) in advanced cancer patients receiving specialist palliative care in a hospice setting. ▪ Sensitivity (cut score of ≥5): 0.78 ▪ Specificity (cut score of ≥5): 0.62	▪ DT: Visual analog with 0 (no distress) to 10 (extreme distress) rating scale for distress ▪ Problems Checklist: Yes or No checklist of practical, family, emotional, spiritual, and physical problems. ▪ Recall period: Past week

ESAS-r: Edmonton Symptom Assessment System-revised[40]	▪ Cut scores ranging from ≥4–5 (moderate-severe) for each item.
	▪ Range across all symptoms:
	  ○ Sensitivity: 0.90–0.96
	  ○ Specificity: 0.53–0.93
		▪ Brief 9-item screening tool for common symptoms in advanced cancer (pain, tiredness, nausea, drowsiness, lack of appetite, shortness of breath, depression, anxiety, and wellbeing).
		▪ Each item is scored on a 11-point numerical rating scale according to symptom severity, with higher scores indicating worse severity.
		▪ Recall period: Current

DEPRESSION AND ANXIETY SCREENING TOOLS		

HADS: Hospital Anxiety and Depression Scale[15]	HADS Total score:
	  ○ Normal: 0–7
	  ○ Mild: 8–10
	  ○ Moderate: 11–14
	  ○ Severe: 15–21
	▪ Recommended cutoff: ≥14–15 (any psychological distress)
	▪ Pooled sensitivity: 0.73
	▪ Pooled specificity: 0.81
	HADS-D cutoff: ≥7–8
	▪ Pooled sensitivity: 0.76
	▪ Pooled specificity: 0.66
	HADS-A cutoff: ≥7–8
	▪ Pooled sensitivity: 0.66
	▪ Pooled specificity: 0.71
		▪ 14-item scale, consisting of two 7-item, 4-point Likert subscales, with one specifically targeted at anxiety (HAD-A) and one specifically targeted at depression (HADS-D) developed to identify distress among non-psychiatric hospital patients
		▪ Recall period: Past week

PHQ-9: Patient Health Questionnaire-9[16]	PHQ-9 cutoff in cancer patients: ≥7 ▪ Pooled sensitivity: 0.83 ▪ Pooled specificity: 0.61	▪ A 9-item measure of depression severity, made in concordance with major depressive disorder as per the Diagnostic & Statistical Manual of Mental Disorder on a Likert scale 0 (not at all) to 4 (almost every day). ▪ Recall: Past 2 weeks
GAD-7: Generalized Anxiety Disorder Scale-7[18]	Recommended cutoff in cancer patients: ≥7 ▪ Sensitivity: 0.77 ▪ Specificity: 0.74	▪ A 7-item measure of anxiety symptoms in concordance with generalized anxiety disorder as per the Diagnostic & Statistical Manual of Mental Disorder on a Likert scale 0 (not at all) to 4 (almost every day). ▪ Recall: Past 2 weeks

Tool	Description	Scoring / Cut-offs

PCL-5: PTSD Checklist for DSM-5[24]	• 20-item, 5-point Likert scale that assesses the severity of each of the 20 B-E symptoms of PTSD outlined in the Diagnostic and Statistic Manual for Mental Disorders (DSM-V)
	• Recall period: Past month
	• Briefer versions of PCL-5: 4-item version of PCL-5 (recommended cut off score of ≥5 validated against full PCL-5 cut score ≥ 32).[23]
	• Assesses only one of each B-E symptom criteria of the DSM-V.
	• Recall period: Past month
		• Cut score recommended ≥31–33 in medical treatment seeking veterans
		  • Sensitivity: 0.88
		  • Specificity: 0.69
		• 4-item version of PCL-5:
		  • Cut score recommended ≥5
		  • Sensitivity: 0.99
		  • Specificity: 0.94

ADNM-20: Adjustment Disorder - New Module[41,42]	• 20-item self-report version of the International Classification of Diseases (ICD)-11 Adjustment Disorder Scale
	• 6 subscales; 8-item version focuses on 2 core subscales of preoccupation and failure to adapt
		• Sum score range: 20–80
		• Cut score >47.5 differentiates high and low risk for adjustment disorder (not validated in medical or palliative populations)
		  • Sensitivity: 0.72
		  • Specificity: 0.82
		• ADNM-8 (recommended cut score ≥18.5):
		  • Sensitivity: 0.97
		  • Specificity: 0.86
		• ADNM-4 (recommended cut score ≥8.5):
		  • Sensitivity: 0.95
		  • Specificity: 0.79

Tool	Description	Scoring / Cut-offs
DS-II: Demoralization Scale revised[25,43]	• 16-item measuring a unidimensional construct of demoralization • 2 subscales: Meaning and Purpose; Distress and Coping Ability	• Score range: 0–32 • Moderate: >10 • Severe: >20 • Sensitivity: 0.82 • Specificity: 0.81
DADDS: Death and Dying Distress Scale[26]	• 15-item measure designed to assesses distress related to loss of time and opportunity, the process of dying, and its impact on others	• Score range: 0–75 • No validated cut-scores
PDI: Patient Dignity Inventory[27]	• 25-item measure to detect end-of-life dignity-related distress • Original 5-factor structure in English[27]: Symptom Distress, Existential Distress, Dependency, Peace of Mind, and Social Support • Factors identified in other populations: Illness-related concerns, Interactions with Others, Psychological Distress, Self-confidence, Anxiety and Uncertainty, Loss of Autonomy[44–48]	• Score range: 25–125 • No validated cut-scores
SAHD-5: Schedule of Attitudes towards Hastened Death short form[35]	• Short form of the 20-item SAHD • Positive screen should be followed up by clinical assessment, either with full SAHD or the DDRS[36]	• Score range: 0–5 • Cut-score ≥2

social work, or chaplaincy). The brevity of the DT and NCCN Problem List has made them appealing for use in palliative care populations.

Another comprehensive distress screening tool is the revised Edmonton Symptom Assessment System (ESAS-r).[10] Originally developed for use in palliative populations, ESAS-r is a 9-item, 11-point rating scale for both physical and psychological symptoms. ESAS-r includes 9 items related to the current severity of physical (i.e., pain, tiredness, drowsiness, nausea, appetite, and shortness of breath) and psychological symptoms (i.e., depression, anxiety, and wellbeing). There is also an optional "Other Problem" item, which can be used to identify other disease-specific concerns (e.g., constipation) not included in ESAS-r. Each item rating score is interpreted independently, with mild, moderate, and severe symptoms being rated as 0–3, 4–6, 7–10, respectively. While there may be significant variation between symptoms, items rated ≥4–5 generally merit further assessment by a clinician. While the single items pertaining to current depression (ESAS-D) and anxiety (ESAS-A) have been used as standalone screening tools for depression and anxiety, the full ESAS-r is generally used because it is both comprehensive and brief. ESAS-D and ESAS-A are similar to the DT in having high sensitivity at a cutoff of ≥4 (sensitivity for depression and anxiety is 0.0.93 and 0.89, respectively), but lower specificity (0.81 and 0.74 for depression and anxiety, respectively). Therefore their use usually requires either secondary screening and/or further assessment by clinicians.

Depression and Anxiety Screening Tools

Several screening tools for depression and anxiety have been validated in palliative care populations, with most studies conducted in patients with cancer receiving palliative care. One of the briefest for depression in palliative care asks a single question: "Are you depressed?" or more accurately, "Are you depressed most of the time?" This item has been shown to have high specificity (74–100%) for depression in palliative care populations.[11,12] However, some patients find this question too nonspecific or simplistic, and it has shown poor sensitivity (~50%) for depression in several studies.[13,14] The addition of a second item, such as anhedonia, has been shown to improve its sensitivity in palliative care populations (sensitivity 90.7%, specificity 67.7%), although this symptom is more strongly associated with a prior history of depression and this item may be less useful for patients with no history of depression.[14] Therefore, measures containing more specific items related to depression in medical illness may be more useful in palliative care.

The Hospital Anxiety and Depression Scale (HADS) is one of the most commonly used mood scales in palliative care settings. It consists of two 7-item, 4-point Likert subscales, one targeted at anxiety (HAD-A) and the other at depression (HADS-D). The HADS has been studied extensively as a case-finding tool for depression and anxiety in medical populations as its intentional exclusion of somatic symptoms was thought to improve its diagnostic accuracy in patients with physical illness. The HADS has utility for screening based on its sensitivity to detect psychological distress with a total HADS cutoff score of 14–15 (pooled sensitivity of 0.73) and its relative brevity compared to other depression screening tools. However, meta-analyses of HADS data suggest that it is insufficient as a case-finding tool for depression, anxiety, or any mental illness in palliative care.[15]

The 9-item Patient Health Questionnaire (PHQ) has been used in routine depression screening in cancer and palliative care settings. This measure assesses the frequency of both somatic and cognitive-affective components of depression, in concordance with the *Diagnostic and Statistic Manual for Mental Disorders* (DSM-5). It has acceptable psychometric properties for major depressive disorder in cancer patients, including in those receiving palliative care.[16] The briefer PHQ-2 is comprised of only the first two items of the PHQ-9, which assess depression and anhedonia. This 2-item measure has been recommended by the American Society of Clinical Oncology as part of a two-step screen, in which patients who screen positive on these two items then complete the full PHQ-9. Such an approach may result in improved patient acceptability due to reduced respondent burden particularly in palliative care, but should be followed by a more comprehensive assessment.

The 7-item Generalized Anxiety Disorder scale (GAD-7) has been well-validated and is commonly used for anxiety screening in oncology and other medical settings.[17] The GAD-7 assesses the frequency of seven core symptoms of generalized anxiety disorder, with sufficient sensitivity and moderate specificity in studies of mixed cancer populations, including those receiving treatment with curative or palliative intent.[18] However, there has been much less research on the validation of anxiety screening measures in end-of-life populations, compared to that conducted on depression screening measures.

Trauma and Stress-Related Screening Tools

Medical illness may be associated with multiple traumatic events that trigger traumatic stress. These events include receiving a diagnosis of advanced disease, undergoing extended periods of illness, health emergencies, and/or major medical interventions. Traumatic stress symptoms are common in palliative care, particularly in response to such events as the diagnosis or recurrence of advanced disease, the exacerbation of physical symptoms, or the discontinuation of active treatment. The severity of these symptoms may range from nonpathological stress response symptoms to those that meet criteria for adjustment disorder, acute stress disorder (ASD), or posttraumatic stress disorder (PTSD). Recognition of these symptoms may be obscured by comorbid dementia, delirium, and pain in palliative care settings, highlighting the potential utility of screening tools to enhance identification of trauma and stress-related syndromes in this context.

Adjustment disorder is the most commonly diagnosed psychiatric disorder in palliative care, but the lack of operational criteria for its diagnosis in DSM-5 has limited the reliability and validity of its assessment. The Adjustment Disorder New Module (ADNM)[19] is a self-report measure based on the proposed ICD-11 definition, developed to address this limitation. The ADNM-20 includes a list of stressors and a list of symptoms that occurred in response to the most distressing events. It has six subscales, although confirmatory factor analyses have demonstrated both a single-factor and two-factor structure (i.e., preoccupation and failure to adapt) which are represented in the brief 8-item ADNM-8 and ultra-brief ADNM-4.[20]

Although there is an extensive research literature using PROMs to study traumatic stress in palliative care, there have been no psychometric validation studies of screening measures for the clinical syndromes of ASD or PTSD specifically in end-of-life settings.

This may be due to the low frequency of PTSD and lack of an operationalized definition near end of life when there may have been multiple, chronic, and anticipatory traumatic events, such as seen with the progression of solid tumors. However, the validity of PROMs such as the Standford Acute Stress Reaction Questionnaire (SASRQ) in palliative acute leukemia populations has not been questioned, as several studies have supported good predictive validity.[21]

The most widely used validated screening tool for PTSD in medical populations and research studies is the PTSD Checklist (PCL-5).[22] The PCL-5 is a 20-item measure that assesses the severity of each of the 20 symptoms of PTSD outlined in DSM-5 on 5-point Likert scale rated from 0–4 for each item. A provisional PTSD diagnosis can be made by rendering items rated ≥ 2 as "present," then following the DSM-5 diagnostic rule that requires the presence of 1–2 symptoms per symptom cluster for PTSD. Given the respondent burden of completing the PCL-5, there have been several attempts at developing briefer versions. The most recent one used machine learning and conventional statistical methods on PCL-5 data from more than 10,000 US army veterans to develop an optimal 4-item version of the PCL-5.[23] This short form of PCL-5 demonstrated psychometric properties similar to the full PCL-5, with a $\geq 5/16$ screening threshold having a sensitivity and specificity of 0.99 and 0.94, respectively, validated against an intermediate definition of PTSD (full PCL-5 $\geq 32/80$). Although both the full and short-form of PCL-5 have excellent psychometric properties (recommended summed threshold score of 31–33 for full PCL-5, with a sensitivity and specificity of 0.88 and 0.69, respectively), more research is needed to determine its validity in palliative care populations.[24]

Existential Distress Screening Tools

Measures that have been used to assess existential distress in palliative care include ones that assess hopelessness, demoralization, meaning, dignity, spirituality, death anxiety, and the WTHD. Many studies have validated such measures in palliative populations, where they demonstrate convergent validity with measures of depression and quality of life. Screening for this domain of distress may be of value to guide psychotherapy for patients with advanced disease (see Part VI). Perhaps the most practical and brief screening tools are the Demoralization Scale revised (DS-II),[25] the Death and Dying Distress Scale (DADDS),[26] the Patient Dignity Inventory (PDI),[27] and the short form of the Schedule of Attitudes Toward Hastened Death (SAHD-5).[28]

The DS[29] was originally developed as a 24-item measure existential distress in patients with cancer. Factor analysis identified five relatively distinct dimensions: loss of meaning, dysphoria, disheartenment, helplessness, and sense of failure, with high internal reliability and convergent validity in multiple international populations and in chronic disease. Rasch analysis was used to refine a 16-item version, with subscales of Meaning and Purpose ($\alpha = 0.84$) and Distress and Coping Ability ($\alpha = 0.82$) (DS-II). The DS-II has been validated in Spanish patients with advanced cancer[25] and, more recently, 13- and 6-item (r = 0.98 and r = 0.95, respectively) versions of the DS have been validated in Italian hospitalized patients using item response theory.[30]

The DADDS is a 15-item measure of death anxiety in advanced disease that has been shown to have good construct validity in patients with advanced cancer, with positive associations with anxiety and depression and negative associations with end-of-life preparation and quality of life. The DADDS has recently been shown to have a two-factor structure, with one factor reflecting distress related to the shortness of time and the other to the process of dying.[31] The DADDS is gaining in use and has now been validated in Western, European, and Asian populations of patients with advanced cancer.

Both demoralization and death anxiety are forms of psychological distress that can underlie requests for palliative sedation or assisted dying in jurisdictions where it is legal (Chapter 8). In as much as assisted dying has been euphemized as death with dignity, the PDI is used as an assessment tool to identify patients who may benefit from end-of-life psychotherapies.[32] The PDI is a 25-item self-report measure of dignity-related distress with strong test-retest reliability and concurrent validity. It measures diverse constructs, with various three- to five-factor structures depending on the population studied, covering domains of physical, psychosocial, existential, and spiritual patient concerns. Its clinical value as a measure of sources of end-of-life distress is demonstrated by its broad international uptake, translated into ten languages to date.

The SAHD[33] is a 20-item self-report true–false measure of the WTHD. It has been validated in patients with cancer and terminal illness and has been shown to have sufficient variability in scores and good utility in large-scale research studies. A cutoff score of 10 has been recommended to indicate a high desire for hastened death. Short forms of the SAHD, including a 6-item version developed through item response theory (SAHD-6)[34] and a 5-item version developed through Rasch analysis[35] have been suggested for use as primary screen for the WTHD, to be followed-up by secondary clinical assessment using the clinician-rated semi-structured interview in the Desire for Death Rating Scale (DDRS).[36]

Future Directions

Routine screening for psychological distress is an emerging standard of practice in palliative care that is fundamentally designed to improve patient outcomes. Further research and novel strategies are needed to address gaps in implementation in palliative care settings. However, there is a surprising paucity of psychometric studies validating screening tools for anxiety and traumatic stress in end-of-life populations. Future psychometric studies should focus on validating briefer versions of existential distress measures given the prevalence and importance of this domain in palliative care.

In the age of technological advances and emergence of Big Data applications in healthcare, remote symptom monitoring is beginning to take flight in medical settings. The deployment of phone-based remote symptom screening programs to screen for treatment toxicities in between clinic visits is currently being studied across the globe,[37,38] providing a unique opportunity to integrate psychological distress screening for outpatients receiving palliative care. Such approaches have health service utility by identifying distress before the clinic visit to assist clinic flow and treatment planning when the patient arrives and can facilitate research on the health outcomes following psychological distress screening in palliative care populations. Patients with advanced illness constitute a unique population in which to study the effect of distress screening on health outcomes such as emergency room visits and hospitalizations and cancer-related survival.

Key Points

- Routine distress screening is an important standard of care to increase the detection of psychological distress, which can otherwise be missed by clinicians in palliative care settings.
- Medical team engagement to ensure a clinical response to elevated scores is the most important part of distress screening; psychiatrists should work collaboratively with palliative care teams to implement screening for distress programs and ensure such responses.
- Two-step screening approaches with an ultra-short tool used first may be optimal, as brevity of screening tools is an important consideration in palliative care populations.
- Screening should be comprehensive, including for psychological distress, physical symptoms, and practical needs.

References

1. Kam LYK, Knott VE, Wilson C, Chambers SK. Using the theory of planned behavior to understand health professionals' attitudes and intentions to refer cancer patients for psychosocial support. *Psychooncology*. 2012;21(3):316–323.
2. Basch E, Deal AM, Dueck AC, et al. Overall survival results of a trial assessing patient-reported outcomes for symptom monitoring during routine cancer treatment. *JAMA*. 2017;318(2):197–198.
3. Basch E, Deal AM, Kris MG, et al. Symptom monitoring with patient-reported outcomes during routine cancer treatment: A randomized controlled trial. *Journal of Clinical Oncology*. 2016;34(6):557.
4. NCCN. Distress management, Version 1. 2022. Accessed December 22, 2021, 2021. https://www.nccn.org/guidelines/recently-published-guidelines
5. Deshields TL, Wells-Di Gregorio S, Flowers SR, et al. Addressing distress management challenges: Recommendations from the consensus panel of the American Psychosocial Oncology Society and the Association of Oncology Social Work. *CA Cancer J Clin*. 2021;17(2):407–436.
6. Li M, Macedo A, Crawford S, et al. Easier said than done: Keys to successful implementation of the distress assessment and response tool (DART) program. *J Oncol Pract*. 2016;12(5):e513–e526.
7. Bickel KE, McNiff K, Buss MK, et al. Defining high-quality palliative care in oncology practice: An American Society of Clinical Oncology/American Academy of Hospice and Palliat Med guidance statement. *J Oncol Pract*. 2016;12(9):e828–e838.
8. Ma X, Zhang J, Zhong W, et al. The diagnostic role of a short screening tool—the distress thermometer: A meta-analysis. *Support Care Cancer*. 2014;22(7):1741–1755.
9. Graham-Wisener L, Dempster M, Sadler A, McCann L, McCorry NK. Validation of the Distress Thermometer in patients with advanced cancer receiving specialist palliative care in a hospice setting. *Palliat Med*. 2021;35(1):120–129.
10. Watanabe SM, Nekolaichuk C, Beaumont C, Johnson L, Myers J, Strasser F. A multicenter study comparing two numerical versions of the Edmonton Symptom Assessment System in palliative care patients. *J Pain Symptom Manage*. 2011;41(2):456–468.

11. Lloyd-Williams M, Dennis M, Taylor F, Baker I. Is asking patients in palliative care, "are you depressed?" appropriate? Prospective study. *BMJ*. 2003;327(7411):372–373.

12. Chochinov HM, Wilson KG, Enns M, Lander S. Are you depressed? Screening for depression in the terminally ill. *Am J Psychiatry*. 1997;154(5):674–676.

13. Warmenhoven F, van Rijswijk E, Engels Y, et al. The Beck Depression Inventory (BDI-II) and a single screening question as screening tools for depressive disorder in Dutch advanced cancer patients. *Support Care Cancer*. 2012;20(2):319–324.

14. Payne A, Barry S, Creedon B, et al. Sensitivity and specificity of a two-question screening tool for depression in a specialist palliative care unit. *Palliat Med*. 2007;21(3):193–198.

15. Mitchell AJ, Meader N, Symonds P. Diagnostic validity of the Hospital Anxiety and Depression Scale (HADS) in cancer and palliative settings: A meta-analysis. *J Affect Disord*. 2010;126(3):335–348.

16. Hartung TJ, Friedrich M, Johansen C, et al. The Hospital Anxiety and Depression Scale (HADS) and the 9-item Patient Health Questionnaire (PHQ-9) as screening instruments for depression in patients with cancer. *Cancer*. 2017;123(21):4236–4243.

17. Spitzer RL, Kroenke K, Williams JB, Löwe B. A brief measure for assessing generalized anxiety disorder: The GAD-7. *Arch Intern Med*. 2006;166(10):1092–1097.

18. Esser P, Hartung TJ, Friedrich M, et al. The Generalized Anxiety Disorder Screener (GAD-7) and the anxiety module of the Hospital and Depression Scale (HADS-A) as screening tools for generalized anxiety disorder among cancer patients. *Psychooncology*. 2018;27(6):1509–1516.

19. Einsle F, Köllner V, Dannemann S, Maercker A. Development and validation of a self-report for the assessment of adjustment disorders. *Psychol Health Med*. 2010;15(5):584–595.

20. Ben-Ezra M, Mahat-Shamir M, Lorenz L, Lavenda O, Maercker A. Screening of adjustment disorder: Scale based on the ICD-11 and the Adjustment Disorder New Module. *J Psychiatr Res*. 2018;103:91–96.

21. Rodin G, Deckert A, Tong E, et al. Traumatic stress in patients with acute leukemia: A prospective cohort study. *Psychooncology*. 2018;27(2):515–523.

22. Blevins CA, Weathers FW, Davis MT, Witte TK, Domino JL. The posttraumatic stress disorder checklist for DSM-5 (PCL-5): Development and initial psychometric evaluation. *J Trauma Stress*. 2015;28(6):489–498.

23. Zuromski KL, Ustun B, Hwang I, et al. Developing an optimal short-form of the PTSD Checklist for DSM-5 (PCL-5). *Depress Anxiety*. 2019;36(9):790–800.

24. Bovin MJ, Marx BP, Weathers FW, et al. Psychometric properties of the PTSD checklist for diagnostic and statistical manual of mental disorders–fifth edition (PCL-5) in veterans. *Psychol Assess*. 2016;28(11):1379.

25. Robinson S, Kissane DW, Brooker J, et al. Refinement and revalidation of the demoralization scale: The DS-II—external validity. *Cancer*. 2016;122(14):2260–2267.

26. Lo C, Hales S, Zimmermann C, Gagliese L, Rydall A, Rodin G. Measuring death-related anxiety in advanced cancer: Preliminary psychometrics of the Death and Dying Distress Scale. *J Pediatr Hematol Oncol*. 2011;33:S140–S145.

27. Chochinov HM, Hassard T, McClement S, et al. The patient dignity inventory: A novel way of measuring dignity-related distress in palliative care. *J Pain Symptom Manage*. 2008;36(6):559–571.

28. Bellido-Pérez M, Crespo I, Wilson KG, Porta-Sales J, Balaguer A, Monforte-Royo C. Assessment of the wish to hasten death in patients with advanced cancer: A comparison of 2 different approaches. *Psychooncology*. 2018;27(6):1538–1544.

29. Kissane DW, Wein S, Love A, Lee XQ, Kee PL, Clarke DM. The Demoralization Scale: A report of its development and preliminary validation. *J Ppalliat Care*. 2004;20(4):269–276.

30. Murri MB, Zerbinati L, Ounalli H, et al. Assessing demoralization in medically ill patients: Factor structure of the Italian version of the demoralization scale and development of short versions with the item response theory framework. *J Psychosom Res*. 2020;128:109889.

31. Shapiro GK, Mah K, Li M, Zimmermann C, Hales S, Rodin G. Validation of the Death and Dying Distress Scale in patients with advanced cancer. *PsychoOncology*. 2021;30(5):716–727.

32. Chochinov HM, McClement SE, Hack TF, et al. The patient dignity inventory: applications in the oncology setting. *J Palliat Med*. 2012;15(9):998–1005.

33. Rosenfeld B, Breitbart W, Stein K, et al. Measuring desire for death among patients with HIV/AIDS: The schedule of attitudes toward hastened death. *Am J Psychiatry*. 1999;156(1):94–100.

34. Kolva E, Rosenfeld B, Liu Y, Pessin H, Breitbart W. Using item response theory (IRT) to reduce patient burden when assessing desire for hastened death. *Psychol Assess*. 2017;29(3):349.

35. Monforte-Royo C, González-de Paz L, Tomás-Sábado J, et al. Development of a short form of the Spanish schedule of attitudes toward hastened death in a palliative care population. *Qual Life Res*. 2017;26(1):235–239.

36. Kelly B, Burnett P, Pelusi D, Badger S, Varghese F, Robertson M. Terminally ill cancer patients' wish to hasten death. *Palliat Med*. 2002;16(4):339–345.

37. Furlong E, Darley A, Fox P, et al. Adaptation and implementation of a mobile phone-based remote symptom monitoring system for people with cancer in Europe. *JMIR Cancer*. 2019;5(1):e10813.

38. Moradian S, Krzyzanowska M, Maguire R, et al. Protocol: Feasibility randomised controlled trial of remote symptom chemotherapy toxicity monitoring using the Canadian adapted Advanced Symptom Management System (ASyMS-Can): A study protocol. *BMJ Open*. 2020;10(6):E035648.

39. Donovan KA, Grassi L, McGinty HL, Jacobsen PB. Validation of the distress thermometer worldwide: state of the science. *Psychooncology*. 2014;23(3):241–250.

40. Selby D, Cascella A, Gardiner K, et al. A single set of numerical cutpoints to define moderate and severe symptoms for the Edmonton Symptom Assessment System. *J Pain Symptom Manage*. 2010;39(2):241–249.

41. Lorenz L, Bachem R, Maercker A. The adjustment disorder–new module 20 as a screening instrument: Cluster analysis and cut-off values. *Int J Occup Environ Med*. 2016;7(4):215.

42. Kazlauskas E, Gegieckaite G, Eimontas J, Zelviene P, Maercker A. A brief measure of the International Classification of Diseases-11 adjustment disorder: Investigation of psychometric properties in an adult help-seeking sample. *Psychopathology*. 2018;51(1):10–15.

43. Belar A, Arantzamendi M, Rodríguez-Núñez A, et al. Multicenter study of the psychometric properties of the New Demoralization Scale (DS-II) in Spanish-speaking advanced cancer patients. *J Pain Symptom Manage*. 2019;57(3):627–634.

44. Mergler BD, Goldshore MA, Shea JA, Lane-Fall MB, Hadler RA. The Patient Dignity Inventory and dignity-related distress among the critically ill. *J Pain Symptom Manage*. 2021;63(3):359–365.

45. Eskigülek Y, Kav S. Validity and reliability of the Turkish version of the Patient Dignity Inventory. *Palliat Support Care*. 2021:1–8.

46. Oh SN, Yun YH, Keam B, et al. Korean version of the Patient Dignity Inventory: Translation and validation in patients with advanced cancer. *J Pain Symptom Manage*. 2021;62:416–424.

47. Sautier LP, Vehling S, Mehnert A. Assessment of patients' dignity in cancer care: Preliminary psychometrics of the German version of the Patient Dignity Inventory (PDI-G). *J Pain Symptom Manage*. 2014;47(1):181–188.

48. Li Y-C, Wang H-H, Ho C-H. Validity and reliability of the Mandarin version of Patient Dignity Inventory (PDI-MV) in cancer patients. *Plos One*. 2018;13(9):e0203111.

13

Communicating with Patients with Advanced Cancer

Patricia A. Parker, Andrew S. Epstein, William E. Rosa, and Smita C. Banerjee

Introduction

Communication between patients, their families, and the healthcare team is a foundation for providing optimal cancer care. Identifying, assessing, and addressing the communication experiences, needs, and goals of patients with any type or stage of cancer is critical. As cancer progresses, what patients want and need from their healthcare team may change. Patients with advanced cancer have diverse and complex physical, psychological, social, and spiritual needs.

Communicating effectively with patients who have advanced cancer is a challenge for many healthcare professionals. As a general rule, when faced with advanced cancer, patients need information to help them understand their illness and plan for their future. In addition to information, many patients also turn to their healthcare team for guidance and support. This chapter describes the communication needs and challenges of patients with advanced cancer and their caregivers and suggest strategies to communicate effectively about these complex issues.

Communication Needs

The communication needs of patients with cancer change over the course of the cancer trajectory. Patients with advanced cancer and their informal caregivers have a variety of needs during their illness, many of which go unmet. For patients with advanced cancer, obtaining information and support are often identified as unmet needs among patients with cancer.

Thorne et al.[1] conducted a qualitative study to examine how cancer patients' information and communication needs change over the cancer trajectory. They asked patients what makes cancer communication helpful and unhelpful across the illness trajectory. They found that patients expressed a need to be known and valued for what they bring to cancer care communication regardless of where they were on the illness spectrum. Patients also described the need for clinicians to frequently assess rather than simply assume what would constitute effective communication for each individual patient at any given point within and across the trajectory. For patients with advanced cancer, the most important need in their communication with their healthcare team was to balance honesty with hope.

Patients typically want their healthcare team to be candid and truthful about their illness while at the same time being compassionate and hopeful. For example, Rainbird et al.[2] assessed the needs of cancer patients who were of varying ages (27–89 years, 53% female) who were determined to have greater than 3 months and less than 2 years to live. Patients reported substantial unmet needs with more than one-third of the patients reported a moderate/high level of need for help on items within the psychological or emotional domain (39–40%), and more than 30 percent had moderate/high needs on the medical communication/information domain (31–35%).

Some studies have identified needs among both patients and their informal caregivers. Wang et al.,[3] for example, conducted a systematic review of unmet needs about both patients and caregivers. The three most commonly reported domains for patients were psychological, physical, and healthcare service and information. The most prominent unmet items of these domains were emotional support (10.1–84.4%), fatigue (18–76.3%), and being informed about benefits and side effects of treatment (4–66.7%). In terms of health system and information, being informed about benefits and side effects of treatment were the most common needs. With regards to patient care and support needs, two prominent unmet needs included "reassurance by medical staff that the way you feel is normal" and "the doctor acknowledges and shows sensitivity to your feelings and emotional needs." Unmet needs of patients with advanced cancer were associated with their physical symptoms, anxiety, and quality of life. Caregivers most commonly reported unmet needs were information needs, including illness and treatment information (26–100%) and care-related information (21–100%).

Collins et al.[4] interviewed caregivers of patients with advanced cancer about how they wanted to talk about palliative care and death and dying. They reported wanting to receive written information supplemented with conversations from the healthcare team. Caregivers also reported that receiving information gradually over time rather than all at once was helpful for them. When their loved one was dying, they wanted to be asked how much information they wanted to have regarding the dying process, have the healthcare team acknowledge that death is imminent, and to be told in direct, simple language rather than in euphemisms.

Healthcare Professionals Perspective on Communication

What do healthcare professionals find challenging about communication with patients with advanced cancer? Less empirical work has focused on the healthcare clinicians' perspective. What is known is that many clinicians feel unprepared to meet the needs of patients with advanced cancer. They rarely receive specific training in how to communicate about challenging topics, such as discussing prognosis and communicating about end-of-life goals of care.

Mok et al.[5] assessed healthcare providers perspective on hope in the palliative care setting. Some of the characteristics that healthcare clinicians perceived as hopeful in their patients was when the patients actively prepared for death, carried on living a normal life, actively achieved goals, or had a vision of life after death. They reported being able to help maintain hope in their patients through strategies such as affirming the patients' worth, their connectedness and partnership with the patient, having religious support, and helping facilitate resolution of unfulfilled family responsibilities. Importantly, participants reported that they needed to have their own hope in order to foster hope in others. Additionally, what is often lacking is knowledge of additional resources for the patient to meet their diverse needs. Often, care is very compartmentalized into specific disciplines and therefore communication across disciplines is essential for providing optimal care to patients.

Discussion of Prognosis

An essential aspect of person-centered care and shared decision-making is optimal two-way communication between clinicians and patients and their families. Such communication is perhaps no more important than when it relates to discussing the prognosis of an advanced cancer and the values, goals, and preferences patients have when navigating such illnesses. Cancer clinicians, particularly medical oncologists, have the experience necessary to estimate a prognosis for a given advanced cancer, while patients and their families are best able to consider their priorities and what's most important to them during an advanced cancer diagnosis.

Data demonstrate that most patients with cancer want to be aware of the details of their medical care, including their prognosis. Prognosis is often discussed and studied as the *amount* of time before which patients will die from their illness. What their life and, ultimately, their death will *look and feel* like is also a crucial aspect of prognosis that must be addressed by clinicians along the cancer care continuum. Patients' prognostic awareness is part of ethically sound care: patients deserve to know information, including about prognosis, when they want to, and be given the space to voice when they may not want to hear prognostic information such as statistical averages or even any information at all. In addition to upholding patient autonomy, clinicians can also achieve beneficence by helping patients to receive prognostic information with which they can plan the rest of their lives. Additionally, clinicians must remain mindful of nonmalfeasance because of the reality for a small but certain minority of patients that disclosure of prognosis for patients who do not want to know, or in a way that may be (unintentionally) upsetting, could have negative consequences.

The concern clinicians have about upsetting patients and families with the disclosure of prognostic information is understandable and likely rooted in the discomfort many clinicians have in talking about death and dying, which itself is likely multifactorial, ranging from insufficient education in how to elicit patient desires for information and how to deliver such serious new information like prognosis in a clear but sensitive way. Pressures on clinician time, as well as a lack of reimbursement structures and institutional recognition for discussions of prognosis, further compound this delicate issue of ensuring patients receive this information in a way that is empathic and as easy to understand as possible.

Prognosis is thus one of several aspects of communication in oncology that needs to be approached by understanding the duality between a patient's need to *know* information and to *feel known* as a person.[6] Namely, patients have a cognitive need to understand information, such as how long they will live and what that remaining time will look like, as well as to be connected with as the unique individuals they are, including through elicitation of their hopes, concerns, and support systems, with such ongoing support rendered from the clinical team to the patient and family throughout the cancer care continuum. Addressing this duality of the patient's need to know and feel known are communication skills tools that clinicians can be trained in and shape in a way that is comfortable to their individual styles of practice and communication.

When approaching the cognitive need patients have to *know* information, the SPIKES model for discussing serious illness is likely the most frequently taught method.[6] The SPIKES model accounts for the medical *Setting*; the patient's *Perspective*; an invitation to share *Information*; the delivery of the medical *Knowledge*/news, such as, in this case, prognosis about a cancer; exploration of *Emotion* and, finally; a *Summary* and discussion of next steps. The exploration of emotion (empathizing) can be seen as the key step for making patients feel *known* and can be approached through its own mnemonic of NURSE: *Naming* emotion, expressing *Understanding* (or lack of understanding) statements, voicing *Respect* for what the patient has endured, endorsing unending *Support* for the patient, and further *Exploring* patients' feelings, perspectives, hopes, and concerns. These mnemonics thus can and should be used together to achieve a balance of responding to the emotional and cognitive needs of the patient.[6]

Despite research demonstrating that these communication skills tools can be learned and used by clinicians who are trained in them, there remains an unmet need to demonstrate if their use both better informs patients about their prognosis (i.e., leads to greater prognostic awareness) and maintains or even improves patient coping (and does not irreparably or majorly upset patients). Prognostic awareness itself represents a major unmet need in oncology, given existing research demonstrating that many patients with advanced cancer are unaware about the incurability of their illness as well as the late stage and terminal nature of it.[7] While many factors explain why patients may appear to be uninformed (e.g., they truly are uninformed or alternatively, know they have a poor prognosis and yet indicate otherwise on surveys because of psychological, cognitive, or other factors), the receipt of nonbeneficial cancer-directed therapy in the days before death is also well documented. Specifically, patients with cancer spend a disproportionate amount of time at the end of life undergoing cancer therapies as well as hospitalizations, ICU admissions, and critical care therapies such as CPR and mechanical ventilation when much literature shows that these things do not return patients to prior states of physical functioning or prolong life by appreciably long periods of time. At the same time, risks of medical procedures are heightened at the end of life, and they can sometimes shorten, instead of extend life. This is likely one of the factors behind why subspecialty palliative care has been shown not only to improve quality of life, but to improve overall survival.

Another key reason that patients should be asked about and then given prognostic information is that there is no research demonstrating significant and/or ongoing harm psychologically to patients who receive information about prognosis. While sometimes upsetting for patients and families to hear, the preponderance of data indicate that while difficult news to receive, prognosis is nonetheless important information to have for future planning, and emotions that arise when discussing difficult news like advanced cancer prognosis can be addressed by clinicians.[8] Because of the ongoing need to help patients in their prognostic awareness and to do so in a way that simplifies this complicated process as much as possible for clinicians, researchers have recognized routine discussions about cancer scan results as an opportune time to discuss prognosis in the setting of advancing cancers. The impact of a cognitive psychology approach (Fuzzy Trace theory) centering on the "gist" or bottom-line information that patients with common progressive cancers (like those of the gastrointestinal tract or lung) have months, not years to live, is being explored.[9] As it relates to healthcare communication and medical decision-making, Fuzzy Trace theory posits that "fuzzy," or broader ("big picture") messaging (e.g., "on average, most people in your situation live months, not years") is needed in addition to or sometimes even in place of quantitative and more detailed data points (e.g., exact measurements of tumor sizes on scans or percentage chance of living 5 more years).

Advance Care Planning and Discussions of End-of-Life Goals of Care

Once adequately equipped with prognostic awareness, patients should also be engaged in discussions about what is important to them as they navigate cancer, particularly ones with poor prognoses. Often labeled as "goals of care" for the end of life, these issues fit into the broader framework of advance care planning (ACP), which is the process by which patients, families, and clinicians plan for future medical care, ideally done early and in an ongoing and bidirectional fashion, including communication of both the medical situation and patients' values (e.g., what is important to them, their concerns, support systems, and goals in a given medical situation). Shortcomings of this process, particularly in end-of-life medical care, have been discussed in the lay press, such as with Atul Gawande's book *Being Mortal*,[10] where he discussed that

> [f]irst, in medicine and society, we have failed to recognize that people have priorities that they need us to serve besides just living longer. Second, the best way to learn those priorities is to ask about them. . . . Medicine has forgotten how vital such matters are to people as they approach life's end. People want to share memories, pass on wisdoms and keepsakes, connect with loved ones, and to make some last contributions to the world. These moments are among life's most important, for both the dying and those left behind. And the way we in medicine deny people these moments, out of obtuseness and neglect, should be cause for our unending shame.

While clinicians arguably should not feel "ashamed" for the lack of exploration of patients' values and goals and priorities at the end of life, this does remain an unmet area for improving quality of care.

The ways in which clinicians can optimize ACP practices, however, is unclear. In oncology, no such gold standard exists despite increasing investigation into different ways ACP can be pursued.[11] Examples of ACP research include video decision aids patients and families can watch to be better informed about advanced cancer topics such as code status and hospice care. The impact of informational booklets about toxicity of chemotherapy has also been studied, as have websites that patients can navigate to indicate their values, goals, and preferences to their clinicians and loved ones. Effectiveness has not clearly been realized, however, for such ACP interventions. A recent editorial[12] presented a sobering opinion that, despite decades of federally and other-funded research support of ACP, there still remain no clear patient benefits seen through ACP. Additionally, studies have shown that in the process of discussing advancing cancer, patients sometimes experience PTSD, distress, or anxiety. While there are no data to suggest that these are significant or long-standing detriments, the lack of clear benefit into the process of ACP on patient-level outcomes such as psychological well-being, prognostic awareness, or healthcare utilization, as well as the possibility that these discussions can be upsetting for patients and families, collectively represent the uncertain current state of affairs of ACP in oncology.

The growing complexity of the oncologic treatment landscape and the ever-enlarging population of patients with cancer, however, behooves researchers to continue investigating the most effective ways to ensure patients' values are elicited and responded to throughout their illness instead of only at the end of life or, as sometimes happens, not at all. While subspecialty palliative care consultation has established an invaluable role in the care of patients with serious illness including cancer, the workforce shortage of palliative care specialists necessitates ongoing investigation into primary palliative care efforts, namely, palliative care delivered at the primary team level. In the case of oncology, this is the palliative care skill set learned and practiced by the medical oncologist and the team that physician works with (e.g., nurse, social worker).

Communication skills training programs have become increasingly available to support this primary palliative care model. Because of needs being highest in patients with advanced cancer, these models often target patients with advanced and/or incurable disease. Because of the risk of stigmatizing patients, a more holistic approach establishes primary palliative care in clinical teams to address needs not just of those with advanced cancer, but any patients for whom they care, regardless of prognosis, stage, and goals of treatment. While this increases the numbers of patients for whom oncology teams must provide support, it normalizes and better systematizes the care process. This has been explored at Memorial Sloan Kettering Cancer Center in the form of the 1-2-3 Program, which routinely assess and responds to symptoms, illness and treatment understanding, and values, all from the start of medical care, for any patient with cancer. Further investigation into the scalability and real-world effectiveness is ongoing after the publications of the process and acceptability, which have been reviewed along with other communication skills training program in oncology.[13]

Discussion of Palliative and Supportive Care

Communication regarding palliative or supportive care should ideally occur in collaboration with the primary care team or provider so the messaging, goals, and intent remain unified across clinicians and teams. When discussing palliative care at any point along the cancer continuum, consistent and concise language is necessary given a number of misconceptions about its role. There are a number of consensus-based definitions that may be helpful.

A global consensus-based definition of *palliative care* describes it as "the active holistic care of individuals across all ages with serious health-related suffering due to severe illness, and especially of those near the end of life. It aims to improve the quality of life of patients, their families, and their caregivers."[14 (p. 761)] It is important to emphasize, where appropriate, that palliative care can be effective in not only addressing physical and symptom management issues, but also mitigating distress resulting from psychological/psychiatric, social, cultural, spiritual/religious/existential, and legal/ethical factors. Although commonly and erroneously associated with end-of-life care, palliative care should be integrated throughout serious illness care, either in conjunction with curative treatment options or as a standalone approach to comfort-focused care per oncology recommendations.

Throughout the conversation, emphasis should be placed on the role of palliative care in improving quality of life and assisting in achieving patient-identified goals. Introducing palliative care options with patients and caregivers should begin with open-ended questions to gather data about their understanding of their clinical condition and palliative care, as well as their emotions, worries, and concerns about next steps.[13] Box 13.1 lists sample questions that are helpful to ask patients.

Conversations that emphasize a person's need for palliative care are not a desirable experience for anyone to have. The consequences of serious illness may incite fears, anxieties, and worries requiring a compassionate presence, deep listening, and verbal and nonverbal responses that communicate support. When palliative care is not integrated throughout the course of serious illness and is reserved for late-stage decision-making or in response to health crises, it is not uncommon for the emotional stakes to be high. The importance of providing both empathic communication and evidence-based clinical information about pragmatic care planning cannot be overstated. Additionally, it may be necessary to have

---

BOX 13.1 Introducing palliative care to patients and caregivers

- What is your understanding about the current plan to manage your cancer?
- Can you tell me a little about what you and your oncologist have discussed regarding your treatment options?
- What is your understanding of palliative care?
- In terms of your illness, what are your biggest challenges right now?
- As we have this conversation, what is most important to you?
- Having described palliative care during our time together, do you see an opportunity for us to partner with you in achieving your goals?

---

several conversations that gradually advance the patient's and family's understanding about palliative care and how it can be valuable in their given circumstances. They may need time to integrate the communication in order make informed decisions. Back and colleagues[15] recommend a number of principles that may be helpful to individualize communication about palliative care (Box 13.2).

Discussion of Hospice

Hospice is a subset of palliative care that focuses on optimizing quality of life and comfort-focused care for seriously ill individuals presumed to be in their last 6 months of life and their caregivers. Hospice teams provide all of the services of palliative care but in the

---

BOX 13.2 Principles to consider to individualize palliative care

- Begin with the patient's agenda to find out where the patient is in their experience and adapt your agenda as needed.
- Regularly assess both the emotional and cognitive experience of the patient.
- Move at the patient's pace, being conscious to only progress the conversation one step at a time.
- Explicitly articulate empathy to support the creation of a safe space.
- Address the things you can do before discussing the things you can't do.
- Talk about big-picture goals before specific interventions and ensure those goals are in alignment with the patient's goals and preferences.
- Spend time giving the patient your undivided attention, particularly when they share something that feels big.

Note: Adapted from Back and Arnold (2009).

---

absence of disease-modifying treatment options. Election of hospice may represent a significant and emotionally challenging transition in the experience of the patient and family. Again, gathering data on the patient/family understanding of hospice and addressing any myths or stigma about what hospice represents is critical. If you are a hospice and palliative specialist who is discussing hospice with a patient and family, it is essential to clarify with the primary team what has been previously discussed and gain an understanding of where the patient and family are emotionally in their decision-making process.

Communication challenges that occur when discussing hospice are not necessarily related to effectively describing what hospice offers but to understanding and addressing what hospice *means* to the patient/family. Common misperceptions include but are not limited to misperceptions of hospice as being a physical setting, the start of patient abandonment, or as an indicator of imminent death. Through thoughtful and open-ended interviewing strategies, clinicians can reveal these misunderstandings and compassionately clarify them.

The clinician may find it helpful to emphasize how hospice can be used to achieve patient- and family-identified goals of care and support them in living their values and preferences through a patient- and family-centered interdisciplinary approach. For instance, some patients may express a desire to die at home as opposed to in a hospital or health facility. Home hospice provides an often feasible and supportive option to achieve this goal. Patients may want to continue receiving cancer-directed treatments that are palliative in nature: hospice reimbursement systems sometimes cover this. Caregivers may be concerned about obtaining the necessary resources to provide support for their loved one (e.g., hospital bed, symptom management medication, education to alleviate patient distress). Hospices provide all of these physical and interpersonal resources. Alternatively, some patients may express a desire for hastened death, and it should be emphasized that hospice is not a method to achieve this aim. Finally, patients and families need to understand that existing treatment relationships, such as with their oncologists, can continue. Even though cancer-directed tests and treatments are no longer the focus during hospice care, intermittent check-ins and even appointments with oncology teams may still occur. Validating and responding to these individual concerns is an important step in fully conveying the benefits and limitations of hospice.

Maintaining Hope

Throughout the cancer care continuum, the maintenance of hope for patients and families as well as clinicians is an important principle. This relates to the threat that cancer poses, particularly to patients but also to family members and the clinicians privileged to care for them. Communications about prognosis and the process of advanced care planning both need to respect the fragility and dynamic nature of hope in situations of serious illness and dying. Patients can be supported by family and clinicians in the characterization and maintenance of hope with the adage of "hoping for the best and being prepared for the worst." While some clinicians argue[10] for a softer tone to this phrase, instead proposing something like "hoping for the best and being prepared, no matter what," both phrases recognize the desire everyone has to live as well and as long as possible, all the while being equipped with the relationships, preparation, and skill sets needed to cope with situations, including dying, should hopes for a better outcome not be realized.

Also particularly challenging to clinicians is when they perceive patient hopes as unrealistic, such as cure of an incurable cancer. Clinicians must support patients in these situations, including when patients have changing hopes throughout a cancer care continuum. Ultimately, the goal is for patients to receive care that is concordant with the values, goals, and preferences that have been elicited earlier in the disease course when they had more time and psychological "space" to process and express their life priorities. All the while, clinicians need to be aware that patient priorities can change. As such, there needs to be a more fluid and "in the moment" approach to goals-of-care discussions, especially when they are revisited at the time of increasing medical complexity, including at the end of life.

Finally, when advancing cancer precludes hope for cure or a longer life with more cancer-directed therapy, clinicians need to work with patients and families in the re-envisioning of hope (e.g., what could be hoped for now given that what was previously hoped for is no longer possible). In this way, patients can be given a chance to make meaning at that time in their lives. The aforementioned communication skills paradigm of ensuring the patient both *knows* as well as *feels known*[7] as a person applies to this very setting as well. For instance, a clinician may say "we wish things were different and that we were able to achieve your hope for a cure and much more time living with this cancer, but because it is no longer controllable with treatments for the cancer, I want to continue to support you by asking what you're now hoping for and feeling during this difficult time." This marriage of information delivery as well as exploration of what the patient is feeling can best help patients travel together with their loved ones and cancer clinicians in identifying where hope can be redirected and what the best possible life might be as cancer advances.

Communicating with Minoritized Persons and Groups

Around the world, structural discrimination has led to health inequities that systematically disadvantage many populations. COVID-19 has increased the global visibility and awareness of these inequities and challenged health systems and clinicians to address disparate care outcomes. In the context of advanced cancer, it is critical to consider how various groups have been historically marginalized across social, economic, and political domains and how these experiences beget subpar health services.

For instance, there is extensive empirical evidence demonstrating cancer pain disparities for Black and African American patients that lead to poor pain-related outcomes, increased health service utilization, and inadequate or inappropriate analgesic treatment.[15] Individuals who identify as lesbian, gay, bisexual, transgender, and/or queer/questioning (LGBTQ+) have endorsed significant distrust of the health system, fear of disclosing sexual and/or gender identity, and homophobic and transphobic behaviors from clinicians.[16] In addition, many persons confront multiple minority stressors due to their intersectional racial, ethnic, cultural, and other minoritized identities. Serious illness inequities extend far beyond the groups previously mentioned and include but are not limited to incarcerated persons, persons experiencing poverty and homelessness, those struggling with mental health challenges or substance use disorder, older populations, and persons with disabilities.

As precision oncology science and practice continue to evolve, clinical trials and cancer care delivery are expected to become more person- and community-centered to enhance inclusivity and increase access to care. Despite these advances, communicating with minoritized persons and other at-risk groups requires that the clinician consider the social and structural determinants of health in a given context as well as the potential power imbalances between the recipient of care and the clinician and/or health system. A number of approaches can assist in preparing to effectively and respectfully engage in culturally inclusive communication with any individual and group.

First, it is important that clinicians are familiar with their own implicit biases about various groups. Implicit bias has been associated with inequitable treatment and poor health outcomes for minoritized persons. These biases may also inform how, what, and why they communicate particular details. Clinicians can evaluate their own implicit biases across a number of social and health domains to identify the ways their biases impact the quality of delivered care (Project Implicit: https://implicit.harvard.edu/implicit/index.jsp).

Next, adopting an approach rooted in cultural humility may be helpful. Cultural humility is "the ability to maintain an interpersonal stance that is other-oriented (or open to the other) in relation to aspects of cultural identity that are most important to the [person or group]."[17 (p. 354)] There are three primary components of cultural humility as identified in Tervalon and Murray-Garcia's[17] seminal work: lifelong practices of self-reflection and self-critique, a commitment to addressing and rectifying power imbalances in the clinician-patient/family dynamic, and fostering mutually beneficial clinical and advocacy partnerships with communities being served.

Finally, concrete strategies are needed to strengthen the quality of patient/family encounters or redirect nonbeneficial communication interactions. Acquaviva[18] offers a seven-step process using the acronym CAMPERS in her work with LGBTQ-inclusive hospice and palliative care that can be adapted for any group at risk of marginalization or inequitable health service delivery. The steps are (1) know your *Clear purpose* for the interaction to ensure clarity about why you are there; (2) know your *Attitudes and beliefs* to be honest about your assumptions, biases, and prejudices about this patient and their identity; (3) know your *Mitigation plan* to decrease power imbalance, enhance patient-centeredness, and promote a patient's self-determination; (4) know the *Patient* as a human being beyond their diagnosis and prognosis in order to best nurture trust and relationship; (5) know your *Emotions* to effectively manage socially undesirable or intense emotions and best serve the experience of the patient/family; (6) know your *Reactions* so that you can quickly self-resolve judgmental or dismissive verbal and nonverbal cues; and (7) know your *Strategy* for self-evaluating patient/family encounters for elements that went well and that could have gone better and then integrating more desirable behaviors into future interactions.

Communication Skills Training Programs

The ability of a clinician to communicate effectively with patients and families is considered an important hallmark of a good clinician. Because communication skills do not improve by experience alone or by observing good role models and mimicking them, considerable effort and expense is dedicated toward communication skills training programs.[19] Research suggests that well-designed communication skills training programs are feasible in healthcare institutions and can improve clinicians' communication skills and patient experience.[19]

Most approaches to teaching communication skills in health care include cognitive, affective and behavioral components, with the general objective of promoting self-awareness and empathy in the clinician.[20] Communication skills training programs that focus on acquiring communication skills and use an experiential component as part of the training have shown to be more effective in clinicians' skill acquisition.[21]

The experiential component in teaching communication skills training programs is achieved by engaging participants in experiential role-play exercises with simulated patients (i.e., trained actors). The simulated patients become a crucial aspect of the training experience and also provide feedback to participants on the quality of interaction they just had with the clinician. This process helps in establishing the experiential component of communication skills training programs.[19,22] It is also important to note that the duration and mode of delivery of communication skills training programs can vary substantially, ranging from 1-hour e-learning to 24-hours in-person trainings.

The latest Cochrane review assesses whether communication skills training is effective in changing behavior of clinicians working in cancer care and in improving clinician well-being and patient health status and satisfaction.[19] The review included 17 randomized controlled trials (RCTs) conducted mainly in outpatient settings. Of the 17 included trials, 11 trials compared communication skills training with no training, 3 trials compared the effect of a follow-up communication skills training intervention after initial communication skills training, 2 trials compared the effect of communication skills training and patient coaching, and 1 trial compared two types of communication skills trainings. The studies used clinician encounters or interactions with real or simulated patients to measure the communication outcomes. The types of communication skills trainings courses evaluated in these trials were diverse and so were the participants. Study participants included oncologists, residents, other doctors, nurses, and a mixed team of clinicians. Overall, the results of the review and meta-analysis indicated that various communication skills training courses appear to be effective in improving communication skills related to supportive skills and to help clinicians to be less likely to give facts only without tailoring or individualizing their responses to the patient's emotions or offering support.[19]

Among the various communication skills training programs available, we focus on the Comskil training program developed by Memorial Sloan Kettering Cancer Center.[22] The Comskil training program includes a menu of different communication skills training courses (or modules) such as sharing serious news, shared decision-making, identifying and addressing palliative needs, responding to patient anger, discussing prognosis, and discussing death, dying, and end-of-life goals of care that have been delivered to physicians since 2005.[22,23] In 2013, the program was adapted to oncology nurses and includes three modules, delivered within 1 day of training: responding empathically to emotions, discussing, death, dying, and goals of care, and managing challenging family interactions.[24]

All communication skills training program courses/modules follow a conceptual model wherein the key components of the clinical consultation are broken up into manageable parts called modules, as described above. Each module has an overarching goal (the intended outcome of a consultation) which is achieved through use of a set of strategies (a priori, step-by-step plans that help achieve the communication goal). Strategies are further broken down into communication skills (discrete verbal utterances) and process tasks (set of verbal and nonverbal behaviors that create a conducive environment for the communication encounter to proceed). Through the process of role-play and reflection, clinicians engage in a lot of experiential learning, the key process that leads to clinician engagement and acquisition of new communication skills and process tasks.[22]

Strategies to Enhance Patient Engagement

The Center for Advancing Health defines patient engagement as the series of actions that individuals must take in order to obtain the greatest benefit from the healthcare services available to them. In discussing patient engagement, it is necessary that clinicians and patients have adequate access to resources, tools, and education that foster engagement skills.[25] The Institute of Medicine (IOM) has a model for a high-quality cancer care delivery system[26] that situates patients in the center with the healthcare workforce surrounding them and patient–staff interaction and communication in the key area in between. Patient engagement is purported to follow once this model is adapted in healthcare.[27]

Some system-level steps that can be undertaken by cancer hospitals to improve patient engagement include the following:[28]

- Make patient engagement a major part of the organization's strategic plan.
- Designate a select group of staff and physicians as "patient engagement champions."
- Review IOM recommendations for steps needed to better engage cancer patients.
- Process map the patient (customer) experience

In the same vein, recommended steps for clinicians to improve patient engagement include the following:[28]

- Adopt a shared decision-making approach.
- Introduce the entire care team early in the treatment process.
- Provide effective patient education.
- Encourage patient involvement in safety and error prevention.
- Develop an up-front care plan.
- Implement survivorship program components.
- Offer support and activity groups.

- Use technology to engage patients.
- Form a Patient and Family Advisory Council.

Similar strategies have been outlined by the Oncology Care Model (OCM), a program initiated by the Centers for Medicare and Medicaid Services (CMS). Two identified modules for patient engagement by the CMS include the Shared Decision-Making Model (SDM Model) and the Direct Decision Support Model (DDS Model). Communication skills training of clinicians is touted as an important strategy for encouraging patient engagement, whereby clinicians can be taught communication skills such as asking open-ended questions, demonstrating empathy to others, eliciting patient's values and preferences, and ensuring understanding of options.[28] More research is paramount to developing oncology infrastructure and processes of care that support patient engagement in meaningful ways and further enable oncology providers to move from policy to practice.[28]

Future Directions

In this chapter, we described some of the communication needs and priorities of patients with advanced cancer. We discussed some of the specific challenges that clinicians may encounter such as discussing prognosis, end-of-life goals of care, palliative care, and hospice care. We also reviewed some specific approaches and strategies for discussing these challenging topics with patients and family members. It is important to remember that communication needs change across the disease trajectory, and there are differences in what would be helpful for individual patients and their caregivers. More work is needed to better understand how to best communicate information about prognosis, the end of life, palliative care, and hospice to patients and what factors might influence what patients want or need to know. These conversations are challenging for clinicians, and studies are needed to examine how having these conversations impacts them. Future studies are also needed to further explore the impact of the training programs and approaches on patients, caregivers, and the healthcare system.

Key Points

- Patients with advanced cancer and their caregivers have unique communication needs.
- The needs of cancer patients differ across the cancer trajectory.
- When discussing topics related to prognosis, advanced care planning and end of life, it is important to find ways to maintain hope.
- There are a variety of programs and strategies that clinicians can learn to communicate effectively with patients with advanced cancer and their caregivers.

References

1. Thorne S, Hislop TG, Kim-Sing C, Oglov V, Oliffe JL, Stajduhar KI. Changing communication needs and preferences across the cancer care trajectory: Insights from the patient perspective. *Support Care Cancer*. 2013;22(4):1009–1015. doi:10.1007/s00520-013-2056-4

2. Rainbird K, Perkins J, Sanson-Fisher R, Rolfe I, Anseline P. The needs of patients with advanced, incurable cancer. *Br J Cancer*. 2009;101(5):759–764. doi:10.1038/sj.bjc.6605235

3. Wang T, Molassiotis A, Chung BP, Tan J-Y. Unmet care needs of advanced cancer patients and their informal caregivers: A systematic review. *BMC Palliat Care* 2018;17(1):96. doi:10.1186/s12904-018-0346-9

4. Collins A, McLachlan S-A, Philip J. How should we talk about palliative care, death and dying? A qualitative study exploring perspectives from caregivers of people with advanced cancer. *Palliat Med*. 2017;32(4):861–869. doi:10.1177/0269216317746584

5. Mok E, Lau K-po, Lam W-man, Chan L-ngor, Ng J, Chan K-sang. Health-care professionals' perspective on hope in the palliative care setting. *J Palliat Med*. 2010;13(7):877–883. doi:10.1089/jpm.2009.0393

6. van Vliet LM, Epstein AS. Current state of the art and science of patient-clinician communication in progressive disease: Patients' need to know and need to feel known. *J Clin Oncol* 2014;32(31):3474–3478. doi:10.1200/jco.2014.56.0425

7. Epstein AS, Prigerson HG, O'Reilly EM, Maciejewski PK. Discussions of life expectancy and changes in illness understanding in patients with advanced cancer. *J Clin Oncol*. 2016;34(20):2398–2403. doi:10.1200/jco.2015.63.6696

8. Derry HM, Epstein AS, Lichtenthal WG, Prigerson HG. Emotions in the room: Common emotional reactions to discussions of poor prognosis and tools to address them. *Expert Rev Anticancer Ther*. 2019;19(8):689–696. doi:10.1080/14737140.2019.1651648

9. Epstein AS, Kakarala SE, Reyna VF, et al. Development of the Oncolo-GIST ("Giving Information Strategically & Transparently") Intervention Manual for oncologist skills training in advanced cancer prognostic information communication. *J Pain Symptom Manage*. 2021;62(1):10–19. doi:10.1016/j.jpainsymman.2020.11.023

10. Gawande A. *Being Mortal: Medicine and What Matters in the End*. New York: Macmillan, 2014.

11. Agarwal R, Epstein AS. Advance care planning and end-of-life decision making for patients with cancer. *Semin Oncol Nurs*. 2018;34(3):316–326. doi:10.1016/j.soncn.2018.06.012

12. Sean Morrison R. Advance directives/care planning: Clear, simple, and wrong. *J Palliat Med*. 2020;23(7):878–879. doi:10.1089/jpm.2020.0272

13. Back A, Arnold R, Tulsky J. Talking about serious news. In: *Mastering Communication with Seriously Ill Patients: Balancing Honesty with Empathy and Hope*. New York: Cambridge University Press; 2009: 21–38. doi:10.1017/cbo9780511576454.004

14. Radbruch L, De Lima L, Knaul F, et al. Redefining palliative care: A new consensus based definition. *J Pain Symptom Manage*. 2020;60(4):754–764.

15. Meghani SH, Byun E, Gallagher RM. Time to take stock: A meta-analysis and systematic review of analgesic treatment disparities for pain in the United States. *Pain Med*. 2012;13(2):150–174. doi:10.1111/j.1526-4637.2011.01310.x

16. "Cultural humility: Measuring openness to culturally diverse clients": Correction to Hook, Davis, Owen, Worthington, and Utsey. *J Couns Psychol*. 2015;62(1):iii–v. doi:10.1037/a0038582

17. Tervalon M, Murray-García J. Cultural humility versus cultural competence: A critical distinction in defining physician training outcomes in multicultural education. *J Health Care Poor Underserved*. 1998;9(2):117–125. doi:10.1353/hpu.2010.0233

18. Acquaviva K. *LGBT-Inclusive Hospice and Palliative Care: A Practical Guide to Transforming Professional Practice*. New York: Harrington Park Press; 2017.

19. Moore PM, Rivera Mercado S, Grez Artigues M, Lawrie TA. Communication skills training for healthcare professionals working with people who have cancer. *Cochrane Database Syst Rev*. 2013. doi:10.1002/14651858.cd003751.pub3

20. Boissy A, Windover AK, Bokar D, et al. Communication skills training for physicians improves patient satisfaction. *J Gen Intern Med*. 2016;31(7):755–761. doi:10.1007/s11606-016-3597-2

21. Wool MS. Teaching and learning communication skills in medicine (2e). *Health Expect*. 2005;8(4):363–365. doi:10.1111/j.1369-7625.2005.00351.x

22. Kissane DW, Bylund C, Banerjee SC, et al. Communication skills training for oncology professionals. *J Clin Oncol*. 2012;30(11):1242–1247.

23. Bylund CL, Banerjee SC, Bialer PA, et al. A rigorous evaluation of an institutionally-based communication skills program for post-graduate oncology trainees. *Patient Educ Couns*. 2018;101(11):1924–1933. doi:10.1016/j.pec.2018.05.026

24. Banerjee SC, Manna R, Coyle N, et al. The implementation and evaluation of a communication skills training program for oncology nurses. *Transl Behav Med.* 2017;7(3):615–623. doi:10.1007/s13142-017-0473-5

25. Ruggiero JE, Robinson CO, Paynter N. *Coordinated Learning to Improve Evidence-based Care: A Model for Continuing Education for the New Healthcare Environment.* 2015.

26. Institute of Medicine. *Delivering High-Quality Cancer Care: Charting a New Course for a System in Crisis.* Washington, DC: The National Academies Press; 2013.

27. Schaeffer C. Talk to me. *Oncology Issues,* 2016;31(1):45–52.

28. Bosworth HB, et al. The future of patient engagement in the oncology setting: How practical patient engagement recommendations and innovative inter-professional education can drive change. *J Particip Med,* 2017;9:e7.

14

Building Interdisciplinary Teams of Excellence

Jaroslava Salman, Juee Kotwal, and Matthew Loscalzo

Introduction

Advances in healthcare in the past several decades have highlighted an increasing need for high-quality palliative and supportive care. The ability of a well-built interdisciplinary team to address patients' supportive care needs and improve their quality of life has been evident. However, a team of experts does not guarantee the creation of a well-functioning team. Institutional culture and leadership's support, thoughtful recruitment of team members, and regular attention to team performance are some of the necessary ingredients required to establish and maintain a high-performing interdisciplinary group of experts. To maximize the benefits of teamwork, it is timely to develop democratic leadership models. One such leadership model, based on the values of courage and compassion and that fosters leadership at every level, is discussed. We would like the reader to become familiarized with not only what it takes to form, but also to sustain a successful interdisciplinary care team.

Brief History

If even in a cursory manner, to understand where palliative care came from, it is essential to understand its visionary founders. Beginning in the 1950s, Dame Cicely Saunders was instrumental in creating a model of hospice care, now more commonly called *palliative* and/or *supportive care*, from the values of hospice. Given her extensive experience with dying patients and prescient concept of "total pain" seen within a wider psychological, social, and spiritual context, the essential presence of coordinated team care was a natural and inevitable outcome. Given that Dr. Saunders was initially a social worker, then a nurse, and finally a physician, perhaps being a one-woman team enabled her to understand the depth, overlap, and unique features of this emerging new field that now went well beyond hospice. The opening of St. Christopher's Hospice in 1967, where patients were cared for inpatient and at home, created a model that would have robust benefits for patients and their grieving families. In Canada, in the mid 1970s, another pioneering giant, Dr. Balfour Mount, surgical oncologist, coined the term "palliative care" for the first time and was extremely influential in further extending the scope and vision of this emerging field. There were, of course, other highly influential pioneers who played critical leadership roles in the vision of palliative medicine and the increasingly accepted term "supportive care." It is important to note that in medicine, a field then dominated almost solely by men, most of these early leaders were women: Drs. Elizabet Kubler-Ross, Kathleen M. Foley, Susan Dale Block, Diane Meier, and, of course, others. Their perspective in seeing the person in context was, and still is, foundational as it relates to health and wellness, but more significantly, to the democratizing of teams. In addition to physicians, there were many others who were essential in creating and expanding this new field, especially from nursing, social work, psychology, pharmacy, spiritual care, and rehabilitation. Since the introduction of board certification in palliative medicine for physicians in 2006, other professions have followed suit and palliative and supportive care programs have proliferated, especially in Europe and North America.[1]

Interdisciplinary Care Team Composition

As outlined in the previous edition of this chapter, every team is uniquely composed to serve a specific purpose.[1] There is no one single definition of an interdisciplinary care team. It is not possible to talk about palliative care without recognizing that the term itself is too limiting and in some cases has become a barrier to greater uptake of such programs.[2] In this chapter, we use the term "palliative and supportive care" to be all inclusive and, for the purpose of this chapter, synonymous with interdisciplinary team care.

We offer this definition for consideration of the palliative and supportive care team:

> A specialist team that seeks to enhance care for patients with serious, complex illness and their families by helping them formulate goals of care, by managing symptoms and by addressing psychosocial and spiritual needs.[1]

A high-functioning team is comprised of a group of experts with diverse skills, abilities, talents, and experiences committed to working together based on shared values in striving to exceed the highest standards of medical, psychological, social, and spiritual care.[3] A comprehensive view of the patient as a whole person within their social context, with an emphasis on maximizing inherent strengths, forms the basis for the work of the team.

In 2004, the *Clinical Practice Guidelines for Quality Palliative Care*, released by the National Consensus Project, established the interdisciplinary team as the standard for delivering palliative care services.[4] The most recent guideline (2018) outlines the criteria for the interdisciplinary team and describes the roles of different team members who contribute their professional skills for the benefit of patients and families.[5] Physicians, advanced practice providers, nurses, social workers, chaplains, and pharmacists are identified as team members. Other specialists, including psychiatrists, psychologists, rehabilitation therapists, and other experts can also have key roles in addressing the comprehensive needs of patients and their families. The interdisciplinary care team works with other clinicians and community service providers supporting continuity of care throughout the illness trajectory and across all settings, especially during transitions of care.[5] Although most of the attention for the interdisciplinary team has been on clinical care, program development, research, and professional education are also major and increasingly important contributions. New requirements for licensing, certification, and continuing education reflect the growth in new and more effective treatment approaches, demand for evidence-based practice, and for teamwork. The result of greater recognition of palliative and supportive care as a specialty has also created expectations that interdisciplinary care teams will enhance quality and continuity of care, reduce costs, and humanize the illness experience. Arguments for the support of interdisciplinary care teams have been primarily financial, focused on savings through reduced pharmacy costs and lengths of stay, but quality, safety, market place competition, and consumer expectations (especially including the referring physicians and healthcare professionals) have also been powerful drivers of comprehensive programs. It is even more important to note that the accumulating evidence has demonstrated both increased quality and length of life as a result of palliative care involvement.[6] Given the breadth of the expectations for interdisciplinary care services, only a well-coordinated team can reach these goals.

Distress Screening: The First Step in Supportive and Palliative Care Integration

Much has been written about distress screening since the promulgation of the American College of Surgeons-Commission on Cancer guidelines were introduced, and since then about 75 national and international organizations have endorsed distress as the sixth vital sign.[7]

Although it is beyond the scope of this chapter to fully discuss distress screening, there are number of significant concerns about the limited range of the content overall: primary focus on psychological factors, unimaginative structure of the instruments to engage patients, struggles with operational implementation, and, not surprisingly, poor patient uptake.[8] Despite these shortcomings, comprehensive biopsychosocial screening has the potential to orient, inform, educate, focus, motivate, and triage patients and their families. In the context of interdisciplinary care, comprehensive biopsychosocial screening has the potential to be the *connective tissue of the healthcare system*.[9] Stover and Basch (2016) have demonstrated that symptom monitoring and management as patient-reported outcomes results in improved communications between clinicians and patients, detection of problematic symptoms, and satisfaction with care.[10] Comprehensive biopsychosocial screening is extremely important in how teams are comprised, function, and evaluated. Precision supportive care needs to be driven by personalized, real-time data, carefully tailored to the patient's strengths and resources, medical situation, treatment burden, and social milieu. The needs of the patient within their social support system and an objective assessment of the most valued preferences in the clinical setting are essential to know how to properly staff any interdisciplinary care team. Treating physicians are the gatekeepers in cancer care, and it is extremely helpful for them to personally experience the benefit of comprehensive biopsychosocial screening, otherwise dissemination and implementation may be a challenge. Screening needs to be integrated into clinic processes without causing disruption or adding to the complexity of the provision of disease-directed care. Benefits to patients and families need to be specific and valued by the treating team by assessing: risk for poor treatment adherence, financial toxicities, perceptions of prognosis, symptom management, available psychological services, tailored education, and need for referrals to consultants. The more integrated into existing processes and preferably automated systems, the better. Ultimately, the most valued asset, time, will almost always be a major influence on whether screening uptake will occur.

Buliding a Successful Interdisciplinary Team

Assembling a team of experts does not guarantee that the team will be successful. Experts, too, are only human, and they bring their personal and professional histories that can shape their interactions with others; this in turn can be influenced by the team itself. In other words, unconscious individual and group dynamics will play a powerful role in the team's life and success. Each team member's educational and professional history colors how they perceive other members on the team. Added influences of age, gender, race, and cultural differences among the team members can be a source of creativity and growth, but also of interpersonal conflict, not uncommonly rooted in unconscious bias. In general, conflict is only a problem when it is not seen as an opportunity for an honest and compassionate discussion.

Applying Team Science to Interdisciplinary Care Teams

Based on a review of the research, the following foundational elements for effective teamwork were identified:[11]

1. *Conditions/context*: Refer to stable team structure, colocation, team culture, defined roles with training and skills to reinforce those roles, standing orders and protocols, workflows, ground rules, modes of communication, etc.
2. *Cognition (shared vision)*: Implies mental models that are shared among team members for *how* and *why* the team works together. Clear goals for the team represent a key element of team cognition and unity in purpose. It is crucial that the team has an explicit and shared "mission and values" system that can serve as a frame of reference for all of team's interactions and task planning/execution, as well as team members' behaviors.

3. *Leadership/coaching*: High-functioning teams require effective leadership. Leadership is critical to establishing team goals and achieving shared understanding of what is needed to accomplish those goals, including how team members will coordinate their activities. Many high-functioning teams use *distributed leadership*, in which various team members have opportunities to enact informal leadership and coaching.

4. *Cooperation*: Represents the *motivational driver of teamwork*; that is, the attitudes, beliefs, and emotions of the team members. The foundation of cooperation is trust. Unresolved, unspoken conflicts subvert cooperation and hamper team performance. Trust involves a strong affective component and requires a climate of psychological safety. Allowing team members to voice and resolve conflict promotes a sense of psychological safety; that is, an interpersonal climate of trust and respect. Psychological safety is strongly linked to improved team performance, improved satisfaction, and lower burnout among team members. Establishing psychological safety is important for encouraging team members to speak up and express differences, for mutual coaching among team members, learning new skills, and assuming new team roles. When psychological safety is absent, team members avoid conflict, hesitate to assume risks, refrain from offering constructive feedback, and react defensively when feedback is given.[12,13] Psychological safety can be developed and enhanced through effective *team debriefs* and leadership communication. During debrief, members are taught to take a learning approach and diagnose areas in need of development and are more likely to feel comfortable speaking up. Practical ways of how to achieve these goals are addressed later in this chapter. Leaders also play an important role in fostering a psychologically safe environment. When leaders admit their own faults, they make others feel that they, too, can safely communicate errors they make.[14]

5. *Coordination*: The process of organizing different individuals' skills, behaviors, and knowledge to meet a combined goal.[14] Coordination is a key driver of outcomes involving the sequencing and timing of team's interdependent actions. Effective coordination requires trust in the abilities of team members to act according to a shared mental model. Structures and processes that facilitate team communication are vital to coordination.

6. *Communication*: Effective and efficient communication facilitates teamwork. Pre-patient huddles, post-session debriefs, and team meetings provide opportunities for face-to-face communication that promotes effective cooperation and coordination. Regular reflection on team performance (What went well? What didn't go well? What can we do to improve?) is critical to improve team coordination and adaptation to changing demands.

The COVID-19 pandemic introduced a plethora of challenges for teamwork, including alternative and virtual methods of meeting with team members. Despite the tragic deaths of so many people as a result of the COVID-19 and a cascade of related social and psychological crises, one of the major benefits for teams is the increased and enhanced use of technologies. Although the physical separation from colleagues can be stressful, people are

TABLE 14.1 Challenges and benefits of integrating technologies to teamwork

Challenges	Benefits/Opportunities
Missing the ritual of being in same space simultaneously	Ability to access the meeting from different workspaces
Inconsistent quality of audio/visual	No geographical limitations
Cost of hardware and programs	Democratizes interactions via Chats, Polls, open microphones
Not a single accepted platform nationally or internationally	Timely information from multiple sources
Difficulty navigating features of different platforms	Immediate access to information and data via screen sharing
Illusion of being able to multi-task and still participate in a meaningful way (i.e., camera turned off)	Ability to simultaneously work together on live documents in real-time

extremely adaptable. Please see Table 14.1 for a brief list of challenges and benefits/opportunities of integrating technologies to support teamwork.

Team Conflict

Difference in opinion leads to inquiry, and inquiry to truth.
—Thomas Jefferson

Healthy teams will inevitably experience varying degrees of creative tension and, at times, outright conflict. The term "conflict" often carries a negative connotation, but not all conflict is harmful. In fact, creative teamwork cannot happen without a healthy conflict of opinions. The avoidance of openly acknowledging and managing conflict as an opportunity for growth will make a problem worse. If the disagreement is acknowledged and respectfully addressed, it can propel the team toward improved decision-making, trust, and performance.

Types of team conflict can be broadly defined as *task-based* (disagreements over ideas and opinions related to the task), *relationship-based* (interpersonal disagreements), or *process-based* (disagreements over responsibilities and how to get the task done). Task conflict of moderate intensity may contribute to effective decision-making and team performance. Process and relationship conflicts are generally found to be negatively related to team outcomes.[15]

Conflict asymmetry refers to the existence of *different perceptions* among group members regarding the amount of conflict in their team. The asymmetry of conflict perception can be detrimental to group functioning. Resolving the conflict can only commence if team members at least agree that a problem exists.

Effective conflict resolution requires teammates to participate in open and honest communication. This can occur only if they do not feel worried about retaliation or being judged or ridiculed. Effective conflict resolution also requires curiosity about team members' perspectives, humility, and an ability to listen and convey understanding. It is amazing to see how quickly the clouds of conflict can part when people are willing to truly hear one another.

Power is the relative ability of an individual to control and influence others. It is a property of relationships between people, rather than a property of an individual. Social perceptions and behaviors are influenced by individuals' respective levels of power. Team members have different personal and professional backgrounds of knowledge and expertise, but they work together with high levels of interdependence on a common task. The diversity of a team can enhance team decision-making and performance by allowing for an exchange of information. But diversity may also raise the possibility—as a result of processes of categorization ("ingroup" and "outgroup") and intergroup bias (different education/training background, gender or age, etc.)—of destructive conflicts. Psychologically, the distinction between "ingroup" and "outgroup" is strong, and social identity theory explains that members of a professional group (e.g., medicine, nursing, or the allied health professions) tend to see the attributes of their group as positive and those of other groups as less desirable.[16] Individuals with strong professional identity are more profoundly driven by the priorities of their profession and more likely to feel threatened by pressure to accommodate alternative perspectives.[17]

Affect regulation refers to the control of team member's emotions during task interactions. It fosters emotional balance and effective coping with stressful demands and frustration. Given the likelihood of negative mood spreading throughout the team, it is important that emotional issues be dealt with in a timely fashion, rather than allowing prolonged and possibly escalating negative affect.[18]

Interpersonal behaviors, such as seeking help, speaking up, and the practice of using different perspectives, are important for intra-team communication, coordination, and conflict resolution. *Help seeking* is facilitated by a psychologically safe environment. *Speaking up* is important for decision-making in interdependent teams, and it, too, requires a psychologically safe environment. *Perspective-taking* behavior implies imagining the world from another's point of view. Persons with a high sense of power are less likely to consider the possibility that another person may not share the same level of knowledge. They are also less accurate in detecting the emotional states of other people. Trying to understand the view of another person promotes collaboration and interpersonal problem-solving ability and lowers interpersonal aggression.[19]

Team members may optimize interpersonal relations by preemptive conflict management, encouraging cooperative behavior and building team morale. Team members help build social support for each other by providing emotional support to other team members, which may be of two types: affective and task related. *Affective* support includes statements of social recognition or encouragement oriented toward providing emotional support. In contrast, *task-related* support consists of instrumental information provided to team members by one another.

Poorly performing teams tend to take an ad hoc approach to managing conflict, rarely correcting the root cause of conflict.[20] They also seldom, if ever, take the strengths-based prospective systematic approach to team building by investing time and psychological

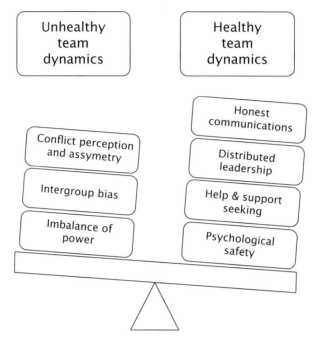

FIGURE 14.1 Balancing healthy and unhealthy team dynamics.

capital to create cohesion and trust by managing and utilizing conflict that is normal and to be expected in any group of individuals, never mind among team members in highly charged emotional environments. *Regular self-reflection practice*—debriefing with focus on specific events/issues on both individual and team levels—is essential for maintaining healthy team interactions and effectiveness in their daily tasks. Team members need to feel aligned around their shared values, benefits, and desired outcomes while supporting healthy interpersonal team dynamics (see Figure 14.1). How to channel conflict for strategic team growth with attention and intention is discussed later in this chapter.

Staff Recruitment

As elaborated in the previous edition of this chapter, choosing staff is the most important part of developing a successful team.[1] There is no shortage of smart people in healthcare. Yet hiring a very smart person is not the same as recruiting a new team member. Thoughtful recruitment of new staff for an interdisciplinary care team encourages the evolving team to elucidate the services they provide and to openly reevaluate and discuss shared values. In a healthcare system where the hiring process is cumbersome and bureaucratic, new positions may remain vacant for extended periods while the search process proceeds. There may be pressure to keep positions unfilled as a strategy to save money. Large caseloads, high stress, and the resulting physical exhaustion will eventually lead to frustration and, in some situations, demoralization. These forces may result in the temptation to hire someone quickly. In our experience, regardless of the reasons or motivations, the desire to engage a

TABLE 14.2 Traits and behaviors to look for when hiring a new team member

Traits	Behaviors
Intellectual curiosity/openness to experience	Reliable and trustworthy
Positive perspective on life	Helpful and supportive to others
Altruism	Willing to be patient and family centered
Emotional Self-awareness	History of functioning well in teams
Commitment to values and ideals of one's discipline	Conscientious and professional
Psychological maturity and ability to self-regulate	Energized by professional accomplishment rather than praise

"warm body" must be resisted. The team needs to support each other in clearly delineating and effectively communicating to hospital administration the negative impact and difficult choices to be made by a prolonged reduction in staff. Unrealistic demands on the team should be openly rejected by the team.

Table 14.2 outlines the ideal personality traits and behaviors important for effective team functioning. This is by no means an exhaustive list of desirable characteristics of a team member, but it is important to consider when forming an interdisciplinary, task-interdependent team.

Because resumes reflect only basic educational and knowledge-based screening requirements of human resource departments, the character traits of candidates must be evaluated through interviewing and careful discussions with references who have directly observed the candidate.

It is prudent to develop systematic approaches that are specifically tailored to the position to be filled. The most important indicator of "team-ness" is past performance. Be sure to talk with former colleagues. Use consensus rather than voting to make hiring decisions. Once recruited, staff needs to be trained for the work, and this must start from day one and be consistent with the recruitment experience. Prospective team members may have been chosen because they have the right orientation, but they may need basic training and education in supportive and palliative care. In addition, continuing education will be required on an ongoing basis. Courses are now offered in many places that are both interdisciplinary and discipline-specific. Time and funding will need to be allotted. Do not expect new team members to just "learn on the job." Clinical attachments to existing palliative and supportive care services in other institutions or hospice programs may provide more than just education and training.

New staff will want to develop mentoring relationships to answer questions and provide support. In addition to the core competencies, new interdisciplinary team staff will need time and support to understand how to address issues related to the culture of the institution. For example, the culture of how physicians communicate with one another is unwritten yet complex. It is likely to be a mystery to a nurse or social worker. It will need explicit explanation and coaching to effectively engage. Similarly, nursing culture and social work culture, as well as the administrative culture in an institution, need explicit deconstruction and coaching for those who have not learned it yet. Time needs to be set aside to assess the developmental process of becoming confident and competent in new roles and with teamwork.

A successful interdisciplinary care team does not work in a vacuum. It is part of a larger department and institution, which also have their organizational dynamics. Basic assumptions (i.e., widely adapted beliefs about the culture of the institution) can powerfully shape the organizational culture and impact the experience of people and teams working within it. These dynamic forces can be implicit and unconscious or more apparent—just as in any organized group of people living and working together. The organization itself must be aligned to support teamwork and collaboration. Institutional leadership is essential in providing structural and cultural support for a well-functioning interdisciplinary care team. It is the top leadership that sends the signal that teamwork matters.[14] However, it does not mean that supportive and palliative care teams cannot create their own culture that actively supports superb teamwork. It does mean that the team must be aware that others in the institution, including the people to whom they report, may not share the skills or values to communicate in such an evolved professional manner.

Culture of Staff Leadership: Making Healthcare Settings Healthier

The previous version of this chapter provided an overview of characteristics of a high-functioning interdisciplinary care team.[1] The staff leadership model is one such democratizing approach to create infrastructure and is described elsewhere.[21]

In this update, the focus is on going deeper into the essential foundational elements to creating healthy team cultures. Healthy teams have the potential to transform healthcare settings by maximizing the diverse strengths of all team members while, with intention, promoting diversity, equity, and inclusion.

The essence of effective team work is building and sustaining high-quality relationships: "None of us are more or less important than anyone else, and ultimately our work is grounded in an ethic of caring for the wellbeing of others and respecting individual self-determination in the context of the collective good."[22] The staff leadership model is a systematic approach to create a culture in which all team members are expected to be leaders in their own areas and actively encourage all colleagues to create healthier environments for teams and healthcare settings.[21] The approach focuses on building trust among team members through personal accountability and providing feedback courageously and compassionately to bring out the best in each other. Interdisciplinary care professionals have the training, skills, and commitment to provide compassionate care by deeply engaging with patients and families. The goal is to leverage these skills and temperament as engagement guideposts with colleagues to maximize wellness and create healthy environments.

To our knowledge, in 2007, the Department of Supportive Care Medicine at the City of Hope National Medical Center developed the first staff leadership model in the country. Courage, compassion, direct and honest one-to-one communication, and commitment to

TABLE 14.3 Systematic cultural transformation: Accountability at individual, team, and leadership levels

Individuals	Teams	Leaders
• Ways of Working I am personally accountable for: **D- Depersonalizing** and letting go of unhelpful personal stories **S-Skills-** Using my active listening and assertion skills, including 3 part "I" statements ("When you . . . I feel . . . Because . . . ") **C- Communicating** directly, respectfully, and honestly **M- Modeling** positive reinforcement and feedback in the moment, while remaining committed to one another's success	• **Value Driven Strategic Small Group Process**[23] o Ground rules are based on Ways of Working o Focus is on agreed upon core values o Each team member gets a turn to speak by going around o Team members take turns running meetings • **Regularly Scheduled Team Check In** o How am I doing on this team? o What can I do (specific behaviors) to be a better team member? o Ongoing feedback on agreed-upon behaviors or commitments • **Brainstorming by specific problem (see Table 14.4)** o Name it, discuss it, and manage it	• **Aspire to inspire**[23] o Aspire to create a shared vision and mission o Inspire team members through role modelling o Invite a deeper level of feedback • **Value Driven Staff Leadership Meeting** o 85% Staff Led/15% Supervisors o "Open mike" format: • Open expression of rational and irrational concerns or fears • Feedback on what we can be doing better • Staff recognition of accomplishments, support to colleagues and valued behaviors • Request to keep cameras on (virtual meeting) • **Staff-planned and led annual department retreat** o Project-focused work teams with clearly stated expectations and outcomes

be one's best self are the foundational values of the staff leadership model. Specific processes and systems implemented to integrate accountabilities at individual, team, and leadership levels are listed (see Tables 14.3 and 14.4).

TABLE 14.4 Brainstorming by specific problems (name it, discuss it, manage it)

Name it	Discuss it	Manage it
Specific problem clearly identified o What do we know about the problem?	**Team brainstorming ways to best manage problem using the small-group meeting process**[3] • **C**reativity • **O**ptimism • **P**lanning • **E**xpert information	**Plan** • Strategies prioritized by least effort and most effective outcome • Team and Individual Commitments to trying specific ways to personally cope and to support the healthiest and courageous parts of each other • Scheduled meetings to track progress

---

BOX 14.1 Channeling conflict for strategic team growth

1. **Courage**
   a. Caring enough about the other person to give them helpful information
   b. Acting on your best judgement, despite the challenges ahead
2. **Compassion**
   a. Connect with curiosity
   b. Taking personal initiative to understand the other person's perceptions and experiences
   c. Owning and sharing your own perspective and feelings using "I" statements
3. **Commitment**
   a. Agreeing on specific behaviors that lead to being proud of ourselves and each other
   b. Inviting ongoing feedback on agreed upon behaviors

Channeling Conflict for Strategic Team Growth

The staff leadership model principles serve as guideposts in unleashing the best and healthiest parts of team members in times of conflict. The goal is to use conflict as a vehicle for self- reflection and mutual growth by creating a no-blame/no-shame environment (see Box 14.1).

Sustaining Staff Leadership Model: Team Deep Dives

The staff leadership model integrates courageous and compassionate honest and direct feedback in all interactions. Regularly scheduled deep-dive check-ins (see Box 14.2) to provide honest/direct feedback on specific behaviors are a sign of a healthy team. Ability to create space and time for deep dives is important to sustain and reinforce staff leadership programs.

Future Directions

High-quality interdisciplinary care is here to stay, and the need for it will only grow in the future. Expanding research in team functioning, organizational psychology, diversity, and unconscious bias will continue to enrich our knowledge about the necessary ingredients of a successful team of experts. Recent advances in technology introduced novel modes of team meetings and care delivery. This will enhance further expansion of care provision, but will also demand flexibility, openness, and more diverse forms of communication within the team. The challenge is to evolve into new ways of working without compromising what is by its very nature a humanistic, rewarding, and emotionally demanding experience.

BOX 14.2 Deep-dive check-in

We are asking that every team member be ready to address the following at the deep-dive session:

1. **The individual**: (up to 2 minutes)
   a. How am I showing up for this team?
      - Please reflect on your strengths and areas of growth in interpersonal interactions and communications within this team.

Following each individual self-reflection:

2. **Each team member responds** (2 min each). **Please identify at least one specific behavior that the individual could benefit from. In addition, please consider the following methods of providing feedback:**
   a. Add a substantive comment on any specific behaviors identified by the individual
   b. Say "I agree" and specify "what" you are agreeing to
   c. Recognize progress related to a specific behavior
   d. Say "pass" if you have nothing substantive to add

Repeat Steps 1 and 2 for each team member.

Key Points

- Supportive and palliative care, like cancer care, is always a team affair. Choosing the right team members is more important than agreeing on lists of what each team member does.
- Role blurring and distributed leadership should be encouraged as part of the high-functioning team.
- There is a need to develop more democratic leadership models that encourage leadership at every level and in which leaders aspire to inspire colleagues.
- A commitment to assessing and addressing team function as a part of routine work will ensure that inevitable tensions and disagreements are openly and honestly discussed and team function enhanced.
- Conflict should not be avoided but expected and used as an opportunity for self-reflection, learning, and team growth.

References

1. Loscalzo MJ, von Gunten CF. Interdisciplinary teamwork in palliative care: Compassionate expertise for serious illness. In: Chochinov HM, Breitbart W, eds. *Handbook of Psychiatry in Palliative Medicine.* 2nd ed. New York: Oxford University Press; 2009:172–185.
2. Jordan K, Aapro M, Kaasa S, et al. European Society for Medical Oncology (ESMO) position paper on supportive and palliative care. *Ann Oncol.* 2018;29:36–43.

3. Arber A. Team meetings in specialist palliative care: Asking questions as a strategy within interprofessional interaction. *Qual Health Res.* 2008;18:1323–1335.

4. National Consensus Project for Quality Palliative Care: Clinical practice guidelines for quality palliative care, executive summary. *J Palliat Med.* 2004;7:611–627.

5. Ferrell BR, Twaddle ML, Melnick A, Meier DE. National Consensus Project Clinical Practice Guidelines for Quality Palliative Care Guidelines, 4th Edition. *J Palliat Med.* 2018;21:1684–1689.

6. Temel JS, Greer JA, Muzikansky A, et al. Early palliative care for patients with metastatic non-small-cell lung cancer. *N Engl J Med.* 2010; 363: 733–742.

7. Bultz B, Loscalzo MJ, Clark KL. Screening for distress, the 6th vital sign, as the connective tissue of health care systems: A roadmap to integrated interdisciplinary person-centered care. In: Grassi L, Riba M, eds. *Clinical Psycho-oncology: An International Perspective.* West Sussex: John Wiley & Sons; 2012:83–96.

8. Fradgley EA, Byrnes E, McCarter K, et al. A cross-sectional audit of current practices and areas for improvement of distress screening and management in Australian cancer services: Is there a will and a way to improve? *Support Care Cancer.* 2020; 28: 249–259.

9. Bultz BD, Loscalzo MJ, Mitchell AJ, Holland JC. Distress, the sixth vital sign: A catalyst for standardizing psychosocial care globally. In: Breitbart W, Butow P, Jacobsen P, Lam W, Lazenby M, Loscalzo M, eds. *Psycho-Oncology.* 4th ed. New York: Oxford University Press; 2021:801–805.

10. Stover AM, Basch EM. Implementation of symptom questionnaires into oncology workflow. *J Oncol Pract.* 2016;12:859–862.

11. Fiscella K, Mauksch L, Bodenheimer T, Salas E. Improving care teams' functioning: Recommendations from team science. *Jt Comm J Qual Patient Saf.* 2017;43:361–368.

12. Nutting PA, Crabtree BF, McDaniel RR. Small primary care practices face four hurdles--including a physician-centric mind-set--in becoming medical homes. *Health Aff (Millwood).* 2012;31:2417–2422.

13. True G, Stewart GL, Lampman M, Pelak M, Solimeo SL. Teamwork and delegation in medical homes: primary care staff perspectives in the Veterans Health Administration. *J Gen Intern Med.* 2014;29 Suppl 2:S632–639.

14. Salas E, Reyes DL, McDaniel SH. The science of teamwork: Progress, reflections, and the road ahead. *Am Psychol.* 2018;73:593–600.

15. Janss R, Rispens S, Segers M, Jehn KA. What is happening under the surface? Power, conflict and the performance of medical teams. *Med Educ.* 2012;46:838–849.

16. Weller J, Boyd M, Cumin D. Teams, tribes and patient safety: Overcoming barriers to effective teamwork in healthcare. *Postgrad Med J.* 2014;90:149–154.

17. Mitchell R, Parker V, Giles M, Boyle B. The ABC of health care team dynamics: Understanding complex affective, behavioral, and cognitive dynamics in interprofessional teams. *Health Care Manage Rev.* 2014;39:1–9.

18. Driskell JE, Salas E, Driskell T. Foundations of teamwork and collaboration. *Am Psychol.* 2018;73:334–348.

19. Bazerman MH, Curhan JR, Moore DA, Valley KL. Negotiation. *Annu Rev Psychol.* 2000;51:279–314.

20. Behfar KJ, Peterson RS, Mannix EA, Trochim WM. The critical role of conflict resolution in teams: A close look at the links between conflict type, conflict management strategies, and team outcomes. *J Appl Psychol.* 2008;93:170–188.

21. Loscalzo M, Clark K, Bultz B, Kotwal J. Building supportive care teams: Working together and self care. In: Breitbart W, Butow P, Jacobsen P, Lam W, Lazenby M, Loscalzo M, eds. *Psycho-Oncology.* 4th ed. New York: Oxford University Press; 2021:775–781.

22. Atkins PWB, Wilson DS, Hayes SC, Ryan RM. *Prosocial: Using Evolutionary Science to Build Productive, Equitable, and Collaborative Groups.* Oakland: Context Press; 2019.

23. Loscalzo M, Clark K, Bultz B, Kotwal J. Integrating interdisciplinary supportive care programs: Transforming the culture of cancer car. In: Breitbart W, Butow P, Jacobsen P, Lam W, Lazenby M, Loscalzo M, eds. *Psycho-Oncology.* 4th ed. New York: Oxford University Press; 2021:775–781.

15

Psychosocial Benefits of Early Palliative Care Intervention

Carrie C. Wu, Jennifer Temel, and William Pirl

Introduction to Early Integrated Palliative and Oncology Care

Palliative care has been a rapidly changing medical specialty in recent decades, undergoing evolution in how it is defined and how it is delivered. In 1990, the World Health Organization (WHO) first characterized palliative care as the active total care of patients whose diseases are not responsive to curative treatment. The main focus of care centered on end-of-life care.[1] However, problems arising at the end of life often originate from an earlier time in the course of illness, and symptoms are more easily managed if treated at onset rather than waiting until the last stages of care. In 2002, the WHO revised its definition of palliative care and recommended its delivery as early as possible for any chronic, ultimately fatal illness and emphasized that it could and should be provided in conjunction with any life-prolonging treatment.[2] Additionally, even among patients who are not struggling with significant symptoms early on, early palliative care could provide anticipatory guidance.

While the WHO definition of palliative care changed, clinical care models needed to evolve before the concept of early palliative care could be applied in practice. Palliative care programs were primary inpatient services which focused on hospitalized patient populations often in crisis or at the end of life, making it difficult to shift care to earlier in the disease trajectory. When Hui et al. looked at the state of availability for palliative care at comprehensive cancer centers, they found that while most cancer centers reported the availability of a palliative care program, many were limited to inpatient care.[3] Less than half of the cancer centers offered outpatient palliative care services. The emergence of more outpatient palliative care clinics allowed for earlier referrals to palliative care and the development of integrated models.

Despite greater availability of outpatient palliative care clinics, several misconceptions regarding palliative care still exist among medical providers. Some may not have clear understandings of how palliative care is different from hospice services. For example, there may be concerns that an early palliative care referral would alarm patients and caregivers or that palliative care providers might prematurely focus on discussions about death. A study on medical oncologists' attitudes and referral practices demonstrates that hematologic oncologists are more likely to hold these misconceptions compared to solid tumor oncologists and that 30% of hematologic oncologists have never referred patients to palliative care.[4] However, several studies have shown that early delivery of palliative care led to improvement in quality of life, symptom relief, psychological outcomes, patient satisfaction, and possibly even survival.[5–11] With growing evidence from multiple randomized clinical trials, the American Society of Clinical Oncology (ASCO) released recommendations that both inpatients and outpatients with advanced cancer should receive dedicated palliative care services early in the disease course, concurrent with active treatment.[12,13]

Delivery of Early Integrated Palliative and Oncology Care

Early integrated palliative and oncology care can be delivered in a variety of ways, and there is immense variation among location, staffing, patient volume, and level of integration.[14] By definition, it occurs earlier in the course of illness and is concurrent with cancer care. While the timing may be a distinguishing factor, the earlier timing of referrals also shape the focus and delivery of care. Models of early integrated palliative and oncology care services described in clinical trials include early consultations with a specialty palliative care team and nurse-led phone interventions.[5] Some models could even be considered co-management of patients by oncologists and palliative care providers. However, across the models, common features include psychoeducation and counseling, particularly regarding prognosis and coping; symptom management; and medical decision-making and end-of-life planning. Not all of these topics are addressed in every encounter. The longitudinal nature of early integrated palliative and oncology care allows these to unfold over time, in the context of a trusting relationship which is built before crises are encountered.

One model of early integrated palliative and oncology care dissected the focus and contents of visits longitudinally from close to metastatic cancer diagnosis to the end of life, to highlight processes of how early palliative care is delivered to patients.[15] Table 15.1 illustrates the elements. The initial visits are primarily social and informational, allowing for relationship and rapport building. During these visits, the palliative care provider establishes patients' understanding of their illness, awareness of their prognosis, and preferences for information and care. Symptom monitoring and coping with illness are key components in both early and subsequent visits. The quality-of-life benefits of early integrated palliative and oncology care have been shown to be mediated by changes in patients' coping styles over time.[16] Later in the course of illness, the visits begin to focus more on changes in illness

TABLE 15.1 Description of key elements of ambulatory PC clinic visits over time

TIMING AND ELEMENTS OF PC VISITS	Description
	INITIAL VISITS
Relationship and rapport building	Learn about patients "who they are" in their social context, their background, support system, work, and interests.
Establishing illness understanding: information preference	Elicit how patients prefer information to be delivered and who should be involved in decision-making.
Establishing illness understanding: prognostic awareness	Elicit from patients their perspective and understanding of their prognosis.
Discussing cancer treatment: effect	Discuss the effect of cancer treatment on patients' lives and address any hopes, worries, or concerns.
	ALL VISITS
Addressing symptoms	Conduct a general symptom review (e.g., nausea, pain, etc.) and address with pharmacologic and/or nonpharmacologic options.
Addressing coping	Check in with patient on their emotional state, discuss coping strategies, and problem-solve. Assess whether patient needs additional mental health support.
Establishing illness understanding: current illness status	Discuss with patient current disease status and elicit understanding of the ongoing surveillance and treatment plan. Elicit from patients their understanding of changing prognosis and illness status if relevant.
Engaging family members	Learn about the patient's support system and assess for caregiver understanding and their own needs. Prepare family members with any resources they might need to support the patient.
	LAST VISITS
Discussing cancer treatment: decision making	Discuss any changes to cancer treatment plans (stop, break, or change), explore rationale, and patients' response.
End of life planning	Explore patients' priorities and preferences for wishes at the end of life. Referral to hospice when appropriate.

Adapted from Yoong et al.[15]

status, patients' understanding of these changes, and evolving decision-making with cancer treatment and end-of-life planning.

Impact of Early Integrated Palliative and Oncology Care on Psychosocial Domains

While specific models of care may vary, randomized clinical trials have demonstrated the impact of early integrated palliative and oncology care across several psychosocial domains, including health-related quality of life and psychological factors. Although healthcare utilization is not traditionally considered as a psychosocial outcome, it has been used as an indicator of the quality of end-of-life care and to further describe final experiences of individuals.

Quality of Life

Quality of life is the primary target of all palliative care interventions, including early integrated palliative and oncology care. With a terminal illness, quality of life tends to decline in the last year of life, with a steep decline in the final 2–3 months. Given that symptoms can amplify over time with chronicity, early integrated palliative and oncology care presents an opportunity to better manage symptoms as early as possible rather than waiting until they are severe or difficult to control.

In 2009, Bakitas et al. led Project ENABLE (Educate, Nurture, Advise, Before Life Ends) II, a randomized controlled trial in which 322 newly diagnosed patients with advanced cancers were assigned to a palliative care intervention concurrent with oncology care or standard oncology care.[5] Using an education and case management approach, the intervention provided by Project ENABLE II involved an advanced practice nurse with palliative care specialty training who followed the patient with periodic assessment and education. Patients had access to group appointments with a palliative care physician and nurse practitioner and could be referred to palliative care team if needed. In this trial, patients who received concurrent palliative and oncology interventions had higher quality of life as measured by the Functional Assessment of Chronic Illness Therapy (FACIT-Pal) compared with patients who received standard oncology care.[5] Subsequently, in a study of 151 patients newly diagnosed with advanced non-small cell lung cancer, Temel et al. randomized patients to receive either early integrated palliative and oncology care or standard oncology care alone.[6] Patients assigned to early integrated palliative and oncology care met with a member of the palliative care team, and additional visits were as needed. In this study, Temel et al. found that patients who received early integrated palliative and oncology care had a better quality of life based on multiple subscales than patients assigned to standard care. At 12 weeks, patients receiving early palliative care interventions scored significantly higher on the Functional Assessment of Cancer Therapy-Lung scale (FACT-L), which assesses multiple dimensions of the quality of life, including physical, functional, emotional, and social well-being; the Lung-Cancer Subscale (LCS), which looks at seven symptoms specific to lung cancer; and the Trial Outcome Index (TOI), which is the sum of the scores on the LCS and the physical well-being and functional well-being subscales of the FACT-L.

The quality-of-life benefits of early integrated palliative and oncology care were shown to extend to other cancers as well. Zimmerman et al. studied the effects of early palliative care on quality of life among those with breast or prostate cancer.[8] They found that, among 461 patients with either stage IV cancer or patients with stage III cancer and poor clinical prognosis, there was a significant improvement in the Quality of Life at the End of Life scale (QUAL-E) that looks at domains of life completion, effect of symptoms, relationship with health provider, and preparation for end of life; the Functional Assessment of Chronic Illness Therapy-Spiritual Well-Being (FACIT-Sp), which measures quality of life including physical, social and family, emotional, functional, and spiritual domains; and the Edmonton Symptom Assessment System (ESAS), which contains numerical anchors for pain, fatigue, drowsiness, nausea, anxiety, depression, appetite, dyspnea, and well-being at 4 months. El-Jawahri et al. found that early integrated palliative and oncology care, in an inpatient setting, improved the quality of life in patients undergoing hematopoietic stem cell transplants.[17] Among 160 adults with hematologic malignancies admitted for stem cell transplants, patients were randomized to either receive inpatient palliative care or standard transplant care. Patients who received inpatient palliative care services scored higher on quality of time measurement based on the Functional Assessment of Cancer Therapy-Bone Marrow Transplant (FACT-BMT) at both 2 weeks after and 3 months after transplant. Temel et al. expanded their original patient population and looked at a larger cohort of patients with varying cancer types, including incurable lung and non-colorectal GI cancers.[10] A total of 350 patients were assigned to either early palliative care intervention or usual care. Across the entire sample, there was a nonsignificant improvement at 12 weeks and a significant improvement at 24 weeks on the FACT-G. When the samples were broken down based on cancer type, lung cancer appeared to have significant improvement in quality of life at both 12 weeks and 24 weeks, while there was no significant improvement noted for the GI cancers.

A trial of early integrated palliative and oncology care by Vanbutsele et al. found significant improvements in quality of life in patients with different types of advanced solid cancers at 12 weeks and 18 weeks based on the global health status/quality of life score by EORTC QLQ C30 and by the MQOL Single-Item Scale, but not at 24 weeks.[11] The loss of significant improvement sustained at 24 weeks was thought likely due to loss of power from patients who died or stopped responding. Additionally, among symptom scales on the EORTC QLQ-C30, there were significant improvement in fatigue and diarrhea at 18 weeks, but no significant differences among other symptoms or other times.

Additional models of early palliative care interventions, such as primary palliative care interventions in which oncology clinicians delivered the palliative care interventions, have also been identified in the ASCO recommendations.[18,19] Using the Functional Assessment of Cancer Therapy-General (FACT-G), Dyar et al. demonstrated significant improvement in quality of life among patients assigned to a palliative care intervention with an oncology advanced registered nurse practitioner compared to those who receive standard oncology care.[18] Ferrell et al. used an interdisciplinary palliative care intervention for patients with non-small cell lung cancer, where a nurse led the baseline assessment and provided education over time, and patients were presented weekly at an interdisciplinary meeting where various team members were able to provide recommendations to the primary treating oncologist.[19] Using this interdisciplinary team approach, Ferrell demonstrated improved quality of life for the intervention group with significantly higher scores on FACT-L, LCS, and the TOI compared to standard oncology care.

Based on the various types of early palliative care intervention models used to improve quality of life, these findings suggest that ongoing quality of life assessments, interdisciplinary care coordination, and patient education are key components to supporting the patient. The palliative care interventions may be provided by either specialty palliative care providers or oncology providers. A team-based or case-management model may be particularly helpful for populations where specialty palliative care providers are limited.

Psychosocial Distress

Psychological and psychosocial distress is also a target for all palliative care interventions, including early integrated palliative and oncology care. Psychological distress is common among individuals with advancer cancer and other serious illnesses. Estimates of clinically meaningful level of depression are reported to be 12.9% among individuals across cancer types and subclinical level of depression to be 29.4%.[20] This is especially pertinent because depression appears to be associated with increased mortality but not disease progression among patients with cancer,[21] and there appears to be an increased suicide risk in the year following cancer diagnosis.[22] Estimated rates of anxiety are even higher, with studies reporting clinically meaningful levels of anxiety in 19% individuals with cancer and subclinical levels of anxiety in 41.6% of individuals with cancer.[20] Early palliative care interventions play an important role in managing psychosocial distress in individuals receiving treatment for serious illnesses by providing additional space and time for relationship-building and more thorough assessment of their coping processes. Palliative care encounters provide key opportunities for clinicians to learn more about the patient, provide counseling, introduce psychosocial resources, and make the appropriate referrals to psychiatry, social work, and spiritual care colleagues, if needed.

The evidence seems to support psychological benefits from early palliative care interventions, although additional studies would be beneficial. For example, the ENABLE II trial demonstrated lower depressed mood using the Center for Epidemiological Studies-Depression (CES-D) scale for those who received early palliative care intervention compared to standard care.[5] The Temel trial from 2010 found that, among all patients, those who received early palliative care services had significantly lower depressive symptoms (measured by the Hospital Anxiety and Depression [HADS-D] and Patient Health Questionnaire [PHQ9]) at 12 weeks compared to patients who received only standard oncology care.[6] Looking specifically at those who met criteria for depression at baseline, patients who received early integrated palliative and oncology care were more likely to have had improvement in their depression at 12 weeks.[23] Rates of antidepressant medication use and mental health referrals were not significantly different among the patients with depression in both trial arms, suggesting that early integrated palliative and oncology care itself might be an intervention for depression. This may be especially meaningful because the distress tends to be the among the highest in the early few months after initial diagnosis. Additionally, El-Jawahri and colleagues also found that early integrated palliative and oncology care led to the development of less depression in patients undergoing hematopoietic stem cell transplantation in a randomized controlled trial.[17] However, the effect of early integrated palliative and oncology care on depression has not been found in all studies. The 2017 trial by Temel and colleagues failed to show significant differences in HADS-D and PHQ9 scores at 12 weeks or 24 weeks, but did show significant improvement in PHQ9 when using the terminal decline model and looking at patients 2 or 4 months before death.[10] Despite an observed increased number of consultations with psychologists, the trial by Vanbutsele and colleagues also found no significant change in depression at 12 weeks, 18 weeks, or 24 weeks in either depression on the HADS-D or PHQ9.[11]

The impact of early integrated palliative and oncology care on anxiety is less clear. While it would seem that the processes involved in early integrated palliative and oncology care would lessen anxiety, there is currently no consistent supporting evidence for that supposition. Notably, neither the two trials by Temel and colleagues[6,10] nor the trial by Vanbutsele and colleagues showed significant changes in anxiety measured the HADS-A.[11] The lack of observed improvement could possibly be related to measurement issues, and future trials should consider additional instruments for anxiety. Of note, the trial by El-Jawahri showed reduction in anxiety at 2 weeks after hematopoietic stem cell transplantation, but the significance of effect was not sustained at 3 months.[17] What is different about the El-Jawahri trial is that the palliative care intervention was provided in the inpatient setting, where the palliative care clinician followed-up on patients at least twice per week while the patient was hospitalized. One possible explanation could be that anxiety disorders tend to be more chronic while mood disorders tend to be episodic in pattern.

Interestingly, early integrated palliative and oncology care might influence the development of posttraumatic stress disorder (PTSD) in patients who survive intensive treatments for serious illnesses. The El-Jawahri trial found lower rates of PTSD symptoms 3 months after hematopoietic stem cell transplantation in patients who received early integrated palliative and oncology care.[17] Based on previous work demonstrating the relationship between quality of life, depression, and anxiety during the hematopoietic stem cell transplant hospitalization and PTSD at 6 months after transplant,[24] better management of the side effects during the transplant, both physical and mental, may have led to the decreased risk of developing PTSD symptoms later.

Coping

Although several trials have included psychosocial distress as an outcome, there has been little attention on how underlying coping skills or styles might be influenced by early palliative care. In a secondary analysis of the 2017 Temel trial, Greer et al. reported that patients with advanced lung and GI cancers who were randomized to early palliative care had greater use of approach-oriented coping at 24 weeks.[16] Approach-oriented coping includes active coping, use of emotional support, positive reframing, and acceptance. Furthermore, in mediational analyses, greater use of approach-oriented coping may have contributed to the observed quality of life improvements from early integrated palliative and oncology care. This is particularly noteworthy because it suggests a potential underlying psychosocial mechanism for the improvement in quality of life from early integrated palliative and oncology care.

Spiritual Well-Being

In addition to the physical and psychosocial, assessment and management of spiritual concerns is a key component of palliative care as defined by the WHO.[2] Spirituality itself may be broadly defined, ranging from religious beliefs to existential issues as a way of seeking meaning to one's experience. Among oncology patients receiving palliative care services, there is evidence to suggest that greater spiritual well-being is associated with better physical, emotional, and functioning wellbeing.[25] Additionally, higher spiritual well-being is associated with lower levels of uncertainty and conflict in medical decision-making. The randomized trial by Zimmerman and colleagues from 2014 on early palliative care interventions specifically used the Functional Assessment of Chronic Illness Therapy-Spiritual Well-Being (FACIT-Sp) scale as a trial outcome that included spiritual domains in additional to physical, social and family, emotional, and functional.[8] While there was no significant difference at 3 months in FACIT-Sp between patients who received early palliative care interventions and patients who received standard oncology care, there was a significant improvement in spiritual well-being as measured by the FACIT-Sp at 4 months for patients who received early palliative care interventions. Spiritual well-being is a particularly relevant measure for patients struggling with life-changing or life-threatening diagnoses in which they are more likely to face existential concerns.

Healthcare Utilization

Through the 1990s, rates of admission for patients with cancer to the hospital, emergency department (ED), and intensive care unit have been increasing, especially in the final month of life.[26,27] Trends in the aggressiveness of care at the end of life continued to climb over the years in a study of Medicare patients from 2006 to 2011[28] and among the VA population from 2009 to 2016.[29]

There is some evidence that early integrated palliative and oncology care may be helpful in curbing aggressiveness of care and improving the quality of end-of-life care without compromising survival.[6,7] Some of the trials have included metrics for quality of end-of-life care as secondary or exploratory outcomes. These quality metrics for end-of-life care, developed with input from providers, patients, and caregivers, focus on the overuse of potentially futile treatments and the underuse of supportive resources in the time immediately before death. These may include no administration of chemotherapy in the last 14 days of life, enrollment in hospice, and length of stay in hospice being greater than 7 days.

Supplementary data from Temel showed that patients with advanced non-small cell lung cancer assigned to early integrated palliative and oncology care compared to standard care alone were less likely to receive any chemotherapy within the last 14 days of life (17.5% vs. 24%), less likely to be admitted (36.7% vs. 53.6%), and less likely to visit the ED (22.4% vs. 30.4%).[6] In the same cohort, Greer et al. found that early palliative care had lower rate of chemotherapy use (0.47 odds ratio) within 60 days of death compared with standard care.[7] More specifically, early palliative care reduced the use of an intravenous chemotherapy regimen within 60 days of death (24.2% vs. 46.3%). Among patients assigned to early palliative care who received intravenous chemotherapy as their final regimen, there was a longer treatment-free interval between patients' last infusion dose and death (median of 64 days vs. 40.5 days), with no negative effect on survival. Patients assigned to early palliative care were also more likely to receive hospice longer than 1 week (60% vs. 33.3%) and received hospice for a longer period time overall (median of 24 days vs. 9.5 days).

Caregivers

Caregivers are an essential part of the team for patients with serious illnesses. They may help with scheduling, transportation, medication administration, and day-to-day tasks like cleaning and preparing meals. The roles are multitude and diverse. Caregivers for those with serious illnesses such as cancer are more likely to struggle with depression and anxiety.[30,31] With its focus on the family and not just the patient, palliative care has the potential to improve outcomes for caregivers as well as patients. Providing early integrated palliative and oncology care services may be a crucial opportunity to provide caregivers education, relieve symptom burden, and facilitate some difficult conversations that caregivers may be too overwhelmed to begin.

Several studies examined the effect of early integrated palliative and oncology care on caregiver outcomes. While significant improvements in the quality of life have not been observed, early integrated palliative and oncology care appears to improve some psychological distress and satisfaction with care in caregivers.[32–34] The nursing-led ENABLE III randomized controlled trial studied the effects on caregivers for patients with various advanced cancers using a caregiver-directed intervention and found that early palliative care interventions led to improvement in caregiver depression and stress burden but no significant improvement on caregiver quality of life.[34] Similarly, based on the 2017 Temel trial, where early integrated palliative and oncology care intervention was provided without a specific caregiver-directed component, El-Jawahri and colleagues found that early integrated palliative and oncology care led to improved total psychological distress among caregivers of patients with lung and GI cancers as measured by the HADS and depression subscale (HADS-depression) at 12 weeks, but not anxiety subscale or quality of life.[32]

Psychiatry and Early Integrated Palliative and Oncology Care

To date, the models of early integrated palliative and oncology care studied in trials have not formally included psychiatry. In those models, psychiatry and other mental health services have served as a referral resource for patients with psychiatric disorders or more complex psychosocial needs. While the identification of, education about, and referrals for psychosocial distress might be prominent in some models, it is unclear if early integrated palliative and oncology care leads to greater utilization of psychiatric and mental health referrals. As mentioned earlier, the number of consultations with psychologists was greater for patients receiving early integrated palliative and oncology care in the trial by Vanbutsele, even though they did not observe significant differences in depression. However, differences in rates of mental health utilization were not found in a trial by Temel and colleagues. Twenty-five percent of patients receiving early integrated palliative and oncology care saw a psychiatrist, which was not significantly different from those who were not receiving palliative care (35%).[23] In fact, even among those with depression, only 44% of those receiving early integrated palliative and oncology care had mental health visits compared to 58% of those who received standard care.

In addition to referrals for psychiatric treatment, psychiatrists might provide some elements of early integrated palliative and oncology care, especially when palliative care resources might be limited. While there are clear differences between psychiatry and palliative care, there is some overlap in the skills and expertise related to certain elements of early integrated palliative and oncology care. Psychiatrists are trained in interpersonal skills and in the diagnoses and management of psychological problems using a biopsychosocial approach. They are also trained in providing psychosocial support to patients with serious medical comorbidities. Additionally, psychiatrists are trained to explore patient narratives and are equipped to carry out goals-of-care conversations. Psychiatry training has the potential to fulfill some areas of palliative care. For example, during the COVID pandemic, one major medical center utilized psychiatry residents and fellows for inpatient palliative care consults that utilized psychiatry trainees' preexisting skills, including carrying out goals-of-care conversations and providing psychosocial support.[35]

Nonetheless, early integrated palliative and oncology care presents an opportunity for psychiatrists to collaborate in the delivery of palliative care. With the longer, longitudinal nature of early integrated palliative and oncology care, psychiatric needs and behavioral issues might become more apparent over time and require specialized intervention. Psychiatry might be particularly helpful in addressing some of the outcomes that may not respond to early integrated palliative and oncology care, such as anxiety. Even if they are not formally part of multidisciplinary palliative care teams, psychiatrists could establish liaison relationships with outpatient palliative care clinics. The liaison relationship could range from serving as a resource for referrals to availability for palliative care providers to discuss challenging patients or receive advice, or even to attending regular ambulatory clinical rounds.

Future Directions

Early integrated palliative and oncology care has emerged as a new standard of care over the past decade. It has many psychosocial benefits, including improvement in quality of life, increased use of active coping skills, reduction in depressive symptoms, and reduced aggressiveness of care at end of life, all without apparent reduction in survival. The longitudinal relationship of early integrated palliative and oncology care allows for patients and caregivers to develop trusting relationships with palliative care providers before major medical crises are encountered. In addition to managing physical symptoms, early integrated palliative and oncology care providers establish patients' understanding of their illness, prognosis, and preferences for treatment and help them cope with their illness throughout the course of the illness. To date, psychiatrists and other mental health professionals have not been part of the early integrated palliative and oncology care models studied in randomized controlled trials. However, given the psychosocial aspects of early palliative care, psychiatrists could play a collaborative role as clinical resources and consultants.

Key Points

- Early palliative care, delivered concurrently with cancer care, is the new standard of care.
- Early palliative care leads to improvement in patient quality of life, symptom relief, psychological outcomes, patient satisfaction, and possibly even survival.

- Early palliative care leads to reduced psychological distress for caregivers, who are essential members of the team.
- There are several models of early palliative care delivery—traditional consultations, team-based population management, psychoeducation sessions—all of them effective for improving psychosocial outcomes.

References

1. WHO. Cancer pain relief and palliative care. 1990:1–76.
2. *National Cancer Control Programmes: Policies And Managerial Guidelines.* 2nd ed. World Health Organization; 2002. https://apps.who.int/iris/handle/10665/42494
3. Hui D, Elsayem A, De la Cruz M, et al. Availability and integration of palliative care at US cancer centers. *JAMA.* Mar 17 2010;303(11):1054–1061. doi:10.1001/jama.2010.258
4. LeBlanc TW, O'Donnell JD, Crowley-Matoka M, et al. Perceptions of palliative care among hematologic malignancy specialists: A mixed-methods study. *J Oncol Pract.* 2015;11(2):e230–e238.
5. Bakitas M, Lyons KD, Hegel MT, et al. Effects of a palliative care intervention on clinical outcomes in patients with advanced cancer: The Project ENABLE II randomized controlled trial. *JAMA.* Aug 19 2009;302(7):741–749. doi:10.1001/jama.2009.1198
6. Temel JS, Greer JA, Muzikansky A, et al. Early palliative care for patients with metastatic non-small-cell lung cancer. *N Engl J Med.* Aug 19 2010;363(8):733–742. doi:10.1056/NEJMoa1000678
7. Greer JA, Pirl WF, Jackson VA, et al. Effect of early palliative care on chemotherapy use and end-of-life care in patients with metastatic non-small-cell lung cancer. *J Clin Oncol.* Feb 1 2012;30(4):394–400. doi:10.1200/JCO.2011.35.7996
8. Zimmermann C, Swami N, Krzyzanowska M, et al. Early palliative care for patients with advanced cancer: A cluster-randomised controlled trial. *The Lancet.* 2014;383(9930):1721–1730. doi:10.1016/s0140-6736(13)62416-2
9. Bakitas MA, Tosteson TD, Li Z, et al. Early versus delayed initiation of concurrent palliative oncology care: Patient outcomes in the ENABLE III randomized controlled trial. *J Clin Oncol.* May 1 2015;33(13):1438–45. doi:10.1200/JCO.2014.58.6362
10. Temel JS, Greer JA, El-Jawahri A, et al. Effects of early integrated palliative care in patients with lung and GI cancer: A randomized clinical trial. *J Clin Oncol.* Mar 10 2017;35(8):834–841. doi:10.1200/JCO.2016.70.5046
11. Vanbutsele G, Pardon K, Van Belle S, et al. Effect of early and systematic integration of palliative care in patients with advanced cancer: A randomised controlled trial. *Lancet Oncol.* 2018;19(3):394–404. doi:10.1016/s1470-2045(18)30060-3
12. Smith TJ, Temin S, Alesi ER, et al. American Society of Clinical Oncology provisional clinical opinion: The integration of palliative care into standard oncology care. *J Clin Oncol.* Mar 10 2012;30(8):880–887. doi:10.1200/JCO.2011.38.5161
13. Ferrell BR, Temel JS, Temin S, et al. Integration of palliative care into standard oncology care: American Society of Clinical Oncology Clinical practice guideline update. *J Clin Oncol.* Jan 2017;35(1):96–112. doi:10.1200/JCO.2016.70.1474
14. Smith AK, Thai JN, Bakitas MA, et al. The diverse landscape of palliative care clinics. *J Palliat Med.* Jun 2013;16(6):661–668. doi:10.1089/jpm.2012.0469
15. Yoong J, Park ER, Greer JA, et al. Early palliative care in advanced lung cancer: A qualitative study. *JAMA Intern Med.* Feb 25 2013;173(4):283–290. doi:10.1001/jamainternmed.2013.1874
16. Greer JA, Jacobs JM, El-Jawahri A, et al. Role of patient coping strategies in understanding the effects of early palliative care on quality of life and mood. *J Clin Oncol.* Jan 1 2018;36(1):53–60. doi:10.1200/JCO.2017.73.7221

17. El-Jawahri A, LeBlanc T, VanDusen H, et al. Effect of inpatient palliative care on quality of life 2 weeks after hematopoietic stem cell transplantation: A randomized clinical trial. *JAMA*. Nov 22 2016;316(20):2094–2103. doi:10.1001/jama.2016.16786

18. Dyar S, Lesperance M, Shannon R, Sloan J, Colon-Otero G. A nurse practitioner directed intervention improves the quality of life of patients with metastatic cancer: Results of a randomized pilot study. *J Palliat Med*. Aug 2012;15(8):890–895. doi:10.1089/jpm.2012.0014

19. Ferrell B, Sun V, Hurria A, et al. Interdisciplinary Palliative Care for Patients With Lung Cancer. *J Pain Symptom Manage*. Dec 2015;50(6):758–767. doi:10.1016/j.jpainsymman.2015.07.005

20. Linden W, Vodermaier A, Mackenzie R, Greig D. Anxiety and depression after cancer diagnosis: Prevalence rates by cancer type, gender, and age. *J Affect Disord*. Dec 10 2012;141(2-3):343–351. doi:10.1016/j.jad.2012.03.025

21. Satin JR, Linden W, Phillips MJ. Depression as a predictor of disease progression and mortality in cancer patients: A meta-analysis. *Cancer*. Nov 15 2009;115(22):5349–5361. doi:10.1002/cncr.24561

22. Saad AM, Gad MM, Al-Husseini MJ, et al. Suicidal death within a year of a cancer diagnosis: A population-based study. *Cancer*. Mar 15 2019;125(6):972–979. doi:10.1002/cncr.31876

23. Pirl WF, Greer JA, Traeger L, et al. Depression and survival in metastatic non-small-cell lung cancer: Effects of early palliative care. *J Clin Oncol*. Apr 20 2012;30(12):1310–1315. doi:10.1200/JCO.2011.38.3166

24. El-Jawahri AR, Vandusen HB, Traeger LN, et al. Quality of life and mood predict posttraumatic stress disorder after hematopoietic stem cell transplantation. *Cancer*. Mar 1 2016;122(5):806–812. doi:10.1002/cncr.29818

25. Rego F, Goncalves F, Moutinho S, Castro L, Nunes R. The influence of spirituality on decision-making in palliative care outpatients: A cross-sectional study. *BMC Palliat Care*. Feb 21 2020;19(1):22. doi:10.1186/s12904-020-0525-3

26. Earle CC, Neville BA, Landrum MB, Ayanian JZ, Block SD, Weeks JC. Trends in the aggressiveness of cancer care near the end of life. *J Clin Oncol*. Jan 15 2004;22(2):315–321. doi:10.1200/JCO.2004.08.136

27. Earle CC, Landrum MB, Souza JM, Neville BA, Weeks JC, Ayanian JZ. Aggressiveness of cancer care near the end of life: Is it a quality-of-care issue? *J Clin Oncol*. Aug 10 2008;26(23):3860–3866. doi:10.1200/JCO.2007.15.8253

28. Wang SY, Hall J, Pollack CE, et al. Trends in end-of-life cancer care in the Medicare program. *J Geriatr Oncol*. Mar 2016;7(2):116–125. doi:10.1016/j.jgo.2015.11.007

29. Smith CEP, Kamal AH, Kluger M, Coke P, Kelley MJ. National trends in end-of-life care for veterans with advanced cancer in the Veterans Health Administration: 2009 to 2016. *J Oncol Pract*. Jun 2019;15(6):e568-e575. doi:10.1200/JOP.18.00559

30. Geng HM, Chuang DM, Yang F, et al. Prevalence and determinants of depression in caregivers of cancer patients: A systematic review and meta-analysis. *Medicine (Baltimore)*. Sep 2018;97(39):e11863. doi:10.1097/MD.0000000000011863

31. Areia NP, Fonseca G, Major S, Relvas AP. Psychological morbidity in family caregivers of people living with terminal cancer: Prevalence and predictors. *Palliat Support Care*. Jun 2019;17(3):286–293. doi:10.1017/S1478951518000044

32. El-Jawahri A, Greer JA, Pirl WF, et al. Effects of early integrated palliative care on caregivers of patients with lung and gastrointestinal cancer: A randomized clinical trial. *Oncologist*. Dec 2017;22(12):1528–1534. doi:10.1634/theoncologist.2017-0227

33. McDonald J, Swami N, Hannon B, et al. Impact of early palliative care on caregivers of patients with advanced cancer: Cluster randomised trial. *Ann Oncol*. Jan 1 2017;28(1):163–168. doi:10.1093/annonc/mdw438

34. Dionne-Odom JN, Azuero A, Lyons KD, et al. Benefits of early versus delayed palliative care to informal family caregivers of patients with advanced cancer: Outcomes from the ENABLE III randomized controlled trial. *J Clin Oncol*. May 1 2015;33(13):1446–1452. doi:10.1200/JCO.2014.58.7824

35. Shalev D, Nakagawa S, Stroeh OM, et al. The creation of a psychiatry-palliative care liaison team: Using psychiatrists to extend palliative care delivery and access during the COVID-19 crisis. *J Pain Symptom Manage*. Sep 2020;60(3):e12–e16. doi:10.1016/j.jpainsymman.2020.06.009

16

Cultural Diversity and Palliative Care

Ayla Pelleg, Cardinale B. Smith, and Leslie Blackhall

Introduction

The US healthcare system serves a diverse population. Due to inequities at all levels of health systems, patients from cultural and ethnic minorities often access and receive healthcare at more severe stages of disease, leading to increased morbidity and mortality. This unequal access to healthcare is particularly seen for patients with serious illness and when it comes to receiving specialty palliative care. Culturally diverse patients may have values and beliefs about end-of-life care (EOLC) which contrast with their providers and difficulties receiving care consonant with those values. Cultural competence is vital in all aspects of medicine, but especially so in palliative and EOLC, to help build rapport and trusting relationships and ensure that patient-centered, culturally sensitive care is provided.

Race and ethnicity have many definitions that often stem from self-identification and social constructs. While cultural diversity is unique to each country and health system, this chapter focuses on cultural diversity within the United States and its health systems. Race and ethnicity, defined by the National Institutes of Health's Office of Management and Budget (OMB), classifies race into five categories (American Indian or Alaska Native, Asian, Black or African American, Native Hawaiian or Other Pacific Islander, and White) and ethnicity into two categories (Hispanic or Latino and Not Hispanic or Latino).[1] The majority of this chapter focuses on health inequalities for Black and Hispanic minority patients, touches on health disparities among Asian minority patients, and highlights geographic or regional variations. A key element of providing culturally sensitive care is understanding the unique challenges of patient populations and adapting medical care to meet those specific needs.

According to the National Institute on Minority and Health and Health Disparities (NIMHD), health disparities can be defined as significant inequality of a particular population's health status compared to the general population in regards to "disease incidence, prevalence, morbidity, mortality, or survival rates."[2] Health disparities are directly linked to social determinants of health (SDOH), which are environmental factors (e.g., economic stability; social and community context; healthcare access and quality; education access and quality; racism, discrimination, and violence; language and literacy skills; neighborhood and physical environment) affecting health, well-being, and quality of life.[3]

Structural racism within health systems has been brought to light by the coronavirus disease 2019 (COVID-19) pandemic. There have been increased COVID-19 diagnoses, hospitalizations, and deaths among Black and Hispanic communities compared to White populations due to health disparities and SDOH factors.[4] Structural racism impacts multiple aspects of healthcare delivery including the timing of when patients seek care and their trust in health systems and its providers.

More specifically, health disparities matter in regard to palliative care as they lead to unequal care provided, decreased utilization of palliative care services, and misperceptions of palliative care by providers, patients, and families. Even with broader education about palliative care at the provider and patient levels, palliative care is still underutilized among certain racial and ethnic groups. Black and Hispanic patients are less likely to use and/or be open to palliative care services.[5] The reason for this is multifactorial, often reflecting misperceptions on what palliative care is, mistrust in the healthcare system and providers, systemic racism, cultural differences, and individual approaches to health and medicine.

This chapter highlights evidence-based data on racial and ethnic health disparities in palliative care in relation to patient values, access to care, and receipt of care. While research on cultural diversity and palliative care exists, limitations remain due to lack of uniform definitions of race and ethnicity and absence of requirements to include race and ethnicity in study designs. This chapter will later identify concrete next steps to move toward reducing health disparities and improving delivery of patient-centered care.

Patient Values

Patient values encompass learning more about patients (e.g., what living well means to them, what worries they may have, what and who are important to them, and what provides them with strength) and knowing preferences on the type of care they want to receive. Personal preferences may be guided by current and/or past healthcare experiences or cultural, religious, family, or community beliefs. Care assumptions made by medical providers based on racial and ethnic identifications can lead to conscious and unconscious biases, miscommunication, disrespect, and patient-discordant care. Cultural competence in palliative care is achieved when medical care meets the cultural, social, and religious needs of patients and their loved ones (Figure 16.1).[6] This section discusses cultural differences as shown in literature, realizing that individual beliefs may vary and generalizations may not apply to every patient with a particular cultural background.

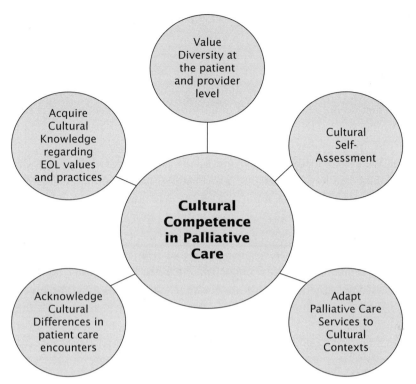

FIGURE 16.1 Cultural competence in palliative care. Key components of cultural competence in palliative care, which is important in mitigating health disparities and providing more equitable care among culturally diverse patients.

Communication of serious illness is fundamental to palliative care. Often, palliative care providers share information on diagnosis and prognosis and come up with care plans that impact care received. Preferences regarding prognostic disclosure may vary from patient to patient and can be driven by cultural preferences. Some patients appreciate hearing the big picture while others prefer detailed information; some want to hear the information directly while others want medical information to be given with loved ones or only to loved ones. Since preferences for how patients want serious news delivered varies greatly, it is imperative for medical providers to ask patients how they want to hear information prior to disclosing any new medical information. In Asian cultures, it can be taboo to talk about death as it may bring bad luck; hospice or palliative care may be seen as giving up on the patient; and some may practice "filial piety," where it is a moral obligation for children to support their parents and elders.[7,8]

Beyond delivering serious illness news and routine patient communication, how patients make decisions may also vary based on racial, ethnic, and cultural differences. Within similar cultures, medical decisions may be made as a family or individually.[9] In some Hispanic families, the *familismo* principle guides decisions, where family needs are prioritized over individual needs.[10] Asian and Hispanic patients have higher family-centered decision-making compared to other culturally diverse patient populations.[11] When it comes to end-of-life decisions, specifically regarding life-sustaining medical interventions (e.g., cardiopulmonary resuscitation [CPR] or mechanical ventilation), religious leaders or communities may make or help make decisions for patients and loved ones.[12]

Patient values may focus on where a patient or their loved ones want a patient to die. The American healthcare system supporting EOLC, including hospice, is built on assumptions that do not meet the needs of all patients—often meeting the needs of those who have more (e.g., easier time accessing medical care, more caregiving support in the home environment) and excluding minority patient populations. When thinking about place of death, it is important to also consider the value of every breath and what quality of life may look like to some patients (e.g., being on life-sustaining interventions like a ventilator, foregoing chemotherapy if side effects may impair independence). Along the lines of the Anglo medical construct, some medical providers may assume that dying at home is preferred, which tends to be truer for White patients. Compared to Whites, Blacks have higher odds of dying in the hospital, which may reflect preferences for life-sustaining interventions, limitations to access of quality care in the home setting, and historical racial injustices in the American healthcare system.[13] Some studies show Hispanics are more likely to die at a relative's home compared to White patients, which may reflect the importance of filial peity.[13,14]

Access to Palliative Care

Palliative care is considered part of standard care for those with serious illness. In the past two decades, annual admissions of hospitalized patients receiving an initial palliative care consult increased from 2.5% (2008) to 5.3% (2017).[15] Within hospitals (>50 size bed hospitals), those receiving initial palliative care consults increased from 658 hospitals (25%) in 2000 to 1,831 hospitals (75%) in 2016.[16] Despite wider access to palliative care, there remain gaps in access to palliative care geographically, across cultural patient populations, and across socioeconomic status (SES) lines.

Geographically disparities in access to palliative care exist within the United States. To better understand the reasoning behind this, Hoeger et al. found palliative care access is reduced in states with more racial diversity and lower SES as well as in rural and Southern states, and in regions with smaller hospitals (<50-bed sized hospital).[17] When it comes to SES, access to palliative care has noticeable differences. Hospitals with most patients of lower SES and hospitals coined as "safety net hospitals" have fewer palliative care teams compared to not-for-profit, large-sized hospitals.[18]

Beyond geography and hospital setting, access to pain assessment and management varies based on cultural differences. Medical providers' subconscious and/or conscious biases impact provider–patient communication and beliefs in how patients report pain, and therefore assessment and treatment decisions regarding pain management among Black and Hispanic patients.[19] This commonly results in pain being undertreated among racial and ethnic patient populations. Additionally, patients' past experiences with the healthcare system impact how pain is perceived and communicated to medical providers. Moreover, fear of addiction is more common among Blacks and Hispanics, which may impact ability to control pain adequately.[20]

There are also systemic causes for pain inequities among racial and ethnic minorities. Access to effective pain medication remains a barrier due to insurance coverage for pain medications, cost of treatment plans, and availability of analgesic medications, specifically opioids.[21] Pharmacies have been found to not stock the same amount of opioids in non-White neighborhoods, making it hard to effectively treat pain for minority patient populations. Black cancer patients who did not graduate from high school and who earned below the federal poverty line had increased trouble getting opioids filled, where some had to wait longer to get their medications or come back to the pharmacy multiple times.[22] This unequal access to adequate pain management impacts quality of life and contributes to increased morbidity among culturally diverse patients.

Even though telemedicine has been present for decades, the COVID-19 pandemic has accelerated the use of telemedicine across all medical disciplines, including palliative care. Cultural differences exist regarding access to and use of telemedicine. Access to technologies for telemedicine (e.g., high-speed internet, computers, smartphone devices) are lower among rural, older, and lower-income adults due to cost and lower technology literacy.[23] The ENABLE CHF-PC (Educate, Nurture, Advise, Before Life Ends Comprehensive Healthcare for Patients and Caregivers) study aimed to evaluate if a 16-week palliative care telemedicine intervention across two hospitals in the Southeast US (55% of study participants were Black) could improve quality of life for patients with advanced heart failure. Using a telemedicine palliative care intervention, symptom management (specifically pain intensity and pain interference with activities of daily living) among minority patients in rural areas was improved.[24] This study shows that, moving forward, integrating telemedicine into palliative care will be vital to increase access to palliative care for culturally diverse patient populations with serious illness.

Receipt of Care

When it comes to receipt of palliative care, healthcare disparities exist for the degree of life-sustaining treatments patients want toward the end of life, advance care planning (ACP), and hospice utilization. These healthcare disparities in relation to receipt of care lead to more aggressive EOLC (e.g., high rates of intensive care unit [ICU] level care, CPR, mechanical ventilation, and hospitalizations), increased symptom burden (e.g., uncontrolled pain, high rates of depression and anxiety), and healthcare system-centered care (e.g., meeting financial and quality metrics, maximizing efficiencies, assessing medical outcomes) instead of patient-centered care (e.g., meeting the wants and needs of individual patients, approaching patients holistically and not by isolated medical diagnoses, prioritizing patients' values when making medical decisions). When thinking about receipt of care, it is important to know that generalizations are made as care within the same health system and by the same healthcare provider can vary based on patient population, specifically among culturally diverse, seriously ill patients.[25]

Many reasons exist for why culturally diverse patients may receive more aggressive treatment or increased life-sustaining treatments toward the end of life. Fragmentation of the US healthcare system can lead to inadequate tools being provided in home settings, resulting in the home not being an option to continue medical care and patients dying in nursing homes or hospitals. Culturally diverse patients, particularly Black patients, tend to have more invasive medical treatments at the end of life and are more likely to deplete personal finances to extend life,[26] which has been linked to reduced prognostic under-standing,[27] distrust of the healthcare system, and concern that care provided is based on one's ability to pay.[28] Additionally, even when similar end-of-life communication prefer-ences were made among White and Black patients, Black patients were less likely to have do not resuscitate (DNR) wishes carried out and received more life-prolonging care at the end of life, which could be due to patient–physician communication, disparity in the translation of preferences to actual care, frequency of end-of-life discussions, and provider racial biases.[29] Higher end-of-life healthcare costs were seen among Black and Hispanic patients when compared to White patients, mostly due to increased intensive care use and life-sustaining interventions.[30] Though the use of feeding tubes among advanced dementia patients in nursing homes has decreased, Black patients when compared to White patients had increased use of mechanical ventilation.[31] Some studies have seen that recent US im-migrants are more likely to want life-sustaining interventions at the end of life and are less likely to engage in ACP conversations compared to those of similar racial and ethnic backgrounds who have lived in the United States longer, indicating that acculturation may impact patient values regarding end-of-life wishes.[32–34]

As discussed above in regard to patient values, when it comes to ACP and end-of-life decision-making, differences in knowledge, attitudes, and communication preferences im-pact completion of ACP among culturally diverse patients. Patient autonomy and anticipa-tory decision-making (i.e., ACP) is primarily a North American construct. Racial, ethnic, and cultural differences exist when it comes to communication; how direct to be when talking about end-of-life preferences (e.g., identifying a healthcare proxy [HCP] or power of attorney [POA] for medical decisions, DNR or do not intubate [DNI] orders, artificial nutrition) and who within a family structure is supposed to know medical information. Data demonstrate that White patients were more likely to engage in ACP conversations and have completed ACP documents compared to Black and Hispanic patients.[35] For some Hispanic patients, the fear of discrimination, language barriers, and specific cultural reli-gious and spiritual influences prevent them from partaking in ACP; this can be mitigated to some extent by using professional translators to help bridge cultural or language barriers.[36]

Health literacy has been identified as another factor that impacts ACP. However, when showing ACP videos on advanced dementia to Black and White patients, both race and health literacy differences (when comparing Black and White patients) dissipated when deciding about preferences regarding aggressive care (i.e., prolonging life at any cost, in-cluding CPR and mechanical ventilation) and limited care (i.e., hospitalization, antibiotics, artificial nutrition and hydration, but not CPR or ICU-level care) versus comfort care (i.e., maximize comfort and relieve pain).[37] Additionally, in some cultures it is considered incon-siderate or taboo to tell patients they are dying since it may be assumed that patients will figure it out for themselves that they are dying.[38] More specifically, in Korean culture, there is a concept of *Nunchi* that emphasizes using nonverbal communication and the assumption that children know the end-of-life preferences of their elders, so ACP conversations do not need to happen overtly.[8]

Though the concept of hospice varies across the world, the underlying principles of hospice are to focus on symptom management and on addressing emotional and spiritual needs at the end of life. Within the United States, health disparities exist when it comes to hospice utilization. As contextual background, hospice within the United States is based on health insurance coverage by Medicare when two physicians believe a patient has less than 6 months to live if a life-limiting illness continues on its disease trajectory. Hospice can be provided in the home, a nursing facility, or in a hospital. Hospice as a benefit, starting in the 1970s within the United States, is indicative of a certain moment in time and a certain patient population that it was set up for and worked best for. Hospice provides minimal custodial care (e.g., helping bathe, feed, toilet patients), so the caregiving mainly falls on family and friends, with this often being a rate-limiting step for some patients, particularly non-White patients and patients of lower SES. Black patients are more likely to be referred to hospice within days of dying, receive hospice in a hospital setting,[39] and are less likely to enroll in hospice overall due to miscommunication, general distrust, and inadequate resources to help keep patients at home.[40] Asian Americans and Pacific Islanders (AAPIs) are less likely to utilize hospice services and on average have a shorter median length of stay within hospice.[41] Patients are more likely to have increased trust, adherence, and satisfaction when there is cultural concordance between provider and patient.[42]

Embracing Cultural Diversity: Next Steps

To ensure cultural diversity is given the attention it needs within palliative care, there are several concrete next steps that can be taken to improve direct patient care (Table 16.1).

TABLE 16.1 Embracing cultural diversity: Next steps

Categories	Actionable steps
Education initiatives	Increase public awareness
	Engage community leaders
	Teach core palliative care skills to all healthcare providers
Policy changes	Provide financial protection to expand palliative care education and skills
	Provide incentives to expand palliative care workforce
	Commit to mitigate health disparities
Palliative care research	Standardize research methods on cultural diversity
	Better understand cultural attitudes, beliefs, and experiences impacting medical care
	Create interventions to reduce health disparities and measures outcomes

Education efforts should be broad and comprehensive. Education on palliative care at the provider, patient, and community levels is important to dispel myths about what palliative care is and how it can help patients and their loved ones. Education efforts should increase public awareness about palliative care services that can be provided in the outpatient and inpatient clinical settings as well as at the community level. An example of this could be a marketing campaign geared toward patient stakeholders to provide education on what palliative care is and how patients can benefit from it. Engaging community stakeholders (i.e., faith-based institutions, local business owners, education providers, local charities) will be important to obtain buy-in for culturally diverse patient populations and to help bridge existing cultural barriers. Given the workforce shortage of specialized palliative care providers, disseminating core palliative care education knowledge and skills (Box 16.1) to all medical providers is crucial to improve the quality of patient care and achieve patient-concordant care (i.e., providing medical care that matches patient preferences and improving communication between clinicians and patients[43]).[44] "All medical providers" includes interdisciplinary team members like social workers and chaplains as well as entry-level nurses, medical students, respiratory therapists. Due to the unknown diversity of the medical workforce and varying degrees of cultural competencies taught to medical trainees, standard curricular education on cultural traditions, beliefs, and practices is imperative. Additionally, to ensure that comprehensive access to medical care is achieved for all patients, educational efforts need to mitigate language barriers. To overcome language barriers, access to language services (e.g., interpreter services in person or via phone or video) where medical care can be translated accurately and in a culturally competent manner into one's first or most comfortable language is essential.

Being able to increase these educational efforts will require large-scale funding and policy changes. One policy measure that was passed by the US House of Representatives in 2019 was the Palliative Care and Hospice Education and Training Act (PCHETA).[45] As of Spring 2021, this bill has not passed both legislative branches of Congress to be completely enacted. If passed, this bill will expand palliative care research programs at the National Institute of Health (NIH), provide palliative care education and awareness campaigns though the Agency for Healthcare Research and Quality (AHRQ), and expand palliative care education by sponsoring the workforce via efforts like financial supports for medical school and career awards through the Department of Health and Human Services (HHS).

BOX 16.1 Core palliative care skills

1. Advance care planning
2. Care coordination
3. Physical and psychosocial assessment and management
4. Spiritual and cultural assessment and management
5. Caregiver support

With PCHETA or future policy changes, it will be necessary to ensure that efforts are made to expand cultural diversity within the palliative care workforce and expand access and education to culturally diverse patient populations.

Beyond policy efforts, when it comes to palliative care research, efforts to standardize research regarding cultural diversity and addressing healthcare disparities should be made. Future palliative care research efforts should be made to understand cultural differences when it comes to disease perception, symptom management, and ACP in order to provide culturally appropriate palliative care clinical services. More specifically, research should continue to assess how racial and ethnic patient populations want to hear medical information, how decisions are made, and how to be more culturally sensitive regarding topics like EOLC.

When thinking about cultural diversity, it is equally important to think about what our current and future palliative care workforce looks like in terms of race and ethnicity. Unfortunately, data are not collected at the fellowship level on current palliative care trainees and their race and ethnicity or at the interdisciplinary team practitioner level (e.g., advanced practice practitioners, physicians, chaplains, and social workers). Increasing the palliative care workforce's cultural diversity is important to ensure that palliative care workforces mirror patient populations in regard to race, ethnicity, and culture. Additionally, acknowledging that healthcare providers bring explicit and implicit biases to the care they provide is important since these biases impact behavioral interactions, clinical decision-making, and patient rapport.[46] There is a lack of standard cultural competencies taught in healthcare curriculums, and this can negatively impact the receipt of care.[47] As discussed above regarding educational next steps, standardization in palliative care training about cultural diversity and unconscious biases is an initial step that can be taken to mitigate racial and ethnic health disparities.

Future Directions

Cultural diversity, especially addressing racial and ethnic health disparities, exists across healthcare, including palliative care. Palliative care is specifically needed for culturally diverse patients in order to improve morbidity and quality of life and provide compassionate care for those with serious illness. When caring for patients, healthcare providers need to consider patient values, access to care, and receipt of care, given that healthcare disparities exist across all aspects of care. Moving forward, to ensure health equity and equality among culturally diverse patients, future palliative care education, policy efforts, and research need to include racial and ethnically diverse patients and realize the complexities of culturally diversity.

Key Points

- Race and ethnic health disparities exist in all aspects of medicine, including palliative care.

- Cultural diversity impacts patient values in regard to communication and how medical decisions are made.
- Racially and ethnically diverse patients often have reduced access to palliative care services and inadequate symptom management.
- When thinking about receipt of care, considering healthcare provider biases and patient preferences is imperative.
- To reduce healthcare disparities in palliative care, education, public awareness, policy changes, and increased research efforts are important next steps.

References

1. US Office of Management and Budget. *Revisions to the Standards for the Classification of Federal Data on Race and Ethnicity*. Washington, DC: General Accounting Office; 1997:58782–58790.
2. Institute of Medicine (US) Committee on the Review and Assessment of the NIH's Strategic Research Plan and Budget to Reduce and Ultimately Eliminate Health Disparities, Thomson GE, Mitchell F, Williams MB, eds. *Examining the Health Disparities Research Plan of the National Institutes of Health: Unfinished Business*. Washington, DC: National Academies Press (US); 2006.
3. Healthy People 2030. Social Determinants of Health. US Department of Health and Human Services. 2022. https://health.gov/healthypeople/objectives-and-data/social-determinants-health
4. Raine S, Liu A, Mintz J, Wahood W, Huntley K, Haffizulla F. Racial and ethnic disparities in COVID-19 outcomes: Social determination of health. *Int J Environ Res Public Health*. Nov 2020;17(21):8115–8145. doi:10.3390/ijerph17218115
5. Johnson KS. Racial and ethnic disparities in palliative care. *J Palliat Med*. Nov 2013;16(11):1329–1334. doi:10.1089/jpm.2013.9468
6. Swihart DL, Yarrarapu SNS, Martin RL. Cultural Religious competence in clinical practice. *StatPearls*; 2021, Stat Pearls Publishing: 2022 Jan. PMID: 29630268.
7. Wei L, Walters J, Guo Q, Fetherston C, O'Connor M. Meaningful and culturally appropriate palliative care for Chinese immigrants with a terminal condition: A qualitative systematic review protocol. *JBI Database System Rev Implement Rep*. Dec 2019;17(12):2499–2505. doi:10.11124/JBISRIR-2017-003867
8. Shin DW, Lee JE, Cho B, Yoo SH, Kim S, Yoo JH. End-of-life communication in Korean older adults: With focus on advance care planning and advance directives. *Geriatr Gerontol Int*. Apr 2016;16(4):407–15. doi:10.1111/ggi.12603
9. Cain CL, Surbone A, Elk R, Kagawa-Singer M. Culture and palliative care: Preferences, communication, meaning, and mutual decision making. *J Pain Symptom Manage*. May 2018;55(5):1408–1419. doi:10.1016/j.jpainsymman.2018.01.007
10. Cervantes L, Zoucha J, Jones J, Fischer S. Experiences and values of Latinos with end stage renal disease: A systematic review of qualitative studies. *Nephrol Nurs J*. 2016 Nov-Dec 2016;43(6):479–493.
11. Kwak J, Haley WE. Current research findings on end-of-life decision making among racially or ethnically diverse groups. *Gerontologist*. Oct 2005;45(5):634–641. doi:10.1093/geront/45.5.634
12. Chakraborty R, El-Jawahri AR, Litzow MR, Syrjala KL, Parnes AD, Hashmi SK. A systematic review of religious beliefs about major end-of-life issues in the five major world religions. *Palliat Support Care*. 10 2017;15(5):609–622. doi:10.1017/S1478951516001061
13. Johnson KS, Kuchibhatala M, Sloane RJ, Tanis D, Galanos AN, Tulsky JA. Ethnic differences in the place of death of elderly hospice enrollees. *J Am Geriatr Soc*. Dec 2005;53(12):2209–2215. doi:10.1111/j.1532-5415.2005.00502.x
14. Teno JM, Gozalo P, Trivedi AN, Bunker J, Lima J, Ogarek J, et al. Site of death, place of care, and healthcare transitions among US medicare beneficiaries, 2000–2015. *JAMA*. 07 2018;320(3):264–271. doi:10.1001/jama.2018.8981

15. Rogers M, Meier DE, Heitner R, et al. The National Palliative Care Registry: A decade of supporting growth and sustainability of palliative care programs. *J Palliat Med*. Sep 2019;22(9):1026–1031. doi:10.1089/jpm.2019.0262

16. Centers to Advance Palliative Care. *Growth of Palliative Care in U.S. Hospitals: 2018 Snapshot (2000–2016)*. New York: Centers to Advance Palliative Care; 2018.

17. Hoerger M, Perry LM, Korotkin BD, et al. Statewide differences in personality associated with geographic disparities in access to palliative care: Findings on openness. *J Palliat Med*. 06 2019;22(6):628–634. doi:10.1089/jpm.2018.0206

18. Morrison RS, Augustin R, Souvanna P, Meier DE. America's care of serious illness: A state-by-state report card on access to palliative care in our nation's hospitals. *J Palliat Med*. Oct 2011;14(10):1094–1096. doi:10.1089/jpm.2011.9634

19. Ghoshal M, Shapiro H, Todd K, Schatman ME. Chronic noncancer pain management and systemic racism: Time to move toward equal care standards. *J Pain Res*. 2020;13:2825–2836. doi:10.2147/JPR.S287314

20. Weiss SC, Emanuel LL, Fairclough DL, Emanuel EJ. Understanding the experience of pain in terminally ill patients. *Lancet*. Apr 2001;357(9265):1311–1315. doi:10.1016/S0140-6736(00)04515-3

21. Shavers VL, Bakos A, Sheppard VB. Race, ethnicity, and pain among the U.S. adult population. *J Healthcare Poor Underserved*. Feb 2010;21(1):177–220. doi:10.1353/hpu.0.0255

22. Jefferson K, Quest T, Yeager KA. Factors associated with black cancer patients' ability to obtain their opioid prescriptions at the pharmacy. *J Palliat Med*. Sep 2019;22(9):1143–1148. doi:10.1089/jpm.2018.0536

23. Calton BA, Rabow MW, Branagan L, et al. Top ten tips palliative care clinicians should know about telepalliative care. *J Palliat Med*. Aug 2019;22(8):981–985. doi:10.1089/jpm.2019.0278

24. Bakitas MA, Dionne-Odom JN, Ejem DB, et al. Effect of an early palliative care telehealth intervention vs usual care on patients with heart failure: The ENABLE CHF-PC randomized clinical trial. *JAMA Intern Med*. Sep 2020;180(9):1203–1213. doi:10.1001/jamainternmed.2020.2861

25. Borum ML, Lynn J, Zhong Z. The effects of patient race on outcomes in seriously ill patients in SUPPORT: An overview of economic impact, medical intervention, and end-of-life decisions. Study to Understand Prognoses and Preferences for Outcomes and Risks of Treatments. *J Am Geriatr Soc*. May 2000;48(S1):S194–198. doi:10.1111/j.1532-5415.2000.tb03132.x

26. Welch LC, Teno JM, Mor V. End-of-life care in Black and White: Race matters for medical care of dying patients and their families. *J Am Geriatr Soc*. Jul 2005;53(7):1145–1153. doi:10.1111/j.1532-5415.2005.53357.x

27. Mack JW, Uno H, Twist CJ, et al. Racial and ethnic differences in communication and care for children with advanced cancer. *J Pain Symptom Manage*. 10 2020;60(4):782–789. doi:10.1016/j.jpainsymman.2020.04.020

28. Blackhall LJ, Frank G, Murphy ST, Michel V, Palmer JM, Azen SP. Ethnicity and attitudes towards life sustaining technology. *Soc Sci Med*. Jun 1999;48(12):1779–1789. doi:10.1016/s0277-9536(99)00077-5

29. Mack JW, Paulk ME, Viswanath K, Prigerson HG. Racial disparities in the outcomes of communication on medical care received near death. *Arch Intern Med*. Sep 2010;170(17):1533–1540. doi:10.1001/archinternmed.2010.322

30. Hanchate A, Kronman AC, Young-Xu Y, Ash AS, Emanuel E. Racial and ethnic differences in end-of-life costs: Why do minorities cost more than whites? *Arch Intern Med*. Mar 2009;169(5):493–501. doi:10.1001/archinternmed.2008.616

31. Sharma RK, Kim H, Gozalo PL, Sullivan DR, Bunker J, Teno JM. The Black and White of invasive mechanical ventilation in advanced dementia. *J Am Geriatr Soc*. Sep 2020;68(9):2106–2111. doi:10.1111/jgs.16635

32. Grace Yi EH. Does acculturation matter? End-of-life care planning and preference of foreign-born older immigrants in the United States. *Innov Aging*. May 2019;3(2):igz012. doi:10.1093/geroni/igz012

33. Tergas AI, Prigerson HG, Shen MJ, et al. Latino ethnicity, immigrant status, and preference for end-of-life cancer care. *J Palliat Med*. Jul 2019;22(7):833–837. doi:10.1089/jpm.2018.0537

34. Pei Y, Zhang W, Wu B. Advance care planning engagement and end-of-life preference among older Chinese Americans: Do family relationships and immigrant status matter? *J Am Med Dir Assoc*. Feb 2021;22(2):340–343. doi:10.1016/j.jamda.2020.06.040

35. Choi S, McDonough IM, Kim M, Kim G. The association between the number of chronic health conditions and advance care planning varies by race/ethnicity. *Aging Ment Health*. Mar 2020;24(3):453–463. doi:10.1080/13607863.2018.1533521

36. Smith AK, Sudore RL, Pérez-Stable EJ. Palliative care for Latino patients and their families: Whenever we prayed, she wept. *JAMA*. Mar 2009;301(10):1047–1057, E1. doi:10.1001/jama.2009.308

37. Volandes AE, Paasche-Orlow M, Gillick MR, et al. Health literacy not race predicts end-of-life care preferences. *J Palliat Med*. Jun 2008;11(5):754–762. doi:10.1089/jpm.2007.0224

38. Thomas RE, Wilson D, Justice CJ, Birch S, Sheps S. A literature review of preferences for end-of-life care in developed countries by individuals with different cultural affiliations and ethnicity. *J Hospice Palliat Nurs*. 2008;10:142–161.

39. Johnson KS, Kuchibhatla M, Tulsky JA. Racial differences in location before hospice enrollment and association with hospice length of stay. *J Am Geriatr Soc*. Apr 2011;59(4):732–737. doi:10.1111/j.1532-5415.2011.03326.x

40. Rizzuto J, Aldridge MD. Racial disparities in hospice outcomes: A race or hospice-level effect? *J Am Geriatr Soc*. 02 2018;66(2):407–413. doi:10.1111/jgs.15228

41. Ngo-Metzger Q, Phillips RS, McCarthy EP. Ethnic disparities in hospice use among Asian-American and Pacific Islander patients dying with cancer. *J Am Geriatr Soc*. Jan 2008;56(1):139–144. doi:10.1111/j.1532-5415.2007.01510.x

42. Street RL, O'Malley KJ, Cooper LA, Haidet P. Understanding concordance in patient-physician relationships: Personal and ethnic dimensions of shared identity. *Ann Fam Med*. 2008 May-Jun 2008;6(3):198–205. doi:10.1370/afm.821

43. Sanders JJ, Curtis JR, Tulsky JA. Achieving goal-concordant care: A conceptual model and approach to measuring serious illness communication and its impact. *J Palliat Med*. 03 2018;21(S2):S17–S27. doi:10.1089/jpm.2017.0459

44. Bickel KE, McNiff K, Buss MK, et al. Defining high-quality palliative care in oncology practice: An American Society of Clinical Oncology/American Academy of Hospice and Palliative Medicine guidance statement. *J Oncol Pract*. 2016;12(9):e828–e838. doi:10.1200/jop.2016.010686

45. H.R.647 - Palliative Care and Hospice Education and Training Act. Congress.gov2019.

46. Marcelin JR, Siraj DS, Victor R, Kotadia S, Maldonado YA. The impact of unconscious bias in healthcare: How to recognize and mitigate it. *J Infect Dis*. 08 2019;220(220 Suppl 2):S62–S73. doi:10.1093/infdis/jiz214

47. Teal CR, Gill AC, Green AR, Crandall S. Helping medical learners recognise and manage unconscious bias toward certain patient groups. *Med Educ*. Jan 2012;46(1):80–88. doi:10.1111/j.1365-2923.2011.04101.x

17

Bereavement in Palliative Care

Wendy G. Lichtenthal, Carol Fadalla, Jonathan Singer, Kailey E. Roberts, William E. Rosa, Amanda Watsula, and Holly G. Prigerson

Introduction

Palliative care professionals witness grief in both patients and their loved ones, often beginning at the time of the patient's diagnosis as the possibility of death is considered. Throughout a patient's treatment trajectory, grief can continue as patients experience multiple losses: physical and mental impairment, unemployment, significant roles, and future plans. Palliative care psychiatrists are instrumental in supporting patients and their caregivers as they navigate these changes and can foster continuity of care from end of life through bereavement.

In order to aid patients and their chosen family (which can refer to relatives, partners, or close friends) as they grapple with grief, psychiatrists working in the palliative care context should be able to recognize the multiple clinical presentations of grief and risk factors for morbid outcomes.[1] They should remain "bereavement-conscious" in their care of the family, maintaining mindfulness about what may stay with the family after the patient dies and helping to mitigate the impact of traumatic stressors and prevent feelings of guilt and regret.[2] Following the patient's death, the ability to identify varied expressions of grief will allow practitioners to make appropriate referrals for individuals who are in need of more specialized or intensive bereavement care.[3] In this chapter, we characterize clinical presentations of typical and pathological grief responses as well as risk factors for poor bereavement outcomes in order to inform clinicians' work with patients and families receiving palliative care.

There are multiple ways to refer to loss, and many terms have been used interchangeably in the bereavement and grief literature. In this chapter, we will refer to the following terms as defined by grief scholars:

- *Bereavement* is the event, referring to the experience of someone significant dying.
- *Grief* is the emotional response to loss, including bereavement, and involves yearning for the lost individual and a variety of related feelings, cognitions, and behaviors.
- *Mourning* is the adaptation to loss influenced by cultural, religious, and social behaviors (e.g., grieving rituals).
- *Anticipatory grief* is the future-oriented emotional response to the impending loss, including feelings related to potential isolation or sadness. It is considered a type of *pre-death grief*.[4]
- *Illness-related grief* is the present-oriented emotional response to current losses (i.e., the patient's physical limitations). It is considered a type of *pre-death grief*.[4]
- *Complications of bereavement* include debilitating bereavement-related psychopathology (e.g., depression, anxiety, prolonged grief disorder, suicidal thoughts and behaviors) that are presumed to occur as a result of a significant loss.
- *Disenfranchised grief* occurs when individual reactions to loss are delegitimatized, unvalidated, and suppressed according to societal norms.
- *Ambiguous loss* occurs when the loss, cognitive or physical, is uncertain, including cases of a missing person or clinical events of dementia.

Grief Trajectories in Palliative Care

Clinicians working in palliative care may witness grieving throughout the illness trajectory, such as when disease progresses, around the time of and following the patient's death, and, in some cases, for a protracted period of time after the loss.

Grief at Bedside: Pre-death Grief

There is extensive literature on grief that emerges before the death of an individual with a life-limiting illness such as advanced cancer and dementia. A recent systematic review found that, across more than 130 studies, there are more than 30 definitions of grief before the loss and that operationalization of the term differs drastically.[4] To consolidate the extant literature and allow for comparison of future findings, Singer and colleagues[4] proposed two terms under the umbrella of pre-death grief to encapsulate the types of grief reactions that commonly occur before a patient's death. *Anticipatory grief* reflects grief occurring in anticipation of the death of the ill person. It often manifests as sadness and worry about a time when the patient will no longer be physically present and thus is considered future-oriented. *Illness-related grief*, on the other hand, is present-oriented, reflecting grief over current losses that the patient faces, such as the loss of roles or functioning. Illness-related grief might involve yearning or longing for characteristics of the patient before they were diagnosed with a life-limiting illness. Clinicians can distinguish and provide validation to individuals experiencing both anticipatory grief and illness-relatedgrief to help patients and families compassionately understand the complexity of their emotional reactions before the patient's death.

There have been multiple risk factors associated with pre-death grief. Risk factors have included increased caregiver burden, low preparedness for the death, increased depression, identifying as female, having a low educational background, the patient being younger in age, and living with the patient.[5] Studies have found downstream effects of heightened pre-death grief during bereavement such as increased risk of depression and prolonged grief disorder (PGD).[4] Therefore, intervening to mitigate grief before the loss might be an essential intervention target for long-term negative outcomes following the loss.

However, there is little research examining changes in grief before the loss over multiple time points. This is despite the effect of recent medical advances that allow people to live longer with a life-limiting illness, which, in turn, may prolong the amount of time that family members could be suffering with grief before the loss. This may be especially true of anticipatory grief, which may intensify as bad news is communicated. Families may be better able to adjust to illness-related grief related current losses. For example, Singer et al.[5] found that illness-related grief in family members of dementia and cancer patients decreased over the course of 1 month for 69% of family members. Of note, those who identified as female and reported greater caregiver burden at baseline had higher rates of illness-related grief at the 1-month follow-up.

Providing support to family members experiencing pre-death grief may not only improve their lives while the patient is still alive, but it also can be an inroad to bereavement care and reduce poor outcomes after the patient's death. This support may include encouragement of open communication with the patient and, when possible, supporting opportunities to address unfinished business, express appreciation for one another, resolve relational issues, and say goodbye. However, members of more dysfunctional families may react with denial, hostility, avoidance, or other maladaptive behaviors, resulting in tension and conflict. Furthermore, in situations in which a patient is noncommunicative, clinicians should be mindful of the role grief may play in the family's medical decision-making. For example, intense anticipatory grief may interfere with the ability of these surrogate decision-makers to effectively make value-congruent decisions, also increasing their risk for challenges in bereavement adjustment.[6]

Acute Grief Following the Death

Following the patient's death, families often appreciate outreach from the patient's care providers. Condolence calls can follow the CARE framework: (1) *communicate* compassionately, (2) *assess* risk for acute bereavement challenges, (3) *refer* when appropriate, and (4) *educate* about resources. Compassionate communication may involve answering family members' questions about the death, offering empathic presence, and ensuring they know that their loved one mattered. An initial screening assessment can involve determining the extent to which their grief and loss are affecting their ability to cope and function and whether they have social support. Referrals for grief counseling and education about resources such as bereavement groups and websites might be offered, thus normalizing the need for support. Additional details can be found in Lichtenthal et al.[3]

Grief reactions may initially be characterized by intense yearning, sadness, guilt, anger, despair, and anxiety. Acute grief manifests in a variety of thoughts, behaviors, and physical changes, and it is important to consider that there may be significant variability in grief reactions within a given family.[7] Surviving family members who have witnessed the patient's suffering through treatment or at the end of life may experience relief in parallel with their grief and sadness. It is not uncommon for grieving family members to experience intrusive thoughts regarding the patient's end-of-life experience or reminisce about the deceased. Family members may exhibit behaviors like searching for the deceased, social withdrawal, or alternatively seeking support and comfort. As family members grapple with the loss, they may also have difficulty sleeping or experience fatigue, anorexia, moderate weight loss, numbness, restlessness, tension, tremors, and sometimes physical pain.[8]

Previous theories posit predictable trajectories of "normal" or adaptive grief, although the evidence to support these consecutive stages has been mixed. One study found that, over time, yearning, shock, and sadness declined, while acceptance of the loss—that is, processing the reality that the loss occurred—gradually increased.[9] While knowledge of such trends is valuable, clinicians should remain cognizant that grief reactions are highly idiosyncratic and nonlinear and mindful not to suggest specific ways to grieve. Bereaved individuals often question or even pathologize their personal grief reactions, especially in the immediate wake of loss. Thus, clinicians should intentionally validate the psychosocial and physical challenges that grievers commonly face and normalize symptom variability and individualized responses to loss. Encouraging the bereaved to compassionately give themselves permission to grieve and offering psychoeducation about contemporary theories of grief may be helpful. For example, the dual-process model of coping highlights how the process of adapting to loss involves a somewhat unpredictable oscillation between coping with loss-oriented stressors, such as memories of the deceased, and restoration-oriented stressors, such as learning to engage in pleasurable activities without the deceased physically present.[10] Thus, bereaved individuals often fluctuate between periods of emotional pain and periods of adaptive engagement in activities as part of their adjustment to their loss. Table 17.1 provides additional details about typical grief.

No stringent timelines for the grieving process have been established, and symptom presentation should be considered in the context of what is culturally sanctioned. Over time, the majority of individuals (80–90%) will find ways to adapt to their loss, deal with reminders with equanimity, and exhibit resilience.[11] While it may be difficult to distinguish adaptive grief from pathological grief reactions, particularly soon after the patient's death, there are certain indicators that professionals can monitor. These include the grieving individual's ability to accept the loss; to re-engage with work, leisure, and creative activities; to connect in other social relationships; and to view life as potentially meaningful and satisfying. Finding ways to remain connected to the deceased (e.g., through conversations or rituals) is considered adaptive. This said, even among bereaved family members who have adjusted to their loss, it is common to continue to deeply miss the deceased individual throughout one's life, with grief typically intensifying during occasions like anniversaries or birthdays.

Bereavement-Related Psychopathology

While psychiatrists should be careful to avoid pathologizing bereavement-related distress, it is equally crucial to recognize when grief symptoms become intolerable and debilitating so that proper intervention and attention can be provided to family members in need of

TABLE 17.1 Considerations for differential diagnosis between typical grief and mental disorders in bereavement

Typical grief/Mental disorder	Symptom distinctions
Typical grief	• Yearning for the deceased, sadness, and disbelief about the loss emerges in waves • Anger; guilt; and sleep, appetite, and concentration disruptions common in the immediate wake of the loss • Intensity and frequency of symptoms decrease over time, though commonly intensifies around reminders of the deceased, anniversaries, holidays, and milestones • Adaptive, transformed relationship with the deceased continues over time
Prolonged grief disorder (PGD)	• Yearning and separation distress related to the lost relationship are intense, persistent, and debilitating • Persistent disbelief, numbness, and difficulty accepting the reality of the loss • Protracted challenges with sense of identity, meaning, and purpose • Distinguished from depression by the focus of sadness being on the relationship with the deceased and the stability and chronicity of symptoms • Distinguished from posttraumatic stress disorder (PTSD) by re-experiencing being more deliberate to connect to the deceased and avoidance focused on triggers of emotional pain related to the absence of the deceased
Bereavement-related major depressive disorder	• Pervasive sadness and anhedonia, not only related to memories of or activities with the deceased • Sadness more prominent than yearning, with less focus on the deceased, and less positive affect than in PGD • Negative cognitions focus on oneself (e.g., sense of worthlessness), the world, and the future rather than focus on the deceased
Bereavement-related posttraumatic stress disorder	• Reaction to witnessing or experiencing a traumatic event such as situations related to the deceased's illness or death, with negative feelings and cognitions emerging after the trauma • Re-experiencing symptoms related to events that threatened the deceased during their illness or death, which are experienced as intrusive and unwanted rather than comforting as with PGD • Avoidance symptoms related to thoughts, feelings, or situations that are reminders of the threatening situation (e.g., end-of-life or death circumstances) rather than reminders of the deceased's absence • Heightened arousal • Greater difficulty experiencing positive affect and fear more dominant than with PGD

Note. Please see https://endoflife.weill.cornell.edu/grief-resources for video vignettes portraying different clinical presentations in bereavement, and Lichtenthal, Roberts, and Prigerson[3] and Zisook and Shear[8] for more information.

support.[8] See Table 17.1 for information to guide making differential diagnoses in bereavement. Among the more common bereavement-related mental health challenges that surviving family members experience is PGD, which occurs in approximately 8% of caregivers and may occur in response to traumatic or non-traumatic losses.[12,13] A core symptom of PGD is yearning for the deceased, and individuals often appear "stuck" in a state of acute grief. They additionally may experience preoccupation with the deceased, disbelief about and avoidance of reminders of the loss, intense emotional pain, numbness, difficulty engaging in life, loneliness, and challenges to their sense of identity and meaning in life. Symptoms of comorbid depression and anxiety may be present, these include dysphoria, changes in appetite or weight, and agitation. Diagnostic criteria for PGD have been included in the International Classification of Diseases-11 (ICD-11) and the Diagnostic and Statistical Manual of Mental Disorders Text Revision (DSM-5-TR).[13,14] Of note, DSM-5-TR specifies that 12 months must have elapsed since death to meet criteria for PGD, as compared to the current criterion of 6 months in the ICD-11, which may change in future editions.[13,14] Expanding the duration criterion may reduce the likelihood of pathologization of typical grief reactions and accounts for the possibility of delayed onset of symptoms while still facilitating identification of individuals with unrelenting grief who may benefit from intervention.[13]

With the removal of the bereavement exclusion criteria in the DSM-5, depression can technically be diagnosed once anhedonia and depressed mood have been present for at least 2 weeks following the loss of a loved one. However, given the frequency and commonality of depressive symptoms such as sadness, anhedonia, and somatic symptoms in the early months of bereavement, clinicians should carefully consider an individual's history and cultural norms of symptom expression and should exercise caution before making such a diagnosis. That said, feelings of regret or perceptions of the patient's pain and suffering, as well as a personal or family history of depression, can increase the risk of developing bereavement-related major depressive disorder,[6] and individuals who are more susceptible may find relief through early diagnosis and treatment with evidence-based interventions.[8]

Bereaved individuals also commonly develop symptoms of persistent and intense anxiety and worry, often beginning while the patient is receiving palliative care. Research has shown that approximately 6 months post-loss, 6% of caregivers meet criteria for major depressive disorder, 2% meet criteria for generalized anxiety disorder, 3% meet criteria for panic disorder, and 3% meet criteria for posttraumatic stress disorder (PTSD).[15] In a palliative care setting, traumatic stress symptoms may develop when the family member perceives circumstances surrounding the patient's illness or death as sudden or traumatic, such as witnessing a patient coding or hemorrhaging. It is not uncommon for the bereaved to experience flashbacks and engage in some avoidance of thoughts or feelings associated with the illness or loss. Clinicians should carefully assess the frequency and persistence of these symptoms to determine whether the family member meets full criteria for PTSD.

Although the loss of a loved one is a clear and identifiable stressor, a diagnosis of an adjustment disorder should be deferred if the clinical symptoms are due to normal bereavement. Bereaved individuals who have a history of substance abuse, such as smoking and alcohol dependence, are at an increased risk of developing PGD symptoms[16] and may be more susceptible to relapse. Increased likelihood of relapse in bereavement is also possible in bereaved individuals with preexisting severe mental illness. Importantly, bereaved individuals are at increased risk of both deliberate self-harm and suicide for up to 10 years following their loss, especially those who have experienced the loss of a child or spouse; however, the risk is highest in the first year.[17] Suicide risk is highest among those with depression and PGD.[13,14]

Risk Factors for Bereavement-Related Psychopathology

While most bereaved individuals will experience an adaptive trajectory of grief in which the intensity of grief decreases over time and they are able to engage in day-to-day life,[11] research has established risk factors that can contribute to individuals developing mental health challenges such as PGD, depression, and PTSD. Bereavement risk factors have been categorized into background characteristics (e.g., being a spouse or parent, insecure attachment style, history of separation anxiety, emotional dependency on the deceased, mental health history), characteristics of the illness or death (e.g., witnessing intensive medical interventions, perceiving the death as traumatic), and experiences in bereavement (e.g., regret, decreased sense of meaning, social isolation).[1]

Certain populations may be particularly at risk for challenges in bereavement. Older adult caregivers are at heightened risk for bereavement-related mental health problems, in part because of the compounding challenges they face related to aging.[1] Not only do older bereaved adults contend with the loss of a significant relationship, they may experience substantial social, financial, and practical support losses, often in the context of preexisting chronic illness, disability, reduced mobility, and cognitive decline.[1] Bereaved parents are also at higher risk and may need specialized support, as the loss of a child is widely considered to be one of the most devastating types of bereavement. In a palliative care context, parents may have had to make extremely difficult end-of-life decisions on behalf of their child and therefore may contend with related feelings of guilt and regret in bereavement. Finally, it is also important to consider that marginalized individuals may be at risk for experiencing disenfranchised grief, meaning their grief is not recognized or validated by those in power, in turn increasing their risk for mental health challenges in bereavement.

Several risk factors may have particular salience in palliative care settings, including the circumstances of the death and preparedness of family members. For example, if family members witness or hear about the patient experiencing uncontrolled pain, having difficulty breathing, seizing, or experiencing delirium, this can put them at risk for developing PTSD in bereavement.[1,3] Additionally, family members may be at risk if end-of-life discussions do not appropriately prepare family members for what they may witness as the patient dies or do not provide them with sufficient support in navigating the practical challenges of death.[1]

Bereavement risk screening has been suggested as one element of palliative care,[18] but the implementation of risk screening has been limited due to a lack of validated, clinically useful screening tools; absence of guidelines for documentation; and insufficient resources put toward bereavement care more broadly.[1] The Bereavement Risk Inventory and Screening Questionnaire (BRISQ) is one tool that shows promise as it has been developed with stakeholder expert and family member input, incorporates significant risk factors identified in the bereavement literature, and is designed to be efficiently administered in palliative care settings to triage resources.[1] Clinicians unable to implement a formal assessment tool may also find use of a mnemonic, such as GRIEF RISK (see Table 17.2), helpful in bringing to mind important bereavement risk factors to consider.[3]

TABLE 17.2 GRIEF RISK mnemonic for assessment of bereavement risk factors

Risk factor	Description
Guilt	• Significant guilt related to the relationship with the deceased or to the deceased's medical care or circumstances of death
Regret	• Significant regret related to the relationship with the deceased or to the deceased's medical care or decision-making
Isolation	• Isolation from sources of positive social support and the subjective experience of loneliness
Experienced multiple losses or other stressors	• Multiple losses (e.g., other death losses, job, etc.) or concurrent stressors
Financial hardship	• Financial problems generally and/or in the context of the patient's illness or death
Relationship dependency or challenges	• High degree of dependence on the deceased person for important tasks (e.g., computer or other technology use, finances) or emotional support • Conflictual relationship with the deceased
Individual history of mental health challenges or trauma	• History of mental health problems (e.g., depression) or prior exposure to trauma • Past evidence of suicidality
Sudden or distressing circumstances of death	• Lack of preparedness for the death • Perception of moments during the patient's illness or circumstances of death as traumatic (e.g., uncontrolled pain, difficulty breathing, delirium)
Kinship type	• Parents, younger spouses, and isolated older adults

Note. Please see Lichtenthal, Roberts, and Prigerson[3] for sample GRIEF RISK assessment questions.

Professional Grief, Mass Bereavement, and COVID-19

Palliative care clinicians should also be mindful of their own reactions to patient loss. Although the clinician–patient relationship is qualitatively different from the attachment relationships between family and patients, clinicians may experience a unique response to loss characterized by sadness, personal responsibility, and guilt.[19] Providers who experience frequent exposure to patient death may face both personal effects (e.g., changes to personality, gaining perspective on life, strain on social relationships) and professional sequelae (exhaustion and burnout, compartmentalization of feelings at work and home, challenges with decision-making).[20] Clinicians have expressed that they value having their grief over patient loss acknowledged, normalized, and validated with opportunities to share their experiences, debrief in group settings, and be supported by mentors.[19]

COVID-19 has amplified a global narrative of loss and bereavement among the healthcare workforce. Research suggests that healthcare providers working during infectious disease outbreaks can experience long-term psychological sequelae, including anxiety and fears, stigmatization, depression, posttraumatic stress, anger and frustration, burnout, and grief.[21] That said, positive growth and transformation has also been observed.[21] A recent systematic review suggested the importance of preparing healthcare providers for the possibility of experiencing grief following a patient's death and of equipping them with information about factors that may compound or alleviate distress related to patient loss.[22]

Future Directions

While there has been some increased attention given to bereavement as part of comprehensive palliative care in recent decades, there remains much to be done to improve continuity of care for grieving families. Investigations should focus on the development of psychometrically sound assessments of both anticipatory grief and illness-related grief and examination of their prevalence and correlates over time. Research on multilevel interventions to evaluate the implementation of standardized bereavement risk screening is needed. Development of guidelines for documentation of bereavement care efforts should be established. Finally, and perhaps most significantly, institutions need to devote resources to effectively implement proposed guidelines for standardizing bereavement care.[18]

Summary

Psychiatrists working in palliative care settings are charged with continuing care through bereavement. While many clinicians may not identify as bereavement specialists, with knowledge of symptom presentations and risk factors, they can be "bereavement-conscious" in their practices prior to the patient's death,[2] offer support and pharmacological interventions in the wake of the loss, and facilitate appropriate referrals when warranted.[3] Details on specific intervention approaches in bereavement can be found in Chapter 41.

Key Points

- Bereavement care is part of psychiatric palliative care. Being a bereavement-conscious clinician means supporting grief from the time of diagnosis and remaining mindful about what experiences and decisions may stay with family members well beyond the patient's death and helping to mitigate the impact of traumatic stressors and feelings of guilt and regret.
- Clinicians can distinguish and validate pre-death grief, including both illness-related grief over current losses and anticipatory grief over the patient's possible death in the future, when working with families at the end of life.
- Grief reactions are highly idiosyncratic and nonlinear, and clinicians should be careful not to pathologize typical grief symptoms in the wake of a loss.
- Prolonged grief disorder, diagnosed when intense and debilitating grief symptoms persist beyond 12 months after the loss, as well as bereavement-related depression, anxiety, and posttraumatic stress disorder may occur in a subset of surviving family members.

- Risk for mental health challenges in bereavement is highest among family members—particularly parents and spouses—who have a mental health history, report significant grief or regret, felt unprepared for the loss, were dependent on the deceased, are isolated, and who face multiple losses, financial challenges, and/or other major stressors.

References

1. Roberts KE, Jankauskaite G, Slivjak E, et al. Bereavement risk screening: A pathway to psychosocial oncology care. *Psycho-oncology.* 2020;29(12):2041–2047.
2. Roberts KE, Lichtenthal WG, Ferrell BR. Being a bereavement-conscious hospice and palliative care clinician *J Hospice Palliat Nurs.* 2021;23(4):293–295.
3. Lichtenthal WG, Roberts KE, Prigerson HG. Bereavement care in the wake of COVID-19: Offering condolences and referrals. *Ann Intern Med.* 2020;173:833–835.
4. Singer J, Roberts KE, McLean E, et al. An examination of family members grief prior to loss of individuals with a life limiting illness: A systematic review. under review.
5. Singer J, Shrout MR, Papa A. Rates and prospective psychosocial correlates of pre-loss grief in cancer and dementia family members. *J Health Psychol.* 2021;27(7):1547–1555. doi:10.1177/1359105321995945.
6. Garrido MM, Prigerson HG. The end-of-life experience: Modifiable predictors of caregivers' bereavement adjustment. *Cancer.* 2014;120:918–925.
7. Parkes CM, Prigerson HG. *Bereavement: Studies of Grief in Adult Life.* 4th ed. Hove, East Sussex, UK: Routledge; 2009.
8. Zisook S, Shear K. Grief and bereavement: what psychiatrists need to know. *World Psychiatry.* 2009;8:67–74.
9. Maciejewski PK, Zhang B, Block SD, Prigerson HG. An empirical examination of the stage theory of grief. *JAMA.* 2007;297:716–723.
10. Stroebe M, Schut H. The dual process model of coping with bereavement: A decade on. *Omega.* 2010;61:273–289.
11. Bonanno GA, Kaltman S. The varieties of grief experience. *Clin Psychol Rev.* 2001;21:705–734.
12. Nielsen MK, Neergaard MA, Jensen AB, Vedsted P, Bro F, Guldin MB. Predictors of complicated grief and depression in bereaved caregivers: A nationwide prospective cohort study. *J Pain Sympt Manage.* 2017;53:540–550.
13. Prigerson HG, Boelen PA, Xu J, Smith KV, Maciejewski PK. Validation of the new DSM-5-TR criteria for prolonged grief disorder and the PG-13-Revised (PG-13-R) scale. *World Psychiatry.* 2021;20:96–106.
14. World Health Organization (WHO). *International Classification of Diseases for Mortality and Morbidity Statistics* (11th revision). Geneva: WHO; 2018.
15. Wright AA, Zhang B, Ray A, et al. Associations between end-of-life discussions, patient mental health, medical care near death, and caregiver bereavement adjustment. *JAMA.* 2008;300:1665–1673.
16. Parisi A, Sharma A, Howard MO, Wilson AB. The relationship between substance misuse and complicated grief: A systematic review. *J Substance Abuse Treatm.* 2019;103:43–57.
17. Guldin MB, Ina Siegismund Kjaersgaard M, Fenger-Grøn M, et al. Risk of suicide, deliberate self-harm and psychiatric illness after the loss of a close relative: A nationwide cohort study. *World Psychiatry.* 2017;16:193–199.
18. Hudson P, Hall C, Boughey A, Roulston A. Bereavement support standards and bereavement care pathway for quality palliative care. *Palliat Support Care.* 2018;16:375–387.
19. Granek L, Mazzotta P, Tozer R, Krzyzanowska MK. What do oncologists want? Suggestions from oncologists on how their institutions can support them in dealing with patient loss. *Support Care Cancer.* 2012;20:2627–2632.
20. Granek L, Ariad S, Nakash O, Cohen M, Bar-Sela G, Ben-David M. Mixed-methods study of the impact of chronic patient death on oncologists' personal and professional lives. *J Oncol Pract.* 2017;13:e1–e10.

21. Chew QH, Wei KC, Vasoo S, Sim K. Psychological and coping responses of health care workers toward emerging infectious disease outbreaks: A rapid review and practical implications for the COVID-19 pandemic. *J Clin Psychiatry.* 2020;81:10–15.
22. Barnes S, Jordan Z, Broom M. Health professionals' experiences of grief associated with the death of pediatric patients: A systematic review. *JBI Evidence Synthesis.* 2020;18:459–515.

18

Family and Couple Issues in Palliative Care

David W. Kissane and Talia I. Zaider

Introduction

A progressive and advanced illness that requires palliative care inevitably needs the partner and/or family to adopt a caregiving role and eventually cope with the death of the patient. Sustaining the well-being of couples and families is a central activity within the philosophy of palliative care. Such a systemic approach can meet complex dynamics, never more so than when relational dysfunction challenges care provision. Special expertise may then be called upon to optimize functioning and strive to prevent morbidity reaching into bereavement.

Progressive illness alters roles and responsibilities, challenges communication, derails plans and routines, and demands time and financial resources to adequately deal with the needs of the ill person. The impact of this predicament can reverberate across the generations, as boundaries of the family group are redefined, and distress is coregulated by the family system. Family members carry high rates of emotional burden and unmet needs, leaving them sometimes unprepared to respond to the caregiving needs of the patient. In this chapter, we examine the impact of palliative and terminal illness on the family, addressing first of all the couple as one potential unit of care, and then the family as a whole, given the inescapable reach of a terminal illness.

Couple-Focused Care

For most adults, the relationship with an intimate partner is the most meaningful and influential social context in which individual distress is expressed and managed. Whether in sickness or in health, marital status is a known protective factor, broadly linked to reduction in mortality risk and improved health practices across a range of chronic illnesses. The health benefits conferred by being in a long-term relationship have been attributed to the multiple ways in which patients and their partners influence one another's well-being. The level of interdependence that characterizes close relationships enables a shared response to stress, allowing couples to access a broader repertoire of adaptive coping strategies than would be available to the individual partner alone. A large body of evidence shows that relationship partners influence one another's stress response, mood, coping behavior, and end-of-life decision-making: in one study, when adults who were widowed subsequently approached their own death, they were twice as likely to use hospice care, advance care planning, or critical care if the same was true for the spouse who died before them.[1]

The high degree of congruence observed in couples suggests that this relationship is a powerful, albeit underutilized, resource that can be leveraged to attenuate distress and support resilience for patients with incurable disease and their caregivers. As would be expected, the extent to which an intimate partnership is a source of strength or strain will depend on the quality of the relationship and its various dimensions (e.g., communication, conflict-management, effectiveness of support provision). Below, we review specific relationship mechanisms that shape and are shaped by the illness course and then provide an overview of empirically tested interventions that target couples coping with advanced disease.

Relational Functions at the End of Life

As couples face the prospect of loss, relational tasks such as saying goodbye, confiding in loved ones, sharing time together, or addressing unresolved emotional injuries become important contributions to a so-called good death. Opportunities for shared meaning-making and an intensification of the attachment bond often coexist with grief, isolation, and existential distress as couples navigate this phase of illness. For couples coping with significant symptom burden or frequent hospital admissions for one partner, usual ways of relating are profoundly altered and it becomes challenging to preserve core aspects of relationship functioning.

Communication

Serious illness often distorts usual communication patterns in couples as partners are driven to protectively buffer themselves and one another from distressing topics. Concerns that may preoccupy each partner privately (e.g., prognosis, end-of-life wishes) become exceedingly difficult to address openly unless by necessity for medical decision-making. Yet communication is also the central means by which patients and their partners co-construct meaning in response to the illness experience, affirm individual and shared priorities, determine and coordinate the patient's caregiving needs, and collaborate on practical tasks. Most dyadic interventions therefore promote constructive communication skills as a major component.

Recent conceptualizations of dyadic communication in the context of illness have encouraged a more nuanced perspective on how and when talking about illness is of benefit to patients and their partners, acknowledging that one size does not fit all in regard to emotional disclosure. When couples coping with advanced disease are observed communicating in the home setting, they appear to balance informational or logistical talk about illness with more routine, non-illness discussions.[2] Although families with poor communication at baseline are predisposed to worse psychosocial outcomes during palliative care and in bereavement, there is evidence that even well-functioning families struggle to talk about end-of-life concerns. Even when prompted to discuss illness concerns as part of a structured dyadic intervention for patients with advanced gastrointestinal cancers, couples were least likely to select the topic "end-of-life preparations" relative to other domains (e.g., pain and symptom management, decision-making).[3] Not surprisingly, sharing anticipatory grief and distress is more likely to be beneficial when partners perceive one another to be responsive to such disclosures (i.e., supportive and accepting).[4] Optimizing communication for a given couple may therefore require a more tailored and nuanced consideration of partners' differential roles and preferences, as well as their capacity for empathic attunement.[2] Negative interaction patterns, such as when one partner's demand for communication is met with the other partner's withdrawal, can worsen tension and should be addressed by normalizing differences in communication styles so that responsiveness can be cultivated. Weingarten (2013) offers an eloquent description of the interplay within couples between acknowledgment of self- versus other-loss and how asymmetries in this process can increase tension and disconnection within relationships.[5]

Intimacy

When there has been a loss of sexual intimacy due to progressive disease and/or its treatment, couples will often shield one another from feelings of embarrassment or shame by withdrawing from physical contact altogether. In doing so, they avoid acknowledging even the most obvious physical changes due to declining health or infirmity. Clinicians follow suit, rarely inquiring about disruptions in sexual functioning or loss of sexual desire in the context of palliative care. Yet the limited research in this area demonstrates that patients are eager to bring these concerns to the fore. In one large study of more than 900 advanced cancer patients, more than half expressed a strong desire for physical intimacy and felt their illness had impaired their ability to sustain sexual closeness.[6] Couples consider it helpful and important to have discussions with their provider about threats to sexual expression and intimacy. Direct assessment of these concerns allows couples to acknowledge the loss of spontaneity and ease with which sexual intimacy was once achieved, revise definitions of intimacy to include the emotional, and identify creative adaptations.

When physical contact is made difficult due to symptom burden, emphasis is placed instead on gestures of emotional intimacy. Couples coping with illness are more likely to experience feelings of closeness when they engage in relationship-enhancing behaviors (e.g., responsiveness and disclosure) and less likely to experience closeness when more compromising behaviors predominate (e.g., criticism, mutual avoidance, pressure-withdraw patterns).[7] The interpersonal processes that contribute to the experience of intimacy in couples are also highly predictive of individuals' psychological adaptation to serious illness. Although these pathways to intimacy and psychological adjustment have not been well tested in the context of advanced disease, their grounding in decades of relationship science suggest broad generalizability.

Communal Coping

The extent to which couples manage cancer-related distress jointly, referred to as "we-ness" or "communal coping," has been consistently linked to better individual adjustment (e.g., self-efficacy, distress) as well as higher relationship functioning.[8] Finding ways to preserve and even amplify the identity and coping capacity of the couple as a unit is an important target for couple therapies. In addition to its implications for joint problem-solving, communal coping assumes a level of congruence in the couples' appraisal of a health threat and recognition of its impact on the family. The couple that is able to externalize the disease is more likely to relate to it collaboratively as opposed to construing it as primarily internal to the individual patient who then carries a sense of burden and guilt in isolation.

Couple-Based Interventions in Advanced Disease

Although supporting the caregiving family is a core tenet of palliative care, relatively few dyadic interventions have been empirically tested for patients with advanced disease and their partners. Broad meta-analyses of couple-based interventions in cancer have demonstrated significant benefits to patient quality of life, reduction in patients' depressive and anxiety symptoms, and improvements in marital functioning.[9] Yet in the context of advanced disease specifically, most of the published data over the last decade come from pilot studies, with preliminary findings that nevertheless offer a strong endorsement for the value and acceptability of such interventions. In a descriptive review of couple and family interventions in advanced cancer, Badr (2014) found that most interventions used educational methods to teach communication, coping, and problem-solving skills jointly to the patient and caregiver.[10] Taken together, intervention studies have yielded moderate effects for patients and caregivers on relationship functioning, patient distress, and caregiver burden, but less impact on global quality of life scores. Although couples generally responded favorably to the content of these therapies, access to couple-based support in the practice setting continues to be a major challenge. Published interventions for couples with advanced illness have therefore tried to minimize burden by limiting session dose[11] or restricting the delivery format to telephone or videoconferencing. Strong endorsement from the medical team and co-location of support with palliative and primary medical care services may facilitate uptake for couples who are contending with complex care regimens and frequent appointments.

One example of an integrated model of dyadic support was implemented by a Danish team[12] who incorporated psychosocial support sessions for couples into a program of home-based, palliative care. Alongside a multidisciplinary palliative care team, a psychologist provided patients and their caregivers with two home-based sessions focused on addressing salient issues of concern to the dyad, with additional strategies used to encourage mutual disclosure, highlight relational strengths, and increase opportunities to respond to disease burden together. Subsequent telephone-based booster sessions were offered to conduct periodic needs assessments and provide couples with continuity of care up to and including early bereavement. Compared with a control condition, the intervention was associated with a significant increase in communal coping efforts among patients and caregivers and increased disclosure of support needs by caregiving partners. Interestingly, in dyads comprised of patients and their adult children, the intervention was associated with *less* communication for the patient-parent, a reminder that any effort to optimize communication must account for family roles and related communication preferences.

The "Me in We" intervention for couples coping with advanced cancer similarly sought to engage the patient–caregiver dyad jointly in palliative care.[13] Whereas usual advance care planning discussions center around the patients' individual values, priorities, and end-of-life wishes, Ketcher and colleagues (2021) developed a two-session intervention in which couples were prompted to identify and define meaningful goals that honored each of their personal and relational priorities at the end of life.[13] Preliminary data demonstrated high acceptability and uptake of the intervention. Contrary to common concerns about the undue influence of the family on patients' expression of end of life goals, participants reported low levels of distress and high satisfaction during these more relationally oriented goals-of-care discussions, in addition to which they reported feeling understood by their partner and more motivated to support their partners' goals.

Whereas the interventions described above were delivered universally to couples facing advanced disease, palliative care services may need to adopt a more targeted approach to ensure that psychosocial resources are being allocated to those with the greatest support needs. Data on differential intervention effects can provide important information on whether dyadic interventions benefit more vulnerable subgroups. For example, a communication skills training intervention for couples coping with advanced gastrointestinal cancers found significant benefits for couples who at baseline featured highly inhibited communication patterns.[3] Badr and colleagues (2015) found that among advanced lung cancer patients who presented with high levels of depression, 71% showed clinically significant improvement in depressive symptoms following a dyadic intervention, as compared with only 33% of depressed patients who received usual medical care.[14] Similar patterns were observed for caregiving partners with high depression scores at baseline. The intervention used a couple-based approach to bolster personal agency and self-competence among patients while simultaneously teaching couples to mobilize support from one another and preserve meaningful aspects of the relationship. It is possible that the inclusion of strategies to support and strengthen personal agency helped to combat depressive symptoms by increasing behavioral activation and self-efficacy. These interventions underscore the value of routine screening to identify couples with greater communication challenges and/ or higher levels of psychological morbidity who may benefit most from couple-based care.

As compared with educational, skill-based models of couple therapy, there has been far less attention given to existential and intimacy-based approaches at the end of life. The need to strengthen connectedness in the face of vulnerability and grief is a central theme of emotion-focused couples therapy (EFT), an attachment-based approach that can be used for couples facing advanced cancer.[15] Implicit in EFT is that communication and problem-solving skills need not be taught, but instead will emerge spontaneously under conditions of safe emotional connection. This intervention is focused on helping couples to recognize destructive or distancing interaction cycles that arise in the context of illness and to generate new ways of interacting that restore closeness and open emotional expression. A randomized controlled trial targeting couples with high relationship distress showed significant improvement in marital functioning for those who participated in the intervention relative to a control group, with 91% of intervention patients meeting criteria for clinically significant improvement in marital distress, compared with only 28% of control patients.[15] Benefits were evident up to 3 months post-treatment, but longer-term follow-up was not obtained. A primary limitation to this approach is that it is more resource-heavy than those described above, requiring more sessions and therapists with more advanced training in systemic and experientially based couple therapy techniques.

Family-Focused Care

The philosophy of palliative care has been both patient- and family-centered from its early origins as this dual approach is both preventive and responsive to needs. Recognizing who constitutes the family is essential. While kinship relationships are often considered, in practice the patient defines their "psychological" family as those who matter, have helped to form part of their world, and contribute to information needs and care provision within the system.

The Psychological Burden of Care Provision

Recent studies have confirmed findings from prior decades and several reviews that palliative illnesses can have a profound impact on the health and well-being of family members. The mean level of distress in family caregivers measured by the distress thermometer was 7.9 (standard deviation [SD] 1.8; range, 2–10), while the prevalence rate for moderate to severe anxiety symptoms on the General Anxiety Disorder (GAD-7) scale was 47% and depressive symptoms on the Patient Health Questionnaire (PHQ-9) was 39%.[16] Being female, having low socioeconomic status, poor sleep, dwelling in a dysfunctional family, and high patient symptom levels profoundly increased the likelihood of developing psychiatric disorders. Morbidity can also take the form of poor quality of life, with fatigue, insomnia, burnout, and social isolation all contributing. Such morbidity among family members transfers into disorders in bereavement, with around 15% developing prolonged grief disorder.[17]

To address such needs, two broad approaches have developed. The first is educational and aims to prepare caregivers and bolster family members during the illness. The second is preventive and seeks to identify and support families at greater risk through a more intensive program of therapeutic care.

Psychoeducation of Caregivers and Families

Providing information in anticipation of needs is seminal to assisting caregivers in their role. The content is proportional to the phase of the patient's illness. Delivery occurs with permission and can be stepped to enable integration. Educational literature that covers the journey of palliative care empowers caregivers to dip into topics as needed.[18]

Interventions can be delivered individually by nurses in the home, or cost-effectively to groups of caregivers to promote competence and preparedness.[19] Topics can range from exercise and nutrition through to use of syringe drivers and the role of breakthrough analgesic medication. Question prompt lists can encourage families to ask questions during consultations to optimize their integration of knowledge and skills.

Conduct of a Routine Family Meeting

This is a frequent and important event in palliative care, where a family meeting is used to (1) assess family needs; (2) educate about the illness and symptom management; (3) understand wishes about end-of-life care, including advance care plans and decision-makers; (4) discuss discharge plans, placement, or continuing goals of care; and (5) assess family coping and concerns about any members.

Families usually clarify prognosis and reach consensus with the care team about ongoing goals of care through discussions in these meetings. They are a critical means to optimize communication, prove to be deeply appreciated by participants, and avoid misunderstandings that can otherwise occur. For many, open discussion of death and dying in a family meeting empowers members to shift from protective or avoidant stances to a greater openness about the present reality.

The presence of the ill or dying family member in such a meeting can present a special opportunity to acknowledge the finite nature of this person's life and help the family to move to words of appreciation and gratitude, paving the way for the family to eventually say goodbye. Frailty of illness can sometimes prevent the sick person from attending, but clinicians do well to remain open to their presence.

Three specific communication skills are used to facilitate a family meeting: agenda setting, circular questions, and integrative summaries.

Agenda Setting

To provide helpful structure, efficiency, and adequate coverage of each family's needs, the process of creating an agenda at the beginning of the meeting proves invaluable. By moving around the circle, each person can be invited to put their questions or concerns on the table, noting commonalities and creating order. The agenda results from this list, which will include the clinician's aims as well. The meeting facilitator needs to ensure that questions are not grappled with prematurely, that problem-solving does not start until the agenda list is complete and agreed to by those present.

Circular Questions

Rather than the facilitator talking and dominating the meeting with a linear dialogue between one person and the facilitator, the circular question invites one family member to express their opinion about the well-being and coping of their relatives, with the facilitator moving around the circle to ask family members to share their perspective in turn. The resultant exchange of views both reveals the family's dynamics and invites empathic interactions between relatives, which fosters mutual care and support. The art of using circular questions to run family meetings is an acquired skill learned through communication skill training.[20]

Integrative Summaries

In working through the agenda, once an issue has been discussed and appears to be resolved, the facilitator summarizes what is understood to be the consensus view of the meeting and checks that this mutual understanding has been agreed to. This ensures readiness to move on to the next issue. From time to time, the caregiver or alternate family member can be invited to offer this summary as a means of confirming that such understanding has been truly achieved.

The sequence of steps for the conduct of a routine family meeting are shown in Box 18.1. Much education and family support can be achieved through the conduct of a routine family meeting in palliative care.

Working with Families in Greater Need

Certain families in palliative care need more formal family support; these are listed in Box 18.2. Let us consider the issues that such families present and approaches to care provision in response to their needs.

Families with a Dying Parent and Adolescent/ Young Children

A psychoeducational approach can guide parents toward open and honest communication with children, sustaining hope and normality of family life.[21] Education is tailored to the

---

BOX 18.1 Sequence of Steps for Running a Routine Family Meeting in Palliative Care

1. *Welcome attendees*, inviting each person to introduce themselves.
2. *Agenda setting*: The leaders offer their reasons for the meeting and invite attendees to add items to a list. Common issues include status of illness, prognosis, goals of ongoing care, family needs and coping, place of future care, wishes about place of death, challenging symptoms, nursing techniques, home supports or placement, and allied health assessments and feedback.
3. *The illness*: Pose circular questions about understanding of illness/prognosis, worrying symptoms, coping of family members, resources, and support needs.
4. *Care plans*: Ask if consensus about goals of care and future plans be agreed to.
5. *Family strengths and coping*: Pose circular questions about how individuals are coping and will cope. What helps? Tasks, roles, and strengths that sustain the family. Any concerns?
6. *Key summaries* are presented of what the meeting has resolved, tasks assigned, and follow-up needs.

BOX 18.2 Families Warranting Family Therapy in Palliative Care

Family therapy is a critical support process for the following families:

Families with adolescent or younger children where a parent is dying

Families with disabled members who may have been dependent on the dying person

Families with older adults in need

Families with poor communication and avoidance of palliative illness issues

Families who are conflictual

Families who lack cohesion and are disengaged, thus uninvolved in care needs

Families of cultural and linguistic diversity with special needs (migrant, refugee, or need for interpreters)

---

developmental age of each child. Use is often made of school counseling services. Treatment of parental depression and family dysfunction is critical because, when untreated, they predict behavioral disturbance in children. Bereaved children in the 8- to 16-year-range have been helped by group sessions.[22] Regular family meetings are a normative approach to management.

Families with a Dying Child

Family conversations need to be realistic, and parents do not regret talking to their child about death, often finding that older children are drawn into the process.[23] Families who are helped to find meaning in the life of the child who is dying or deceased end up adjusting satisfactorily. Regular meetings with the parents at one level and the family as a whole from time to time prove invaluable in guiding the family through this experience.

Families with Older Adults

Availability for care provision becomes a major factor for adult children whose parent becomes frail and elderly, necessitating home help or use of a residential care facility. Family meetings empower more open discussion of these topics, which otherwise cause awkwardness and embarrassment. Questions involve how to overcome loneliness, social devaluation, or disenfranchisement.

Families with Disabled Members

When parents have been long-term caregivers for children with Down's syndrome, chronic schizophrenia, or cerebral palsy, as examples, future care planning with community systems, group homes, and related organizations becomes crucial. Issues of emotional dependence and care transition can be addressed across several family meetings.

Low-Communicating Families

Studies across Western cultures have revealed that around 20% of families carry restricted communication, often based on avoidant coping, reduced education or health literacy, or lower interpersonal confidence. Inviting them to talk in family sessions about the illness, prognosis, and journey ahead can quickly open up conversation, but what becomes crucial is continued family sessions across the months lest they resort to the status quo pattern. Cancer centers and tertiary medical centers do well to operate a Family Therapy Clinic that normalizes the use of this model of family centered care.

Conflictual Families

For this type of family, the genogram will typically reveal a pattern across generations of separations, cutoffs, or bitter fractures. Some 5–6% of families in palliative care resemble this pattern. Engagement is the challenge as the clinician must reach out to and engage with individual members to invite their help with the ill relative. They will fear conflict breaking out in a family meeting. They require a facilitator who commits to maintaining a safe gathering, one that fosters respect, tolerance, and a search for practical solutions and which empowers some cooperation among family members. Regular sessions become crucial to establish a holding frame that sustains improved cohesion across many months.

Uninvolved Families

In families with long-established patterns of noncontact, the die may be firmly cast and motivation for anything different is absent. Another 5–6% of families in palliative care resemble this pattern, which can prevent the family as a whole from attending a family meeting. The clinician has to accept their choice of distance, which often avoids unbridled conflict, and so therapy can only occur with that segment of the family still in contact with the sick relative. Goals of care may need to be more modest; clinicians might see opportunities for reunion, yet these families usually maintain their status quo.

Migrant or Refugee Families

Trauma may be an important feature of the narrative for these families, with loss and grief needing acknowledgment alongside acclamation of the courage and determination that has built a new life. The resilience and strengths of the family become a model for future generations. Parents may have preferred to not talk about the hardship and indignity of their past, yet a skilled facilitator can reframe this into a story of triumph to celebrate. Curiosity about traditions and customs of the mother country, religious rituals, or family mottos can facilitate fresh understanding that nurtures pride and a sense of accomplishment.

Where language is an apparent barrier to the conduct of a family meeting, the use of a skilled interpreter who can sit just outside the circle of clinician and family members and provide a simultaneous background translation of what is being said allows the dynamics of the family to remain apparent to the facilitators.[24] This contrasts markedly with the use of less skilled interpreters who cannot offer simultaneous translation, extend the time needed considerably, and stop facilitators working in real time with the relational dynamics.

Model of Family-Centered Care for "At-Risk" Families

Empirical studies of families in the palliative care setting have identified a method to either assess or screen families to identify frank dysfunction or, alternatively, those "at-risk" of poorer adaptation and complicated bereavement outcomes.

Assessment can be based on three questions about family relationships: the three "C's" of relational life: communication, cohesion, and conflict resolution.

- How easily do you communicate as a family?
- How well do you support one another as a team?
- How effectively do you tolerate differences of opinion without conflict?

Should a family acknowledge concern with any of these elements, it becomes a clinical hook on which to offer regular family meetings to support the family and guide them through the illness.

Screening with a simple questionnaire is an alternative approach to recognize those in need. The Family Relationships Index (FRI) is a well validated, 12-item, true–false measure, which includes four items about cohesion, four about communication, and four about conflict resolution. Scores of 9 or less out of 12 carry a high level of sensitivity to identify family dysfunction.[25] The FRI can be completed by the patient, caregiver, or any available family member. Averaging scores is unwarranted as any person who declares concern for family relationships acts as a spokesperson on behalf of the family. When screening is used, the family is not labeled negatively. Generally, the therapist can either confirm family concern for their communication during the opening, agenda-setting phase of a meeting or make gentle reference to a clinical impression that communication can be challenging for many families in palliative care, highlighting the value of meeting together as a family as a whole.

Empirical Evidence from Family Therapy Studies

An initial randomized controlled trial as "proof of concept" was conducted with 81 palliative care families (363 family members) selected by screening with the FRI as carrying some risk of complicated grief outcome. The patient was present in the early family meetings, which were then continued into bereavement. Sixteen social workers maintained fidelity to the manualized model of therapy. Family members who were depressed at baseline revealed a significant improvement at 6 and 13 months of bereavement, while overall distress in family members improved for treated families across these 13 months post death.[26] Families received sufficient therapy as deemed necessary by their therapists, with low-communicating families averaging seven and dysfunctional families averaging nine sessions across 18 months. This trial proved promising as a preventive palliative care intervention.

A larger hybrid efficacy-effectiveness trial was then conducted using 32 therapists, 170 families, and 620 family members, wherein families were randomized to receive either usual care or 6 or 10 sessions of family therapy, a dose testing intervention. Screening was again used with the FRI to select families deemed to be carrying some risk through dint of an FRI score equal to or less than 9 out of 12. Families were stratified by these FRI scores across the arms of this randomized controlled trial. Using the abbreviated Complicated Grief Inventory as a primary outcome measure, both a significant treatment effect and a treatment by family type interaction were found.[27] Ten sessions of therapy delivered better outcomes for low-communicating and conflictual families, but not for uninvolved families. When families received standard palliative care, 15.5% of the bereaved developed a prolonged grief disorder by 13 months of bereavement, compared to 3.3% of those who received 10 sessions of therapy. Evidence for this prevention of complicated grief was evident by 6 months of bereavement.

In this larger replication study, although prevention of depression was not achieved as a main effect of intervention, at 13 months of bereavement 21% of those receiving standard care exceeded critical diagnostic thresholds to become Beck Depression Inventory "cases" of depression compared to 11% of those receiving the family intervention. Again, fidelity of the model of therapy was well maintained by the therapists. These studies show the protective benefit of family therapy commenced during palliative care in reducing the effects of complicated grief, which is a disorder of attachment and subject therefore to the influence of care aimed at the quality of family relationships. The greater the level of dysfunction in the family, the larger the dose of therapy needed to gain this benefit. However, families who have already chosen distance as their solution to unbridled conflict prove less amenable to help, a reality which can reassure clinical services when members of some families decline to meet together.

In detailed process studies of what proves to be therapeutic in family therapy in this palliative care setting, Zaider and colleagues tracked families painstakingly, session by session.[4] The establishment of open family communication about matters generally hard to discuss emerged as the significant process that guided families toward improvement. This, *par excellence*, becomes the important goal of family centered care: to initiate safe conversations within the family of topics usually deemed taboo. To talk about loss and death, frailty and disability, themes both ugly and distressing, poignant and healing, the hurts and wrongs alongside love and forgiveness—when families begin these conversations, human life can be celebrated and its meaning deeply appreciated by those who matter most. Family-centered care is powerfully meaning-focused in the coping it encourages and the adaptation it achieves.

Future Directions

Couple- and family-centered care warrants further research to adapt to the potentially limited time available, implement as a routine service, and offer continuity of care into bereavement. Studies of the processes that optimize outcomes will continue to enhance care delivery. In these ways, the gap that still exists between the rhetoric of family-centered care as integral to palliative care and the reality of care delivery will be reduced.

Key Points

- Promoting couple communication, intimacy, and communal coping enhances relational functioning and sustains the sense of "we-ness" that can empower couples to celebrate their shared years, express gratitude, and begin the process of farewell that unfolds during a terminal illness.
- Couple sessions may need to be brief (2–3 sessions), promote mutual disclosure and emotional connection, honor relational strengths, and offer continuity of support for the surviving partner into bereavement.
- Key skills used to facilitate a family meeting include agenda setting, use of circular questions, and integrative summaries, while important outcomes from a family meeting are consensus about the goals of care and mutual support needs to enhance adaptation to the transitions inherent in palliative care.
- Family therapy can be offered to families with greater needs, dependent children or adolescents, disabled members, or patterns of low communication and some conflict to optimize family coping and bereavement outcomes for survivors. It can prevent prolonged grief disorder in bereavement.

References

1. Kotwal AA, Abdoler E, Diaz-Ramirez LG, Kelley AS, Ornstein KA, Boscardin WJ, Smith AK. Til death do us part: End-of-life experiences of married couples in a nationally representative survey. *J Am Geriatr Soc.* 2018 Dec;66(12):2360–2366.
2. Reblin M, Otto AK, Ketcher D, Vadaparampil ST, Ellington L, Heyman RE. In-home conversations of couples with advanced cancer: Support has its costs. *Psycho-oncology.* 2020 Aug;29(8):1280–1287.
3. Porter LS, Keefe FJ, Baucom DH, Olsen M, Zafar SY, Uronis H. A randomized pilot trial of a videoconference couples communication intervention for advanced GI cancer. *Psycho-oncology.* 2017 Jul;26(7):1027–1035.
4. Zaider TI, Kissane DW, Schofield E, Li Y, Masterson M. Cancer-related communication during sessions of family therapy at the end of life. *Psycho-Oncology.* 2020 Feb;29(2):373–380. https://doi.org/10.1002/pon.5268
5. Weingarten K. The "cruel radiance of what is": Helping couples live with chronic illness. *Family Process.* 2013 Mar;52(1):83–101.
6. Bond CB, Jensen PT, Groenvold M, Johnsen AT. Prevalence and possible predictors of sexual dysfunction and self-reported needs related to the sexual life of advanced cancer patients. *Acta Oncol.* 2019 May;58(5):769–775. https://doi.org/10.1080/0284186X.2019.1566774
7. Manne S, Badr H. Intimacy and relationship processes in couples' psychosocial adaptation to cancer. *Cancer.* 2008 Jun 1;112(S11):2541–2555.
8. Traa MJ, Braeken J, De Vries J, Roukema JA, Slooter GD, Crolla RM, et al. Sexual, marital, and general life functioning in couples coping with colorectal cancer: A dyadic study across time. *Psycho-Oncology.* 2015 Sep;24(9):1181–1188. https://doi.org/10.1002/pon.3801
9. Hu Y, Liu T, Li F. Association between dyadic interventions and outcomes in cancer patients: a meta-analysis. *Support Care Cancer.* 2019 Mar;27(3):745–761.
10. Badr H. Psychosocial interventions for patients with advanced cancer and their families. *Am J Lifestyle Med.* 2016 Jan;10(1):53–63.

11. Milbury K, Engle R, Tsao A, Liao Z, Owens A, Chaoul A, Bruera E, Cohen L. Pilot testing of a brief couple-based mind-body intervention for patients with metastatic non-small cell lung cancer and their partners. *J Pain Sympt Manage.* 2018 Mar 1;55(3):953–961.

12. von Heymann-Horan A, Bidstrup PE, Johansen C, Rottmann N, Andersen EA, Sjøgren P, von der Maase H, Timm H, Kjellberg J, Guldin MB. Dyadic coping in specialized palliative care intervention for patients with advanced cancer and their caregivers: Effects and mediation in a randomized controlled trial. *Psycho-oncology.* 2019 Feb;28(2):264–270.

13. Ketcher D, Thompson C, Otto AK, Reblin M, Cloyes KG, Clayton MF, Baucom BR, Ellington L. The Me in We dyadic communication intervention is feasible and acceptable among advanced cancer patients and their family caregivers. *Palliat Medi.* 2021 Feb;35(2):389–396.

14. Badr H, Smith CB, Goldstein NE, Gomez JE, Redd WH. Dyadic psychosocial intervention for advanced lung cancer patients and their family caregivers: Results of a randomized pilot trial. *Cancer.* 2015 Jan 1;121(1):150–158.

15. McLean LM, Walton T, Rodin G, Esplen MJ, Jones JM. A couple-based intervention for patients and caregivers facing end-stage cancer: Outcomes of a randomized controlled trial. *Psycho-oncology.* 2013 Jan;22(1):28–38.

16. Oechsle K, Ullrich A, Marx G et al. Psychological burden in family caregivers of patients with advanced cancer at initiation of specialist inpatient palliative care. *BMC Palliative Care.* 2019;18:102. https://doi.org/10.1186/s12904-019-0469-7

17. Zordan RD, Bell ML, Price M, et al. Long-term prevalence and predictors of prolonged grief disorder amongst bereaved cancer caregivers: A cohort study. *Palliat Support Care.* 2019 Oct;17(5):507–514. https://doi.org/10.1017/S1478951518001013

18. Hudson P, Aranda S. The Melbourne Family Support Program: Evidence-based strategies that prepare family caregivers for supporting palliative care patients. *BMJ Supportive & Palliative Care* 2014;4:231–237. https://doi.org/10.1136/bmjspcare-2013-000500

19. Holm M, Arestedt K, Carlander I, Fürst CJ, Wengström Y, Öhlen J, Alvariza A. Short-term and long-term effects of a psycho-educational group intervention for family caregivers in palliative home care: Results from a randomized controlled trial. *Psycho-Oncology* 2016;25(7):795–802. https://doi.org/10.1002/pon.4004

20. Kissane DW, Hempton C. Conducting a family meeting. In: DW Kissane, BD Bultz, PN Butow, CL Bylund, S Noble, S Wilkinson, eds. *Oxford Textbook of Communication in Oncology and Palliative Care,* 2nd ed. Oxford: Oxford University Press; 2017:109–117.

21. Muriel AC. Care of families with children anticipating the death of a parent. In: DW Kissane DW, F Parnes, eds. *Bereavement Care for Families.* New York: Routledge;2014:220–231.

22. Sandler IN, Ayers TS, Wolchik SA, et al. The family bereavement program: Efficacy evaluation of a theory-based prevention program for parentally bereaved children and adolescents. *J Consult Clin Psychol.* 2003;71(3):587–600. https://doi.org/10.1037/0022-006x.71.3.587

23. Schonfeld D. Providing support for families experiencing the death of a child. In: J Wolfe, PS Hinds, BM Sourkes, eds. *Textbook of Interdisciplinary Pediatric Care.* Philadelphia: Elsevier; 2012:223–230.

24. Lubrano di Ciccone B, Brown RF, Gueguen JA, Bylund CL, Kissane DW. Interviewing patients using interpreters in an oncology setting: Initial evaluation of a communication skills module. *Ann Oncol.*2010 Jan;21(1):27–32. https://doi.org/10.1093/annonc/mdp289

25. Edwards B, Clarke V. The validity of the Family Relationships Index as a screening tool for psychological risk in families of cancer patients. *Psycho-Oncology.* 2005;14(7):546–554. https://doi.org/10.1002/pon.876

26. Kissane DW, McKenzie M, Bloch S, Moskowitz C, McKenzie DP, O'Neill I. Family focused grief therapy: A randomized controlled trial in palliative care and bereavement. *Am J Psychiatry.* 2006 Jul;163(7):1208–1218. https://doi.org/10.1176/appi.ajp.163.7.1208

27. Kissane DW, Zaider TI, Li Y, et al. Randomized controlled trial of family therapy in advanced cancer continued into bereavement. *J Clin Oncol.* 2016 Jun;34:1921–1927. https://doi.org/10.1200/JCO.2015.63.0582

19

Cancer Caregivers

Allison J. Applebaum and Hannah-Rose Mitchell

Introduction

The impact of cancer extends beyond the patient to family, friends, and community members who often serve as informal caregivers and assist with the patient's cancer experience in a variety of ways. Increased cancer prevalence and shifts to outpatient cancer care have resulted in additional burden on informal caregivers. Exact definitions vary, but an *informal cancer caregiver* is herein defined as any individual who provides uncompensated care and support to a person with cancer with significant time and energy costs. The numerous responsibilities placed on cancer caregivers are linked to an enormous psychological and physical health burden. Caregivers' poor health outcomes are associated with their own healthcare costs, as well as with difficulty with providing patient care and subsequent risk to the patient. The onerous public health problem of cancer caregiving has come into increasing focus over the past decade and has been particularly highlighted in the setting of the COVID-19 pandemic.

The purpose of this chapter is to describe the prevalence and characteristics of cancer caregivers; the developmental, social and cultural context which shapes the caregiving experience; and the burden of caregiving on physical and psychological health outcomes. The chapter also describes current empirically supported interventions designed to address the unique needs of cancer caregivers and implications for clinical practice and policy to improve caregiver and patient health outcomes.

Who Are Caregivers?

Caregiver Characteristics

Limited national data exist on the prevalence of individuals who are providing care for a loved one with cancer and estimates vary, but at least 2.8 million American adults are currently serving as a caregiver for an adult with cancer,[1] though the number is likely higher as a result of the COVID-19 pandemic. Cancer incidence, prevalence, and mortality rates vary by sociodemographic factors including age, race/ethnicity, and socioeconomic status (SES). However, caregiving does not discriminate: all demographic groups partake in caregiving. According to the *Cancer Caregiving in the U.S.* 2016 report, most adult cancer caregivers are women (58%), with a mean age of 53.1 (median of 52). Approximately 65% of cancer caregivers reported non-Hispanic White ethnicity, followed by Hispanic (16%), non-Hispanic Black (11%), and Asian (8%). Cancer caregivers reported a median household income of $55,500, and 40% have a college or graduate degree. The majority provide care for a relative (88%), largely parents or parents-in-law (44%) and including spouses and partners (16%). Around 10% care for friends or community members.[1]

Compared to caregiving for patients with other chronic medical illnesses, cancer caregiving is shorter due to cancer's acute and episodic nature. Nonetheless, cancer caregiving presents a sustained challenge lasting 2 years on average. Moreover, cancer caregiving is more intense compared to caregiving for individuals with other chronic illnesses; cancer caregivers tend to endorse a high frequency of hours of care provided, reporting an average of 32.9 hours, and 32% of cancer caregivers provide at least 41 hours of care per week. This time commitment is often juggled with other roles and responsibilities, as 50% of caregivers reported being employed while caregiving.[1]

Caregiving Tasks

The roles and responsibilities of cancer caregivers are vast and present unique challenges. Cancer caregivers assist with a variety of tasks, including helping with activities of daily living (ADLs). Almost half of cancer caregivers reported helping with at least three different ADLs such as dressing, transferring in and out of bed, using the bathroom, and eating. Cancer caregivers also report assisting with instrumental ADLs (IADLs), such as housework or grocery shopping, preparing meals, and providing transportation. Caregivers also often provide emotional support and assist with problem-solving and decision-making.[1]

Cancer caregivers increasingly assist with medical and nursing tasks, such as administering medication, tube feeding, catheter/colostomy care, or helping to use medical equipment. Importantly, cancer caregivers providing medical and nursing tasks often have little to no training to do so, and 43% report helping with a medical or nursing task without receiving any preparation.[1] Caregiving tasks may also vary throughout the treatment trajectory. During active treatment, caregivers often help manage symptoms and side effects due to chemotherapy, radiation, immunotherapy, or biologics; when patients are no longer receiving curative care, caregivers often provide more direct care and assistance with ADLs and IADLs.[1]

Caregiving Across the Lifespan

Cancer caregiving spans the life course, and while caregivers across the developmental spectrum have many common experiences, there are also unique challenges at each life stage.

For example, role changes throughout life, such as starting a career, becoming a parent, losing a parent, entering "empty nest," or retirement result in shifts that could impact preparedness for and consequences of the caregiver role.

Nearly half of cancer caregivers in the United States (44%) are age 18–49,[1] which approximately represents the early adult stage. In contrast to the typical independence and self-actualization characteristic of early adulthood, caregiving is frequently restrictive and involves self-sacrifice, resulting in experiences that are not developmentally normative. Early adult caregivers also often perceive a deficiency of resources (e.g., emotional, financial, informational, social) to manage their caregiving responsibilities, especially as they may be less socially connected to other informal caregivers.[2]

Early adult caregivers as well as middle-aged caregivers (age 50–64), who comprise 31% of adult cancer caregivers in the United States,[1] frequently face competing demands of providing care for their own children and for the patient with cancer. Middle-aged caregivers also tend to be at the peak of their career. Caregiving duties may interrupt employment, which is particularly challenging given that middle-aged caregivers often depend on employer-provided health insurance. Both groups of early and middle-aged adults providing cancer care for spouses may face heightened stress given the nondevelopmentally normative stressors of facing widowhood and uncertainty for the entire family.[2]

Older adults (age 65 or older) comprise 25% of cancer caregivers in the United States.[1] Older adulthood is a time of change and often renewed independence after adult children leave the home. Older adult caregivers may have more time to devote to caregiving responsibilities. Caregiving is more expected or normative during later life, and older adult caregivers may have greater access to resources to assist with caregiving. However, later life presents its own challenges, and older adult caregivers may face strained finances and normative age-related health challenges that hinder their ability to help with the physical demands of caregiving and present the need to manage competing medical appointments. However, because the experience of facing illness and existential threats are normative in older age, this group of caregivers may be more prepared to handle the demands of caregiving, hence reducing the extent to which they perceive caregiver strain.[2]

Finally, a growing literature recognizes the caregiving responsibilities of children and adolescents involved in multigenerational involvement of caregiving for parents, grandparents, and other relatives. Child and adolescent caregivers are likely particularly isolated by such a non-normative experience and vulnerable to negative impact on their development. Indeed, cancer caregiving can occur at any stage in the life course, and developmental factors are likely to influence the adjustment to the caregiver role.[2]

Sociocultural Factors Impacting Caregiving

Sociocultural factors influence the experience of caregiving, including the initial uptake of the role and caregivers' subsequent perceptions of their roles. *Familism* is a cultural construct referring to prioritizing the needs of the family over the needs of individuals and the accompanying feelings of loyalty and connection to the family. Those from cultures high on familism may expect to provide care for relatives and may be more likely to accept and embrace the caregiver role. In the United States, high levels of familism have been identified in Black, Asian, and Latinx individuals, for whom providing care for the family is culturally expected. Familism has generally been viewed as protective against caregiving-related burden, but it can also result in less use of formal support services and additional demands on caregivers feeling that their primary responsibility is to provide care for their loved one.[3]

The role of chronic discrimination in the experiences of cancer caregivers has not been well studied. However, caregivers who perceive discrimination, such as being mistreated or disrespected by other people, are likely more vulnerable to elevated caregiving-related stress, as perceived discrimination has been a significant predictor of poor quality of life, independent of the effects of ethnicity/race. Caregivers in marginalized groups are also more vulnerable to the negative health consequences of cancer caregiving, and structural racism may complicate the challenges of caregiving. Indeed, Black and Latinx caregivers reported greater difficulty taking time from work to attend to caregiving responsibilities compared with White counterparts.[4]

SES is another factor that shapes the caregiving trajectory. Lower SES and less access to care and resources is associated with intensified caregiving responsibilities and heightened vulnerability to financial and employment loss. Low-SES caregivers spend more hours per day engaged in caregiving-related responsibilities, which has been attributed to caring for sicker parents and inaccessibility to hired help. Financial burden is often incurred directly due to cancer, which can be compounded by additional financial strain if caregivers are required to take time off from work to provide care.[5]

Gender has also been shown to influence the experience of caregiving. In many cultures, there is an expectation that women assume the caregiver role, and women represent 75% of caregivers in the United States.[1] With this expectation, and often providing care in isolation, women caregivers tend to report greater burden and lower self-esteem from providing care than men.[6] For men, taking on a role not traditionally assumed may enhance their esteem, suggesting adherence to traditional gender roles is associated with higher caregiving-related stress. Together, the extant literature suggests that sociocultural factors may be central to the experience of family cancer caregivers.

The Negative Impact of Caregiving on Caregivers

As a result of the many responsibilities and challenges discussed above, the majority of caregivers will experience caregiver burden. This is a multidimensional response that refers to all the ways in which the caregiving role can potentially negatively impact the caregiver, including psychological, medical, spiritual, and financial outcomes.

Many caregivers experience psychological distress, including diagnostic levels of anxiety and depression that are often more severe than rates seen among the patients for whom caregivers provide care.[7] Importantly, such psychological distress is associated with increased risk for poor physical health consequences such as cardiovascular disease, poor immune functioning, sleep disturbances, impaired immune responses, neuroendocrine dysregulation, chronic back pain, and arthritis. Caregivers also engage in higher rates of poor health-related behaviors, such as increased substance use and decreased exercise, and are less likely to use preventative healthcare services and delay their own screening or follow-up care.[8] All of these factors put caregivers at increased risk for poor health outcomes.

Caregiving may also result in spiritual and existential distress. Regardless of the patient's prognosis, the caregiving trajectory naturally evokes thoughts about death. Caregivers are often faced with balancing a desire to focus on the present moment and on the patient's recovery with feelings of hopelessness about an uncertain future.

The financial toxicity associated with caregiving is significant, and cancer caregiving is in fact more financially onerous compared to other types of caregiving.[5] Caregivers are often forced to give up work responsibilities or take leaves of absence to provide care, and the whole family may also incur costs related to the patient's treatment. Importantly, the financial toxicity of cancer and caregiving may be experienced for years after the patient's death.[5]

Unmet needs are well-documented among caregivers, who frequently endorse areas in which they feel inadequate, insecure, unprepared, or unsupported to provide patient care. These include psychosocial, cognitive, financial, medical, and daily activity. Younger caregivers, spouses, and women tend to report greater unmet needs. Moreover, greater unmet needs earlier in the treatment trajectory in turn are associated with lower levels of mental and physical health quality of life.[9] As such, addressing caregiver unmet needs may be one approach to reduce caregiver burden.

Interventions

Over the past decade there has been a proliferation of empirically supported interventions developed to address the unique needs of cancer caregivers.[10] Here we present an overview of several such interventions and encourage readers to take note of the systematic review referenced above for a more comprehensive review of caregiver-specific psychosocial interventions.

Psychoeducation

Psychoeducation is a therapeutic approach in which practitioners help individuals gain more in-depth knowledge and fact-based understanding of an illness in order to self-reflect on its impact on their overall well-being and day-to-day life.[11] There are three core techniques comprising psychoeducation: building a therapeutic alliance, educating about fact-based and "how to" topical content, and facilitating self-reflection and adaptive coping.[11] The goal is to enhance comprehension and self-awareness that will activate individuals to engage in healthy, constructive behaviors to optimize their circumstances and self-care. In a secondary analysis of 50 randomized trials of cancer family caregiver interventions, 36 (72%) primarily employed psychoeducation.[12] In these interventions, the content of psychoeducation was wide-ranging and focused on enhancing the family member's comprehension of cancer and its basic pathophysiology; treatments, procedures, and tests; local, state, and national resources; communication; and frameworks of stress management, coping, problem-solving, and self-care.

One psychoeducational intervention for caregivers of patients with cancer is the Educate, Nurture, Advise, Before Life Ends (ENABLE) Caregiver intervention,[13] which focuses on enhancing caregivers' knowledge, improving skills in problem-solving and coping, and providing home-based support to patients with newly diagnosed advanced cancer. Caregivers are paired with a palliative care-trained nurse coach who facilitates a series of 3 weekly one-on-one telephone-delivered sessions that address problem-solving coping and problem-solving support (Session 1), partnering effectively to improve patients' self-care and symptom management (Session 2), and enhancing communication skills, leveraging social support, and implementing advance care plans (Session 3). These sessions are supplemented with a Charting Your Course-Caregiver informational guide. After receiving core sessions, caregivers receive check-in calls monthly to identify new issues and reinforce prior content until the patient's death, after which they receive a bereavement call. A "fast track" or wait list randomized controlled trial of 122 family caregivers of newly diagnosed advanced cancer patients, that compared immediate versus delayed initiation (12 weeks later) of ENABLE, found that the early group caregivers had significantly fewer depressive symptoms and lower stress burden at 12 weeks compared to the delayed arm. These same benefits were also noted in the early group 36 weeks from the patient's death.

Cognitive Behavioral Therapy

Cognitive behavioral therapy (CBT) is an evidence-based therapy used to treat anxiety, depression, substance use disorders, insomnia, and stress management and is finding relevance within the context of cancer caregiving. CBT focuses on altering individuals' interpretation of a stressor to influence the emotional response in the presence of that stressor, thus promoting problem-solving skills. There is growing evidence for the efficacy of CBT for use with patients and caregivers, though a recent meta-analysis of CBTs for caregivers of both patients with cancer and survivors suggests the approach may be more effective for caregivers who are younger and female.[14]

The majority of CBT studies with cancer caregivers focus on psychological distress and caregiver adjustment during the acute phase of treatment, from diagnosis to 1–2 years post-diagnosis. Very few CBT interventions are tailored to address challenges during later phases of caregiving, and fewer still have addressed topics of bereavement in family caregivers using CBT. This may reflect, in part, the sensitivity required in delivering traditional CBT to caregivers. The traditional cognitive-behavioral model emphasizes the existence of an individual's unrealistic or unhelpful automatic thoughts and the benefit of CBT to reframe these cognitions to be more realistic or accurate. In the oncology setting, these methods may lack appropriate validation of the lived experience of caregivers who are coping with patients' changing needs and prognoses, and therefore the delivery of CBT must be flexible and sensitive to caregivers' needs.

To address the limitations of traditional CBT and more focally target distress among cancer caregivers, a "new wave" CBT intervention—Emotion Regulation Therapy for

Cancer Caregivers (ERT-C)—has been developed. ERT-C is a theoretically grounded, evidence-based treatment that incorporates principles from traditional and contemporary CBTs with findings from affective science. ERT-C offers a framework for improving regulatory skills of caregivers who have high psychological distress, engage in perseverative negative thinking (e.g., rumination, worry, self-criticism), and evidence poor behavioral responding (e.g., withdrawal, emotional numbing). There is preliminary support for the utility of ERT-C in treating distress among cancer caregivers and for ERT-C as a conceptual model and treatment modality for distressed cancer caregivers.[15]

Dyadic Interventions

Dyadic interventions are delivered by a therapist or clinician to a patient–caregiver dyad (pair) and are designed to simultaneously address the needs of the patient with cancer, their caregiver, and the relationship between them. Dyadic interventions help patients and caregivers work together to manage the demands of illness, problem-solve important treatment decisions, and support one another as they cope with the stress of illness. Several key factors are typically addressed in dyadic interventions, including effective communication, relationship issues that are affected by the illness (e.g., role changes), and dyadic coping, a form of stress management in dyads.

An exemplar of a dyadic intervention is the FOCUS Program, an empirically supported[16] intervention designed to help patients and caregivers cope with cancer and maintain their quality of life. F-O-C-U-S represents the five content areas of the program: *Family* involvement, which promotes open communication, support, and teamwork to manage cancer-related stress; *Optimistic* attitude, which addresses each person's outlook and helps them work together to maintain hope and find meaning in the illness; *Coping* effectiveness, which promotes effective dyadic coping and encourages active rather than avoidant coping; *Uncertainty* reduction, which provides psychoeducation about cancer etiology and treatments and assists patients and caregivers to live with illness-related uncertainty; and *Symptom* management, which helps patients and caregivers learn strategies to manage symptom distress. FOCUS has been delivered to patient–caregiver dyads as a face-to-face home-based program, a web-based program, and a small-group program, and it has had positive outcomes on both patient and family caregiver outcomes, including higher quality of life, self-efficacy, coping effectiveness, and more perceived benefits of illness.

Meaning-Centered Psychotherapy

Although many psychosocial interventions have been developed to target various elements of caregiver burden, few attend to existential distress or the potential to connect to a sense of meaning, purpose, and growth despite the challenges of caregiving. Based on an empirically supported intervention that has demonstrated efficacy in improving the quality of life of patients with advanced cancer, breast cancer survivors, and bereaved parents,[17] Meaning-Centered Psychotherapy for Cancer Caregivers (MCP-C) is the first psychotherapeutic approach to target existential concerns commonly experienced by caregivers of patients with cancer. MCP-C helps caregivers connect—or reconnect—to various sources of meaning in their lives. Over the course of seven hour-long sessions that involve both didactic components and experiential exercises, caregivers come to understand the benefits of connecting with meaning in their lives and how these sources of meaning (i.e., historical, attitudinal, creative, experiential) may serve as resources, buffer common symptoms of burden, and diminish despair, especially as patients transition to end-of-life care. In addition to being delivered in person, MCP-C has been adapted for delivery over the internet to address the documented barriers to engaging caregivers in in-person support.[18]

Caregiving in the Time of COVID

The experience of providing care to a patient with cancer is more demanding in the setting of the COVID-19 pandemic than ever before. The burden, distress, disparities, and unmet needs discussed in this chapter have all been exacerbated as a result of this pandemic. Historically, caregivers have been able to depend on support from extended family care networks, home health aides, and visiting nurses, whereas now, at the time of this writing (December 2020), most have been providing care in isolation and even from afar. The separation of caregivers from patients receiving care in inpatient settings has had a devastating impact on families, and undoubtedly, we have seen significant trauma when caregivers and patients are separated as patients take their last breaths.

The widespread delivery of psychosocial support to caregivers over telehealth modalities has been a potential silver lining of this pandemic. Historically, there have been many barriers to psychosocial service use documented among caregivers, including the time and financial cost associated with traveling to and from our treatment centers, the guilt that caregivers feel when taking time away from patients and in taking time for themselves, and what remains to this day a stigma associated with mental health service utilization. Our ability to provide high-quality psychosocial support to caregivers in need across the country via telehealth addresses these barriers to care and likely has set a new standard for the type of care that caregivers should have access to moving forward.

Future Directions

Cancer caregivers are an essential extension of the healthcare team. A significant burden of responsibility is placed on caregivers, many of whom have little to no preparation for this role. Without adequate training and support, the health and well-being of caregivers is challenged, as is the quality of the care that is provided to patients.

A decade of research,[19] combined with the significant toll on caregivers in the setting of the COVID-19 pandemic, has highlighted caregiving as a national public health crisis. As such, steps must be taken to ensure that caregivers are supported in their critical roles on healthcare teams. It is necessary for our field to understand how our changing public policy landscape will impact cancer caregivers and to advocate for additional policies that will improve the capacity of caregivers to serve in this crucial role. For example, the American Association of Retired Persons (AARP) drafted model legislation that would standardize hospital procedures and help caregivers as their family members make the transition from the hospital back to home. This legislation, the Caregiver Advise Record Enable (CARE) Act, requires hospitals to formalize the procedures by which they identify and document the existence of caregivers, which represents a cultural shift to one where caregivers are being recognized as partners in a patient's recovery and improved health outcomes.[20] As of this writing (December 2020), 43 states have approved the CARE Act, but we still have a ways to go. It is not clear whether there is widespread adoption of the provisions of the Care Act (i.e., documenting the name of the caregiver in patients' medical records and providing caregivers with education in advance of discharge planning), and, as such, additional steps are needed to ensure that the CARE Act is implemented. The CARE Act also represents an opportunity for healthcare teams to screen caregivers for distress and engage them in psychosocial support.

Additionally, we must make it a priority to address the financial toxicity of caregiving. According to the AARP, caregivers spend, on average, nearly $7,000 of their own funds annually on caregiving, which is almost 20% of their income.[1] The recognition of caregiving as a life course issue is essential for maximizing the impact of caregiving resources. Specifically, some available support is tied to the age of the caregiver or patient and/or the patient's health condition(s), such as the National Family Caregiver Support Program, which provides services to caregivers who are 55 years of age or older themselves or who are caring for someone 60 years of age or older (or someone with dementia, regardless of age). Other programs such as Medicare and Medicaid provide additional mechanisms of financial support based on life stage (e.g., eligible individuals in receipt of Medicare are age 65 or older, or, in the case of Medicaid, those who are elderly or permanently disabled may qualify even if they do not meet the income restrictions). These programs, therefore, exclude younger and middle-adulthood caregivers who may be, due to competing demands of caregiving and childcare, in significant need of financial support but are ineligible to receive such support because of their age. We must systematically examine groups of caregivers who fall through these financial support cracks and create new ways to support them, which likely will include changes in policy. Toward this end, the AARP has proposed legislation called the Credit for Caring Act, which would create a federal, nonrefundable tax credit of up to $3,000 for family caregivers who work while also financially supporting their loved ones.[19] This type of legislation would help alleviate the financial strain that many caregivers are facing.

Finally, while our field has made considerable progress in intervention development over the past decade, dissemination and implementation efforts are necessary to ensure that our psychotherapeutic technologies reach caregivers in the greatest need of support. Research is needed to understand why some interventions may be appropriate for some caregivers versus others and which interventions may be appropriate for caregivers based on factors such as life stage, relationship to the patient, cultural background, and coping capacity. This work will help us to further adapt and tailor our interventions to enhance outcomes and meet the needs of this incredibly vulnerable population. The COVID-19 pandemic and our field's subsequent transition to a model of primarily telehealth-delivered care underscores the importance of our continuing to capitalize on the rapidly advancing telehealth technologies to deliver interventions to diverse groups of caregivers across the country and the world. In effect, this work will move us toward accomplishing precision and individualized medicine for cancer caregivers.

Key Points

- Cancer caregiving, or providing care for family and friends with cancer, is a fundamental part of the cancer experience. A growing number of family members and friends are tasked with serving as cancer caregivers and providing multiple complex care tasks.
- Caregiver needs and outcomes vary across the lifespan and by the relationship to the patient and are influenced by myriad sociocultural factors.
- The demands on cancer caregivers throughout the cancer trajectory often result in caregiver burden, including negative psychological, medical, spiritual, and financial outcomes.
- Several evidence-based interventions targeting cancer caregivers show promise in improving both caregiver and patient psychological and physical health outcomes.
- As the United States increasingly depends on out-of-hospital care, policies must be implemented that support caregivers in serving as critical members of healthcare teams.

References

1. Hunt G, Longacre M, Kent E, Weber-Raley L. Cancer caregiving in the US: An intense, episodic, and challenging care experience. *A Research Report from the National Alliance for Caregiving*; June 2016.
2. Litzelman K. The unique experience of caregivers based on their life stage and relationship to the patient. In: Applebaum AJ, ed. *Cancer Caregivers*. Oxford University Press; 2019:34–49.
3. Pharr JR, Dodge Francis C, Terry C, Clark MC. Culture, caregiving, and health: exploring the influence of culture on family caregiver experiences. *Int Scholarly Res Notices*. 2014;2014:Article ID 689826, 8. https://doi.org/10.1155/2014/689826
4. Siefert ML, Williams A-L, Dowd MF, Chappel-Aiken L, McCorkle R. The caregiving experience in a racially diverse sample of cancer family caregivers. *Cancer Nurs*. 2008;31(5):399.
5. Bradley CJ. Economic burden associated with cancer caregiving. *Semin Oncol Nurs*. 2019;35(4):333–336.
6. Hagedoorn M, Sanderman R, Bolks HN, Tuinstra J, Coyne JC. Distress in couples coping with cancer: A meta-analysis and critical review of role and gender effects. *Psychol Bull*. 2008;134(1):1.
7. Geng H-M, Chuang D-M, Yang F, Yang Y, Liu WM, Liu HL, et al. Prevalence and determinants of depression in caregivers of cancer patients: A systematic review and meta-analysis. *Medicine (Baltimore)*. 2018;97(39):e11863-e11863.
8. Stenberg U, Ruland CM, Miaskowski CJ. Review of the literature on the effects of caring for a patient with cancer. *Psycho-oncology*. 2010;19(10):1013–1025.
9. Kim Y, Carver CS. Unmet needs of family cancer caregivers predict quality of life in long-term cancer survivorship. *J Cancer Survivorship*. 2019;13(5):749–758.
10. Treanor CJ, Santin O, Prue G, et al. Psychosocial interventions for informal caregivers of people living with cancer. *Cochrane Database Syst Rev*. 2019(6). doi:10.1002/14651858.CD009912.pub2
11. Brown N. *Conducting Effective and Productive Psychoeducational and Therapy Groups*. New York: Routledge; 2018.
12. Dionne-Odom J, Bakitas M, Ferrell B. Psychoeducational interventions for cancer family caregivers. In: Applebaum A, ed. *Cancer Caregivers*. New York: Oxford University Press; 2019:105–129.

13. Dionne-Odom JN AA, Lyons KD, et al. Benefits of early versus delayed palliative care to informal family caregivers of patients with advanced cancer: Outcomes from the ENABLE III randomized controlled trial. *J Clin Oncol.* 2015;33(13):1446–1452.

14. O'Toole MS, Zachariae R, Renna ME, Mennin DS, Applebaum A. Cognitive behavioral therapies for informal caregivers of patients with cancer and cancer survivors: A systematic review and meta-analysis. *Psycho-oncology.* 2017;26(4):428–437.

15. Applebaum AJ, Panjwani, A.A., Buda, K, et al. Emotion regulation therapy for cancer caregivers: An open trial of a mechanism-targeted approach to addressing caregiver distress. *Translat Behav Med.* 2020;10(2):413–422.

16. Northouse L, Kershaw T, Mood D, Schafenacker A. Effects of a family intervention on the quality of life of women with recurrent breast cancer and their family caregivers. *Psycho-oncology.* 2005;14(6):478–491.

17. Breitbart WS. *Meaning-Centered Psychotherapy in the Cancer Setting: Finding Meaning and Hope in the Face of Suffering.* New York: Oxford University Press; 2016.

18. Applebaum AJ. Meaning-centered psychotherapy for cancer caregivers. In: Applebaum AJ, ed. *Cancer Caregivers.* New York: Oxford University Press; 2019:237–256.

19. Applebaum AJ. *Cancer Caregivers.* New York: Oxford University Press; 2019.

20. Reinhard SC, Young HM, Ryan E, Choula RB. *The CARE Act implementation: Progress and promise.* Washington, DC: AARP Public Policy Institute; 2019.

20

Care for the Healthcare Provider

Daniel C. McFarland and Mary L. S. Vachon

Introduction

Clinicians face numerous daunting tasks in their work with patients at the end of life. Work environments and clinician lifestyle choices can deteriorate their quality of life and lead to adverse patient outcomes. The implications for palliative care are quite significant given the interpersonal stressors of dealing with end-of-life issues, boundary excursions, difficult family dynamics, and the need for emotional openness and relatedness in this setting. The medical setting in which palliative care is delivered also puts demands on timeliness, coordination of care (e.g., logistics such as patient disposition), urgent symptom management, and interdisciplinary stress from other medical colleagues who may not feel comfortable, competent, or adequately prepared to tackle these issues. The unpredictability and need to be available or ever present for one's patients result in ongoing and potentially cumulative stress.

The primary issues of mental health in healthcare clinicians vary in scope, intensity, and dysfunction. In addition, the root causes of these work-related issues vary and should be addressed in determining their treatments. Work-related stress syndromes such as burnout, compassion fatigue, empathy fatigue, and moral distress are tied directly to the work environment and overlap with other mental health maladies such as depression and substance abuse, which are more highly prevalent in medical professionals but not necessarily directly tied to work environments. In other words, mental health phenomena should be considered in their entirety for the differential diagnosis of clinician dysfunction. This chapter addresses mental health conditions in clinicians directly tied to the work environment. Major depression, suicide, substance abuse, and other psychiatric disorders in clinicians are discussed elsewhere. Briefly, issues concerning physician well-being are not new and are well-documented in the historical literature. For example, increased rates of suicide among clinicians have been documented since antiquity.[1]

In the current era, increasing attention is given to the phenomena of burnout in clinicians. Hospitals and healthcare organizations incur large losses in revenue from physician turnover and lack of work efficiency related to burnout. Also, reimbursement is increasingly tied to patient satisfaction, which is adversely affected by clinician burnout. The World Health Organization (WHO) now recognizes the burnout syndrome in its classification of disorders. Historically, burnout and its related conditions were essentially covered up and physicians who were struggling were seen as deficient or undeserving of the privilege of being allowed to administer medical care. Stoicism was the only option and remains a well-trodden approach for many medical professionals and clinicians.

It has become clear that many of the work-related mental health issues stem from systemic or organizational problems. At the same time, the end of the Golden Era of Medicine by the 1980s brought about less physician autonomy and ability to control many aspects of medical practice. While there are many individual factors that can predispose a clinician to burnout and other conditions, it is important to also evaluate the workplace-worker relationship as well. Clinicians who are single, female, younger, type A, committed, diligent, seeking to gain approval or advance professionally (e.g., taking on more and more responsibilities), and willing to cross personal work-related boundaries (e.g., working late instead of spending time with family) are typically considered to be at a higher risk for burnout.[2] While these risk factors are important, all clinicians are at risk, as demonstrated by high prevalence rates of burnout across medical specialties. Palliative care and other fields that frequently encounter and manage end-of-life care, such as oncology, do not have the highest burnout rates. This is likely due to some of the rewarding aspects of the work. It turns out the administrative burdens, along with finding oneself repeatedly doing less than desirable aspects of one's job, are the leading culprits in terms of burnout. Palliative care physicians have relatively more time spent with patients and families, which may bolster the meaningfulness of their work but creates other stressors and problems for these clinicians.

At the same time, the historical term "hardiness" or the modern one, "resilience" connotes the human propensity toward adaptability and those characteristics that allow clinicians to thrive despite adversity.[3] These factors are equally important when considering burnout and its related conditions. Understanding protective factors is key to figuring out how to prevent and treat burnout and to provide effective coping mechanisms. Many palliative care and oncology clinicians find end-of-life work, or at least aspects of it, rewarding. They may draw on previous experience to confront adversity, think creatively to adapt to a given situation, accept certain losses, or undergo a change of perspective. While resilience tends to focus on individual factors, the culture of the work environment can certainly bolster resilient workers and teach many skills and habits that increase resilience (i.e., resilience can be learned). For example, reducing stigma around mental health phenomena in clinicians is paramount, along with providing adequate mental health services for clinicians and immediate debriefing strategies for tense or disturbing clinical situations (e.g., Code Lavender allows for a clinician "huddle" directly after a distressing clinical encounter as a form of psychological first aid typically for inpatient clinicians).[4] For physicians, state licensing boards should rethink questions pertaining to history of mental health disorders and treatments, which dissuade many physicians from seeking needed care.

Resilience comes in many forms. The enhancement of clinician wellness should consider resilience attributes that were effective for clinicians at other times and why they may not work in a new or novel employment situation. In their research with prisoners of war, military personnel, Holocaust survivors, and trauma survivors, Dennis Charney and Steven Southwick identified key protective factors associated with posttraumatic growth and resilience. Those resilience factors are the following: the confrontation of fear, maintaining an optimistic outlook, seeking and accepting social support, imitation of sturdy role models, relying on an inner moral compass, embracing spiritual or religious practice, accepting what cannot be changed, attending to health and well-being, creating meaning and opportunity from adversity, and accepting personal responsibility for emotional well-being.[5]

The effects of poor clinician well-being are not only disastrous for individual clinicians, their families, colleagues, and patients, but also for healthcare organizations. The economic losses may be reflected in suboptimal performance as well as physician turnover, which can cost organizations over a million dollars in recruitment, onboarding, and ramping-up practices. These metrics, along with patient satisfaction, and a general trend toward enhancement of work life balance, have created organizational commitments toward clinician well-being. Some organizations have created new executive roles for Chief Wellness Offices, for example. Not only is paying attention to clinician well-being an ethical imperative, but it is also good business.

Key Concepts

The key concepts involved in clinician wellness tend to be dichotomized and exist along a spectrum. For example, the opposite of burnout is engagement, the opposite of compassion fatigue is compassion reward, and the opposite of moral distress is moral success. Many of these domains overlap such that clinicians may experience various conditions on the same side of the spectrum. For example, a clinician who becomes more engaged and less burned-out also helps mitigate moral distress and compassion fatigue.

Engaged but over-committed, driven, and disciplined clinicians may become burned-out. Burnout is defined by its three component parts: emotional exhaustion, depersonalization (or cynicism, which is more common in males), and a depleted sense of professional accomplishment. Of these domains, the first two are the most important as depletion of professional accomplishment may be secondary to the other two domains. The Maslach Burnout Inventory (MBI) is the most widely used scale to measure burnout and incorporates those three domains. It was the first scale to measure burnout and was developed in 1981.[6] The Copenhagen Burnout Inventory (CBI) was developed in 2005, and consists of three scales measuring personal burnout, work-related burnout, and client-related burnout that can be used in these different domains.[7] Many of the symptoms of burnout mimic depression, and some researchers posit that burnout is only secondary to underlying depression. But the key distinction is its relationship with the work environment such that changes in the work environment directly affect the presence or absence of burnout but do not affect depression. Burnout allows for disengagement from work by distancing through exhaustion, depersonalization (i.e., treating clients as objects, lacking humanity), and a belief in not being effective. Its opposite is feeling and acting engaged with one's work as a statement of mental health. Burnout and engagement exist on a spectrum. Engagement depends on alignment of work environment and personal attributes but can also be cultivated as a tool to prevent burnout.

> When we are engaged, we feel nourished by our work. We have personal agency and the means to affect outcomes. We have the sense that our work makes a difference to others ourselves and perhaps even the world.[8 (p. 174)]

Conversely,

> When our engagement gets off balance and our work seems driven by fear, escapism, or compulsion, we are vulnerable to *burnout*—that bleak experience of fatigue, pessimism, cynicism, and even physical illness, accompanied by the sense that our work is of little or no benefit to anyone, including ourselves.[8 (p. 180)]

First-hand accounts of burnout are often helpful for clinicians to understand and appreciate the insidiousness of burnout and how the disengagement with work can occur, especially in the palliative care setting where the rewards are tinged with bittersweet emotions. Dr. Michael Kearney, a palliative care physician (2018) reported the following:

> While I loved the people I was working with, I noticed that I was no longer excited, as I had been in those early days at St. Christopher's, to go to work each morning. Instead, I was feeling emotionally and physically run down most of the time. I no longer had that inner "hum" that had been there in the past that came with knowing that I was in and doing the right work. Even after a restful weekend, my energy felt flat. More often than not I felt unhappy with the quality of my work. I had the pervasive feeling that I was not doing what I really wanted to do and was doing too much of what I did not want to do, and I frequently found myself fantasizing about leaving medicine. I remember the moment I realized one evening, as I was reading a paper on the symptoms of burnout, that I was experiencing every symptom on the list. I was burned out.[9 (pp. 35–36)]

Burnout rates are consistently high across healthcare sectors, but disciplines most immediately involved with end of life have average rates of burnout that are not especially high.[10] A recent comparison of physician burnout and satisfaction with work–life integration between 2011 and 2017 found that 43.9% had at least one symptom of burnout on the Maslach Burnout Inventory (MBI) in 2017 compared with 54.4% in 2014 and 45.5% in 2011.[11] A study of 1,357 palliative care clinicians (physicians, nurses and advanced practice nurses, social workers, chaplains, and others) who belonged to the American Academy of Hospice and Palliative Medicine, found that 38.7% reported burnout with rates being higher in the non-physicians.[12] In addition, clinicians working in smaller organizations, working longer hours, being younger than 50, and working weekends were associated with burnout.[12] These work-related and individual factors are perhaps more relevant than medical discipline. Although each discipline engenders unique stressors that may lead to burnout. For example, burnout in psychiatry has been linked to having experienced violence on the job (e.g., battered by patient), which is surprisingly common. The high rates of burnout in emergency medicine (roughly 75% in 2014) are likely related to unpredictability of workload and structure.[13]

Burnout is associated with neurobiological changes. Uncontrollable stress, but not controllable stress, impairs the functioning of the prefrontal cortex, which regulates thoughts, actions, and emotions. The prefrontal cortex governs many cognitive operations essential to physicians, including abstract reasoning, higher-order decision-making, insight, and the ability to persevere through challenges.[14] The prefrontal cortex is reliant on arousal state and becomes impaired under conditions of fatigue or incontrollable stress. In short, reduced prefrontal cortex self-regulation may explain several challenges associated with burnout in physicians, including reduced motivation, unprofessional behavior, and suboptimal communication with patients.[14] Morphologic changes in the prefrontal cortex are noted in highly stressful occupations where burnout is common. Thinning of the prefrontal cortex and recruitment of larger volumes of prefrontal cortex may be needed to retain the same level of cognitive performance as someone who is not experiencing burnout.[14] Burnout is related to poor patient care and may affect best practices (e.g., standard of care), medical errors, patient outcomes with treatments, quality, and safety.[15]

Compassion fatigue stands on the other side of compassion satisfaction. Compassion fatigue results from vicarious traumatization occurring through patients whose stories and clinical situations directly affect their professional caregivers. It has many similarities with posttraumatic stress disorder (PTSD) and is also called *secondary traumatic stress*.[16] Although compassion fatigue has been described extensively, its overlap with burnout and occupational stress is not entirely clear. Emerging evidence suggests that there is an inverse relationship between compassion and fatigue since compassion is not a commodity that becomes depleted but a perspective or clinical attitude that facilitates meaningful clinical encounters.[17] Compassion satisfaction results from the rewarding feeling of caring for another and a sense of accomplishment.[18] Compassion satisfaction has been defined as the pleasure derived from doing clinical work well. It stands in sharp contrast to compassion fatigue, where work is a source of negativity for the clinician. Compassion satisfaction may result from the feeling that the clinician is able to provide a reflection of how they believe the world should be in terms of patient care, when one's work aligns with the clinician's belief system.[10] A large Canadian study found that when clinicians were involved with multiple compassion-requiring tasks they became more likely to report compassion fatigue and burnout, but no significant difference was seen in levels of compassion satisfaction.[19] The study authors hypothesized that even staff who did not provide direct clinical care derived compassion satisfaction from their work.

The concept of *edge states* has been described by Roshi Joan Halifax, an anthropologist and Zen Buddhist teacher who has been teaching and writing about compassion and dying for many years. She collaborated with neuroscientists and social psychologists in compassion-based projects working with dying patients.[8] She describes edge states as "five internal and interpersonal qualities that are keys to a compassionate and courageous life, and without which we cannot serve, nor can we survive." The edge states are altruism, empathy, integrity, respect, and engagement. These assets exemplify caring, connection, virtue, and strength. However, these peak states can result in emotional suffering, "we can also lose our firm footing on the high edge of any of these qualities and slide into a mire of suffering where we find ourselves caught in the toxic and chaotic waters of the harmful aspects of an Edge State."[8] [(p. 3)] Altruism can become pathological and harmful, empathy can turn into distress, integrity can lead to moral suffering; respect can shift to disrespect, and engagement can result in overwork and burnout.[8]

Altruism can become *pathological altruism.* Selfless actions that serve to benefit others are essential to society and the natural world. "But sometimes, our seemingly altruistic acts harm us, harm those whom we are trying to serve, or harm the institutions we serve in."[8] [(p. 3)] For example, a palliative care clinician may make a promise that cannot be kept, such as preventing suffering or other adverse events, and the altruistic act becomes pathological for the clinician and possibly for the patient. Numerous examples arose during the height of the COVID-19 pandemic when overworked and exhausted clinicians turned to suicide to alleviate their emotional burdens. In this way, altruism and underlying stoicism may undermine the clinician who does not pay enough attention to their individual needs or is in a situation that precludes any work–life balance. Individual clinician needs should not be supplanted by the altruistic pursuit of the communal common good.[2]

Empathy can slide into *empathic distress.* "When we are able to sense into the suffering of another person, empathy brings us closer to one another, can inspire us to serve, and expands our understanding of the world."[8] [(p. 3)] Halifax reports the following:

> When we identify too strongly with someone who was suffering, our emotions can push us over the edge into distress that might mirror the anguish of those we are trying to serve. If our experience of his or her suffering overwhelms us, empathic distress can also cause us to go numb, to abandon others to protect ourselves from suffering.[8] [(p. 68)]

Empathic distress may be related to secondary, vicarious trauma and compassion fatigue. Both may be regarded as a "disruption" in empathy. *Empathic strain* may be experienced as intrusive when the clinician over-identifies with the patient, which may ultimately result in avoidance and antipathy.[20] In these situations, the objective aspects of empathy are underdeveloped, while the affective components are no longer imagined but are derived from self-experience (i.e., sympathy). The imaginative component of the other's experience is crucial for empathic practice because otherwise the empathy is not experienced as authentic by the patient because the affective component has been substituted with one's own experience (i.e., the clinician's personal experience). Empathy denotes a clear delineation between self and other and therefore can be protective against burnout, whereas sympathy conflates the patient's feelings with one's own feelings (i.e., self-experience) effectively revisiting one's past traumas.[21] Thus, the patient's situation feels "intrusive" and can cause the clinician to retreat as a necessary precaution or survival mechanism.

Integrity can become *moral suffering*. "When we cause suffering to others or to ourselves, our integrity is violated. When we alleviate the suffering of others our integrity is affirmed . . . To have integrity is to have a conscious commitment to honor strong moral and ethical principles."[8 (p. 94)]

Respect can shift to *disrespect*. "There are three aspects to respect: respect for others; respect for principles and values, and self-respect. To have respect for another means to acknowledge their worth and value."[8 (p. 135)] *Engagement* can shift to *burnout*. This concept was described earlier and is likely a protective response to a mismatched work environment.

Another concept that exists on a spectrum and is relevant for palliative care clinicians is moral distress. *Moral distress* arises when the clinician is aware of a moral problem, can determine a remedy, but is unable to act on it because of internal or external constraints.[10] This inability to act ethically makes the clinician feel compromised in their duties, usually imposed upon by an authority who is creating or perpetuating the source of moral distress. "*Moral injury* is a psychological wound resulting from witnessing or participating in a morally transgressive act: it's a toxic festering mix of dread, guilt, and shame."[8 (p. 101)] "*Moral apathy* occurs when we simply don't care to know or when we are in denial about situations that cause harm."[8 (p. 101)] Moral injuries leave a "moral residue" that is cumulative and erodes the clinician's sense of well-being over time.[22] Dr Cynda Hylton Rushton, a nurse and bioethicist working in palliative care, writes about moral resilience and moral suffering in health care as

> An anguish experienced as a threat to our composure, our integrity, the fulfillment of our intentions, and more deeply as a frustration to the concrete meaning that we have found in our personal experiences. It is the anguish over the injury or threat to the injury to the self and thus the meaning of self that is at the core of suffering.[23 (p. 2)]

Clinical Case

A patient with cancer was given an overdose of chemotherapy. The oncologist knew that the problem was irreversible and that the patient would die. The patient was told that he would have to stay in the hospital for a few extra days and that his nurse would continue to provide the psychosocial support she had been giving to the patient. The nurse did not know if the patient had been informed of the overdose and understood its fatal ramifications. The nurse experienced significant moral distress as her moral agency was compromised by a clinical situation wrought with moral compromise (i.e., providing end-of-life care to a patient who did not understand the goal or the palliative nature of the situation). She did not have the necessary means or tools to rectify the situation. She did not feel empowered to raise her concerns.

Moral resilience is the potential for moral distress to be a catalyst for beneficial outcomes and growth. That is, addressing the moral issue through open communication may effectively mitigate the moral distress. This has been described as *ethical environments*, where ethical concerns are freely shared, communicated, and investigated. It is a collective learning process that may be implemented in clinical communities of patient care. Ethical environments that inspire communication and the free flow of ethical information provide an anecdote to moral distress that has been termed moral success and is also derived from the Kantian concept of self-contentment (i.e., *Selbstzufriedenheit*).[24] In the case above, the nurse should feel empowered to express her feelings or concerns, raise ethical concerns, and begin a dialogue to gain multiple clinical perspectives, facilitate honest disclosure, and acknowledge shortcomings.

Unique Stressors in Palliative Care and Psychiatry Related to Burnout:

Stressors in Palliative Care

Palliative care clinicians have identified several key factors that result in increased stress: constant exposure to death, inadequate time with dying patients, growing workload and increasing numbers of deaths, inadequate coping with one's own emotional response to dying patients, the need to carry on "as usual" in the wake of patient deaths, communication difficulties with dying patients and relatives, identification with or developing friendships with patients, inability to live up to one's own standards (e.g., internalized responsibility to provide a "good death"), and feelings of depression, grief, and guilt in response to loss. Time commitment or workload is a consistent risk factor for burnout, which is also seen in the work of oncologists and palliative care clinicians.[10] When clinicians experience greater autonomy and acknowledgment, they are more satisfied with their jobs and able to find more meaning in their work, and when they have less control, they are less satisfied.[12]

The collegial community plays an important role in palliative care but can also be a source of stress. Teamwork has multiple benefits for palliative care but relationships with colleagues may engender certain stresses. The need to meet emotional demands is associated with burnout; however, generally care of the dying has not been a major stressor in palliative care, in part because of the choice to enter the field. A sense of connectedness with others, part of compassion, is a source of the meaning in our work and sustains us. Another source of stress can be found in the success of palliative care as a discipline. Managing a clinical program that is in high demand but understaffed, addressing the multiple and complex needs of patients and caregivers who are often in crisis, and facilitating resolution of conflicts between any combination of patients, caregivers, and the healthcare system brings multiple stresses.[12] Evidence suggests that palliative care clinicians are challenged by several factors in their environments that may be summarized by the following: struggling, changing mindset, adapting, and resilience, which may be enhanced by self-awareness, reflection, and continued growth or evolution.[25]

Stressors in Psychiatry

Interpersonal dynamics, boundaries, and personality disorders are within the purview of psychiatry. While these issues can be stressful, especially in their most severe forms, psychiatrists are trained and well-prepared to deal with them in comparison with other medical professionals. As a discipline, psychiatry does not have the highest rates of burnout. But emotional exhaustion may be higher among psychiatrists given the nature of the work, the vicarious trauma involved in continuous exposure to psychologically laden content, and the belief that becoming emotionally exhausted is just part of the job.[26] Emotional exhaustion can negatively impact patient care and the clinician's health, but it may also serve a protective role. It allows for escape from many impossible and emotionally draining situations. In fact, aspects of burnout (e.g., depersonalization) were originally described by Freudenberg as homeostatic mechanisms that protect against depletion of emotional resources.[27] Attitude changes (e.g., reduced work goals), heightened self-interest and emotional detachment, and becoming less idealistic are forms of coping as well. These changes collide with many personality factors among psychiatrists. As a group, psychiatrists score higher on items of neuroticism but also openness and agreeableness.[28] Higher levels of neuroticism may explain reportedly higher levels of emotional exhaustion, depression, addiction, and even suicide among psychiatrists.

As a discipline, psychiatrists are more prone to experience violence from patients in clinical situations (e.g., being battered from a disruptive patient), which has been associated with burnout.[26] While the risk may appear to be more relevant for general psychiatry, it is also relevant for psychiatrists working with elderly patients with cognitive impairment or patients who become delirious. In addition, psychiatrists who are working in palliative care and hospice may not receive as much direct training or experience with end-of-life issues unless they undertake specialized training. Despite having skills to understand patient dynamic (transference-countertransference, for example), having limited experience working directly with patients at the end of life may be a source of frustration and burnout for some psychiatrists.

The Role of Attachment in Patient Care and Its Heightened Importance at the End of Life

Attachment plays a significant role in how a person relates to others throughout the lifecycle. Attachment and its psychological implications were originally described by Mary Ainsworth. Her work focused on child–parent attachment and has been used to describe attachment throughout the life span. The spectrum of attachment described by Mary Ainsworth and her colleagues in *Patterns of Attachment: Assessed in the Strange Situation and at Home*, spanned from secure attachment to insecure-avoidant or insecure-ambivalent attachments. It should be emphasized that these categories were descriptive and that children and adults may exhibit elements of each category but tend to utilize one more than others.[29]

Attachment is a far-reaching concept that is paramount for humans, non-human primates, and other animal species. Its applicability to work in end-of-life care reflects its essential humanistic qualities that are generally enhanced in patients, and caregivers throughout vulnerable life transitions. At the same time, clinicians have their own attachment styles that may be adapted or reflected throughout clinical encounters. For clinicians, attachment may be experienced as rewarding (i.e., secure attachment) but may also become threatening (i.e., avoidant) or confusing (i.e., ambivalent clinician attachment). Typically, clinicians adapt to patients' varied attachment styles but may not be aware of their own attachment styles, especially to patients and their work. In other words, clinicians may be aware of patients' varied approach to connectedness; they may embrace the clinical situation and the support from their clinicians, or they may be more reserved, cautious, or even incredulous, or skeptical in their approach to the clinical relationship. Patients who have a trauma history may be particularly vulnerable to complicated relationships with clinicians in illness situations. Clinician attachment style may impact the patient experience to some extent but also may predict how the clinician is affected by difficult patient situations in which they are involved. Clinicians with maladaptive attachment may not be able to adapt to patients varied attachment needs.

In caregiving or care-eliciting relationships those who are securely attached can give clear and coherent accounts of their experiences, including painful and difficult ones. They are curious about how they came to be the people they are. Insecurely attached individuals find attachment relationships stressful because they stimulate internally insecure attachment systems. There are a variety of ways of conceptualizing insecure attachment patterns along the secure to insecure attachment dichotomy. In addition to secure attachment, Ciechanowski describes three additional forms of insecure attachment as "cautious," "support seeking," and "self-reliant."[30] Insecure patterns of attachment resist change over time, tend to dismiss negative emotion or overemphasize the cognitive aspects of experience, and emphasize psychological normality, independence, and strength, or they may be preoccupied with their emotional needs and oscillate between seeing others as either wonderful or dreadful.

In essence, a clinician with an insecure attachment style (i.e., ambivalent or avoidant) has a challenging base from which to deal with negative feelings and emotions that arise in patients confronting the end of life. Clinicians who are prone to becoming overwhelmed in an emotionally intense clinical environment may use an ambivalent attachment style, which typically oscillates from enmeshment to emotionally distant. Alternatively, clinicians with an avoidant attachment style remain emotionally distant to patients and are limited in their ability to enter emotionally intense relationship with patients. Both groups struggle to cope with negative feelings. Insecure ambivalent (or enmeshed) individuals may seek help for relational difficulties but may not be able to use it effectively.[31]

In a 1977 article in the *British Journal of Psychiatry*, John Bowlby, pioneer in attachment theory, hypothesized that pathological caregiving behavior was characteristic of insecure attachment. This biopsychological vulnerability may not manifest itself until the individual is stressed, which may come in the form of burnout or other work-related stress. Specific attachment and personality traits may be functional in one scenario but not others. For example, professionals with a dismissive attachment style tend to "negate personal distress, emphasize personal strength and invulnerability, and denigrate dependence on others. They may be reluctant to acknowledge distress or seek help and will attempt to be self-reliant in dealing with stress."[31] This type of approach may be helpful in situations that require perseverance but not in chronic situations that require a thoughtful, self-determinant, grounded, reflective approach. Also, attachment styles may predict which aspects of work are meaningful for clinicians and may be intimately tied to how clinicians cope with stress. Among several groups of nurses, it was found that a secure attachment style was associated with less burnout while an insecure attachment style was associated with burnout.[31]

Among fourth-year medical students, 60% had a secure attachment style to their relationships while 40% exhibited an insecure form of attachment; with self-reliant (20%), cautious (10%), and support-seeking (10%), similar in ratio to the general population. Attachment styles were reflected in their specialty choices. Securely attached students were more likely to choose patient-centered specialties and were less likely to choose specialties based on career rewards (financial rewards, job opportunities, comfortable lifestyle, prestige, and independence). Students with a self-reliant style were significantly more likely to match in a nonprimary care specialty. A study of hospice nurses found that more than half had insecure attachment styles (higher than other studies of health professionals or the general population), which was also associated with having more stress.[31] Hospice nurses with a fearful or dismissing style of attachment were less likely to seek emotional social support as a means of coping with stress than were those with a secure or preoccupied attachment style.[31]

Compassion and Clinical Empathy at the End of Life

The relationship between caring or caregiving and burnout and its related conditions is complicated. There appears to be a dose-dependent relationship between work intensity (e.g., hours worked) and burnout This implies that more caring or deeply caring puts the clinician at risk of burnout. Yet other data suggest that becoming more caring, empathic, or compassionate can be protective against burnout.

"Caring" implicates several related but disparate concepts. Once defined, their relationships become more apparent in terms of how they relate to burnout. The key concepts are compassion, empathy, and sympathy. The latter, "sympathy," was once a term used to describe a person's sensibilities or feelings about specific topics (e.g., poverty, illness). This use of sympathy has fallen out of favor. It is now associated with pity or shallow, self-centered feelings since the beginning of the 20th century once empathy was established as a concept. Sympathy can be thought of as "feeling with" whereas empathy is described as "feeling into," placing oneself in another person's shoes. This implies that sympathetic feelings are one's own while empathic feelings are representations of another's feelings. This key distinction means that sympathy calls up one's own feelings without necessarily gaining the other's perspective, which is why it can be received as superficial or shallow. The patient who experiences an empathic clinician feels "heard" and understood. In other words, the self versus other distinction is clear; the clinician is not conjuring up their own past experiences but has an accurate representation of the patient's experience. Sympathy refers to "feeling" but without direct reference to an objective grounding in the other's experience. Essentially, vicariously induced feelings run the risk of not being in synch or compatible with the other and may be more consistent with revisiting a known mental state (of the clinician). For this reason, people are skeptical of being "sympathized with" and do not want to have someone's pity. Providing sympathy is exhausting because it conjures up one's own emotional repertoire while empathic listening is difficult but more accurately resonates with the patient's experience and worldview, enhances clinical accuracy, and is meaningful for both clinician and patient. Emotional resonance is generally rewarding for the clinician, but it is strenuous and hard work. The term "clinical empathy" described by Judith Halpern is a useful concept because it captures empathy as work along with its clinical meaningfulness for patient and clinician.[32] Interventions used to enhance empathy may also decrease burnout given the implied engagement associated with empathic listening and an empathic stance toward caregiving.[33] "Empathy fatigue" implicates the affective parts of empathy and sympathy, where one is more specifically "feeling with" rather than "feeling into."

Compassion operates from a caring stance, or philosophical perspective, and a personal missive. It has implied behaviors and morality but without the necessarily implied knowledge of another person's experience, which is an irreducible aspect of empathy but can lead to empathic distress. Compassion is a powerful clinical tool that is highly motivating and also protective against clinician burnout.[19] Halifax has defined compassion as the capacity to be attentive to the experience of others, to wish the best for others, and to sense what will truly serve others.[8] Four conditions make compassion possible. They are the capacity to attend to the experience of others, feel concern for others, sense what will serve others, and interact intending to enhance the well-being of others.[8]

Compassion and empathy share many essential features but diverge in their particular emphasis. It could be argued that both enhance clinical care but may threaten clinician well-being to a certain extent. Both have maladaptive counterparts: compassion fatigue and empathy fatigue or empathic distress. Yet training for empathy or compassion enhancement is associated with reduction in burnout. This is counterintuitive and may depend on their definition, along with the quantity and quality of these attributes. A study evaluated brain function initially after empathy training and then after compassion training and found that compassion training reversed brain function associated with negative affect and other non-overlapping regions. The authors concluded that compassion training in place of empathy training may provide additional benefits for clinicians in burnout reduction.[34] Compassion training is further described below.

Death and end-of-life care are challenging for all clinicians, and especially when these situations conjure up personal experience that may not have been dealt with or processed adequately. Of course, death and end-of-life care are challenging to witness irrespective of one's prior experiences. The universal experience of mortality creates a sense of greater purpose that resonates with compassion. At the same time, many of the emotional challenges of caring for patients at the end of life come from obtaining an accurate representation of their experiences. A primary challenge of clinical empathy in the context of end-of-life care is to deal with mortality and mortality salient experiences in one's life so that the clinician's interpretation of the patient's experience is informed objectively without too much interference from one's own experiences with mortality.

Interventions for Burnout and Related Conditions

Interventions should address the root causes of burnout or other clinician maladies. While there are many types of interventions, they can be divided into those that address the individual clinician or the organization or institution. Some interventions address both, and some may be adaptable depending on the situation. Meta-analyses show that organization-based interventions not only induce a greater reduction in burnout but also exhibit a longer duration of response.[35,36] In terms of burnout, even reduction of a few points on the MBI is clinically meaningful. Among the individual-based interventions, those that incorporate mindfulness-based stress reduction or cognitive behavioral therapy tend to be most efficacious.[35] In general, drawing awareness into the clinical encounter and moment-by-moment interactions tends to reduce symptoms of burnout.

Specific interventions to reduce burnout and related conditions in the palliative care or end-of-life clinical setting should address its inherent stressors and the workplace environment. Clinicians working in palliative care settings may benefit from interventions directed at the unique environment of end-of-life care as well as other general burnout reduction interventions. This following section focuses on interventions specific to palliative care.

Connectedness and Spirituality

Clinicians working with patients at the end of life generally find that connectedness and spiritual aspects of this work are meaningful and rewarding but, at the same time, feeling connected to patients may be uniquely stressful and burnout-inducing. In other words, it may be difficult for a clinician experiencing burnout to decide whether to enhance her engagement with work or disconnect from work, perhaps for a respite and internal reflection away from patient care. While either may be effective in the short term, learning ways to engage and cope with work stressors offers not only strategy but durability in terms of burnout prevention. Clinicians working in palliative care with higher levels of individual and collective spirituality had greater compassion satisfaction and less burnout. Medical residents who practiced greater self-care had more empathy toward patients.[10]

Dr. Balfour Mount, a pioneer in the palliative care field, has lived with metastatic esophageal cancer for many years and posited "healing connections" as a therapeutic endeavor for patients that resonates with clinicians.[37] He and his colleagues found that isolation and feeling disconnected were most associated with suffering and anguish. Many participants suffering from burnout and related conditions described an existential vacuum, a crisis of meaning, and an inability to find solace or inner peace. Patient participants often expressed feelings of victimization and a need for control, which can be similarly expressed by burned-out clinicians. Ruminations about unsettling issues of the past and anxieties about the uncertain future consistently removed them from the potential of the present moment. Interestingly, these coping patterns frequently had their roots in early childhood, which speaks to how ingrained these patterns are and the necessary tenacity to fix or change them.

> These individuals tended to find a sense of meaning and connectedness in the context of their illness. They also tended to experience a greater acceptance of their

illness. This might even be expressed as a degree of sympathetic connection to their disease.[37]

Healing connections are meaningful for not only the patient, but for caregivers as well. This is reflected in the fact that caregivers in oncology and palliative care with a greater sense of spirituality had greater compassion satisfaction and less burnout, and medical residents who practiced greater self-care had more empathy toward patients.[10] The time is right for connections to be formed, rebuilt, or repaired in surprising ways as patients contemplate and make peace with their lives. In the words of Dr. David Kerr,

> Dying is more than the suffering we either observe or experience. Within the obvious tragedy of dying are unseen processes that hold meaning. Dying is a time of transition that triggers a transformation of perspective and perception. If those who are dying struggle to find words to capture their inner experiences, it is not because language fails them but because it falls short of the sense of awe and wonder that overcomes them. They experience a growing sense of connectedness and belonging. They begin to see with their unlocked souls.[38]

Therefore, the identification, cultivation, and perpetuation of healing connections benefits patients, families, and caregivers by providing meaning and purpose. These relationships may manifest themselves through subtle moments or ways and may be transient. It is helpful to acknowledge that the dying process can feel individualized despite its universal aspects. It is important to not impart judgment in terms of what "should be" as this is most often tinged with the clinicians' ideals of "good death," which may or may not be in line with what the patient is experiencing and her own assessment of the situation. Healing connections built on patients' needs are the most meaningful and effective.

Last, healing connections apply to the healers as well. Clinicians may work to cultivate those meaningful connections in their lives inside and outside of the work environment. The clinician's understanding of her own necessary connections for healing may empower her to invoke those connections for her patients facing the end of life as well. Replenishment can be found within this inner voice that is asking for wholeness and wellness. Sensitivity to it will help clinicians guide their patients in finding it for themselves as well.[9] Compassion practices and recognizing the need for self-compassion can reduce burnout.

Interventions Targeting Individual Clinicians or Institution/Organization

This distinction is fundamentally important when one considers that burnout is a mismatch of worker to workplace. Therefore, it may not be surprising that organizational or structural changes tend to be more effective and of longer durations. Commonly, these systemic changes are straightforward, such as duty hour restrictions for residents or coverage changes, but may involve leadership changes or other more profound arrangements.[35,36] Clinicians can feel blame (i.e., stigma) for not doing enough on an individual level to prevent burnout. But attention at the individual level (e.g., yoga or exercise practices, etc.) will have limited efficacy when the root cause of burnout is not addressed or in the setting of organizational dysfunction.

Mindfulness-Based Stress Reduction and Other Mindfulness Practices

Mindfulness-based stress reduction (MBSR) is a protocolized intervention that teaches mindfulness and stress reduction techniques over approximately eight weekly sessions. Its benefits are numerous as it enables perspective taking and enhances new ways of thinking and feeling about anxiety-provoking situations. While many interventions may incorporate mindfulness techniques, MBSR is a specific form of mindfulness training that has the most robust data behind it in terms of burnout prevention and reduction to date.[39] Attention to mindfulness along with compassion in the end-of-life setting was found to be effective in reducing clinician distress and enhancing clinician self-care.[40]

Meaning-Based and Compassion-Based Interventions

Meaning-centered therapy (MCP) is a protocolized prescriptive, time-limited group or individually based therapy that has proved efficacy for patients experiencing existential distress.[41] It is based on the work of Viktor Frankl, an Austrian psychoanalyst and Holocaust survivor. It has been adapted for use in many disease-related settings and for clinicians. The restoration of meaning in clinicians working in palliative care settings is highly effective in reducing and preventing burnout.[42]

Joan Halifax developed two related models of compassion that are useful for developing and cultivating compassion. The first was the ABIDE Model of Compassion.[8] *Attention and affect* (A) refers to the ability to hold attention without distraction. *Balance* (B) refers to the mindfulness needed to perceive the reality of suffering without being overwhelmed by the magnitude or intensity of it. *Intention* refers to the drive or motivation to relieve suffering. *Insight* (I) refers to perceptual knowledge, which is integral to cultivate *discernment* (D) in difficult situations as part of a cognitive process. *Embodiment, engagement, and equanimity* (E) speak to the innate drive to connect with other people. Of note, intention (to alleviate suffering) is the feature that differentiates compassion from empathy, where the motivational or behavioral component is contested. Subsequently, Halifax developed the GRACE model as an active contemplative practice focused on cultivating compassion as we interact with others.[8] GRACE is an applied model and stands for *Gathering* attention, *Recalling* intention, *Attunement* (to self and others), *Consideration* (open to insights and discernment of what will benefit the patient), and ethically *Engaging/Enacting, and Ending* the interaction. This process works to engender compassion as caregivers fully engage in interactions with patients and families.

Future Directions

There is increasing attention drawn to clinician well-being and the effects of work environment. Its application to palliative care for clinicians who treat patients at the end of life presents a challenge but also an opportunity where both generalized and specific interventions to address stressors working with end-of-life patients can be integrated into care. Mitigating the effects of mortality salience and cultivating sustained engagement with patients at the end of life are examples of what may be addressed in the future. In addition, attention should be given to understanding how clinicians will be best able to adapt wellness changes to their clinical practices. Research in this area has been instrumental in moving the field forward as studies are gathering disparate data to answer these questions. Interventions will be best designed by incorporating what is known from the evidence thus far and expanding upon it in ways that are adaptive and collaborative. There is not a one-size-fits-all solution to burnout and its related conditions. Interventions will need to be applied within the bounds of medical practices and administration. Stressful situations are frequently encountered in palliative and supportive care settings and can become overwhelming for patients, families, and the clinicians. Stress is particularly detrimental to communication, and the clinician is expected to take the lead in opening effective lines of communication. Therefore, attention to clinician needs and emotions is paramount to providing effective end-of-life care. Self-care should include not only respite but also a coordinated effort to meaningfully engage with one's work in a way that is healthy in mind and body and sustains the clinician. Attention to how clinical work is affecting well-being as caregivers is also instrumental for the calibration of the field as one that provides quality and value alongside other disciplines. Part of the appeal to supportive and palliative care is the expectation to emulate and cultivate wellness among other clinicians. In short, preventing or treating burnout and its related conditions is a basic need and assumption of the field. It benefits patients, families, clinicians, and colleagues. This understanding is becoming increasingly commonplace across medical disciplines. Expectations for burnout prevention and wellness may become increasingly expected in the future as this bodes well for patients, clinicians, and medical practices.

Key Points

- Care for the healthcare provider is a multipronged endeavor that largely depends on the root cause of occupational stress along with identification of specific work-related conditions (e.g., burnout, moral distress).
- Prevention and treatment of burnout and other work-related conditions can leverage clinician predisposition toward adaptation, coping, and resilience while also addressing the insidious nature of factors that perpetuate these conditions (e.g., asking about mental health as part of board licensure, organizational structures).
- Attachment styles influence not only how patients relate to their clinicians but also how clinicians relate to them and may be susceptible to interpersonal work-related distress.
- Concepts such as healing connections and methods to facilitate compassion (e.g., ABIDE, GRACE models) may be particularly helpful for clinicians working with patients at the end of life.

- Interventions to reduce burnout and related conditions can be divided into individual or organizationally targeted interventions. The latter are more efficacious and durable, but optimal interventions depend on root causes of these conditions and the needs of individual clinicians
- Mindfulness-based stress reduction (MBSR) and other interventions that incorporate mindfulness or components of cognitive behavioral therapy led to greatest reductions in burnout and related conditions.

References

1. Legha RK. A history of physician suicide in America. *J Med Humanit.* 2012;33(4):219–244.
2. McFarland DC, Hlubocky F, Susaimanickam B, O'Hanlon R, Riba M. Addressing depression, burnout, and suicide in oncology physicians. *Am Soc Clin Oncol Educ Book.* 2019;39:590–598.
3. Zwack J, Schweitzer J. If every fifth physician is affected by burnout, what about the other four? Resilience strategies of experienced physicians. *Acad Med.* 2013;88(3):382–389.
4. Johnson B. Code Lavender: Initiating holistic rapid response at the Cleveland Clinic. *Beginnings.* 2014;34(2):10–11.
5. Southwick SMC, Dennis S. *Resilience: The Science of Mastering Life's Greatest Challenges.* New York: Cambridge University Press; 2012.
6. Maslach C JS. *The Maslach Burnout Inventory* Palo Alto, CA: Consulting Psychologists Press; 1981.
7. Kristensen TS BM, Villadsen E, Christensen KB. The Copenhagen burnout inventory: A new tool for the assessment of burnout *Work Stress.* 2005:152–207.
8. Halifax J. *Standing on the Edge: Finding Freedom Where Fear and Courage Meet.* New York: Flatiron Books; 2018.
9. Kearney M. *The Nest in the Stream: Lessons from Nature on Being with Pain.* Berkeley, CA: Parralax Press; 2018.
10. Vachon MLS, Huggard PK, Huggard JA. Reflections on occupational stress in pallaitive care nursing: is it changing? In: Ferrell B. CN, Paice J., ed. *Textbook of Palliative Care Nursing.* 4th ed. New York: Oxford University Press; 2015:215–229.
11. Shanafelt TD, West CP, Sinsky C, Trockel M, Tutty M, Satele DV, et al. Changes in burnout and satisfaction with work-life integration in physicians and the general US working population between 2011 and 2017. *Mayo Clin Proc.* 2019;94(9):1681–1694.
12. Kamal AH, Bull JH, Wolf SP, et al. Prevalence and predictors of burnout among hospice and palliative care clinicians in the U.S. *J Pain Symptom Manage.* 2020;59(5):e6-e13.
13. Moukarzel A, Michelet P, Durand AC, et al. Burnout syndrome among emergency department staff: Prevalence and associated factors. *Biomed Res Int.* 2019;2019:6462472.
14. Arnsten AFT, Shanafelt T. Physician distress and burnout: The neurobiological perspective. *Mayo Clin Proc.* 2021;96(3):763–769.
15. Tawfik DS, Scheid A, Profit J, et al. Evidence relating health care provider burnout and quality of care: A systematic review and meta-analysis. *Ann Intern Med.* 2019;171(8):555–567.
16. Figley C. *Compassion Fatigue: Coping with Secondary Traumatic Stress Disorder.* New York: Brunner/Mazel; 1995.
17. Sinclair S, Raffin-Bouchal S, Venturato L, Mijovic-Kondejewski J, Smith-MacDonald L. Compassion fatigue: A meta-narrative review of the healthcare literature. *Int J Nurs Stud.* 2017;69:9–24.
18. Neville K, Cole DA. The relationships among health promotion behaviors, compassion fatigue, burnout, and compassion satisfaction in nurses practicing in a community medical center. *J Nurs Adm.* 2013;43(6):348–354.

19. Slocum-Gori S, Hemsworth D, Chan WW, Carson A, Kazanjian A. Understanding compassion satisfaction, compassion fatigue and burnout: A survey of the hospice palliative care workforce. *Palliat Med.* 2013;27(2):172–178.

20. Neumann M, Bensing J, Mercer S, Ernstmann N, Ommen O, Pfaff H. Analyzing the "nature" and "specific effectiveness" of clinical empathy: A theoretical overview and contribution toward a theory-based research agenda. *Patient Educ Couns.* 2009;74(3):339–346.

21. Thirioux B, Birault F, Jaafari N. Empathy is a protective factor of burnout in physicians: New neurophenomenological hypotheses regarding empathy and sympathy in care relationship. *Front Psychol.* 2016;7:763.

22. Jameton A. Dilemmas of moral distress: Moral responsibility and nursing practice. *AWHONNS Clin Issues Perinat Womens Health Nurs.* 1993;4(4):542–551.

23. Rushton CH. *Moral Resilience: Transforming Moral Suffering in Healthcare.* New York: Oxford University Press; 2018.

24. Walshchots M. Kant on moral satisfaction. *Kantian Rev.* 2017;22(2):281–303.

25. Koh MYH, Hum AYM, Khoo HS, et al. Burnout and resilience after a decade in palliative care: What survivors have to teach us. A qualitative study of palliative care clinicians with more than 10 years of experience. *J Pain Symptom Manage.* 2020;59(1):105–115.

26. Rotstein S, Hudaib AR, Facey A, Kulkarni J. Psychiatrist burnout: A meta-analysis of Maslach Burnout Inventory means. *Australas Psychiatry.* 2019;27(3):249–254.

27. Freudenberger HJ. Burnout: contemporary issues, trends, and concerns In: Farber BA, ed. *Stress and Burnout in the Human Services Professions* New York: Pargamon; 1983:46–58.

28. Fond G, Bourbon A, Micoulaud-Franchi JA, Auquier P, Boyer L, Lancon C. Psychiatry: A discipline at specific risk of mental health issues and addictive behavior? Results from the national BOURBON study. *J Affect Disord.* 2018;238:534–538.

29. Bretherton I. Emotional availability: An attachment perspective. *Attach Hum Dev.* 2000;2(2):233–241; discussion 249–250.

30. Ciechanowski PS, Walker EA, Katon WJ, Russo JE. Attachment theory: A model for health care utilization and somatization. *Psychosom Med.* 2002;64(4):660–667.

31. Vachon ML. Targeted intervention for family and professional caregivers: Attachment, empathy, and compassion. *Palliat Med.* 2016;30(2):101–103.

32. Halpern J. What is clinical empathy? *J Gen Intern Med.* 2003;18(8):670–674.

33. Kelm Z, Womer J, Walter JK, Feudtner C. Interventions to cultivate physician empathy: A systematic review. *BMC Med Educ.* 2014;14:219.

34. Klimecki OM, Leiberg S, Ricard M, Singer T. Differential pattern of functional brain plasticity after compassion and empathy training. *Soc Cogn Affect Neurosci.* 2014;9(6):873–879.

35. West CP, Dyrbye LN, Erwin PJ, Shanafelt TD. Interventions to prevent and reduce physician burnout: A systematic review and meta-analysis. *Lancet.* 2016;388(10057):2272–2281.

36. Panagioti M, Panagopoulou E, Bower P, et al. Controlled interventions to reduce burnout in physicians: A systematic review and meta-analysis. *JAMA Intern Med.* 2017;177(2):195–205.

37. Mount BM, Boston PH, Cohen SR. Healing connections: on moving from suffering to a sense of well-being. *J Pain Symptom Manage.* 2007;33(4):372–388.

38. Kerr C, Mardorossian, Carine *Death Is But a Dream: Finding Hope and Meaning at Life's End.* New York: Penguin Random House; 2020.

39. Lamothe M, Rondeau E, Malboeuf-Hurtubise C, Duval M, Sultan S. Outcomes of MBSR or MBSR-based interventions in health care providers: A systematic review with a focus on empathy and emotional competencies. *Complement Ther Med.* 2016;24:19–28.

40. Orellana-Rios CL, Radbruch L, Kern M, et al. Mindfulness and compassion-oriented practices at work reduce distress and enhance self-care of palliative care teams: A mixed-method evaluation of an "on the job" program. *BMC Palliat Care.* 2017;17(1):3.

41. Breitbart W, Pessin H, Rosenfeld B, et al. Individual meaning-centered psychotherapy for the treatment of psychological and existential distress: A randomized controlled trial in patients with advanced cancer. *Cancer.* 2018;124(15):3231–3239.

42. Fillion L, Vachon M, Gagnon P. Enhancing meaning at work and preventing burnout: The meaning-centered intervention for palliative care clinicians. In: Breitbart W, ed. *Meaning-Centered Psychotherapy in the Cancer Setting.* New York: Oxford University Press; 2017:168–181.

21

Prognostic Understanding in the Terminally Ill

Laura C. Polacek, Leah E. Walsh, Melissa M. Duva, Login S. George, and Allison J. Applebaum

Introduction

For patients with serious or life-limiting illnesses, providing high-quality care to reduce burden and distress while improving quality of life throughout the disease course is of the highest importance. While palliative care is available to patients across the spectrum of their diagnosis, it is primarily utilized by those whose illnesses have progressed to advanced stages and require more extensive symptom management and coordinated care. Providing a "good death" is a primary aim of palliative care, which is often defined as a death which is concordant with patient and family wishes and cultural expectations through early idenfication of medical and psychological needs, avoiding unecessary distress and suffering.

To provide care that is concordant with patients' wishes and values, palliative care should be offered and utilized early on in the care trajectory. However, providing patient-centered care requires the patient to accurately and thoroughly understand their prognosis. The provision of care that is overly aggressive or discordant with patient values is often due to suboptimal communication, including both provider prognostic disclosure and patient prognostic understanding. Therefore, studying how patients understand their prognosis has become a focus within palliative care research.

This chapter provides an overview of progonstic understanding across various diseases which commonly utilize palliative care, although cancer will be a primary focus as it encompasses a majority of the research literature. We review how the construct has evolved, as well as current research into its multidimensional structure. The chapter pays particular attention to the relationship between prognostic understanding and psychological outcomes, coping skills, patient–provider communication, how prognostic understanding may be improved, and cultural nuances in patients' understanding of prognosis. It concludes with recommendations for future directions in both research and clinical practice.

Defining Prognostic Understanding

Prognostic understanding is a multifaceted construct which has assumed various definitions over time. Gathering a more nuanced understanding of how patients understand their prognosis and utilize the term is important to help healthcare professionals communicate effectively with patients and their loved ones. Applebaum and colleagues[1] conceptualized prognostic understanding in a systematic review of patients with advanced cancer. Thirty-seven studies were qualitatively analyzed, eliciting structured, semi-structured, and unstructured methods to understand patients' understanding of their prognosis. In these studies, prognostic understanding was defined in many ways, from awareness of the advanced or metastatic nature of the cancer, to likelihood of survival, to plans for the future. Importantly, some studies lacked a clear definition altogether.

Masterson and colleagues[2] sought to characterize prognostic understanding through the viewpoint of 15 healthcare professionals in the fields of psycho-oncology, medical oncology, and palliative care utilizing semi-structured interviews. Five themes arose throughout the qualitative analysis: an understanding of the current medical state of the disease, approximate life expectancy, perceived disease curability, anticipated decline over the disease course, and available treatment options. Patient information preferences and the extent to which physicians have communicated prognostic information were also identified as separate but related constructs that impact a patient's level of prognostic understanding. Together, these five facets provide the first multidimensional conceptualization of the construct of prognostic understanding, laying the foundation for the establishment of a multifaceted, structured measure of prognostic understanding that may serve as a "gold standard." Although there is not yet a gold standard for defining prognostic understanding, in this chapter we define prognostic understanding according to Masterson and colleagues'[2] recent work.

Measuring Prognostic Understanding

The definition of prognostic understanding invariably affects the way it is measured and, by extension, how we interpret the research on this topic. In the review conducted by Applebaum and colleagues,[1] specific approaches to measuring prognostic understanding were also examined, and the authors found that those approaches differed vastly. However, most studies focused on a single facet of prognostic understanding, often utilizing a single-item measure. For example, one of the most widely used single-item measures of terminal illness acknowledgment (TIA) asks patients to identify their current health status as (1) relatively healthy, (2) seriously but not terminally ill, or (3) seriously and terminally ill.[1] This measure addresses a central facet of prognostic understanding—the patient's understanding of the terminal nature of their disease—but ignores many other potentially important domains. Other single-item methods used to measure prognostic understanding have addressed a patient's understanding of the intent of treatment (palliative vs. curative in nature) or estimation of their proximity to death.[1]

However, many of the measures identified by Applebaum et al.[1] have had limited research to support their utility. For example, the Brief Illness Perception Questionnaire (IPQ)[3] is a 9-item measure with three items assessing prognosis: "How long do you think your illness will continue?", "How much do you think your treatment can help your illness?", and "How well do you feel you understand your illness?" Each of these questions is rated on a 0–10 scale, but the extent to which they effectively measure prognostic understanding is not clear. Nevertheless, this scale, which was originally developed for patients with myocardial infarction, has been used in more than 188 studies of patients with various advanced illnesses including diseases of the nervous system, musculoskeletal and connective tissue disorders, and infectious diseases, and it has been shown to predict patient involvement in their medical decisions.[3] Still, much of the scientific literature on prognostic understanding continues to rely on single-item measures that address only one element of this multifaceted construct.

Ideally, the measurement of prognostic understanding should capture patients' knowledge across the disease continuum. A patient's desire for information about their disease and its treatment likely changes over time and as their illness changes or progresses. As such, the measurement of prognostic understanding should be sufficiently flexible to apply to patients at each point along the illness trajectory. A multifaceted quantitative measure of prognostic understanding would allow researchers to better determine how varying levels of prognostic understanding relate to a patient's healthcare communication, decision-making, and psychological functioning at each stage of their disease. By doing so, clinicians will be better equipped to tailor prognostic discussions to the individual needs and information preferences of their patients.

Importance of Prognostic Understanding
Psychological Outcomes

It is well-understood that prognostic understanding can have a significant impact on a patient's healthcare decision-making and thus one's physical health and wellness.[4] However, prognostic understanding has also been linked to important psychological outcomes, such as depression, anxiety, and quality of life,[5,6] although the direction of those associations is equivocal. A recent review of factors associated with accurate prognostic understanding among patients with advanced care[7] found that depression, anxiety, and quality of life were positively associated with accurate prognostic understanding in some studies, while other researchers found accurate prognostic understanding to be associated with greater psychological distress. Therefore, accurate prognostic understanding does not appear to have benefits that are universal for all patients and all times in the cancer trajectory, highlighting the need for additional research to better understand when and for whom accurate prognostic understanding is psychologically beneficial and when it may be detrimental.

Fortunately, research on healthcare information preferences has highlighted the importance of considering individual preferences for healthcare information when discussing prognostic information with patients and families. For example, Innes and Payne[8] identified wide variation in the degree of information that patients desired about important aspects of their diagnosis and treatment trajectory. Although prognostic awareness has generally been positively associated with hope, feelings of control, trust in their physician, satisfaction with care, and spiritual well-being, Innes and Payne[8] found that patients at the most extreme ends of the spectrum (patients who preferred full prognostic disclosure or no prognostic disclosure) reported higher levels of distress than those patients who stated preferences for a moderate amount of prognostic disclosure from their healthcare providers. This finding highlights the importance of attention to individualized patient preferences for information and challenges the assumption that full disclosure is always optimal. Thus, research supports the notion that patients' preferences for prognostic disclosure should be identified and attended to during these difficult conversations. Doing so will increase the likelihood of patients feeling confident and empowered to make important healthcare decisions consistent with their information preferences and level of prognostic understanding.

While optimally patients are provided with the type and quantity of prognostic information desired, delivery of prognostic information does not ensure prognostic understanding. It is vital that patients and family members can come to a place of understanding and acceptance of this information. In a review of prognostic communication preferences, Trice and Prigerson[9] differentiated between *cognitive* and *emotional* understanding and acceptance of illness. They described cognitive acceptance as a factual understanding of the illness, while emotional acceptance occurs on a deeper, more spiritual or relational level. Both cognitive and emotional acceptance are important and related to different aspects of end-of-life decision-making. Specifically, cognitive acceptance of one's prognosis has been positively associated with engagement in advance care planning, while emotional acceptance has been positively associated with quality of life. The goal of a "good death" appears to require both cognitive and emotional understanding and acceptance. The nuances inherent in a patient's preference for prognostic information and the various ways in which a patient can come to understand and accept his or her prognosis highlight the need for clear communication between physician and patient to determine what type(s) of information is desired by the patient and/or family members, how detailed that information should be, and when the information should be delivered.

Research on prognostic understanding has occasionally distinguished between the ways that a patient internalizes information. For example, Thompson and colleagues[5] assessed patients with advanced cancer who had an estimated life expectancy of less than 6 months, examining prognostic acceptance and its relationship with psychological outcomes. They found that among patients who understood their prognosis (i.e., a "cognitive understanding") but still experienced difficulty accepting that their disease was terminal (i.e., lacked "emotional acceptance"), almost half met diagnostic criteria for a depressive or anxiety disorder. This finding demonstrates what many clinicians experience: patients can acknowledge the "facts" associated with their illness but nonetheless struggle to accept this information. In short, conveying prognostic information is an important first step in the process, but ensuring that a patient understands and appreciates their prognosis on both a cognitive and emotional level is a vital second step.

Coping Styles

Coping styles play a critical role in adjusting to a life-threatening medical illness. Coping styles can be divided into active or passive approaches, where active coping is oriented in problem-solving to manage stressors and passive coping uses avoidance to minimize the stress itself. As coping with the information relayed is a key element of the process of understanding one's prognosis, coping strategies likely impact a patient's understanding of the prognostic information provided.

In one study that examined the link between coping and prognostic understanding, Nipp and colleagues[10] found that both coping style and accuracy of prognostic understanding impacted patients' mood and quality of life. Patients who indicated an awareness of terminal illness and relied on active coping strategies, such as positive reframing in response to increased distress, reported better quality of life and mood than patients who did not acknowledge that the illness was incurable, even when they used those same active coping strategies to navigate the illness. On the other hand, patients who relied on passive coping strategies such as behavioral disengagement reported more depressive symptoms than those using positive reframing. These findings, and those of others,[3] suggest that adaptive coping skills may help buffer against the negative psychological reaction that is often associated with the understanding that one's life is limited.

Prognostic Communication

Information Preferences

Patients can vary widely regarding the type and amount of prognostic information they desire. Such differences can be due to both patient- and disease-related factors, including the type of disease, the patient's point in the disease trajectory, what the patient expects or requests to know, or cultural and religious factors. For example, Ellis and Varner[11] studied information preferences in patients with cancer to better understand how it may impact patient-centered care. In their sample of 176 patients with heterogeneous cancers, more than three-quarters said they wanted "a lot" of information about their diagnosis and prognosis, and more than half of the sample was satisfied with the amount of information they received about the chances of a cure and their life expectancy. However, about a third of the sample wanted *more* information regarding these two parts of prognosis, which suggests that while many patients get an adequate amount of information, a substantial amount feel dissatisfied and want to know more about their disease trajectory. Less than 5% of the sample wanted less information about curability and life expectancy, which again highlights the importance of openly and thoroughly communicating about prognosis.

Innes and Payne[8] reviewed the literature on information preferences for patients with advanced cancer and identified 13 studies which focused on patient preferences. Overall, they found that patients often preferred qualitative versus quantitative or statistical information about their prognosis; however, some studies noted a greater level of interest in time-oriented information than others. Furthermore, a recent review of prognostic communication found higher patient satisfaction with quantitative versus qualitative estimates of survival, suggesting that some types of quantitative information may be more useful in some contexts.[12] Studies also found patients did not want information presented in an indisputable way, but rather in a manner that acknowledged the potential for individual variation among patients with similar prognoses. Importantly, patients emphasized that hope was extremly important to instill throughout the conversation even if the patient's prognosis was poor. However, patients preferred information about prognosis that was straightforward or nonparadoxical and that was delivered at their level of health literacy to prevent misunderstandings around prognostic information.

Because prognostic information is heterogeneous across and within certain illnesses, it becomes increasingly difficult for physicians to anticipate when and how such information should be disclosed. As such, it is vital for physicians to thoughtfully and sensitively deliver prognostic information and gather an understanding of what and how the patient hopes to receive prognostic information as early as possible. This can subsequently guide providers in how they navigate communication across the illness trajectory, from diagnosis through a transition to purely palliative care.

Understanding patient preferences for prognostic information is not the only challenge healthcare providers face when disclosing prognostic information. In fact, Brighton and Bristowe,[13] in their review of the importance of communication in palliative care, identified a number of other challenges clinicians face. One issue in discussing prognosis and end-of-life care is that patients often expect clinicians to initiate such conversations, while clinicians often wait for patients to ask about prognosis before initiating the conversation. When clinicians do disclose prognostic information, they may discuss it in a manner that is vague or overly optimistic, which impedes patients from getting a clear and accurate understanding of their prognosis[13] and can lead to care decisions that are incongruent with patient preferences.

The uncertain nature of prognosis can also make discussing prognosis difficult. Since disease trajectories can change and prognostication can be imprecise, clinicians may be hesitant to share prognostic information before they are sure it is the "best time" to do so.[13] While delivering information when patients are ready and able to comprehend it is important, it is also important to understand the dynamic nature of prognostication throughout the trajectory of a given illness. For example, within oncology, this is particularly important in the age of individualized medicine, where the number and type of available treatments are consistently growing and becoming more specialized, making it difficult to predict how one's cancer will respond to a given intervention.

Another barrier to prognostic communication is the perceived potential impact of this news on patients' psychological well-being. Physicians often worry about damaging rapport with patients and their families during the prognostic discussion, which can make transparency difficult.[12] Physicians may be concerned with shattering hope or causing psychological harm, and together these factors can obstruct their willingness to discuss prognosis. However, research has shown that patients are able to hold hope and accurate prognostic information at the same time, and this emphasizes the importance of delivering prognostic information plainly.[13] Additionally, research has shown that, in the context of advanced illness, the object of one's hope often shifts from cure or survival to a good death for oneself and positive psychosocial outcomes for loved ones facing bereavement.[14] Furthermore, a systematic review of the literature on prognostic communication in advanced cancer suggests that prognostic disclosure does not actually harm patients; while it may cause immediate distress, over time it may not negatively affect patients psychologically.[12] This might be explained by the concept of "middle knowledge," which describes prognostic understanding and denial as a dialectic in which one is able to both deny their terminal diagnosis and engage in end-of-life planning such that, over time, one is able to come to terms with one's death at an emotionally manageable pace.[15] Prognostic communication, though difficult and nuanced for each patient, can therfore help patients and their families better prepare for their future.

Finally, delivering prognostic information can be challenging for professionals. Clinicians may feel unprepared to have discussions about prognosis and may feel unsure about the "right way" to discuss the stage of the illnes, its impact on life expectancy, and the patient's physical and psychological functioning.[4] In fact, many clinicians have attributed their feeling of unpreparedness to a lack of formal training in end-of-life communication, ultimately rendering prognostic disclosure a daunting and uncomfortable task.[4] Training for healthcare professionals regarding how to communicate information about prognosis can both help clinicians feel more confident in these discussions and normalize the value of having these conversations often as the disease changes or progresses (see Chapter 13).

Improving Prognostic Understanding

To date, several interventions have been developed to improve prognostic understanding among patients with terminal illness.[16–18] Tested interventions have taken a variety of forms and approaches, including the incorporation of decision aids (e.g., information booklets or audio files) into routine oncologic consults to enhance patients' understanding,[16] palliative care consultations with a focus on enhancing illness understanding,[17] and targeted discussions with dedicated healthcare providers centering specifically on discussions of prognosis and end-of-life care planning.[18] At the heart of most interventions is the provision of information regarding prognosis and available treatment/care options.[17] However, as information alone may not lead to improved prognostic understanding, most tested interventions also feature additional components such as emotional and decisional support (e.g., eliciting fears and worries; providing emotional validation; assisting with value clarification) and assistance with concrete aspects of end-of-life care planning.[18] These components assist patients in understanding and accepting potentially difficult prognostic information and taking concrete steps to facilitate goal-concordant end-of-life care.

Some research suggests that prognostic understanding may be improved through intervention. One randomized controlled trial evaluated the effect of a multicomponent advance care planning intervention among patients with a terminal cancer diagnosis.[18] The intervention consisted of repeated visits with a nurse that focused on prognostic and end-of-life care discussions up until the patient's death. Compared to a sham control, participants who received the intervention had higher odds of accurate prognostic understanding earlier in their illness trajectory, and this understanding was associated with a lower likelihood of receiving cardiopulmonary resuscitation (CPR) in the final month of life. Another randomized controlled trial examined the impact of early integrated palliative care among patients with metastatic non-small cell lung cancer.[17] Patients had repeated meetings until death with a palliative care physician or advanced practice nurse that focused on addressing illness understanding, treatment decision-making, symptom management, and coping. Results showed that the intervention group patients were more likely to either remain or become accurate in their perception of curability, relative to participants in the control group receiving standard oncology care.

While only a handful of interventions have been evaluated in terms of a demonstrated effect on patient prognostic understanding, numerous others have also been developed over the past two decades.[6] These interventions aim to increase the prognostic information received by patients, which presumably would improve patients' understanding of their prognosis. A recent systematic review found 17 randomized controlled trials of interventions aiming to increase delivery of prognostic information.[6] These interventions consisted of efforts to increase clinician education, provide patient coaching, and/or coordinate care (e.g., consultation with specialty palliative care). One example of a recently evaluated prognostic communication intervention is the Serious Illness Care Program, a communication quality-improvement project consisting of clinical tools, clinician training, and system changes.[19] As part of the intervention, clinicians received training in communication and a structured communication guide; patients received a pre-conversation letter introducing the patient–clinician discussion and a "family guide" to help them continue the conversation with their families thereafter; and system-level changes were implemented, including clinician assessment of prognosis, email reminders to have prognostic discussions, and a structured electronic medical record (EMR) template for documenting the conversation. Analysis of the medical record after patients' death demonstrated that patients in the intervention group were more likely to have documented prognostic conversations, and these occurred earlier in the illness course.[19]

Existing research thus suggests that interventions hold the potential to improve patients' receipt of prognostic information and their prognostic understanding.[18,19] Additional future research is needed to determine what components of existing interventions are most potent in increasing prognostic understanding. Such research would inform widespread dissemination and implementation of prognostic understanding interventions into routine practice.

Cultural Influences on Prognostic Understanding

A growing body of literature explores how one's sociodemographic background shapes one's understanding of the construct of prognosis and its impact on health information preferences. As such, it is essential that healthcare professionals are aware of their patients' cultural background. For example, a study of 221 patients with advanced cancer in South Africa surveyed patient's perceived health status and life expectancy to assess illness understanding.[20] Only 5.8% of patients acknowledged that they were terminally ill, and more than three-quarters were unable to estimate their life expectancy. Importantly, most patients expressed disinterest in knowing their physician-estimated life expectancy, which highlights the importance of eliciting patients' prognostic information preferences rather than assuming that more (or less) disclosure is desired. Interestingly, more than two-thirds of this sample endorsed a preference for comfort care over life-extending measures at the end of life, and more than three-quarters had already made funeral plans. Even patients with poor illness understanding still had identified end-of-life preferences and engaged in some form of advance care planning (e.g., preferring comfort care, preferring to die at home, executing funeral plans and arrangements).

A qualitative study in the Netherlands sought to characterize what comprised "good palliative care" for 33 Turkish and Moroccan immigrant patients with cancer and 30 of their family members.[21] Additionally, the authors examined how Dutch treatment providers handled the challenges surrounding intra-family differences in thinking around end-of-life care. The authors found that family members often preferred curative or more invasive care than did patients, even at the end of life when the likelihood of cure was low. Importantly, family members felt providers should avoid discussing a negative prognosis to maintain an "optimistic outlook" for the patient, both in terms of a hope for recovery and to preserve the patient's strength to fight the illness. The Dutch healthcare providers, however, reported often feeling that openly discussing negative aspects of the patient's prognosis was an important and necessary component of high-quality palliative care as it facilitated greater shared decision-making, which they believe served to optimize patient quality of life. Physicians acknowledged an awareness of their migrant patients' information preferences, and some acknowledged difficulty upholding those preferences due to their own belief in the need for clear and comprehensive prognostic communication.

Similarly, cultural and religious factors unique to Asian cancer patients may impact how (and how much) prognostic information is provided to them. Specifically, filial piety might dictate who receives prognostic information and whether or how that information is delivered to the patient. One study interviewed 24 Chinese physicians to understand information sharing about a patient's cancer diagnosis and prognosis.[22] Results suggested that physicians felt they had to share information with the family first so they could then determine what to share with the patient. Together, these studies highlight the need for physicians to recognize the impact of a patient's and their family's culture on prognostic communication and decision-making, which may help them avoid making assumptions or imposing their own healthcare beliefs onto the patient. While the majority of research on prognostic understanding and end-of-life decision-making is conducted with Western samples, these studies emphasize the need for researchers and clinicians to approach such topics from a patient-centered perspective that first understands their culturally influenced preferences and means of engaging with end-of-life care.

Future Directions

Prognostic understanding is a complex, multidimensional construct that has gained increased attention among palliative care researchers and clinicians over the past two decades, particularly for its role in end-of-life decision-making and its impact on patients' psychological well-being. Physicians have often struggled with how to best discuss prognostic information with patients and their families because prognosis is often inherently uncertain. Furthermore, researchers have yet to establish a gold standard measure of prognostic understanding that would enable researchers to comprehensively and uniformly assess prognostic understanding among patients with advanced illness and result in more robust research on which clinical recommendations can be made. Fortunately, research has focused on how to improve prognostic communication by emphasizing the importance of eliciting a patient's information preferences, goals, and values for end of life. As a result, many emerging interventions aimed at improving prognostic understanding are beginning to incorporate elements of patient-centered emotional and decisional support, including the incorporation of families and multidisciplinary providers into the conversation. Further research is needed to understand at which point in the disease course it is most useful to first initiate such discussions, how often they should occur, and how much information should be communicated at each discussion.

Clinicians and researchers in Western countries are increasingly aware of the complexity and individualized nature of prognostic health information preferences, prognostic understanding, and end-of-life decision-making. However, much less research has been conducted on these constructs among non-Western patient populations, including immigrants and those of ethnic, religious, or social minority groups. As a result, physicians risk making inaccurate assumptions about the information needs and preferences about prognosis for minority and non-Western patients, which could ultimately lead to the provision of goal-discordant care for those individuals. Therefore, continued research is needed into the intersection of culture, race, religion, and acculturation with information preferences and prognostic understanding.

Research has highlighted the delicate balance required between "maintaining hope" and providing realistic prognostic information to help foster patient's psychosocial well-being. Patients who know their prognosis yet struggle with accepting the severity of their illness may benefit from timely referrals to mental health services. Moreover, a treatment focusing on the development of active emotional coping skills may help facilitate better prognostic understanding that considers both its cognitive and emotional components. At the same time, it is equally important to train physicians to help patients identify and articulate life goals and values in the context of advanced disease to ensure the provision of goal-concordant care. Inevitably, there may be conflicts between what physicians believe is the best medical care and the wishes of the patient or their families, and guidelines for exactly how to navigate such challenges are still needed. The field of prognostic understanding in patients with advanced illness has grown considerably as knowledge of palliative care has expanded. However, as highlighted in this chapter, there remain significant difficulties in measuring prognostic understanding and transferring knowledge gathered from its assessment to high-quality research and clinical care.

Key Points

- Prognostic understanding is a complex, multifaceted construct that currently lacks a consensus definition and "gold standard" quantitative measure.
- Prognostic understanding is important for end-of-life medical decision-making and the provision of goal-concordant, patient-centered care.
- Patient preferences for prognostic information vary across cultures and individuals, thus requiring a personalized, individualized approach to eliciting prognostic information preferences.
- The research on the relationship between prognostic understanding and psychological well-being is mixed, and further research is needed to better understand when and for whom accurate prognostic understanding is useful.
- A variety of interventions have been developed to improve prognostic understanding, ranging from decision aids to palliative care consults and including the provision of information, emotional and decisional support, and assistance with practical end-of-life care matters.
- Existing interventions are insufficient, and additional interventions that allow for patients to process and absorb aversive prognostic information while alleviating psychological defenses are needed.

References

1. Applebaum AJ, Kolva EA, Kulikowski JR, Jacobs JD, DeRosa A, Lichtenthal WG, et al. Conceptualizing prognostic awareness in advanced cancer: A systematic review. *J Health Psychol.* 2014;19(9):1103–1119.
2. Masterson MP, Applebaum AJ, Buda K, Reisch S, Rosenfeld B. Don't shoot the messenger: Experiences of delivering prognostic information in the context of advanced cancer. *Am J Hosp Palliat Care.* 2018;35(12):1526–1531.
3. Broadbent E, Wilkes C, Koschwanez H, Weinman J, Norton S, Petrie KJ. A systematic review and meta-analysis of the Brief Illness Perception Questionnaire. *Psychol Health.* 2015;30(11):1361–1385.
4. Glare PA, Sinclair CT. Palliative medicine review: Prognostication. *J Palliat Med.* 2008;11(1):84–103.
5. Thompson GN, Chochinov HM, Wilson KG, McPherson CJ, Chary S, O'Shea FM, et al. Prognostic acceptance and the well-being of patients receiving palliative care for cancer. *J Clin Oncol.* 2009;27(34):5757–5762.
6. Selim S, Kunkel E, Wegier P, et al. A systematic review of interventions aiming to improve communication of prognosis to adult patients. *Patient Educ Counsel.* 2020;104(9):1850–1855.
7. Vlckova K, Tuckova A, Polakova K, Loucka M. Factors associated with prognostic awareness in patients with cancer: A systematic review. *Psycho-Oncology.* 2020;30(9):1449–1456.
8. Innes S, Payne S. Advanced cancer patients' prognostic information preferences: A review. *Palliative Medicine.* 2009;23(1):29–39.
9. Trice ED, Prigerson HG. Communication in end-stage cancer: Review of the literature and future research. *J Health Commun.* 2009;14 Suppl 1:95–108.

10. Nipp RD, Greer JA, El-Jawahri A, et al. Coping and prognostic awareness in patients with advanced cancer. *J Clin Oncol.* 2017;35(22):2551–2557.

11. Ellis EM, Varner A. Unpacking cancer patients' preferences for information about their care. *J Psychosoc Oncol.* 2018;36(1):1–18.

12. van der Velden NC, Meijers MC, Han PK, van Laarhoven HW, Smets EM, Henselmans I. The Effect of prognostic communication on patient outcomes in palliative cancer care: A systematic review. *Curr Treatm Opt Oncol.* 2020;21:1–38.

13. Brighton LJ, Bristowe K. Communication in palliative care: Talking about the end of life, before the end of life. *Postgrad Med J.* 2016;92(1090):466–470.

14. Rousseau P. Topics in review: Hope in the terminally ill. *West J Med.* 2000;173(2):117.

15. Weisman AD. *On dying and denying: A psychiatric study of terminality.* New York: Behavioral Publications; 1972.

16. Leighl NB, Shepherd HL, Butow PN, et al. Supporting treatment decision making in advanced cancer: A randomized trial of a decision aid for patients with advanced colorectal cancer considering chemotherapy. *J Clin Oncol.* 2011;29(15):2077–2084.

17. Temel JS, Greer JA, Admane S, et al. Longitudinal perceptions of prognosis and goals of therapy in patients with metastatic non-small-cell lung cancer: Results of a randomized study of early palliative care. *J Clin Oncol.* 2011;29(17):2319–2326.

18. Chen CH, Chen JS, Wen FH, et al. An individualized, interactive intervention promotes terminally ill cancer patients' prognostic awareness and reduces cardiopulmonary resuscitation received in the last month of life: Secondary analysis of a randomized clinical trial. *J Pain Symptom Manage.* 2019;57(4):705–714.e707.

19. Paladino J, Bernacki R, Neville BA, Kavanagh J, Miranda SP, Palmor M, et al. Evaluating an intervention to improve communication between oncology clinicians and patients with life-limiting cancer: A cluster randomized clinical trial of the serious illness care program. *JAMA Oncol.* 2019;5(6):801–809.

20. Shen MJ, Prigerson HG, Ratshikana-Moloko M, et al. Illness understanding and end-of-life care communication and preferences for patients with advanced cancer in South Africa. *J Glob Oncol.* 2018;4:1–9.

21. de Graaff FM, Francke AL, van den Muijsenbergh ME, van der Geest S. "Palliative care": A contradiction in terms? A qualitative study of cancer patients with a Turkish or Moroccan background, their relatives and care providers. *BMC Palliat Care.* 2010;9:19.

22. Hahne J, Liang T, Khoshnood K, Wang X, Li X. Breaking bad news about cancer in China: Concerns and conflicts faced by doctors deciding whether to inform patients. *Patient Educ Couns.* 2020 Feb;103(2):286–291.

PART IV

Ethical, Existential, and Spiritual Issues in Palliative Care

22

Ethical Issues in Palliative Care

Kari L. Esbensen and Daniel P. Sulmasy

It is as much the business of the physician to alleviate pain and smooth the
avenues of death, when inevitable, as it is to cure disease.
—John Gregory (1725–1773), *On the Duties and Qualifications*
of Physicians

The care of incurably ill persons has always presented moral challenges. For families,
friends, and society, these challenges reside in the burdens of ministering to the decline
of fellow human beings. For physicians and other caregivers, these challenges lie in the
apparent impotence of medicine in the face of inevitable death and in the need to shift the
focus of the medical art from seeking *cure* to providing *healing*—by providing care, comfort, consolation, and support to those confronting imminent mortality. In short, medical
professionals have a duty to continue seeking healing even when cure is no longer possible.
They often seek assistance in fulfilling this duty by engaging the expertise of interdisciplinary palliative care teams.

In truth, the ethical issues surrounding the practice of palliative care are no different
from those encountered in the care of *all* patients. Yet these issues find added poignancy
and urgency—and often elicit added moral distress or anxiety for healthcare providers—in
the care of terminally ill patients, who are particularly vulnerable and whose impending
confrontation with death weighs heavily on each decision that must be made.

First Principles: The Good of the Patient and the *Telos* of Medicine

Becoming a patient signals one's entrance into a new form of existence characterized by
dis-ease, need, and a special state of vulnerability. When, in addition to becoming a patient, a person is confronted with a terminal diagnosis, a new order of magnitude is added

to this vulnerability. The vulnerable patient who seeks healing must enter into an unequal relationship with the doctor or other caregiver and, therefore, must rely on that caregiver's expertise and moral character. The patient must trust that the doctor possesses the requisite knowledge and skills to recommend and carry out what will serve the patient's best interests. Likewise, the patient must rely on the implicit promise that, in agreeing to help, the doctor will make the good of the patient, rather than the doctor's own interests, the central and primary concern.

The patient's good has a four-fold, hierarchical character: (1) the biomedical good, (2) the good as it is understood by the patient in the particular circumstances, (3) the good of the patient as a human being, and (4) the patient's highest good, as understood by the patient.[1 (pp. 73–91)] All four dimensions must be served.

In providing healing by acting for the good of the patient, the doctor is obliged not only to address the biomedical, but also to respect the patient's dignity as a human being and respect the autonomy that is integral to the good of the patient. It is particularly important to respect a patient's conception of his or her own *highest* good, which may come into most distinct focus as a person faces imminent mortality and confronts the "ultimate" questions of meaning at the end of life. Many fear the process of dying—and the anticipated pain and suffering thought to be unavoidable aspects of dying—more than death itself. Terminally ill persons may experience significant symptoms, worry about burdening others, fear a loss of self-worth or value in the sight of others, question the meaning of their lives or relationships, or feel alienation from their own bodies, among other sources of suffering. To provide healing, caregivers must attend to the many dimensions of suffering experienced by patients and seek to serve their four-fold good, even as the biomedical good may be less and less attainable for terminally ill patients.

Healing, in its deepest sense, always entails the *restoration of right relationship and wholeness*.[2] This expansive notion of healing specifies the guiding aim, or *telos*, of medicine. It points to the reality that a patient's good lies beyond the biomedical good. A genuinely holistic approach to healing, therefore, is not exhausted when it is no longer possible to restore biological health. Illness also affects relationships between mind and body and between the patient, family, society, and whatever the patient regards as the source of transcendent value (e.g., the divine). If we understand healing in this broader sense of restoring wholeness and establishing a *new* balance, then healing may occur even when the patient is dying. Healing, here, means to recompose the person as a being-in-right-relationship even while that person must face death as an imminent, inevitable, and palpable reality.

This *telos* of providing healing determines what actions should be taken and which treatments should be provided (or ceased), as well as the duties incumbent on physicians, nurses, and other caregivers in caring for their patients. Healthcare professionals have a profound moral obligation to render healing care that attends to the multifaceted dimensions of a patient's good, particularly when we encounter patients in such existentially vulnerable states.

Historical Context and the Contemporary Social Milieu

The historical roots of the moral obligation of physicians to care for the terminally ill can be traced as far back as Hippocrates, but the duty to alleviate the suffering of dying patients gained prominence with the advent of Christian communities dedicated to the care of the sick, the poor, and the dying, which gave birth to the first hospitals.[3] A fusion of Hippocratic ethics and Judeo-Christian solicitude for the sick subsequently shaped the ethical codes adopted by Western medical societies, which espouse the dual obligations to cure and to care for the incurable.[4]

Ethical issues in palliative care must be contextualized in terms of the social milieu within which patients experience illness and dying. Unfortunately, much of modern medical practice and training appears to allow the goal of seeking cure to overshadow the equally important duty to provide healing care when cure is no longer possible. Added to this is the fact that, within modern Western societies, death is no longer seen as an inevitable, public, and social event, but rather as a private, hidden affair.[5] The modern patient frequently denies the inevitability of death and regards dying as a medical failure. Nonetheless, the patient may well fear the prospect of suffering and dying alone in a hospital rather than at home surrounded by loved ones. Moreover, modern society frequently ostracizes the seriously ill, regarding dying persons as unwelcome reminders of our shared mortality and the imperfection of medical science. The concerns, thoughts, and feelings of the dying are often left unspoken and unheard because we no longer have the experience and vocabulary to know how to approach the transition from life to death. Within this milieu, the dying person often faces death in relative isolation. In short, our contemporary Western culture often provides yet another source of suffering for those facing terminal illness. Medicine's frequent failure to provide healing when cure is no longer possible compounds the terminally ill patient's sense of vulnerability, abandonment, and diminished self-worth.

Intensive Comprehensive Palliative Care

Against this phenomenological, historical, and sociological backdrop, we advocate for what we call *intensive comprehensive palliative care* (ICPC). To *palliate* means to ease or lessen the *burden* of a disease while often recognizing medicine's inability to change the natural course of illness; to palliate is to follow the Hippocratic injunction to "lessen the violence" of disease and to "do away with suffering."[6] This requires much more than relief of pain or other symptoms, although this is an important first step in many cases.

The care provided must be tailored to the multifaceted good of the individual patient, taking into account the highly personal and unique response of *this* patient to the predicament of *this* sickness. The care must be *comprehensive,* encompassing not only physical, but also psycho-social-spiritual, needs. ICPC is also *intensive*; it brings to bear all the capacities of available medical care to achieve palliation. Palliative care to alleviate suffering must be pursued just as energetically, purposefully, and forcefully as care in the intensive care unit to extend life. The goal of ICPC is still to restore or protect the multidimensional good of the patient *as vigorously as possible*. The difference is that the primary goal of *cure* is replaced or augmented by the goals of providing *healing*, easing suffering, and (often) preparing for death. When successful, ICPC provides *healing*—by serving the holistic good of the patient—*even while the patient is dying*.

Ethical Issues in Intensive Comprehensive Palliative Care

Addressing Pain, Other Symptoms, and Suffering

The first moral obligation of any palliative care physician is to be competent in providing optimal relief of pain and other symptoms. This is so obvious as hardly to need mention, were it not for the fact that many physicians still do not treat pain appropriately. Measures for pain relief are available today such that no patient need die in pain. Not to use pain medication well is a moral failure that is inexcusable and may be considered a violation of a patient's rights.[7]

Patients should participate in decisions about pain medications, including optimal tradeoffs between sedation and pain relief. Some patients accept any degree of sedation required to attain relative comfort whereas others prioritize unimpaired alertness and choose to tolerate greater pain in order to optimize cognition, to maintain interaction with family and friends, or to preserve decision-making ability. Such informed tradeoffs serve the best interests of the patient, as determined by his or her own conception of the good. Freedom from pain—like any other medical aim—is not an absolute good apart from the patient's goals of care and personal values.

Medications should be used in doses sufficient to control pain, as aligned with the patient's goals. Opioids should not be withheld or used sparingly for fear of making the patient an addict, particularly when death is imminent. Nor is fear of respiratory depression a good moral argument against adequate analgesia. According to the moral principle of *double effect*, so long as (1) the intention is not to hasten death but to relieve pain, (2) no other less risky measure is available to relieve pain, (3) the patient's relief of pain is not dependent on the death of the patient, and (4) there is a proportionate reason for running the risk, then increasing doses of opioids can be provided until adequate pain relief is achieved, even if hastening death might be a foreseen, though unintended, consequence.[8] In reality, the risk of respiratory suppression and hastening death in patients being treated appropriately with opioids for pain or dyspnea is often exaggerated.[9] Patients treated chronically with opioids—or patients for whom opioid doses are appropriately titrated—develop rapid tolerance to their sedating and respiratory depressant effects. In many cases, opioids actually extend life by decreasing stress-related physiological demands while providing comfort.[9] Our focus, from the perspective of ethics, is the moral reasoning (the principle of double effect) that justifies providing pain-relief *even if* the unintended outcome were to be hastened death. Such justification, however, is rarely required. In short, it is a moral failing that many patients are deprived of appropriate pain relief as they approach the end of life on the basis of unfounded clinical fears and faulty ethical reasoning.

Pain management is necessary, but not sufficient, for ICPC. Dying patients experience a myriad of symptoms for which effective treatments are available, and it is both a medical and moral mistake to neglect to treat other symptoms such as nausea, constipation, dyspnea, or fatigue. Likewise, psychiatric syndromes such as anxiety, depression, insomnia, and delirium should not be regarded as "normal" aspects of the dying process; they, like all treatable symptoms, are appropriate targets for ICPC.

However, even vigorous *symptom* relief is not morally sufficient for truly ICPC. Care of the whole person, or *healing,* also entails an obligation to relieve *suffering,* a much more complex phenomenon. Neurocognitive phenomena such as pain, dyspnea, anxiety, delirium, or depression can certainly occasion suffering and should be treated.[10] Yet the scope of suffering is much wider than the biological and also consists of "agent-narrative" forms of suffering. *Agent-narrative* suffering occurs when a person's sense of self, agency, narrative history, or relationships with others are perceived to be damaged or threatened. Such suffering may become particularly profound as a person faces the end of life.[8] Agent-narrative suffering includes phenomena such as loneliness, guilt, despair, fear, and a host of other experiences often referred to as "spiritual" or "existential." In agent-narrative suffering, it is not the medical condition as such that occasions distress, but patients' *beliefs* about how illness affects their *personhood,* especially their ability to see themselves as agents living coherent life stories characterized by continued meaning, value, and affirming relationships. Such suffering occurs when patients see their personhood damaged by their own or others' beliefs about the *meaning* of their illness and impending mortality. Agent-narrative suffering also requires healing. Family, friendship, religion, philosophy, the arts, natural beauty, and even the patient–clinician relationship can provide solace for agent-narrative forms of suffering.[8] Multidisciplinary ICPC teams ought to help assure such care.

Distinguishing between neurocognitive and agent-narrative aspects of suffering is important because one has a moral obligation to employ means of treatment that are appropriate to the source of suffering. Just as one ought not treat the pain of bony metastases with psychotherapy, so one ought not treat despair and loneliness with high doses of morphine or sedative medications.[10] Concern, love, listening, family meetings, and referrals to psychiatry, pastoral care, or social workers are examples of the appropriate responses to agent-narrative suffering.

Spiritual and Existential Care

Whether a patient embraces a specific religious faith, a more personal spirituality, or rejects any such beliefs, dying inevitably raises questions that may aptly be described as spiritual: questions of meaning, questions of value, and questions of relationship.[11] These questions, if pursued seriously, all have a transcendent form, regardless of whether the patient believes that they can be answered in spiritual terms. They reflect the patient's understanding of his or her *highest* good, which may include profound elements including hope, dignity, and reconciliation.

Hope, on which so much of the human capacity to face the future depends, may be threatened in the face of death. Dying persons may ask: Did my life have meaning and does it still? Is there any meaning in my suffering and dying? Will anything of myself persist beyond the grave? Palliative care providers frequently focus on providing comfort by trying to "reframe hope" in dying patients—redirecting hope toward important, still-attainable goals, such as attending family events, living the last days as well as possible, mending or strengthening relationships, preserving legacy, and achieving personal growth. However, *ultimate* hope can only be found in a source of meaning that transcends death.[12] Thus, in pursuing the laudable goal of preserving hope, one should use caution against the danger of subverting or failing to support the transcendent, guiding, and sustaining hope that many patients have for an enduring existence that transcends death and which gives their continued living, their dying, and their relationships both profound meaning and enduring value, even in the midst of suffering and dying.

Dignity, in its intrinsic sense, means the value that a person has simply by virtue of being a human being.[13] In the end, this is often the only sense of self-worth to which the dying might cling, as everything else is eventually stripped away. Dying may raise doubts about a person's ultimate value, since what society "counts" as valuable—independence, appearance, productivity, cognition, and the ability to communicate—is typically diminished or lost in the dying process. An important spiritual task for the dying is to recover, rediscover, or affirm their own continued intrinsic worth as their capacities decline, even in the throes of death. The ethical task of healthcare professionals is to respect and reaffirm that intrinsic worth, most importantly when patients struggle to see (or deny) the continued value of their own lives.

Reconciliation is another important aspect of the highest good frequently sought by dying persons. Brokenness in body has a tendency to remind persons of brokenness in their relationships. Dying patients often struggle to forgive those who have hurt them or to ask for forgiveness from others. Reconciliation provides healing by restoring the wholeness of the patient-in-relationship-with-others. Healthcare providers can help to facilitate reconciliation by being sensitive to this need and by providing honest communication around prognoses.

Although addressing spiritual and existential aspects of suffering is an important component of ICPC, it raises additional ethical issues. For example, some patients might reject attempts to delve into their psychological, personal, family, or sexual lives or their spiritual beliefs and concerns. Acceptance of palliative care into one's medical care does not imply acceptance of every facet of its multidisciplinary approach. Respect for patient autonomy requires respecting patient privacy and honoring patient refusal of services regarded as intrusive or unwanted.

For many patients, however, the spiritual dimension may be the most important way to find meaning in suffering and death. Therefore, regardless of a healthcare provider's own views on religion, there is an obligation to offer patients opportunities to receive help in confronting spiritual issues. Psychiatrists and palliative care physicians are not, by virtue of their training, experts in spiritual counseling and should refer to the patient's own clergy or to pastoral care experts if significant spiritual or religious issues are uncovered. Most interdisciplinary palliative care and hospice teams include (or are affiliated with) specially trained spiritual health providers who can assist in addressing these sources of suffering or in supporting a patient who relies on spirituality for maintaining hope and meaning in the face of illness and impending death.

Truth-Telling and Bad News

Patients are unable to prepare for, or participate authentically in, their own care and their dying unless they know the truth. There is an ethical obligation to discuss dying with patients, and patients have a right to know about their expected prognoses. Clinicians, unlike patients and families, may have more insight into what to expect as death draws near and should, therefore, help patients and families prepare for this unfamiliar and likely feared event. Unless patients know that they are dying, they lose important opportunities for trying to make sense of their lives, their suffering, and their dying. They lose the ability to set realistic priorities for the time that remains, and they may lose opportunities for doing and saying the things that matter most. Furthermore, feelings of isolation, helplessness, and despair can be most profound when patients feel that they are dying but no one is willing to talk honestly with them about their experiences. With some exceptions, therefore, truth-telling is an essential component of providing good ICPC.

The ethical challenges surrounding truth-telling arise largely from uncertainty regarding how the truth should be communicated, cultural differences that may influence preferences about how (and to whom) information is delivered, and clinicians' fear of inflicting further harm.

Communication, particularly the delivery of "bad news" is a highly personal interaction, and each discussion is a unique event. However, there are some common elements of effective communication that serve to express care, encourage deeper understanding, strengthen the caregiver-patient relationship, and provide healing (rather than cause harm, as is often feared). *Listening* is the most fundamental aspect of effective communication. Listening enables one to discover what patients already understand about their illness and prognosis, their preferences and values, hopes and fears, what helps them cope, their most important goals, and how one can tailor care to best serve their individual conceptions of the good. Although patient preferences should guide how much, with what specificity, and to whom information is conveyed, such information-sharing about prognosis should invariably use unambiguous language (including words such as death) and be clear (avoiding medical jargon) while maintaining prognostic humility. One must allow time for patients and families to process the information given and their corresponding emotions. It is important to let patients guide further discussion and express what they understand, what they want to know, what they fear, and what they need. This opportunity to achieve a *shared understanding* of the patient's experience allows the patient to play an active role in his or her own care, builds trust, and opens the door to further discussion. Finally, when conveying "bad news," it is important to emphasize that one's care, concern, and efforts to ensure the patient's comfort and healing will continue even as death approaches.

For many patients, including loved ones in these difficult conversations provides important support, yet most patients would not want information conveyed to family without their own presence. In some cultures, however, it is customary not to disclose a poor prognosis to the patient on the grounds that this might destroy hope and increase suffering.[14] Clinicians ought to respect patients' cultural values, but it is important to confirm how the patient prefers to have the truth disclosed and to whom. The clinician may, for instance, ask the patient, "Would you prefer to hear everything from me directly, or would you prefer that I talk first with your family and allow them to guide what information is shared with you?" Provided that such a choice is genuine and made freely, it ought to be respected.

To harm a patient by conveying "bad news" in an abrupt, rushed, harsh, or unkind manner is as much a breach of the caregiver's moral obligations as it would be to perform a procedure without allowing sufficient time, without taking appropriate care and concern to avoid error, or while lacking the required expertise or training. Nonetheless, despite the harms that may accompany *poor* communication, there are very few instances in which patients are genuinely harmed by knowing the truth itself, even when that truth involves the fact that the patient is dying. Delivering the truth with skill and compassion is a fundamental moral obligation of all healthcare providers.

Informed Consent and Decision-Making Capacity

While this is not the place to review in detail the requirements for an ethically valid informed consent, in broad strokes, a valid consent must be (1) informed, (2) understood, (3) free of coercion, and (4) made by a patient with intact decision-making capacity. Here, we wish to underscore some ethical issues in informed consent peculiar to the care of patients who are in the existential state of being terminally ill and, therefore, particularly vulnerable.

Patients' decision-making capacity may be adversely affected by disease itself, by disease-specific treatments and their side effects, or by treatments used to palliate symptoms. Decision-making capacity should be clearly distinguished from competency. *Competency* refers to a *legal* determination that a person is wholly incapable of managing his or her own affairs and needs someone appointed to make decisions—financial, medical, and personal—on his or her behalf. *Decision-making capacity* is a *clinical* judgment that the patient has sufficient cognitive capacity to exercise appropriate judgment about a *particular* decision (or set of decisions) about his or her medical care. Although the responsibility for determining a patient's decision-making capacity lies with the attending physician, psychiatrists are often consulted when this capacity is uncertain or contested. Decision-making capacity requires that one can (1) understand the nature, risks, benefits, and alternatives to a proposed treatment (or non-treatment), (2) make a decision, (3) express that decision, (4) explain the reasons for that decision (whether the physician agrees with those reasons or not), and (5) consistently maintain that decision (e.g., not vacillate, as in delirium). Capacity may vary over time as one's condition changes and is also a variable-threshold concept, determined relative to the gravity of the decision at hand. For instance, a patient may not have sufficient decision-making capacity to make an informed decision regarding whether to undergo a high-risk procedure or initiate a high-burden treatment but may still maintain adequate decision-making capacity to appoint a durable power of attorney for healthcare (DPAHC) to make treatment decisions on his or her behalf or refuse certain non-critical interventions. Importantly, decision-making capacity should be ascertained apart from the content of the patient's decision itself. For example, it is not morally appropriate to contest a patient's decision-making capacity simply because he or she chooses against a therapeutic course that the physician deems to be in the patient's best interest. As noted earlier, the good of the patient is multidimensional, entails respect for patient autonomy, and encompasses far more than the biomedical good that may be the narrow focus of the physician when proposing various treatments. Likewise, it is morally objectionable to overlook potential deficits in a patient's decision-making capacity simply because he or she agrees to accept recommended treatments.

It is important to note that, even if the patient has been determined to lack capacity, what the patient says and does should not be completely discounted in making treatment decisions. A patient may be too demented or delirious to be capable of deciding to forgo a feeding tube, but if the patient yells and pulls out a tube that the family thinks ought to be used, the patient's active refusal and distress should factor into one's deliberations about whether to replace it. Likewise, if a patient with limited decision-making capacity refuses non-critical labs or medications, this may be reason enough to seriously reconsider (ideally, in partnership with the patient's surrogate decision-maker) which nonessential tests or treatments might be eliminated to better align care with the patient's own perception of the good, as balanced against his or her biomedical good.

Again, decision-making capacity is not a global or static determination but rather relative to the complexity of the decision at hand and may vary depending on the patient's current clinical condition. The obligation to respect patient autonomy entails preserving the patient's agency to make those decisions for which he or she remains capable, and it requires frequent reassessing of patient capacity throughout the clinical course.

Aside from cognitive dysfunction that may limit decision-making capacity in terminally ill patients, these patients may face other threats to their ability to make decisions in line with their authentic values and preferences. For example, valid informed consent might be compromised in patients who grasp at unrealistic hope for cure or engage in denial even when treatment is described as solely palliative rather than curative in nature. Providers must be highly attuned to this danger, avoid medical jargon, not offer false hope, and revisit goals of care at regular intervals to ensure that ongoing treatment remains consistent with the patient's beliefs, values, and preferences, which will likely continue to evolve over time. Similarly, patients who are particularly vulnerable or desperate may be highly influenced by the suggestions of those around them, including well-meaning family and caregivers, and they may be unduly inclined to pursue alternative or experimental therapies. Such patients are often eager to become research subjects, in hopes that an untried treatment might alter the fatal thrust of their illness. Patients with full decision-making capacity can legitimately participate as research subjects if they give informed consent, if the therapy is not expected to cause them significant harm, and if it is potentially of value for the patient or for others similarly afflicted.[15] However, given that terminally ill patients may be more readily swayed than others, clinicians must be particularly careful not to suggest more benefit than can realistically be expected from an experimental therapy nor to encourage participation in research to further their own agendas. Patients should understand that the primary purpose of research is to help *others* and not be encouraged to believe that the primary purpose it to provide benefit to the patient (the so-called *therapeutic misconception*).[16]

Advance Care Planning and Surrogate Decision-Makers

Since many terminally ill patients will eventually lack decision-making capacity, especially in the late stages of illness, it is important to respect patient autonomy by encouraging patients to engage in advance care planning early in their illness and to revisit their wishes—preferably in conjunction with their appointed surrogate decision-maker(s)—as their illness progresses. Later, when the patient no longer has decision-making capacity, abiding by preferences the patient expressed when he or she *did* have capacity is one way to honor the patient's authentic values.

There are various means of legally documenting a patient's wishes regarding end-of-life care, some of which have been introduced only in recent years and all of which vary from state to state. They all serve two basic functions. (1) They may specify which treatments a patient would prefer to be used or withheld in the event of decisional incapacity and terminal decline. (2) They may appoint a DPAHC—the surrogate decision-maker chosen to make *healthcare* decisions for the patient when he or she no longer has decision-making capacity. Advance planning documents that serve only the first function were historically called *living wills*, but specifications regarding treatment decisions are now often incorporated into documents that serve *both* functions (often called *advance directives*) or into documents such as *physician orders for life-sustaining therapy* (POLST), which attempt to make such treatment decisions more enforceable by giving them the force of explicit physician orders.

All documents outlining a patient's future treatment decisions have several disadvantages. Such documents are relatively inflexible but yet vague, cannot anticipate all potential clinical scenarios, and require contextual interpretation in light of nuances of a patient's clinical condition. Typically, they provide merely a rough guide that may be difficult to interpret and apply in a given context, and they fail to provide the certainty one seeks that one is honoring a patient's wishes. Furthermore, there is evidence that most patients prefer a model of *shared* decision-making, which would include their physicians' advice and the judgment of loved ones, as well as their own expressed values and preferences—rather than a strict reliance on the treatment preferences outlined in an advance directive—to guide decisions about their future care.[17]

In light of these concerns, we suggest emphasizing the importance of surrogates, ideally those appointed as DPAHCs. We believe that identifying a surrogate decision-maker—and encouraging honest and robust conversations between the patient and surrogate(s) about what the patient would want under various circumstances—is by far the most important step in advance care planning, and clinicians should focus their efforts on facilitating this as much as possible. DPAHCs have the advantage of allowing for flexibility and context sensitivity. The person whom the patient entrusted to uphold his or her values and preferences can be told the specifics of the patient's condition and play an instrumental role in shared decision-making. The surrogate can, ideally, provide insight into what the patient has always valued, how the patient has lived and confronted challenges, what beliefs and commitments have defined the patient as a person, what the patient most hoped and feared, and what has given the patient's life meaning. With these insights into the patient's authentic values and real interests, the clinician can help guide care in a way that fosters the patient's good, as understood beyond simply the biomedical good, and help surrogates to make the best choices.[18] Unfortunately, many patients have no advance directives or appointed DPAHCs, so decision-making falls to the next-of-kin as specified by a legal hierarchy. Some patients have no one who can speak for them, so decisions regarding their care require the additional oversight of an ethics committee or other institutional mechanism.

A surrogate's authority is not absolute. In all cases, the physician remains morally bound to protect the good of the patient and may challenge a surrogate's decisions if they appear to be in conflict with the patient's well-being or known values and preferences. The physician has an obligation, within reasonable limits, to ascertain the moral validity of a surrogate by judging whether the surrogate actually knows the patient, has a significant conflict of interest, or is failing to represent either the patient's wishes or best interests.[1] (pp. 164–167) Ethics consultants can often play a significant role in ameliorating these sorts of conflicts.

Patients maintain the prerogative to change their treatment preferences at any time, even in opposition to their own prior advance directives. In such cases, it is best to revisit and update the legal documents, if possible, and include surrogates in these discussions. Nonetheless, the patient's most current wishes ought to be respected, even if only expressed verbally, so long as it can be established that the patient has decision-making capacity to revise his or her prior choices.

Palliative care providers, psychiatrists, ethicists, and other caregivers should be alert to the strain and stress experienced by surrogate decision-makers. Clinicians should be prepared to offer emotional and spiritual support as well as to correct misconceptions, including reaffirming that the *illness*—rather than decisions made by surrogates or the patient's caregivers—is the cause of the patient's dying. It is important to acknowledge and assist loved ones with their feelings of anxiety, guilt, and grief surrounding decision-making.

Withholding and Withdrawing Life-Sustaining Treatments

A systematic ethical framework should be used when analyzing the appropriateness of any therapy, examining whether the proposed treatment is *medically effective, beneficial for the patient*, and *not excessively burdensome*.[19] *Medically effective* treatments are those that slow, stop, or reverse the natural progression of an illness or alleviate an important symptom. If it is determined that a treatment is medically effective, the next question is whether it is also *beneficial for the patient* in that it promotes the complete four-fold good of the patient (beyond simply the biomedical good). Finally, one must determine that the proposed treatment is *not excessively burdensome* (i.e., that its burdens, broadly construed to include physical, financial, emotional, interpersonal, and spiritual, do not outweigh its benefits, also broadly construed). A therapy is *inappropriate* when it fails to meet any of these conditions, and it should be withheld or withdrawn once this shared judgment is reached between the healthcare team and the patient (or surrogate). This framework is particularly morally salient when considering the withholding or withdrawing of life-sustaining treatments (LSTs).

Well-established moral, medical, and legal norms hold that there is no ethical or legal distinction between withdrawing and withholding LSTs. However, it is common for decisions about withdrawing LST to create significant anxiety, stress, guilt, and moral distress for healthcare providers, surrogates, and families when confronting decisions about the discontinuation of LST for incapacitated patients. One significant source of moral distress is the oft-reported "felt moral difference" between *withdrawing* LST (discontinuing ongoing therapies) and *withholding* LST (choosing to forgo therapies before they are initiated). However, *heightened* concerns about *withdrawing* LST (vs. less concern about *withholding* non-beneficial or excessively burdensome treatment) appear to rely on unexamined moral intuitions about moral agency and responsibility that cannot withstand closer scrutiny. These common moral intuitions tend to view acts of *commission* (withdrawing ongoing therapy) as bearing greater moral weight and potential culpability than acts of *omission* (not initiating therapy). However, ethical analysis reveals that it is just as morally egregious to fail to perform an action that is morally obligatory (omission) as it to perform an action contrary to our moral obligations (commission). Thus, the "felt moral difference" between withdrawing and withholding treatment is illusory and should not be accepted as a reliable guide to ethical conduct.[20] Healthcare providers should be held morally accountable if they allow treatment that no longer has benefit for the patient, or is excessively burdensome, to continue (i.e., a *failure* to withdraw inappropriate LST), just as they should be held accountable if they choose to employ a treatment that does not serve the patient's good or creates excessive burdens. It is, therefore, morally incumbent on caregivers to re-examine ongoing LST at regular intervals to combat the dual threats of "clinical inertia" and these unreliable moral intuitions which can lead to clinician reluctance to *withdraw* LST once started, thus prolonging therapies long after they cease to serve the good of the patient.

Caregivers have deep moral commitments to protect their vulnerable patients from further harm. Acknowledging and *redirecting* these moral motivations toward a more critical examination of ongoing treatments—and an appropriate desire to protect patients from the harms entailed by therapies once they become excessively burdensome—may be the crucial element in resolving conflicts surrounding the withholding and withdrawing of LST.[20] This is particularly important when clinicians struggle to recognize that *refraining* from further LST might actually best serve the holistic good of the patient and, therefore, best promote healing.

Despite these concerns, a desire to minimize excessively burdensome therapies should not overshadow the importance of allowing for "time-limited trials" of LST when such therapy might serve the multidimensional good of the patient. Even when facing end-stage terminal illness, patients (or surrogates) might request a trial of LST in order to allow for attempts at restoring function, treating reversible acute illness or complications of the terminal illness, clarifying prognosis, or achieving other important goals, such as surviving long enough for family to gather or to complete tasks deemed important to fulfilling the patient's notion of what a "good death" might require.[20] The best approach is to engage in ongoing conversations with the patient (while the patient has decision-making capacity) and surrogate regarding goals of care to avoid initiating treatments that *should* be withheld—because they do not promote the patient's goals—and to avoid prolonging therapies once they no longer serve the patient's good.

Artificial Nutrition and Hydration

The same moral considerations discussed in relation to withholding or withdrawing LST in general apply to deliberations about artificial nutrition and hydration (ANH). Yet it is common for even experienced healthcare providers to experience heightened moral distress in relation to withholding or withdrawing ANH than with other forms of LST, even when patients' wishes to forgo ANH are clear, due to an additional overlay of moral concerns regarding the cessation of ANH.[20] Such concerns arise partially from an appropriate ethic of care, which views caregivers as advocates and protectors of their vulnerable patients. In addition, there is a frequent misperception that providing ANH is an "ordinary" form of care and, therefore, does not require the same level of justification as the provision of "extraordinary" means of LST that could only be offered in an ICU. Moreover, the act of feeding often carries with it deep symbolism as an act of care and compassion, even when the feeding is carried out through medical means. However, the crucial moral distinction— as with *all* forms of LST—is whether the treatment satisfies the conditions of being medially effective, beneficial, and not excessively burdensome. Any treatment, including ANH, that fails to meet these criteria no longer provides healing, comfort, or care. Caregivers' moral obligations of care and advocacy then must turn to other means of providing healing, including through ICPC.

Despite evidence that ANH generally provides little, if any, benefit at the end of life and may pose significant burdens,[21] a time-limited trial of ANH may sometimes be useful and ethically justified—when in keeping with the patient's preferences or the surrogate's view of what best serves the good of the patient—to ensure that all reversible conditions have been addressed, clarify any prognostic uncertainty, and assuage any lingering doubts on the part of the patient or family that ANH might change the course of illness. However, ANH should be discontinued if it becomes excessively burdensome or no longer serves the good of the patient.[20]

Responding to Requests for Futile and Potentially Inappropriate Treatments

When it can be determined that a treatment will not achieve the biomedical goals of therapy, that treatment can be deemed "futile" and should be withheld or withdrawn.[22] There is no moral obligation to provide an intervention that cannot meet its biomedical goals; in fact, we are morally obligated to *refrain* from causing harm or imposing unnecessary burdens by discontinuing or withholding futile therapies. A treatment should be deemed *biomedically futile* (even though it may produce some *physiological effect*) if it can be ascertained, to a reasonable degree of medical certainty, that it will be continuously or repeatedly required and yet still be ineffective in preventing the patient from dying in a very short time despite the intervention. Only in these narrow circumstances can an intervention be unilaterally withheld on the grounds that it is futile. Importantly, decisions about futility should be judgments solely about the effectiveness of treatment in achieving its biomedical goals, *not* judgments about whether the patient's quality of life is such that it is "worth prolonging." [23]

Requests for treatments that are futile are uncommon. Clinicians more often face requests for treatments that are *potentially inappropriate*, a term that has gained favor, in part, due to an influential policy statement (the "ATS Statement," for short).[24] It suggests that the term "potentially inappropriate" be used "to describe treatments that have at least some chance of accomplishing the effect sought by the patient, but clinicians believe that competing ethical considerations justify not providing them."[24 (p. 1318)] While valuable, the ATS statement centers more on offering a process for addressing intractable disagreements rather than providing insight about *how* to determine whether a treatment should be judged inappropriate within a particular patient-specific context; it appears to defer to clinician discretion to make such judgments on an unclear basis and leaves important questions unaddressed, like which "competing ethical considerations" ought to count.

We caution against allowing considerations such as resource allocation to play a role in these decisions concerning the care of particular patients, sometimes referred to as "bedside rationing," except in very extreme cases of resource scarcity. For reasons beyond the scope of this discussion, even in such exceptional circumstances, it is best for limits on the provision of LST to be determined by social and political policy processes appropriately informed by medical and bioethical expertise.

We also caution against allowing clinician judgments about patient quality of life to play a role in decisions about whether a treatment is appropriate. To guard against problematic value judgments about disability or dependency, it is always important to discuss the goals of care with the patient (or surrogate), including short-term goals, even when a treatment is judged to offer minimal *biomedical* benefit. As noted earlier, so long as a treatment is anticipated to have some biomedical benefit, time-limited trials of the therapy may be warranted. Finally, we again emphasize that *palliative treatment* to relieve pain and suffering is *always appropriate* and should never be withheld, even in situations where appropriate symptom management may hasten patient death (as discussed earlier).

The most common treatment to be withheld due to the above considerations is cardiopulmonary resuscitation (CPR). CPR should not be offered to patients who are clearly dying and for whom CPR would be biomedically futile. However, a patient's decision whether to forgo attempts at resuscitation should be regarded as merely a small component of much broader discussions with dying patients and/or surrogates regarding a plan for end-of-life care. There is a moral obligation to respect any limits on treatment on which the physician and patient (or surrogate) agree, and there remains a duty to comprehensively attend to all the domains of the patient's palliative care needs regardless of decisions made about LSTs. Finally, there is a moral imperative to ensure that a patient's choice to enact a do-not-resuscitate (DNR) request is not misconstrued to preclude other forms of care that the patient still desires, such as antibiotics, blood transfusions, parenteral fluids, or other treatments that should be negotiated individually based on considerations of whether the treatment is medically effective, beneficial for the patient, and not excessively burdensome.

Euthanasia and Physician-Assisted Suicide

As of 2021, both euthanasia and physician-assisted suicide (PAS) are legal in the Netherlands, Belgium, Canada, and Luxembourg, and PAS is legal in Switzerland, Germany, Finland, and eight states and the District of Columbia in the United States.[25,26] While a robust discussion of PAS and/or euthanasia (PAS/E) is beyond the scope of this chapter, we believe that these practices subvert the very *telos* of medicine—to cure, when possible, and *to provide healing always*, even when death becomes inevitable. As we have argued, this moral obligation to provide *healing* to patients in need can still be profoundly effective and is perhaps most urgently required for vulnerable, dying patients. Such care should be continued, right up until the time of death. We fear that the acceptance of PAS/E will lead to even greater vulnerability for patients who are already particularly vulnerable and in need of healing due to the existential circumstance of being terminally ill. Moreover, fear of the "slippery slope" is well-founded, already having been demonstrated in places where euthanasia has progressed from a practice reserved for those who have decision-making capacity to one that can be performed on the decisionally incapacitated,[27] from a practice for adults to one that includes children,[28] and from one permitted only for the terminally ill to one that has been performed for chronic psychiatric disorders, "loneliness," and being "tired of living."[29] Given fears about the expansive nature of PAS/E, there is strong opposition among disability groups,[30] who argue that these practices threaten to perpetuate biases against those living with disabilities and reinforce judgments that some lives "are not worth living," with the risk of subtly influencing those persons who are already suffering to feel that they *should* end their lives to avoid being a burden on others.[31] For these reasons and others not discussed here, although we acknowledge that PAS and euthanasia remain deeply morally controversial, we concur in the *opposition* to the legalization of these practices voiced by multiple US professional organizations,[29,32] the World Medical Association,[33] and the International Association for Hospice and Palliative Care.[34]

We believe that increased availability and improved implementation of ICPC and hospice and freeing patients from excessive therapy are the appropriate ethical responses to the perceived need for PAS/E. These steps may not eliminate *all* requests for PAS/E, but should go a long way toward decreasing them.

The moral philosophy of intention is a neglected subject in ethics, yet intention is an essential element in evaluating the moral status of any human act.[35] It is important to carefully distinguish between withdrawing disproportionately burdensome LST and *intentionally* hastening death through PAS/E.[36] As noted by the International Association for Hospice and Palliative Care, withholding or withdrawing futile or inappropriate LST "does not constitute euthanasia or PAS because it is not intended to hasten death, but rather indicate[s] the acceptance of death as a natural consequence of the underlying disease progression."[34] [(p. 11)] It is crucial to preserve a similar distinction when justifying palliative treatments, which may *unintentionally* hasten death as an unintended (though possibly foreseen) side effect of therapies intended *only* to provide comfort, as is justified under the rule of double effect discussed earlier. Intentionality is not only "internal" to the moral agent, but can often also be inferred from the means employed. For example, the intention manifest in the careful, gradual titration of medications only as required to achieve symptom control without further escalation (consistent with the rule of double of effect and good medical practice) is markedly different from the intention exhibited by administering likely lethal doses or the further escalation of doses beyond those required to achieve comfort.

Psychiatrists may sometimes be asked to certify the decision-making capacity of patients who are requesting assistance in legal PAS/E. A psychiatrist who is morally opposed should not be compelled to certify that the patient has the capacity to request PAS/E, which would make such psychiatrists morally complicit in what they judge to be immoral. Governments, professional societies, and healthcare institutions should all protect the rights of physicians and other healthcare providers not to cooperate in PAS/E, even though protecting conscientious objection does not truly address fundamental ethical objections to these practices.[29]

Regardless of their moral beliefs about PAS/E, if the patient is known to lack capacity, a psychiatrist or other healthcare provider should intervene to try to stop the PAS/E to the best of his or her ability. Clinicians have a moral duty to try to uncover and address all sources of distress and suffering that might cause patients to request to end their own lives. Terminally ill patients requesting PAS/E, whether due to fears of losing their autonomy, social isolation, becoming a burden, or losing their sense of dignity and self-worth,[37] are as equally deserving of suicide prevention strategies, treatment, and support as any other patients. Yet, in Oregon, for example, out of 188 (reported) patients who died from ingesting a lethal dose of medication under the Death with Dignity Act (DWDA) in 2019, only *one* was referred for psychiatric evaluation.[37] To neglect obligations to provide appropriate psychiatric care simply because of patients' terminal illnesses is not only discriminatory toward these patients but is even more morally problematic given their increased vulnerability and need.

The means necessary to provide enough support for dying patients may well extend beyond the realm of healthcare, palliative care, or hospice, but if increased societal engagement or novel models of support for those who suffer are required to eliminate hopelessness and despair, then our moral obligations to the terminally ill require us to work diligently toward such solutions rather than to take the easier path of succumbing to pleas for assistance in dying.

Palliative Sedation and Terminal Sedation

Given ambiguous and inconsistent usage of the term "palliative sedation," we begin by defining it as *intentionally* bringing about *sedation* (or *unconsciousness*) as *the goal of therapy*, with the aim of thereby relieving intractable suffering. This is both medically and morally distinct from what might be called "*double effect sedation*," where sedation may arise as a *foreseeable* but *unintended side effect* of therapies aimed solely at the palliation of symptoms.[8] We will argue that palliative sedation, as opposed to double effect sedation, is morally and medically unsound.

From the moral standpoint, consciousness is recognized as an objective, though not absolute, human good that serves as a necessary condition for many central elements of the patient's good, including a person's capacities for reason, choice, imagination, communication, love, and aesthetic appreciation of the world around them, among others. Consciousness remains a good even for dying patients. Thus, even though sedation may be morally justified, such as in double-effect sedation, the loss or diminishment of consciousness should *always* be regarded as bad—a true human "cost" that should be avoided or minimized, whenever possible.[8]

According to the rule of double effect, it is morally permissible to escalate doses of opioids or other drugs required to alleviate symptoms—even to the point of causing sedation, unconsciousness, or, perhaps, hastening death—provided that this is done in accordance with the intention solely to relieve symptoms rather than to cause sedation or death, which one would avoid, if possible. Thus, if the symptom in question were to be adequately relieved by a particular dose of the drug, but the patient were not yet sedated, one would not increase the dose further to bring about sedation. Properly understood, the aim of therapy is symptom relief, and the level of sedation tolerated should only be what the patient (or surrogate) has agreed to as an acceptable tradeoff—in terms of diminished consciousness— as a side effect of the treatment(s) required to provide comfort. The therapeutic agents employed to achieve such symptom relief do not themselves distinguish double-effect sedation from palliative sedation. Anxiolytics such as benzodiazepines can be used to treat symptoms such as nausea, anxiety, dyspnea, panic, myoclonus, and seizures as well as be used specifically for their sedative properties, as when used for palliative sedation. When used in accordance with the principle of double effect, these drugs are used with the intention of alleviating symptoms while producing the *least sedation possible* as an unavoidable side effect of therapy. This intention demarcates the clear distinction between double-effect sedation and those practices of palliative sedation in which *sedation* (or *unconsciousness*) is intentionally sought as the purported *means to the end* of relieving suffering.

From the medical standpoint, it appears that the practice of palliative sedation is built on the (false) premise that causing sedation or unconsciousness thereby alleviates suffering by "dissociating" the patient from the awareness of his or her symptoms. This belief is not borne out by clinical experience. Numerous validated assessment tools to measure pain in unresponsive patients rely on the fact that patients still exhibit subtle pain behaviors even when unconscious. Clinicians need only observe their own patients, whose terminal illnesses have rendered them unresponsive, to see that unconscious patients may still continue to suffer from pain, dyspnea, or other symptoms which continue to require treatment despite unconsciousness. Likewise, the practice of providing anesthesia during surgical procedures demonstrates that even deeply sedated patients experience pain and require adequate concomitant analgesia (via systemic opioids, nerve blocks, or local anesthetics) when using sedatives that produce only unconsciousness without analgesia, such as benzodiazepines or more potent sedatives like propofol, which might be employed for palliative sedation. Whereas patients in a surgical setting can be assessed for unrelieved pain by meticulous monitoring of various parameters in response to known painful stimuli and therefore have analgesia titrated appropriately, this is not the case for patients undergoing palliative sedation at the end of life. Thus, in providing palliative sedation, we run the profound medical and moral risk of trapping patients in a state of being too sedated to communicate their needs for further symptom relief without adequately addressing the symptoms themselves. In short, sedation—even to the point of unconsciousness—is not a panacea for suffering, and palliative sedation is a misguided therapeutic approach. In fact, producing profound sedation in dying patients with severe, unrelieved symptoms may do more to ease the distress of care providers and families who feel helpless and distraught at *witnessing* the patient's suffering than to alleviate the patient's suffering itself. When suffering is "intractable" and no other options remain, the solution is not to aim for *sedation* as a goal—which may simply mask suffering by removing the patient's ability to communicate—but, rather, to aim for as much *palliation* as is required to alleviate symptoms, although this may cause sedation and even hasten death as an unavoidable side effect of treatment. A clearer understanding and acceptance of double-effect sedation is the morally and medically appropriate response to unrelieved neurocognitive suffering, as opposed to palliative sedation.

Likewise, we reject the practice of *terminal sedation*—intentionally maintaining sedation (usually unconsciousness) until death. To accede to a patient request to "make sure I never wake up again" is to agree to forgo any attempts at preserving or restoring the good of consciousness, even if this could be achieved at a later point once symptoms were alleviated sufficiently. Such promises to permanently end all conscious awareness of oneself or others until death should be rejected for all the reasons we would do so in non-dying patients and for the same moral reasons that led us to oppose PAS/E. If one can provide comfort while still maintaining some consciousness, then one should do so.

Of course, patients may experience profound existential or spiritual suffering even in the absence of (or despite good control over) pain or other symptoms. However, it is a misunderstanding of the power and scope of medical practice to assume that there is a pharmacological solution to all forms of suffering or a moral mandate to "fix" the many sources of agent-narrative suffering that frequently arise as a person is forced to confront his or her own mortality. Palliative sedation should not be undertaken in an attempt to relieve such agent-narrative suffering since doing so eliminates any possible pathways for overcoming or reconciling the sources of spiritual or existential distress, all of which require enough consciousness and coherence to address these issues. Ethical and evidence-based psychiatric care would not condone the use of a drug-induced state of deep sedation as a means to help *non-dying* patients "escape" agent-narrative forms of suffering, such as despair, loneliness, broken relationships, grief, emotional trauma, existential angst, guilt, or fear.[8] Therefore, those who support the use of palliative sedation to ease agent-narrative suffering must meet a very large burden of justification—both to explain why doing so is warranted *only* in terminally ill patients and to define the threshold of "imminently dying" that would satisfy this justificatory burden. Expressions of continued care, concern, listening, advocacy, support, pastoral care, referrals to psychiatric counselling, or efforts to enlist additional psychosocial support through family, friends, or hospice services are the morally appropriate responses to agent-narrative suffering.

Finally, treatment for the psychiatric aspects of suffering (such as anxiety, insomnia, or depression) in dying patients should follow the same ethical and therapeutic principles as should guide care for *any* patient; for example, treatment should be as minimal as necessary to achieve the desired effect, restore or preserve cognitive functioning insofar as possible, and utilize medications with the best safety profiles. The doses of medications required to adequately address these issues do not cause profound or permanent sedation, and to further increase doses in order to intentionally produce sedation or unconsciousness as a means of "dissociating" the patient from his or her existential, spiritual, or psychosocial concerns is a morally and medically distinct endeavor for which adequate ethical justification has not been provided.

Future Directions

Ethical challenges surrounding the care of terminally ill patients continue to present countless opportunities for ethical investigation, both normative (theoretical) and descriptive (empirical). Some particularly rich areas include the following: (1) Should primary care, emergency, critical care, hospitalists, and other clinicians be required to become proficient in providing "primary palliative care," using palliative care consultants only for difficult cases? (2) What are the moral considerations that arise in ensuring the provision of adequate pain relief for terminally ill patients within a medical culture now more hesitant to use opioids as a result of the "opioid crisis" in the United States? (3) What is the appropriate role of the surrogate in decision-making at the end of life? Should a surrogate strive to *guess* the patient's unknown prior wishes ("substituted judgment"), despite evidence of the inaccuracy of surrogates in predicting patient preferences?[38,39] Or should a surrogate's task be to convey his or her best understanding of the patient's known values, interests, and personal notions of the good in order to join clinicians in shared decision-making about how to best provide healing for the incapacitated patient?[18]

Key Points

- The terminally ill patient's existential condition of increased vulnerability, medicine's moral obligation to serve the four-fold good of the patient, the *telos* of medicine as providing healing by restoring wholeness even when cure is no longer possible, and the many domains of suffering experienced by patients as they face imminent mortality all justify intensive comprehensive palliative care (ICPC) as the appropriate response to these realities.
- An important aspect of serving the good of patients is enabling patients to guide their care according to their own authentic values and interests. Thus, engaging patients in decision-making as fully as possible, ensuring informed consent, assisting with advance care planning, and fostering crucial conversations between patients and their surrogate decision-makers (to facilitate authentic choices on the patient's behalf, even as

the patient's decision-making capacity deteriorates) are each important moral tasks for healthcare providers.

- The appropriateness of any therapy should be assessed by examining whether it is *medically effective, beneficial for the patient* (according to the patient's conception of his or her own good) and *not excessively burdensome*. Therapies that fail to meet these criteria should be withheld or withdrawn. There is no moral distinction between withholding and withdrawing treatments. Ongoing therapies (including life-sustaining therapies) should be reassessed regularly and should be discontinued when they no longer serve the patient's goals of care.

- Treatment of pain and other symptoms is *always* appropriate and should be undertaken as vigorously as required for comfort, even if there is reasonable fear that doing so may *unintentionally* impair consciousness or hasten death. However, neither profound sedation nor hastening death should ever be sought as the *intended aim* of therapy, even under the misguided notion that these are appropriate means to relieve suffering. We thus argue that physician-assisted suicide, euthanasia, and certain forms of palliative sedation are morally unjustified.

- A commitment to providing palliative care that is *intensive* (i.e., as vigorous as life-saving efforts in the ICU) and *comprehensive* (including spiritual and existential care) and to making such care more widely available is the appropriate moral response to the many dimensions of suffering that may be experienced by persons who face terminal illness.

Acknowledgments

We are grateful to the late Dr. Edmund D. Pellegrino, teacher and mentor to both of us, and the original author of the first edition of this chapter. His wisdom and spirit live on in these words.

References

1. Pellegrino ED, Thomasma DC. *For the Patient's Good: The Restoration of Beneficence in Health Care.* New York: Oxford University Press; 1987.

2. Sulmasy DP. A biopsychosocial-spiritual model for the care of patients at the end of life. *Gerontologist.* 2002;42(suppl 3):24–33.

3. Amundsen DW. *Medicine, Society, and Faith in the Ancient and Medieval Worlds.* Baltimore: Johns Hopkins University Press; 1996.

4. Pellegrino ED. Percival's medical ethics: The moral philosophy of an 18th-century English gentleman. *Arch Intern Med.* 1986;146:2265–2269. Also reprinted in Barondess JA, Roland CG, eds. *The Persisting Osler II: Selected Transactions of the American Osler Society 1981–1990.* Malabar, FL: Krieger Publishing Company; 1994:9–21.

5. Aries P. The reversal of death: Changes in attitudes toward death in western societies. In: Stannard DE, ed. *Death in America.* Philadelphia: University of Pennsylvania Press; 1974:137–138.

6. Hippocrates. *The Art.* English translation by W. H. S. Jones. Loeb Classical Library, vol. 2. Cambridge: Harvard University Press; 1981:193.

7. Burt RA. The Supreme Court speaks: Not assisted suicide but a constitutional right to palliative care. *N Engl J Med.* 1997;337:1234–1236.

8. Sulmasy DP. The last low whispers of our dead: When is it ethically justifiable to render a patient unconscious until death? *Theor Med Bioeth.* 2018;39(3):233–263.

9. Fohr SA. The double effect of pain medication: Separating myth from reality. *J Palliat Med.* 1988;1(4):315–328.

10. Jansen LA, Sulmasy DP. Proportionality, terminal suffering and the restorative goals of medicine. *Theor Med Bioeth.* 2002;23:321–337.

11. Sulmasy DP. *The Rebirth of the Clinic: An Introduction to Spirituality in Health Care.* Washington, DC: Georgetown University Press; 2006:197–212.

12. Sulmasy DP. *A Balm for Gilead: Meditations on Spirituality and the Healing Arts.* Washington, DC: Georgetown University Press; 2006:116–130.

13. Sulmasy DP. Dignity and the human as a natural kind. In: Taylor CR, Dell'Oro R, eds. *Health and Human Flourishing.* Washington, DC: Georgetown University Press; 2006:71–87.

14. Surbone A. Information, truth, and communication: For an interpretation of truth-telling practices around the world. In: Surbone A, Zwitter M, eds. *Communication and the Cancer Patient: Information and Truth.* New York: New York Academy of Sciences; 1997:7–16.

15. National Commission for the Protection of Human Subjects of Biomedical and Behavioral Research. *Ethical Principles and Guidelines for the Protection of Human Subjects of Research (The Belmont Report),* April 18, 1979. https://www.hhs.gov/ohrp/regulations-and-policy/belmont-report/read-the-belmont-report/index.html

16. Henderson GE, Churchill LR, Davis AM, Easter MM, Grady C, Joffe S, et al. Clinical trials and medical care: Defining the therapeutic misconception. *PLoS Med.* 2007;4(11):1735–1738.

17. Sulmasy DP, Hughes MT, Thompson RE, Astrow AB, Terry PB, Kub J, Nolan MT. How would terminally ill patients have others make decisions for them in the event of decisional incapacity? A longitudinal study. *J Am Geriatr Soc.* 2007;55(12):1981–1988.

18. Sulmasy DP, Snyder L. Substituted interests and best judgements: An integrated model of surrogate decision making. *JAMA.* 2010;304(17):1946–1947.

19. Sulmasy DP, Pellegrino ED. Medical ethics. In: Warrell DA, Cox TM, Firth JD, Benz EJ, eds. *Oxford Textbook of Medicine.* 4th ed. Oxford: Oxford University Press; 2003:14–16.

20. Esbensen KL. A closer look at health care providers' moral distress regarding the withdrawal of artificial nutrition and hydration. *AJOB Neuroscience.* 2016;7(1):1–4.

21. Bruera E, Hui D, Dalal S, Torres-Vigil I, Trumble J, Roosth J, et al. Parenteral hydration in patients with advanced cancer: A multicenter, double-blind, placebo-controlled randomized trial. *J Clin Oncol.* 2013;31:111–118.

22. Pellegrino ED. Futility in medical decisions: The word and the concept. *HEC Forum.* 2005;17:308–318.

23. Sulmasy DP. Futility and the varieties of medical judgment. *Theor Med.* 1997;18:63–78.

24. Bosslet GT, Pope TM, Rubenfeld GD, Lo B, Truog RD, Rushton CH, et al. An official ATS/AACN/ACCP/ESICM/SCCM policy statement: Responding to requests for potentially inappropriate treatments in intensive care units. *Am J Respir Crit Care Med.* 2015;191:11:1318–1330.

25. ProCon.org. Euthanasia and physician-assisted suicide (PAS) around the world. Revised December 3, 2020. https://euthanasia.procon.org/euthanasia-physician-assisted-suicide-pas-around-the-world/

26. ProCon.org. States with legal physician-assisted suicide. Revised July 25, 2019. https://euthanasia.procon.org/states-with-legal-physician-assisted-suicide/

27. Mangino DR, Nicolini ME, De Vries RG, Kim SY. Euthanasia and assisted suicide of persons with dementia in the Netherlands. *Am J of Geri Psych.* 2020;28(4):466–477.

28. Samanta J. Children and euthanasia: Belgium's controversial new law. *Diversity Equality Health Care.* 2015;12(1):4–5.

29. Sulmasy LS, Mueller PS, for the Ethics, Professionalism and Human Rights Committee of the American College of Physicians. Ethics and the legalization of physician-assisted suicide: An American College of Physicians position paper. *Ann Intern Med.* 2017;167:576–578.

30. Disability Rights Education and Defense Fund. National disability organizations that oppose the legalization of assisted suicide. Accessed April 24, 2021. https://dredf.org/public-policy/assisted-suicide/national-disability-organizations-that-oppose-the-legalization-of-assisted-suicide/

31. Golden M, Zoanni T. Killing us softly: The dangers of legalizing assisted suicide. *Disability Health J.* 2010;3:16–30.

32. American Medical Association. AMA code of medical ethics: Caring for patients at the end of life. Revised June 24, 2019. https://www.ama-assn.org/system/files/2019-06/code-of-medical-ethics-chapter-5.pdf

33. World Medical Association. WMA declaration on euthanasia and physician-assisted suicide. Revised November 13, 2019 https://www.wma.net/policies-post/declaration-on-euthanasia-and-physician-assisted-suicide/

34. De Lima L, Woodruff R, Pettus K, Downing J, Buitrago R, Munyoro E, et al. International Association for Hospice and Palliative Care position statement: Euthanasia and physician-assisted suicide. *J Palliat Med.* 2017;20:8–14.

35. Donagan A. *Choice: The Essential Element in Human Action.* London and New York: Routledge and Kegan Paul; 1987.

36. Sulmasy DP, Courtois, MA. Unlike diamonds, defibrillators are not forever: Why it is sometimes ethical to de-activate implanted cardiac electric devices. *Camb Q Healthc Ethics* 2019;28: 338–346.

37. Public Health Division, Center for Health Statistics. Oregon death with dignity act 2019 data summary. Revised February 25, 2020. https://www.oregon.gov/oha/PH/PROVIDERPARTNERRESOURCES/EVALUATIONRESEARCH/DEATHWITHDIGNITYACT/Documents/year22.pdf

38. Sulmasy DP, Terry PB, Weisman CS, Miller DJ, Stallings RY, Vettese MA, Haller KB. The accuracy of substituted judgments in patients with terminal diagnoses. *Ann Intern Med.* 1998;128:621–629.

39. Shalowitz DI, Garrett-Mayer E, Wendler D. The accuracy of surrogate decision makers: A systematic review. *Arch Intern Med.* 2006;166:493–497.

23

Palliative Aesthetics

B. J. Miller, Johanna Glaser, and Justin Burke

We can forgive a man for making a useful thing as long as he does not admire it.
The only excuse for making a useless thing is that one admires it intensely.
—Oscar Wilde, *The Picture of Dorian Gray*

Introduction

Since its inception, palliative care has recognized existential suffering as a key dimension of the experience of serious and terminal illness. If death's proximity and the uncertainty of living with serious illness have a way of eliciting big questions about the nature and purpose of existence, a lack of answers to such questions can just as easily give rise to crises of *meaning*. It follows, then, that many of the tools developed within palliative care to assuage existential distress, including existential psychotherapy, logotherapy, meaning-centered therapy, and dignity therapy, are aimed at least in part to promote *meaning-making*. By helping to answer existential questions with narratives of purpose, legacy, personhood, and capacity for transformation, meaning-making goes a long way in providing practical ways for patients to deal with existential distress. The spirit of such efforts is well captured by Victor Frankl's retelling of Friedrich Nietzche's words: "He who has a *why* to live for can bear with almost any *how*."[1,2]

But what if, despite our best efforts, the *why* of suffering remains elusive? Indeed, experiences of the *meaning-less* are common in the setting of palliative care and need not give rise to despair. Rather, we believe that such experiences are opportunities to employ a different set of therapeutic tools not yet structured as a coherent practice. In this chapter we draw on philosophy, historical and current medical practices, integrative medicine, the arts, design, and clinical and personal experiences to offer a novel therapeutic approach that can be applied to various forms of suffering and that may be particularly useful when solutions to existential problems cannot be found. We term this approach "palliative aesthetics" (i.e., the philosophy of aesthetics applied to the aims, practices, and therapeutic modalities of hospice and palliative medicine). We begin with an introduction to the philosophical concept of aesthetics, then outline some of the ways in which the aesthetic has historically been applied in medical and end-of-life care. We then explore how modern therapies aimed at mollifying existential distress draw on and could further integrate aesthetics and the evidence behind aesthetically focused interventions in integrative medicine. We end by discussing the concept of *aesthetic knowing* and some of the therapeutic potentials of the aesthetic within palliative care, with an emphasis on its self-sufficiency, experiential nature, immediate accessibility, and its capacity to enliven, establish connection, and provide a sense of wholeness. Perhaps most astounding is the unique ability of aesthetics to inform what constitutes a meaningful life while freeing participants of the need for meaning in the first place.

Evolution of Philosophical Aesthetics

The Greek root of the word "aesthetic" is *aisthētikós*, meaning "perception." It was first used in the context of Western philosophy in the 18th century by a German philosopher, Alexander Gottlieb Baumgarten (1714–1762).[3] In contrast to modern, more narrow conceptions of the aesthetic as that which is beautiful or visually pleasing, Baumgarten described the aesthetic as encompassing *all that is perceived or apprehended by the senses*, which is how we apply the word throughout this chapter. Baumgarten argued for the need to incorporate the human capacity for aesthetic experience and expression into the purview of philosophy, expanding philosophy's traditional scope beyond the limits of logic and reason. In so doing, Baumgarten laid the foundation for 18th- and 19th-century British and German aesthetic traditions, in which philosophers including Hume, Kant, Hegel, Schopenhauer, and Nietzsche dealt with questions of art, taste, beauty, and the sublime.

Among the more famous works addressing philosophical aesthetics is Immanuel Kant's *Critique of the Power of Judgment* published in 1790.[4] In this work, Kant (1724–804) argues that aesthetic experiences offer an important respite in the course of our daily lives in which nearly everything is done for the sake of something else. Submersion in an aesthetic experience halts a ceaseless striving, if only momentarily, by means of engaging with something that is complete in and of itself. The effect of such engagement can be an enlivened state—a quickening or an animation, captured in Kant's use of the word *belebten* from *leben*: "to live," or "to be alive." Kant thus helped to establish aesthetic experiences as "purposive" but without any definite purpose. In other words, such experiences are unique in that they are valuable in themselves, rather than for their utility or output; their purpose is simply to be. Feeling something—taking life in, realizing it, participating in it—is accomplishment enough. In this way, the aesthetic is an elegant source of self-sufficiency and senses of adequacy, fullness, and wholeness.

In the 20th century, the study of aesthetics was taken up by John Dewey (1859–1952), an American philosopher, psychologist, and educator, who published his influential work, *Art as Experience*, in 1934. He criticized Kant and other philosophers for restricting the aesthetic domain to lofty works of fine art and marvels of the natural world and instead emphasized the ways in which the aesthetic operates in everyday life. He argued that *any* experience or activity in which a person is "carried forward . . . by the pleasurable activity of the journey itself" and which "intensifies the sense of immediate living" may be considered aesthetic.[5] For Dewey, this activity or experience might be as common as attending a baseball game or as rare as viewing Botticelli's *Birth of Venus*. If Kant established the aesthetic as a source of self-sufficiency, Dewey made that wellspring accessible to almost anybody, anywhere. *Art as Experience* continues to influence aesthetic contemplation of readily accessible aspects of modern life, including popular culture,[6] the built and natural environment,[7] and the objects and experiences of everyday living.[8–10]

Though Dewey often wrote about "aesthetic experience," the concept is most closely associated with another American philosopher, Monroe Beardsley (1915–1985). Inspired by Dewey, Beardsley analyzed and wrote about aesthetics throughout his life, helping to furnish aesthetics with a systematic organization that was previously lacking. His final statement of aesthetic experience, published only a few years before his death, includes five criteria:[11]

1. *Object directness*: This is simply the act of attending to an object present to the senses, such as a painting, sunrise, or piece of music, or an object present to the imagination, such as a poem.
2. *Felt freedom*: Beardsley describes "felt freedom" as something we might experience if we were to turn on the radio in the middle of a string quartet by Mozart. He uses music as an example of an aesthetic encounter that can cause a "sudden dropping away of thoughts and feelings" currently occupying our minds, instead drawing us into a self-contained world of harmony and counterpoint, dissonance and resolution. Experiences such as this are purely *felt*; they contain no overlying narrative constructed by the mind. They are also *freeing*, insofar as they provide a "sense of release from the dominance of some antecedent concerns about past and future, a relaxation and sense of harmony."
3. *Detached affect*: Aesthetic appreciation requires a distance that allows for the object to be appreciated in a detached manner. We must be *disinterested* but not *uninterested*, attending to an object without being overly bound up in it. (As it happens, this aptly describes the goal of symptom management.) Thus, "even when we are confronted with dark and terrible things, and feel them sharply," Beardsley says, "they do not oppress but make us aware of our power to rise above them." Taken together, Beardsley's description of felt freedom and detached affect resembles the concept of mindfulness.
4. *Active discovery*: Beardsley describes our role in aesthetic engagement as one "actively exercising constructive powers of the mind." This recalls Kant's articulation of aesthetic contemplation as a "state of free play,"[4] which requires both understanding and the active engagement of one's imagination. Active discovery entails open-ended connection with the object of aesthetic contemplation that prioritizes process and eschews attachment to

any particular endpoint. It points to a sense of unfurling or becoming or creation in real time, even if entirely in the mind's eye. In this way, the aesthetic tends to pique curiosity more than resistance.

5. *Wholeness*: Beardsley's final criterion of aesthetic experience is wholeness in two senses: first, in terms of "the coherence of the elements of the experience," and second, "the coherence of the self [having that experience]." Aesthetic experience, he says, provides a "sense of integration as a person, of being restored to wholeness from distracting and disruptive influences . . . and a corresponding contentment, even through disturbing feelings, that involves self-acceptance and self-expansion." Here, Beardsley is describing what may be palliative medicine's highest and most elusive therapeutic endeavor.

To summarize this overview of philosophical aesthetics: the value of the felt human experience was first introduced into modern Western thinking with the use of the word *aesthetics* by Baumgarten in the 18th century. Kant then helped to establish aesthetic experiences as being self-sufficient, requiring no utility or output to be valuable, and capable of engendering an enlivened state of being. Dewey argued that practically anything we experience as *an* experience, whether lofty or mundane, is aesthetic in nature and therefore enlivening. Finally, Beardsley articulated criteria that demonstrate the potential therapeutic benefits of the aesthetic, such that any aesthetic experience involves a self-contained, actively engaged, disinterested relationship with an actual or mental object that engenders freedom from unhelpful narratives, a sense of wholeness, and connection to the present moment.

These phenomena should resonate with anyone seeking a sense of well-being in the face of life's challenges and the limitations of time and capacity. What is more, the aesthetic realm is always and immediately accessible to us, and it provides a way to appreciate our material circumstances without becoming indentured to them. In aesthetics we have a third major branch of human experience, something not quite thought and not quite emotion, but underlying and inclusive of both.

Historical Medical Applications of the Aesthetic

Though we offer palliative aesthetics as a novel therapeutic approach, the value of applied aesthetics has historically, if not explicitly, been recognized in medical and end-of-life care. In early medicine, attention to aesthetic experience largely focused on the built environment of care. Hospitals and clinics today are designed primarily to be safe, sterile, and efficient: important priorities to be sure, but almost entirely lacking in attention to the felt experience of patients. Bland food, untouchable surfaces, harsh lighting, lack of access to greenery and the natural world, and the constant noise of monitors and overhead systems are all too familiar to those who have worked in or been cared for in the modern healthcare system.

In contrast, one of the most renowned healing centers of antiquity was the Sanctuary of Asklepios at Epidaurus. This vast complex of temples and hospital buildings in the Greek countryside included statuary, libraries, baths, fountains, and one of the largest theaters in the classical world. In designing the hospital and grounds to actively engage the senses and imagination, the ancients demonstrated an appreciation for the fact that the built environment can be an active participant in the process of healing. In a more modern example, Massachusetts General Hospital was designed in the early 1800s with the intent of being "ornamental to the town, and gratifying to the sight and feelings."[12] In the mid-19th century, Florence Nightingale discussed numerous aesthetic aspects of healthcare in her famous book, *Notes on Nursing*, including the effects of music, laughter, artwork, nature, and other sensory experiences on patients in her care.

> People say the effect is only on the mind. It is no such thing. The effect is on the body, too. Little as we know about the way in which we are affected by form, by colour, and light, we do know this—that they have an actual physical effect.[13]

Nightingale was writing at a time of largely pre-scientific medicine, when lack of understanding of the etiology and pathophysiology of disease often rendered palliative rather than curative treatments more likely to provide benefit to patients. While medical intervention today is significantly more effective in treating disease states, it has, for the reasons mentioned above, also been criticized for being unnecessarily unpleasant and dehumanizing and even unhealthy. Or, to use the language central to our argument, modern medical environments might best be described as *anaesthetic*, more numbing—deadening—than invigorating. We suggest that the focus on safety, sterility, and efficiency, without proportionate attention paid to aesthetic value, means that our medical advances have come at the expense of valuable healing practices. In many ways, it is possible to see hospice and palliative medicine as a way to bridge current medical sciences with the wisdom of earlier periods of medical history, including applied aesthetics, to promote healing and well-being alongside the marvel of modern disease-focused therapies.

Fittingly, to find more recent examples of applied aesthetics, we need look no further than the progenitor of the modern hospice movement, Dame Cicely Saunders. In designing St. Christopher's Hospice in London, she imagined numerous odes to aesthetic experience, including space to present "live entertainments," a day room adorned with comfortable chairs and an open fire, and buildings "grouped round a courtyard" with a fountain and landscaped foliage visible from patients' windows and visitable by wheelchair or gurney. In addition, she wrote that "there must be a piano in the ward," that patient beds should be equipped with "pillow headphones," and that "imaginative and colourful" decorations should be visible throughout the premises.[14] In its final form and to this day, St. Christopher's Hospice partners with the Royal Academy of Arts to offer a comprehensive menu of "arts and complementary therapies," and the facility builds-in numerous nods to the primacy of aesthetic experience, including extensive bathing facilities, a hair salon, and liquor available every afternoon and evening. At first glance, these might appear to be pleasantries or the otherwise inessential stuff of distraction. Through the aesthetic lens, however, such attention to the senses can be seen as a skillful way to promote a sense of aliveness and well-being—no small service to those who are otherwise dying. Surely, in the face of a prognosis measured in days, anything instantiating *a sense of immediate living* is to be considered invaluable.

Aesthetics in Psychotherapy

While not named explicitly as such, elements of palliative aesthetics are already utilized in established practices aimed at diminishing existential suffering, including in meaning-centered therapy and existential psychotherapy. For example, Breitbart offers exercises designed to foster connections with life through "experiential sources of meaning" as one of eight sessions covered in meaning-centered group therapy.[15] Such immersive sources of meaning are accessed via a "sensory engagement with life," with a focus on such themes as love, beauty, and humor.

Likewise, Irvin D. Yalom, a pioneer of existential psychotherapy, emphasized the need to cultivate comfort with uncertainty and mystery, staying close to raw experiences without the overlay of meaning-full narratives. He conceptualized the search for meaning as being conducted obliquely—better achieved by engaging in activity that is worthwhile in and of itself (read: aesthetic engagement) than by pursuing meaning outright. It is as if the attribution of a particular goal to an experience has the untoward effect of crimping the full capacity or expression of that experience, especially if imposed too soon in the series of events and responses evoked. In this regard, one of the valuable aspects of the aesthetic is its potential to supply raw material and an expansive sense of possibility for the construction or discovery of meaning—serving as a kind of *pre-meaning*—which both meaning-centered therapy and existential psychotherapy can draw on for therapeutic fodder.

There is also ample opportunity to integrate palliative aesthetics into dignity therapy. The dignity model, which already includes such concepts as dignity-conserving perspective (e.g. continuity of self, legacy, and role preservation) and social dignity,[16] could easily accommodate *aesthetic dignity*. If dignity is defined as "the quality or state of being worthy, honored or esteemed,"[17] aesthetic dignity could, in the Kantian spirit, explicitly recognize the very act of experiencing being alive as worthy and esteemed. In other words, any output or meaning made is secondary or irrelevant. Indeed, life reviews often evince memories that have prominent aesthetic components, and sense-memories may be the most profound of that life in review. In addition, dignity itself has its own aesthetic. Anyone who has been long ill or consumed by the rigors of treatment or hospitalization will attest to the simple powers of bathing, wearing one's own clothing in place of hospital gowns, and tasting familiar food brought by friends or family to bolster one's mood and restore a sense of individual humanity. The same may be said for the conferral of respect between persons, which is often mediated by aesthetic exchanges such as eye contact, handshakes, and consensual touch. For those caring for loved ones who are too ill for conversation or engaged interaction, the ability to offer respect and honor by attending to the body, such as through grooming or holding hands, becomes especially important. Between clinician and patient, aesthetic dignity recognizes the value of the physical exam as providing not only diagnostic information to the provider but an enhanced sense of esteem to the patient, owing to this palpable conveyance of attention, care, and respect. And by virtue of this exchange, a strengthened bond is also in the making, to everyone's betterment. This is reminiscent of Abraham Verghese's work to reestablish the primacy of therapeutic touch, the bedside chat, and informed observation as foundational to clinical medicine,[18] all of which are fundamentally aesthetic experiences.

Aesthetics in Integrative Medicine

In addition to modes of psychotherapy, integrative medicine recognizes the sensory and perceptive capacities of the body as an important therapeutic focus. There is growing evidence for the benefits of treatments with an aesthetic element. For example, art therapy techniques, involving either the creation or aesthetic contemplation of works of art with the aid of an art therapist, have been shown to decrease global distress as well as specifically reduce symptoms of pain, anxiety, depression, fatigue, breathlessness, and poor appetite in seriously ill patients.[19–21]

There is also good evidence supporting the benefits of guided imagery. Guided imagery is a form of focused relaxation that uses recall and imagination of somatic sensations and mental images associated with feelings of comfort and peace to ameliorate physical and psychological discomfort. Studies have shown that guided imagery is effective in reducing abdominal pain in children with functional gastrointestinal disorders,[22] as well as diminishing stress, fatigue, and pain for those undergoing cancer treatments.[23–26]

Biofeedback is another therapeutic tool increasingly used in integrative medicine. This practice uses monitors to assess and display certain physiological parameters such as heart rate, muscle tension, and skin temperature and electrical conductance. Practitioners guide patients in modifying mental and physical states to produce physiologic changes, which affect the measured parameters and are then reflected back to the patient. By observing these parameters, patients can learn to better attune to their bodies and aesthetic realities, practice beneficial cognitive and behavioral responses to distressing symptoms, and eventually to affect therapeutic physiological shifts without the assistance of monitors. Limited evidence exists to evaluate the effectiveness of biofeedback, though one study demonstrated a statistically significant improvement in cancer-related pain in palliative care patients using electromyography (EMG)-assisted biofeedback techniques.[27]

Bodywork is a form of integrative medicine that includes aesthetic interventions focusing on posture, body alignment, and therapeutic touch. Massage therapy is a particularly popular form of bodywork, though the evidence is mixed as to its efficacy. Studies suggest that massage can reduce pain and anxiety as well as improve mood and relaxation in patients with cancer pain[28–30] and advanced illness,[31,32] though not all achieve a statistically significant effect. Few studies have evaluated other forms of bodywork, so the effectiveness of such interventions remains formally unknown though anecdotally encouraging.

Finally, music therapy, the most studied aesthetic intervention, has been shown to be effective in reducing pain, fatigue, and other distressing symptoms in the context of palliative care,[33–35] as well as to promote relaxation, positive mood, and feelings of well-being.[36–38]

Multiple studies have also demonstrated that music provides emotional and behavioral benefits for people living with dementia.[39–42]

What we have listed above represents only a smattering of the literature base of aesthetically focused interventions in integrative medicine. Though not a comprehensive take, we offer an overview of these modalities to highlight their potential and to suggest that such interventions are ripe for further research. We also note that these forms of applied aesthetics offer therapeutic benefit not only by ameliorating symptoms, but also by actively enhancing well-being. To accurately accommodate this bigger effect, studies will need to expand their endpoints to include beneficial outcomes such as a sense of wholeness or animation or the cessation of striving, for example. Research methodologies will likewise need to grow to suit. Borrowing from Kant's language, we are seeking the capacity to *enliven*, a profound impact heretofore considered incidental by clinicians if considered at all.

A dramatic example of enlivenment through music can be seen in the 2013 documentary film, *Alive Inside: A Story of Music and Memory*.[43] In it, we meet Henry, a nearly catatonic 94-year-old nursing home resident with dementia. At first, Henry is slumped over in a wheelchair with a baseball cap covering his eyes. Neurologist Oliver Sacks is interviewed in the film, and he describes Henry as "inert, maybe depressed, unresponsive, and almost unalive." When headphones are placed over Henry's ears, we watch as he is transformed by the sound of the music he hears. Sacks comments: "Immediately, he lights up. His face assumes expression; his eyes open wide. He starts to sing and to rock and to move his arms. He's being animated by the music." Then, citing Kant, Sacks says: "Henry is being 'quickened'; he is being brought to life." After the headphones are removed, the "quickening" persists as Henry is able to interact with people around him and engage in rudimentary conversation. Sacks describes Henry as having been "restored to himself; he has remembered who he is, and he's reacquired his identity, for a while, through the power of music." If this is not medicine, then what is? What is less clear is how to capture, study, and routinize these kinds of experiential, qualitative interventions.

Aesthetic Knowing

So the field of aesthetics holds more therapeutic promise than simply as material for meaning-making or by offering a toolset for symptom suppression. Another important example of its therapeutic potential is how the aesthetic engenders a particular kind of *knowing*. In times of existential distress, the body, where life and death are meted out, is ultimately the site of consequence. It makes sense, then, that attunement to the body is a critical though often overlooked component of graduating knowledge into wisdom and in judging what is right for oneself. We would argue that for a truth to register as authentic, it must be felt.

Insight is important to the human experience and for informed decision-making, especially when navigating complex terrain, such as illness, or counterintuitive systems, like healthcare. One of the central aims of palliative medicine is goal concordance (i.e., making choices that support one's wishes and well-being, with the least potential for regret).

If helping patients to achieve goal concordance often feels difficult, it may be because we are not playing with a full deck. To date, helping patients and families make decisions that best serve their values has largely been an exercise of communicating pertinent information, answering questions, and taking care to acknowledge emotions that arise. While kind, honest information-sharing is important, it is insufficient. Patients classically defer to their doctors on medical decisions no matter what information is transmitted. We also know that people, physicians included, don't always make choices in their own best interest. To say that humans are not governed by reason alone is not new, but the retort that humans also make decisions based on emotion is also incomplete. We are suggesting that people make choices based on aesthetic considerations, too. Self-awareness and good judgment are not to be taken for granted, and, as processes, they could use some help. By uploading aesthetics into our ways of understanding and connecting, we might feel our way with our patients into sounder and sturdier decisions. This, perhaps, is more a process of discernment than of determination.

Though aesthetic experience has largely to do with what we take *in*, this does not negate the important role that aesthetic knowing can have on our outputs, including our decisions, actions, narratives, and creative pursuits. The so-called *flow state*, for example, a construct of positive psychology, can be understood as an aesthetic experience and points to the heightened performance that can flow freely from such presence. The totality of our aesthetic awareness in any given moment is related to the concept in neuroscience of *interoception*, which is defined as the mind's collective conscious and unconscious representation of internal sensation. In an influential 2017 paper, Lisa Feldman Barrett outlines a new theory of "constructed emotion" based on two decades of modern scientific research in which interoception plays a central role.[44] She argues that brains did not evolve for rationality, but rather to achieve allostasis (i.e., efficiently anticipating and ensuring resources for physiological systems within the body). She goes on to cite numerous studies suggesting that allostasis requires an internal model of the body in the form of interoception, and she argues that this felt perception of the world and ourselves affects our emotions and identity, guides our actions, and influences how we construct meaning from experience. In Barrett's view, the brain evolved in service of the body, rather than the other way around. Or, as neuroanatomist and author Jill Bolte Taylor puts it, "Most of us think of ourselves as thinking creatures that feel, but we are actually feeling creatures that think." Indeed, there is growing interest in this area, as evidenced by the emerging discipline of *neuroaesthetics*, which aims to explore the neurobiological bases of aesthetic experience and cognition. Aesthetic knowing and improved interoception can thus provide insight and enhance self-integration, allowing people to make decisions more aligned with their personal truths, prior to or in absence of a narrative generated by the mind. Perhaps the aesthetic helps to make our unconscious conscious, lending further fidelity to our judgments.

Similar to the idea that the aesthetic offers a sort of pre-meaning, aesthetic knowing is different from and often precedes understanding or comprehension. This kind of knowing is rich with possibility—part of everything and not yet declared as any one thing. It cannot conjure nor does it rely on proof; rather, the proof is in the feeling itself. In this way, aesthetic awareness likely has much to do with *intuition* and our relationship with mystery. It also relates to *faith* and the often-powerful choice to heed what cannot be objectively justified. Awe and the sublime have long been recognized as poignant examples of aesthetic experience. Religious traditions, especially so-called charismatic sects and those committed to self-actualization or transcendence, rely heavily on aesthetic experience as a means to knowing God, Creation, the Absolute, etc. Certainly, ritual leans on aesthetics, too. If we define existential suffering as a loss of *meaning* and spiritual suffering as a loss of *connection to something greater than oneself*, we begin to see how applied aesthetics may offer a salve in both cases. For the former, as a source of raw material for meaning-making, for experiencing one's life and daily interactions as worthy in and of themselves, for grounding in the present moment, and for shedding the yoke of unhelpful narratives. For the latter, as a way to connect with an object of aesthetic contemplation, for feeling with others, for honoring intuition and faith, and for accessing experiences of wonder.

Another way of getting at the importance of aesthetic knowing is to consider how much trouble is caused by the *misapplication* of meaning or significance—either where there is none, or where some other, fuller, or truer meaning gets missed. This is a regular occurrence in daily life: a missed word that changes the nature of a sentence, eye contact held or dropped at the wrong moment, chasing distinctions of no difference, confusing absolutism for relativism or objectivity for subjectivity, projecting residual emotion where it does not belong, mistaking association for causation, forcing dichotomies onto spectrums, overidentification with incomplete or no-longer-relevant personal and interpersonal narratives, and choosing compelling stories over accurate ones. Indeed, the misapplication of meaning is no less rampant within healthcare: anchoring bias, framing and availability heuristics, symptoms ignored or perseverated upon, misdiagnoses, the pursuit of futile treatments, and all manner of other energy-consuming detours from truth. Symptoms of all stripes are, at base, aesthetic experiences; whether or not those cues are read correctly is much the game of medical science and patient care. Indeed, the act of *coming to a conclusion* is a fraught and error-prone enterprise, but we believe it could be less so if we learned how to affectively recognize and appropriately utilize our felt ("gut") sense as part of the diagnostic toolset. For many of us, the mode has long been to override our aesthetic knowing or to bypass it altogether—itself a kind of willful fracture or self-abnegation that can lead to a particular type of unnecessary suffering.

For Building Upon

Accessibility

Building on Dewey's concepts, a key element of the therapeutic potential of palliative aesthetics is its remarkable accessibility. As long as a person possesses any degree of consciousness and an intact sensory pathway, it is possible to turn attention to that which is perceived. To form narratives of meaning requires high levels of neurological processing, at a minimum, taking in complex information, filtering for relevance, reconciling with preceding understandings, followed by processes of synthetization and articulation. Aesthetic experiences, in contrast, do not demand much of the thinking mind. The difference may be that of *reflecting on* a thing as opposed to *being* a thing; reflections can be warped or obscured or halted, while being is always itself and always happening. This makes aesthetic therapeutics particularly valuable in times of distress or cognitive compromise. Of equal importance is the fact that, since sensations are practically immediate, aesthetic experiences do not require much time. A lived experience unfolds in real time, measured in moments rather than minutes. Even with advancing dementia or within the countdown to what we may suppose is the end of conscious existence, a person can access some connection to the world through their senses and feel alive.

Sharable Ground

It is not complicated to have an aesthetic experience. If illness is discombobulating, then aesthetics offers a source of orientation and presence, as well as a mode of inquiry and engagement that can be leveraged in clinical practice. At the ready is a suite of sensations to discuss, validate, and share. It is telling that therapeutic engagement often begins with the question, *how are you feeling?* And what is empathy—acknowledged both as a diagnostic tool in clinical practice as well as a therapeutic offering in and of itself—if it is not sensed? Empathy is, at base, an aesthetic experience for both clinician and patient. Similarly, the critical difference between pity and compassion can be understood as an aesthetic one. And there's no doubt that people choose partners or doctors or friends based on how they feel in the other's company. People bond over their tastes, and, even when not shared, per se, personal preferences offer rich subject matter for exploration and appreciation. This is part of how we come to know one another, and it's also how we share reality, with a higher correspondence than with emotion or reason alone. This gets at the more nuanced and thorough truth of *intersubjectivity*, over the clunky classical Cartesian separation of subject and object.

Style

Something like *style* may in fact be an important component of care, or at least not as irrelevant as the word implies. For starters, as a distillate of culture and conditioning and individuation, style conveys a great deal about a person. Second, *how* we do things, more than *what* we do, is foundational to any therapeutic exchange. Especially given the purview of palliative care to address issues that are not fixable, per se, the way in which we mete out care is likely to have outsized importance. In other words, when outcome is preordained—advancing illness, death—then the details of the route to getting there become nearly everything. Texture, timbre, tone, et al. As the medium, aesthetics is much the domain of *how*.

Relational Dynamism

The field of palliative care places a great deal of importance on relationships, often presuming that human–human relationships are the only ones of consequence. Yet consider animals and our relationship with them. Less governed by reason or thought, and often with outrageous sensory capacity compared to ours, non-human animals may be entirely or nearly entirely aesthetically motivated. Animated! This also accounts for our bonds with animals. We do not just value animals for food or labor. They compose, with us, a relationship that supplies its own significance and requires no justification. Anyone who has ever bonded with an animal will attest to the power of these connections. Indeed, in addition to animals, we foster substantial connections with objects, places, activities, nature, and ourselves. Such relationships may even be safer forms of attachment for some people than human–human relationships, making the aesthetic domain an especially important consideration in attending to loneliness. These connections are not so much forged by recall or language or performance; they rely instead on perception and sensed modes of communication and real-time entwinement. If we can uptick and honor the relevance of these heretofore-sidelined relationships, we have more to work with and new avenues of healing to explore.

Interdisciplinarity

One of the joys of practicing palliative medicine is the opportunity our subject matter affords us to look out across myriad disciplines and join other fields of study in conversation. Palliative care has many tools to help diminish suffering, but this is only half of the equation. As a field we must not only strive to help patients have *less painful* lives but rather to have *more wonderful* lives and, importantly, realize the relationship between the two. A mandate to treat suffering and catalyze quality of life is enormous, endless even, and an excuse to mix more wildly than cure- and disease-focused healthcare typically allows. It's not hard to imagine aesthetics-focused projects involving anthropologists, sociologists, designers, architects, linguists, neuroscientists, behavioral economists, philosophers. And, just like that, with phrases like *holistic* and *whole-person* and *person-centered care* on the table, human priorities such as love, sexuality, sensuousness, beauty, craft—and other states we humans pursue very much for their own sake—gain purchase within healthcare.

Set and Setting

Consider the environment of care and how we affect and are affected by it. Consistent with Dame Cicely's vision for St. Christopher's, or Florence Nightingale's exposition on the role of the senses in convalescence, or Epidaurus with its statuary and enormous amphitheater, we know that the clinical environment can either help or hinder healing. Psychedelics are the latest therapeutic frontier to prove the importance of set and setting. It seems that a psychedelic experience is, at root, indistinguishable from an aesthetic one. This bears out in subjects' descriptions of their personal experiences, consistently noted as both ineffable and supremely effective. As human beings ourselves, we clinicians need look no further than to our own lives for evidence of the import of setting: consider the precision and deliberation and effort we expend on our own built environments, accessing the arts, cuisine, and traveling to remarkable places. We either must accept our own pursuits as idiosyncratic, or we must elevate these basic impulses into best practice.

Inspiration

Then there is the issue of inspiration. What a fitting word: literally, breathing in, taking *in*. Reception precedes output. As clinicians, we can lay out exquisite treatment plans, researched to the hilt, bolstered by hard-earned experience, and know with certainty that they would provide benefit to the patient in front of us. These well-laid plans, however, amount to nothing without the patient's participation. So, how to evince and support the patient's will to try? How to foment confidence and a sense of trust and safety? Clinicians typically take for granted that patients want nothing more than to live another day, falsely presuming an unyielding will to live on. What may look like giving up or noncompliance or mental illness, however, may simply be a flagging sense of inspiration. Certainly, the aesthetic offers something to this good end. Nietzsche's converse is just as true: He who has a *how* to live for can bear with almost any *why*. Try listing the reasons you want to live another day, and you will likely name wholly or partially aesthetic experiences.

Expansion

An increasingly common patient encounter centers around the complaint, *I do not want to be a burden*. It is a telling and consequential statement, often preceding a request to hasten death. This statement is as much about the dominant worldview of our times as it is a comment about the patient's condition. Our notions of health and our ideas of a meaningful life may be too narrow for our own good, leaving many of us feeling irrelevant or with important parts of ourselves cordoned off. Medicine, as powerful a tool as it has become, is a model, and, as such, it is incomplete. If we are not careful, *we* become the source of reduction in a patient's life and options, even more so—or differently so—than illness itself. It seems likely that oppositional problems such as self *versus* other, pathological *versus* normal, death *versus* life, suffering *versus* well-being, all speak to shortcomings in our constructs rather than to truths of nature.

Future Directions

We acknowledge a dialectic between the world of the well and the world of the sick—that they are, in fact, not two worlds, but rather two aspects of the *same* world, however difficult it may be at times to tell. Patients and providers alike suffer for trying to separate the two. Happily, there is much more to tap into, much more with which to work, and it's already among us all the time. Aesthetics gives us the material to bridge divides, reconnect us to ourselves, honor our myriad relationships, and draw on the wisdom of other fields of study and ways of knowing. All of this to great purpose, or to no purpose whatsoever—yet always a vital part of feeling alive until we actually die. With palliative aesthetics, the means *are* the ends, and a human who is being is doing enough.

Key Points

- *Aesthetics* means far more than "pretty." Aesthetics refers broadly to perception—life as presented to the senses (the felt or embodied or "lived" experience)—and is inherently neutral, neither good nor bad per se. Aesthetics is also a field of study with a rich tradition and body of knowledge, typically associated with philosophy; more recently, it is part of the neurosciences and other disciplines seeking to describe and evince the full human experience. The aesthetic has the added conceptual or philosophical significance of affecting a sense of enlivenment.

- Humans are compelled by the pursuit of meaning, whether discovered or constructed. But meaning-making is not the ultimate or only human impulse, and narratives of meaning are not required to feel alive. Aesthetics helps inform what and how meaning is gleaned, but it also allows for a person to linger with an experience irrespective of whether an external sense of purpose or greater meaning follows. This attribute makes aesthetics especially valuable in the face of existential and spiritual crises.

- Aesthetics also offers a refined way of knowing. This sort of knowing resides in the body and has much to do with concepts such as intuition, "gut" sense, and interoception. This attribute may help advance the pursuits of self-awareness, orientation, presence, and sound decision-making.

- Aesthetics offers an opportunity to reach out across a wider array of disciplines to realize a deeper and more durable "quality of life," including the arts, architecture, design, philosophy, anthropology, and neuroscience, to name a few. Aesthetic interventions tend to be readily accessible, immediately effective, and inexpensive, and there is no need for a prescription pad or advanced degree to manifest them.

- To fully serve its mission, palliative medicine must learn how to transcend the trappings of construct and convention to more fully depathologize and realize the human experience (including the very normal human states of illness and death). Aesthetics offers a ground upon which to link the aims of mitigating suffering and optimizing aliveness, of doctor and of patient.

References

1. Frankl VE. *Man's Search for Meaning.* New York: Washington Square Press, Simon and Schuster; 1963.
2. Nietzsche F. Large D, trans. *Twilight of the Idols: Or How to Philosophize with a Hammer.* Oxford: Oxford University Press; 1998.
3. Baumgarten AG. *Reflections on Poetry.* Berkeley: University of California Press; 1954.
4. Kant I. Guyer P, trans. *Critique of the Power of Judgment.* Cambridge: Cambridge University Press; 2000.
5. Dewey J. *Art as Experience.* New York: Penguin Group; 2005.
6. Shusterman R. *Pragmatist Aesthetics: Living Beauty, Rethinking Art.* 2nd ed. Lanham, MD: Rowman & Littlefield; 2000.
7. Berleant A. *The Aesthetics of Environment.* Philadelphia: Temple University Press; 1992.
8. Kupfer J. *Experience as Art: Aesthetics in Everyday Life.* Albany: State University of New York Press; 1984.
9. Saito Y. *Everyday Aesthetics.* Oxford: Oxford University Press; 2010.
10. Leddy T. *The Extraordinary in the Ordinary: The Aesthetics of Everyday Life.* Ontario: Broadview Press; 2012.
11. Beardsley MC. *Aesthetics: Problems in the Philosophy of Criticism.* 2nd ed. Indianapolis, IN: Hackett Publishing Company; 1981.
12. Eaton LK. Charles Bulfinch and the Massachusetts General Hospital. *Isis.* 1950;41(1):8–11.
13. Nightingale F. *Notes on Nursing: What It Is and What It Is Not.* New York: Dover Publications; 1969.
14. Cicely Saunders, unpublished "Scheme" for an experimental hospice unit (c. 1959), London: Halley Stewart Library, St. Christopher's Hospice.

15. Applebaum AJ, Kulikowski JR, Breitbart W. Meaning-centered psychotherapy for cancer care-givers (MCP-C): Rationale and overview. *Palliat Supprt Care*. 2015;13(6):1631–1641. doi:10.1017/S1478951515000450

16. Chochinov HM. Dignity-conserving care: A new model for palliative care: Helping the patient feel valued. *JAMA*. 2002;287(10):2253–2260. doi:10.1001/jama.287.17.2253

17. *Webster's International Dictionary*. 2nd ed. Springfield, MA: Merriam; 1946:730.

18. Costanzo C, Verghese A. The physical examination as ritual: Social sciences and embodiment in the context of the physical examination. *Med Clin North Am*. 2018;102(3):425–431. doi:10.1016/j.mcna.2017.12.004

19. Lefèvre C, Ledoux M, Filbet M. Art therapy among palliative cancer patients: Aesthetic dimensions and impacts on symptoms. *Palliat Supprt Care*. 2016;14(4):376–380. doi:10.1017/S1478951515001017

20. Collette N, Güell E, Fariñas O, Pascual A. Art therapy in a palliative care unit: Symptom relief and perceived helpfulness in patients and their relatives. *J Pain Symptom Manage*. 2021;61(1):103–111. doi:10.1016/j.jpainsymman.2020.07.027

21. Nainis N, Paice JA, Ratner J, Wirth JH, Lai J, Shott S. Relieving symptoms in cancer: Innovative use of art therapy. *J Pain Symptom Manage*. 2006;31(2):162–169. doi:10.1016/j.jpainsymman.2005.07.006

22. Youssef NN, Rosh JR, Loughran M, Schuckalo SG, Cotter AN, Verga BG, et al. Treatment of functional abdominal pain in childhood with cognitive behavioral strategies. *J Pediatr Gastroenterol Nutr*. 2004;39(2):192–196. doi:10.1097/00005176-200408000-00013

23. Coelho A, Parola V, Sandgren A, Fernandes O, Kolcaba K, Apóstolo J. The effects of guided imagery on comfort in palliative care. *J Hosp Palliat Nurs*. 2018;20(4):392–399. doi:10.1097/NJH.0000000000000460

24. Roff L, Schmidt K. A systematic review of guided imagery as an adjuvant cancer therapy. *Psycho-Oncology*. 2005;14(8):607–617. doi:10.1002/pon.889

25. Syrjala KL, Donaldson GW, Davis MW, Kippes ME, Carr JE. Relaxation and imagery and cognitive-behavioral training reduce pain during cancer treatment: A controlled clinical trial. *Pain*. 1995;63(2):189–198. doi:10.1016/0304-3959(95)00039-U

26. Lee MH, Kim DH, Yu HS. The effect of guided imagery on stress and fatigue in patients with thyroid cancer undergoing radioactive iodine therapy. *Evid Based Complement Alternat Med*. 2013;2013:130324. doi:10.1155/2013/130324

27. Tsai PS, Chen PL, Lai YL, Lee MB, Lin CC. Effects of electromyography biofeedback-assisted relaxation on pain in patients with advanced cancer in a palliative care unit. *Cancer Nurs*. 2007;30(5):347–353. doi:10.1097/01.NCC.0000290805.38335.7b

28. Kutner JS, Smith MC, Corbin L, Hemphill L, Benton K, Mellis BK, et al. Massage therapy versus simple touch to improve pain and mood in patients with advanced cancer: A randomized trial. *Ann Intern Med*. 2008;149(6):369–379. doi:10.7326/0003-4819-149-6-200809160-00003

29. Lopes-Júnior LC, Rosa GS, Pessanha RM, Schuab SIPC, Nunes KZ, Amorim MHC. Efficacy of the complementary therapies in the management of cancer pain in palliative care: A systematic review. *Rev Lat Am Enfermagem*. 2020;28:e3377. doi:10.1590/1518-8345.4213.3377

30. Ernst E. Massage therapy for cancer palliation and supportive care: A systematic review of randomised clinical trials. *Support Care Cancer*. 2009;17(4):333–337. doi:10.1007/s00520-008-0569-z

31. Mitchinson A, Fletcher CE, Kim HM, Montagnini M, Hinshaw DB. Integrating massage therapy within the palliative care of veterans with advanced illnesses: An outcome study. *Am J Hosp Palliat Care*. 2014;31(1):6–12. doi:10.1177/1049909113476568

32. Zeng YS, Wang C, Ward KE, Hume AL. Complementary and alternative medicine in hospice and palliative care: A systematic review. *J Pain Symptom Manage*. 2018;56(5):781–794. doi:10.1016/j.jpainsymman.2018.07.016

33. Gutgsell KJ, Schluchter M, Margevicius S, DeGolia PA, McLaughlin B, Harris M, et al. Music therapy reduces pain in palliative care patients: A randomized controlled trial. *J Pain Symptom Manage*. 2013;45(5):822–831. doi:10.1016/j.jpainsymman.2012.05.008

34. McConnell T, Porter S. Music therapy for palliative care: A realist review. *Palliat Support Care*. 2017;15(4):454–464. doi:10.1017/S1478951516000663

35. Gallagher LM, Lagman R, Walsh D, Davis MP, Legrand SB. The clinical effects of music therapy in palliative medicine. *Support Care Cancer*. 2016;14(8):859–866. doi:10.1007/s00520-005-0013-6

36. Schmid W, Rosland JH, von Hofacker S, Hunskår I, Bruvik F. Patient's and health care provider's perspectives on music therapy in palliative care: An integrative review. *BMC Palliat Care.* 2018;17(1):32. doi:10.1186/s12904-018-0286-4

37. Warth M, Keßler J, Hillecke TK, Bardenheuer HJ. Music therapy in palliative care. *Dtsch Arztebl Int.* 2015;112(46):788–794. doi:10.3238/arztebl.2015.0788

38. Curtis SL. Music therapy and the symphony: A university-community collaborative project in palliative care. *Music and Medicine.* 2011;3(1)20–26. doi:10.1177/1943862110389618

39. Moreno-Morales C, Calero R, Moreno-Morales P, Pintado C. Music therapy in the treatment of dementia: A systematic review and meta-analysis. *Front Med (Lausanne).* 2020;7:160. doi:10.3389/fmed.2020.00160

40. Lyu J, Zhang J, Mu H, Li W, Champ M, Xiong Q, et al. The effects of music therapy on cognition, psychiatric symptoms, and activities of daily living in patients with Alzheimer's Disease. *J Alzheimers Dis.* 2018;64(4):1347–1358. doi:10.3233/JAD-180183

41. García-Casares N, Martín-Colom JE, García-Arnés JA. Music therapy in Parkinson's disease. *J Am Med Dir Assoc.* 2018 Dec;19(12):1054–1062. doi:10.1016/j.jamda.2018.09.025

42. Chu H, Yang CY, Lin Y, Ou KL, Lee TY, O'Brien AP, et al. The impact of group music therapy on depression and cognition in elderly persons with dementia: A randomized controlled study. *Biol Res Nurs.* 2014;16(2):209–217. doi:10.1177/1099800413485410

43. Roassato-Bennet M. *Alive Inside: A Story of Music and Memory.* New York: Projector Media; 2014.

44. Barrett LF. The theory of constructed emotion: An active inference account of interoception and categorization. *Soc Cogn Affect Neurosci.* 2017;12(1):1–23. doi:10.1093/scan/nsw154

24

Compassion

Alleviating Multifactorial Suffering in Palliative Care Through the Art and Science of Compassion

Daranne Harris and Shane Sinclair

Introduction

Compassion is a defining characteristic of quality palliative care. Patients and families expect to receive and deserve compassion from their healthcare providers. Decisions to pursue a career in palliative care and psychiatry are often motivated by compassion. A growing body of research has begun to provide clarity on this vital, seemingly simple, but complex construct. As a result, increasing clinical guidance is available to support healthcare providers in improving compassion in clinical practice, addressing an essential patient need in the process. This chapter explores the importance and fundamental role of compassion in palliative care, identifies defining features that distinguish it from empathy and sympathy, delineates and illustrates the key domains of compassion using an empirical model, and describes the inhibitors and facilitators that healthcare providers face in providing compassion.

The Importance of Compassion in Palliative Care

The imperative for compassion is embedded in the practice of palliative care and has been a guiding principle since the beginning of the modern palliative care movement.[1,2] In addition to compassion's explicit role in patient–provider healthcare interactions, compassion is implicit within palliative care guidelines and the World Health Organization's definition of palliative care, which aims to alleviate multifactorial suffering in order to optimize the quality of life for patients and their families living with or dying from an incurable illness.[3] Compassion, with its central focus on not only acknowledging but also understanding, engaging, and taking action aimed at alleviating patient and family suffering, is arguably the most salient care medium for the provision of high-quality palliative care.

Patients' experiences of compassion are largely defined by the therapeutic presence and actions that healthcare providers exhibit to address and alleviate multifactorial suffering—"the state of severe distress associated with events that threaten the intactness of the person."[4 (p. 32)] Palliative care patients and family members value healthcare providers who can address their suffering through both their technical skills and their shared humanity.[5] Studies also demonstrate that patients and families prioritize components of compassion, such as a genuine emotional connection, trust, and open, honest clinical communication as central indicators of quality end-of-life care.[5,6] Patients and families indicate that they want their healthcare providers to not only attend to their physical needs, but also to their mental, social and spiritual suffering.[7,8]

What Is Compassion

Distinguishing Between Sympathy, Empathy and Compassion

While there are notable differences between the constructs, the terms "compassion," "empathy," and "sympathy" are often used interchangeably within palliative care and medicine in general. Recent research suggests that patients can not only discern between these care mediums but also prefer compassion.[9] Understanding both the historical roots of sympathy, empathy, and compassion and how patients experience them in current clinical care is essential in not only understanding the construct but optimizing person-centered care.

Sympathy. Etymologically, the word sympathy comes from the Greek word *sympatheia*, which literally means "with feeling."[10] In medicine, the term was first used to describe biophysical resonance between pathology in different parts of the body—namely, where diseases (*pathé*) resonate and create symptoms (*symptómata*) in other parts of the body.[11] In the 16th century, the biophysical roots of sympathy began to expand to include the affective element of attuning to the feelings to another.[12] By the 18th century, this emotional resonance was employed as a mechanism for prosocial behavior and social reform.[12] In this way, the historical understanding of sympathy is very close to contemporary understandings of compassion. However, with the emergence of the construct of empathy in the 20th century, this understanding of sympathy was eclipsed by the contemporary notion of empathy.[12] As a result, conceptualizations of sympathy devolved over the 20th century to a more pejorative, pity-based response to suffering.[9,12]

Empathy. The term "empathy" is a translation of the late-19th-century German term *Einfühlung*, which literally means "in feeling"—describing the ability to project one's self into an aesthetic experience like a painting or another person's experience.[12] Translations of Freud's works into English employed the term empathy for *Einfühlung*, giving rise to a long lineage of the term's usage within psychoanalytic schools of the 20th century.[12] Initially, empathy emerged as a more objective, emotionally detached way of relating; a vicarious, cognitive experience of mentalizing another person's situation that attempted to avoid the more intimate sense of "feeling with" another that is associated with modern conceptualizations of sympathy.[13] This is the perspective that informed Heinz Kohut's definition of empathy as "vicarious introspection," which through observation unlocks an inner experience that allows the observer to vicariously position themselves in the experience of another.[13] In recent decades, this more objective understanding of empathy was augmented with the concept of *affective empathy*, reintroducing the affective elements of sympathetic resonance and the ability to attune to another person's feelings.[14] While conceptual variance exists, including conceptualizations of empathy that attempt to include a behavioral domain, current definitions of empathy imply an attempt to objectively and affectively understand another's feelings.[9] A number of limitations of empathy have been identified by researchers, including its predication on the perceived deservedness of the person in need and their relatedness to the responder, along with the fact that it does not require a prosocial desire to help.[9,15]

Compassion. "Compassion" derives from the Latin word *compassio* combining the root *pati*, which means "to suffer" and the prefix *com,* which means "with."[10] In contrast to the origins of sympathy and empathy, which were largely restricted to the physical and social realms, compassion was rooted in an existential or spiritual worldview that compassion was not only the deepest form of care that could be shared between human beings, but between humanity and the Universe, God, a Higher Power, Nature, or Life Force.[12] This is reflected in the words of both the Dalai Lama who said "Our prime purpose in life is to help others,"[16] and Albert Einstein's reflection that "Our task must be to free ourselves by widening our circle of compassion to embrace all living creatures."[17] Thus, whether one ascribes to the evolution of the species or the path to enlightenment, compassion was conceptualized as a metaphysical conduit connecting humanity and humanity's connection to a Higher Purpose.[18] While contemporary definitions of compassion are divergent, with some scholars restricting it to an emotion, a motive, or a trait,[19,20] most researchers understand it to be a multidimensional process culminating in action.[15,21] Despite its esoteric roots and dynamic nature, compassion is inherently relational and pragmatic, involving engaging the suffering of another with action aimed at alleviating it. The definition of compassion utilized herein, derived from direct accounts of palliative care providers and their patients, is "a virtuous and intentional response to know a person, to discern their needs and ameliorate their suffering through relational understanding and action."[22 (p. 5)]

The Relationship Between the Constructs of Sympathy, Empathy, and Compassion: Insights from Palliative Care Patients

Dying patients' perspectives on the relationship between sympathy, empathy, and compassion offer valuable insights for healthcare providers, ensuring that healthcare providers' expressions of compassion and patients' experiences of compassion align.[9] In a large qualitative study, palliative care patients (*n* = 53) described sympathy as "a pity-based response to a distressing situation that is characterized by a lack of relational understanding and the self-preservation of the observer."[9] [(p. 440)] Sympathy was considered unhelpful, lacking in understanding, and relationally distant, and it was felt to be primarily focused on the self-preservation of the healthcare provider rather than the needs of the patient, with expressions of sympathetic care or emotion being described as exaggerated and superficial. In contrast, patients found that the affective nature of empathy promoted a closer connection with their healthcare providers and thereby facilitated a better understanding of a patient's needs and preferences.[9] However, patients felt that compassion subsumed many of the positive attributes of empathy and extended the care relationship beyond understanding and emotional resonance to action that was felt to be motivated not only by a sense of duty but by the personal virtues of their healthcare providers.[9,15] While there was consensus among patients that sympathy was unwelcome, unhelpful, and misguided because it did not align with patients' emotional needs, the affective qualities of both empathy and compassion were appreciated by patients.[9] Compassion's action-oriented nature and virtuous motivators, however, were felt to have a much more salient and transformative effect on patients' multifactorial suffering, and, as a result, compassion was felt to be the most impactful and preferred form of care by individuals experiencing suffering—patients.[22]

Conceptualizing Compassion in Healthcare

The widespread inclusion of the term "compassion" in healthcare organization mission statements, policies, patient bills of rights, and experience surveys further reflects the value patients and families assign to compassion in healthcare.[2] In medicine, the Canadian Medical Association Code of Ethics lists compassion as the first quality exemplified by an ethical physician "A compassionate physician recognizes suffering and vulnerability, seeks to understand the unique circumstances of each patient and to alleviate the patient's suffering, and accompanies the suffering and vulnerable patient."[23] Likewise, compassion is embedded in the first principle of medical ethics for the American Medical Association, "A physician shall be dedicated to providing competent medical care, with compassion and respect for human dignity and rights."[24] The increasing recognition of compassion's importance to future healthcare providers is evident in recent reports[25] calling for the integration of compassion into medical education, including the development of compassion curricula.[26]

The Healthcare Provider Compassion Model

While the historical roots, contemporary understandings, and perspective of patients provide valuable insight on the nature of compassion, a fulsome understanding of compassion requires the perspective of healthcare providers, those individuals who desire but are often challenged in delivering compassion within complex, resource-constrained, and high-pressure clinical environments. The Healthcare Provider Compassion Model[22] is the first empirical model to incorporate the conceptualizations of healthcare providers (Figure

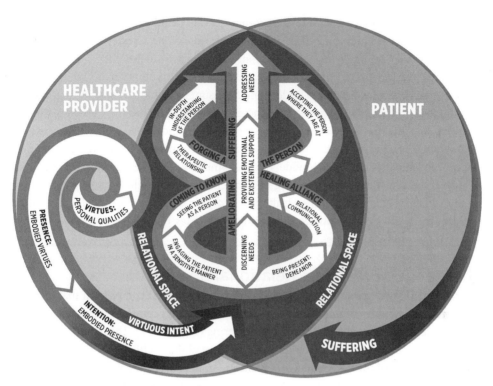

FIGURE 24.1 Healthcare provider compassion model.

24.1). While being largely congruent with the patient compassion model distilled from the perspective of patients,[15] the Healthcare Provider Compassion Model provides further clarity and insight on the key elements of compassion and their relationship to one another that were outside the purview of patients. The model was developed by synthesizing the perspectives and experiences of interdisciplinary palliative care providers (*n* = 57), depicting the key domains of compassion and how they relate to one another.[22]

Motivation and Attitudes: Virtuous Intent

Both healthcare providers and patients point to innate human qualities embedded in the character of healthcare providers as the underlying motivators of compassion (Figure 24.1).[15,22] In this sense, compassion begins with the intent to embody and express one's good and noble personal qualities in professional practice. When expressions of care flow through virtues of love, acceptance, honesty, genuineness, humility, and kindness they are perceived more readily as compassionate compared to routine care, sympathy, or empathy.[9,22] How these virtues are expressed to others shapes the way a healthcare provider behaves at the bedside and the ensuing therapeutic relationship. Importantly, patients report being able to distinguish between care that flows from healthcare provider virtues and routine care that is typically motivated by a sense of duty and prescribed actions.[15] Through self-awareness, healthcare providers can become aware of their virtues, refining and tailoring their therapeutic presence toward patients accordingly.[22]

Developing an awareness of one's presence or what healthcare providers bring to the clinical encounter is common within psychosocial professions. Concepts like therapeutic presence,[27] the core conditions,[28] and the contextual model[29] identify the presence of the therapist as instrumental to the therapeutic relationship. This ability to attune to the moment in order to deeply listen and understand a person[27] was foundational to Rogers's core conditions of congruence, empathy, and unconditional positive regard,[28] emphasizing the necessity for therapists to be aware of both their feelings and the feelings of their patients in the clinical encounter. Furthermore, the impact of the therapist's presence is a defining feature of Wampold's contextual model of psychotherapy, which emphasizes the therapist effect over treatment effect, highlighting how the character of the therapist shapes the therapeutic alliance.[29] Likewise, in the Healthcare Provider Compassion Model, the virtuous intent of the healthcare provider engenders and mediates the relational space where the other components of compassion occur.

Therapeutic Presence: Relational Space

The relational space ensconces the three additional domains of compassion that occur as the healthcare provider begins to engage a person's suffering: coming to know the person, forging a healing alliance, and ameliorating suffering (Figure 24.1). The quality of the relational space is contingent on a willingness on the part of the healthcare provider to engage with the suffering of the patient and an openness, on the part of the patient, to receive the compassion offered within it.[22] This movement from virtues to action catalyzes a transformative interpersonal experience that parallels Geller's notion that therapeutic presence is a conduit to a deeper, more authentic wisdom and healing within the therapeutic relationship.[27] In relation to compassion, this relational space is where compassion is engendered, serving as the gateway for the other domains of compassion to flow and flourish. Within the depth and breadth of relational space, healthcare providers engage in three concurrent processes: relational understanding, coming to know the person, forging a healing alliance, and ameliorating suffering.[22] Rather than being a systematic or linear process, compassion in palliative care involves healthcare providers traversing each of these domains based on both the clinical situation and patients' immediate needs in an ongoing, reflexive manner.

Relational Understanding: Coming to Know the Person

The third domain of the healthcare provider compassion model, coming to know the person, involves healthcare providers seeking to engage, see, and understand the patient as a person in order to accept the person where they are at (Figure 24.1). Through this process, a fuller picture of the patient emerges, including their broader life story, common humanity, and personhood beyond their disease, which is accompanied by a nonjudgmental approach on the part of healthcare providers. Practically, this involves behaviors like using the patient's preferred name, responding to their individualized needs and wants, respecting patient autonomy, and also, while sometimes the most challenging part, seeking to understand how difficult behaviors (or perhaps "compassion-seeking behaviors") are related to a patient's past and present suffering.[22]

Relational understanding by healthcare providers in the face of patient suffering and challenging behaviors echoes Kohut's trauma theory which connects unmet longings and fragility with circumstances that overtax and undersupport the individual.[30,31] This understanding allows the clinician to remain an objective observer and respond from a place of shared humanity that rejects a tendency to pathologize or blame and shame.[30,31] Furthermore, cultivating relational understanding mitigates *iatrogenic suffering*[32] (suffering patients experience that originates from the actions or inactions of their healthcare providers) by being thoughtful about the experiences and perspectives of the patient. While healthcare providers are encouraged to attune to their own experiences of suffering in relating to patients, this needs to always be tempered with the question of "How would the patient like to be treated?", recognizing that patient's experiences of suffering and how they optimally experience compassion may be different from the healthcare provider's personal experiences and preferences.

Clinical Rapport and Communication: Forging a Healing Alliance

Being fully present with the patient and actively listening to them are two essential components of forging a healing alliance and producing a deeper understanding of the person and their individualized needs.[22] Building rapport, in relation to compassion, forges a path for a deeper therapeutic relationship, which healthcare providers described as "human-to-human connection facilitated through the mutual sharing of stories, feelings and expressions of care between healthcare providers and their patients in order to promote healing."[22] (p. 8) Compassionate communication is more than just saying the right words; rather, it is about conveying them in a genuine tone and actively listening to the patient as a fellow human being.[22] Active listening involves healthcare providers being sensitive to what is said and also what is unsaid so they can create opportunity and safety for the patient to talk about hidden suffering.[27,28] Acknowledging this *existential suffering*, suffering related to an individual's underlying sense of meaning, has been identified as a significant element of healing even when cure is not possible.[33]

The term "healing alliance" was used by Raymond to emphasize active collaboration between patients dealing with mental illness, their families, and their mental health professionals.[34] Raymond hoped to forge a more cooperative and empowering relationship, one that replaced the alienating distrust, isolation, powerlessness, and defeat that often accompanied these circumstances, separating the patient from familiar surroundings and close relationships.[34] In relation to compassion, a healing alliance extends this understanding beyond simply the therapist–client relationship to a relationship based in shared humanity— requiring vulnerability on the part of healthcare provider to engage the patient in this manner and be professionally and personally affected by their suffering.

Addressing Needs: Ameliorating Suffering

Healthcare providers and patients agree that the end outcome and a defining feature of compassion is "ameliorating suffering,"[9,15,22] which involves tangible acts aimed at alleviating actual or anticipatory threats to the patient's physical, social, emotional, and/or spiritual well-being.[22] Clinically, having established an in-depth understanding of the patient, ameliorating suffering involves proactively discerning a person's needs based on this understanding, which may be different from the needs of healthcare providers if they were in the patient's shoes. While often involving addressing physical needs, patients and healthcare providers both emphasized that compassion included addressing emotional and existential needs associated with living with a life-limiting illness.[15,22]

Facilitators and Inhibitors of Compassion

Healthcare providers who desire to provide compassion in palliative care face a number of inhibitors and facilitators within healthcare systems that are increasingly complex, resource-constrained, and overly focused on efficiencies and economics (Table 24.1).[35,36] While compassion is a growing expectation of patients and families, is increasingly mandated by governments and healthcare organizations, and is associated with various patient health outcomes and healthcare provider well-being, research and policies to address the facilitators and inhibitors of compassion are still in their infancy.[2] Emerging research has identified three broad facilitators and inhibitors to improving compassion in healthcare: workplace and systems, relational, and personal factors.[37] While workplace and systems inhibitors of compassion have received the most scholarly attention and were identified by healthcare provider participants as being signficant,[38–40] healthcare providers identified personal factors as being the greatest facilitators and inhibitors of compassion.[37]

While recognizing and addressing inhibitors to compassion is essential for improving compassion in palliative care, healthcare providers cautioned against treating these inhibitors as excuses or barriers to compassion.[37] In fact, healthcare providers felt that compassion, by its very nature, was resilient and dynamic in overcoming these inhibitors and identified a number of adaptive responses that healthcare providers could employ in allowing compassion to flow more freely in spite of these challenges.[37] Adaptive responses include, but are not limited to remembering that small acts of compassion can be expressed to the most challenging patients, engaging in intentional acts of compassion to create momentum when compassion is lacking, and practicing self-care.[37]

The Myth of Compassion Fatigue

The term "compassion fatigue" is commonly employed to describe a decrease in compassion for others arising from the cumulation of work-related stress specifically among healthcare providers.[41,42] Despite the majority of healthcare providers being highly motivated to care, it is speculated that compassion is a finite resource and inherently tiring, requiring healthcare providers to regulate their compassion in order to preserve their well-being.[42] While compassion fatigue has received widespread endorsement as a specialized form of burnout unique to healthcare, multiple and conflicting theories about the nature of the concept have begun to emerge,[42] including its conflation with occupational stress, burnout, and vicarious suffering. Recent reports have concluded that the correlation between compassion and

TABLE 24.1 Summary of compassion facilitators and inhibitors across three domains

Domains	Facilitators	Inhibitors
Workplace and systems factors	• Feeling supported by colleagues, leaders who model compassion and organizational values that reflect compassion • Measuring compassion on a routine basis as a quality care indicator that is monitored, reported, and integrated within the healthcare system organization • Supporting healthcare providers and senior leaders to attend ongoing evidence-based compassion training	• A culture of practice that does not value and lacks compassion • Restrictive institutional and practice guidelines and policies that stifle compassion • Work environments described as stressful, negative, resistant to change • Competing professional demands • Limited resources, lack of time, being short-staffed, and economic constraints • Inflexible schedules • Overly outcome driven or task-orientated healthcare systems • Overly biomedical model of care • Focus on knowledge-based competencies with little value or time dedicated to cultivating skills and practices related to compassion
Relational factors	• Opportunities to develop meaningful relationships with patients and families • Expressions of gratitude from patients and families to help healthcare providers know their compassion made a difference • Exposure to patient suffering	• Implicit bias and judgment toward patients • Patients who are perceived as resistant, aggressive, violating boundaries, or demanding • Perceived lack of receptivity to compassion from patient and family • Contempt toward patients, disregard, negativity, and having a pre-existing poor clinical relationship with patient
Personal factors	• Personal virtues • Previous experience of suffering like personal health issues, grief, hardship • Personal experiences if compassion • Exposure to compassionate clinical role models • Exposure to patient suffering • Self-care, including contemplative practice	• Egotistic caregiving or self-serving attitudes on the part of healthcare providers • Unresolved issues or personal frustration • Healthcare provider personal or family issues • Feeling incompetent • Feeling disregard, disrespect, or hostility toward patients • Being overly focussed on "fixing" situations • Perceiving compassion to be weak

From Sing et al.[37]; Brown et al.[38]; Dewar and Mackay[39]; and Fernando and Consedine.[40]

fatigue is unsubstantiated, with some scholars suggesting that there is, in fact, an inverse relationship between the provision of compassion and burnout.[42]

The term "compassion fatigue" was first used in healthcare in 1992, by Carol Joinson, a nurse, who adopted it from Doris Chase, a crisis counselor, to explain burnout or the "loss of the ability to nurture" in emergency room nurses.[43] Charles Figley later adopted the term to describe the "cost of caring" in psychotherapists who were vicariously impacted in supporting veterans suffering from posttraumatic stress disorder.[44] Figley acknowledges that his use of the term "compassion fatigue" was intentional and not empirically based, providing a less stigmatizing and more sympathetic term to describe the empathic reaction to secondary traumatic stress and its manifestations in trauma workers and healthcare providers.[44] Researchers critical of the term argue that it implies a causal relationship, implying that there is something inherent within compassion that is fatiguing or that compassion has a more detrimental effect on healthcare providers than other forms of caring. Recent research, however,[45,46] has refuted these claims, acknowledging that while there are growing rates of burnout in healthcare providers, these are due to other factors such as moral distress and empathic distress.[45]

Finally, recent scientific evidence indicates that compassion, rather than being fatiguing, may actually have a sustaining effect on healthcare providers, serving as a valuable resource for buffering against vicarious suffering, occupational stress, and burnout.[42,46,47] In fact, ongoing neuroscience research shows that engaging in practices intended to elicit compassion actually activates endorphins,[48] reward pathways,[49] and regions of the brain associated with positive affective states of warmth, love, reward, affiliation, and concern for another.[47] Compassion also seems to have a buffering effect against stress, activating the parasympathetic nervous system through increased activity in the vagus nerve[50] and by boosting circulating neuromodulators such as oxytocin which triggers feelings of calm and closeness.[51]

Thus, while compassion in healthcare is rooted in healthcare providers' personal virtues and requires vulnerability and a willingness on the part of healthcare providers to be both professionally and personally effected by suffering, this does not necessarily make them more susceptible to burnout. Rather, opportunities to cultivate and practice compassion in a care culture where it is valued, supported, and encouraged seems to be beneficial to not only healthcare providers but also to the patients they serve.

Conclusion

Compassion, with its primary aim to alleviate suffering through intentional action arising from an in-depth understanding of a person and their personal needs, is a hallmark of quality palliative care.[5-8] Patients and families who describe their healthcare providers as compassionate have higher quality care ratings, higher satisfaction, and better patient outcomes.[2] Though healthcare providers desire to provide compassion, they often struggle in delivering it.[22,37] Recent research delineating the key domains of compassion provides healthcare providers with the basic building blocks to begin to incorporate an evidence-based and patient-informed approach to compassion in practice, even in the most challenging conditions.[22]

Future Directions

Empirical models of compassion in healthcare from both patient and healthcare perspectives provide a foundation for future palliative care research, practice, education, and policy development. However, focused research is needed on the role of compassion for palliative care psychosocial professionals specifically and its therapeutic effect on patients' suffering from mental, social, and existential issues. Likewise, while compassion in palliative care needs to be practiced by all members of the interdisciplinary team, identifying which aspects of compassion are ideally and optimally addressed by psychosocial professionals is needed. Finally, due to the centrality of compassion to quality palliative care, integrating compassion competencies in both medical school and continuing medical education is needed and should be routinely assessed and potentially adopted as a standard of care.

While healthcare providers are the primary conduits of compassion, focusing exclusively on ways to improve healthcare provider compassion is short-sighted, emphasizing the need for focused research on factors related to how the health system inhibits or improves compassion. In order to improve compassion at a health systems level, compassion needs to be routinely assessed alongside other measures of psychosocial distress and pain and symptom management in order to give healthcare providers the ability to improve compassion in real time. Importantly, governments and healthcare authorities, should consider including compassion as a component of patient experience and satisfaction surveys, requiring healthcare institutions to report, monitor, improve, and be accountable for the delivery of compassion to the patients they serve.

Key Points

- Compassion is a virtuous and intentional response to know a person, discern their needs, and ameliorate their suffering through relational understanding and action.
- Compassion in palliative care transcends a single discipline and requires each team member to attend to each of the domains of compassion when conducting routine care.
- While the terms "compassion," "empathy," and "sympathy" are often used interchangeably, patients can distinguish between them and prefer compassion due to its being rooted in the personal virtues of their healthcare providers and its predication on action.
- Compassion is not inherently fatiguing, and, as such, the term "compassion fatigue" needs to be reconceptualized in clinical practice. Emerging research shows compassion may actually be a protective or restorative resource for buffering against the vicarious suffering, occupational stress, and burnout experienced by healthcare providers.

References

1. Saunders C. *The Management of Terminal Illness*. London: Edward Arnold; 1967.
2. Sinclair S, Norris JM, McConnell SJ, Chochinov HM, Hack TF, Hagen NA, et al. Compassion: A scoping review of the healthcare literature. *BMC Palliative Care.* 2016;15(6):1–16.
3. World Health Organization. *Planning and Implementing Palliative Care Services: A Guide for Programme Managers.* Geneva: World Health Organization; 2016.

4. Cassell EJ. *The Nature of Suffering and the Goals of Medicine.* 2nd ed. New York: Oxford University Press; 2004.

5. Heyland DK, Dodek P, Rocker G, Groll D, Gafni A, Pichora D, et al. What matters most in end-of-life care: Perceptions of seriously ill patients and their family members. *Can Med Assoc J.* 2006;174(5):627.

6. Cherlin E, Schulman-Green D, McCorkle R, Johnson-Hurzeler R, Bradley E. Family perceptions of clinicians' outstanding practices in end-of-life care. *J Palliat Care.* 2004;20(2):113–116.

7. Vedel I, Ghadi V, Lapointe L, Routelous C, Aegerter P, Guirimand F. Patients', family caregivers', and professionals' perspectives on quality of palliative care: A qualitative study. *Palliat Med.* 2014;28(9):1128–1138.

8. Chochinov H. Dignity and the essence of medicine: The A, B, C, and D of dignity conserving care. *Br Med J.* 2007;335:184–187.

9. Sinclair S, Beamer K, Hack TF, McClement S, Raffin Bouchal S, Chochinov HM, et al. Sympathy, empathy, and compassion: A grounded theory study of palliative care patients' understandings, experiences, and preferences. *Palliat Med.* 2017;3(5):437–447.

10. Hoad T, ed. *Oxford Concise Dictionary of English Etymology.* New York: Oxford University Press; 1996.

11. Holmes B. Galen's sympathy. In: Schliesser E, ed. *Sympathy: A History.* New York: Oxford University Press; 2015:61–69.

12. Soto-Rubio A, Sinclair S. In defense of sympathy, in consideration of empathy, and in praise of compassion: A history of the present. *J Pain Sympt Manage.* 2018;55(5):1428–1434.

13. Kohut H. Introspection, empathy and psychoanalysis. *J Am Psychoanal Assoc.* 1959;7:459–483.

14. Halpern J. What is clinical empathy? *J Gen Intern Med.* 2003;18:670–674.

15. Sinclair S, McClement S, Raffin-Bouchal S, Hack TF, Hagen NA, McConnell S, et al. Compassion in health care: An empirical model. *J Pain Sympt Manage.* 2016;51(2):193–203.

16. The Fourteenth Dalai Lama His Holiness Tenzin Gyatsi. A talk to western Buddhists (1990). In: Pilburn S, ed. *The Dalai Lama: A Policy of Kindness: An Anthology of Writings by and about the Dalai Lama.* Delhi: Motilal Banarsidass Publishers; 1997:89.

17. Ricard M, Thuan TZ. *The Quantum and the Lotus: A Journey to the Frontiers Where Science and Buddhism Meet.* New York: Three Rivers Press; 2001.

18. Armstrong K. *Twelve Steps to Lead a Compassionate Life.* London: Bodley; 2011.

19. Goetz JL, Keltner D, Simon-Thomas E. Compassion: An evolutionary analysis and empirical review. *Psychol Bull* 2010;136(3):351–374.

20. Shantz M. Compassion: A concept analysis. *Nursing Forum.* 2007;42:48–55.

21. Eckman P. *Moving Toward Global Compassion.* San Francisco: Paul Eckman Group; 2014.

22. Sinclair S, Hack TF, Raffin-Bouchal S, McClement S, Stajduhar K, Singh P, et al. What are health-care providers' understandings and experiences of compassion? The healthcare compassion model: A grounded theory study of healthcare providers in Canada. *BMJ Open.* 2018;8(3):e019701.

23. Canadian Medical Association. *Code of Ethics and Professionalism.* 2018.

24. American Medical Association. *Code of Medical Ethics: Principle 1*; 2001.

25. Institute of Medicine. *Improving Medical Education: Enhancing the Behavioral and Social Science Content of Medical School Curricula.* Washington, DC: National Academies Press; 2004.

26. Sinclair S, Kondejewski J, Jaggi P, Dennett L, Roze des Ordons A, Hack T. What is the state of compassion education? A systematic review of the content, methods and quality of compassion training in health care. *Acad Med.* 2021;96(7):1057–1070.

27. Geller SM, Greenberg LS. *Therapeutic Presence: A Mindful Approach to Effective Therapy.* Washington, DC: American Psychological Association; 2012.

28. Rogers CR. *Client-Centered Therapy: Its Current Practice, Implications and Theory.* Boston, MA: Houghton Mifflin; 1951.

29. Wampold B, Imel Z. *The Great Psychotherapy Debate.* 2 ed. New York: Routledge; 2015.

30. Kohut H, Goldberg A, Stepansky PE. *How Does Analysis Cure?* Chicago: University of Chicago Press; 1984.

31. Kohut H, Tolpin P, Tolpin M. *Heinz Kohut: The Chicago Institute lectures.* Hillsdale, NJ: Analytic Press; 1996.

32. Kuhl D. Facing death: Embracing life. *Can Fam Physician.* 2005;51(12):1606–1608.

33. Boston P, Bruce A, Schreiber R. Existential suffering in the palliative care setting: An integrated literature review. *J Pain Sympt Manage.* 2011;41(3):604–618.

34. Raymond ME. *The Healing Alliance.* New York: Norton; 1975.

35. Francis R. *Report of the Mid Staffordshire NHS Foundation Trust Public Inquiry.* London: The Stationery Office; 2013.

36. Department of Health. More care, less pathway: A review of the Liverpool care pathway. 2013. https://www.gov.uk/government/uploads/system/uploads/attachment_data/file/212450/Liverpool_Care_Pathway.pdf

37. Singh P, Raffin-Bouchal S, McClement S, Hack TF, Stajduhar K, Hagen NA, et al. Healthcare providers' perspectives on perceived barriers and facilitators of compassion: Results from a grounded theory study. *J Clin Nurs.* 2018;27(9-10):2083–2097.

38. Brown B, Crawford P, Gilbert P, Gilbert J, Gale C. Practical compassions: Repertoires of practice and compassion talk in acute mental healthcare. *Sociol Health Illness.* 2014;36(3):383–399.

39. Dewar B, Mackay R. Appreciating and developing compassionate care in an acute hospital setting caring for older people. *Int J Older People Nurs.* 2010;5(4):299–308.

40. Fernando AT, Consedine NS. Barriers to medical compassion as a function of experience and specialization: Psychiatry, pediatrics, internal medicine, surgery, and general practice. *J Pain Sympt Manage.* 2017;53(6):979–987.

41. Boyle DA. Countering compassion fatigue: A requisite nursing agenda. *Online J Issues Nurs.* 2011;16(1):Manuscript 2.

42. Sinclair S, Raffin-Bouchal S, Venturato L, Mijovic-Kondejewski J, Smith-MacDonald L. Compassion fatigue: A meta-narrative review of the healthcare literature. *Int J Nurs Stud.* 2017;69:9–24.

43. Joinson C. Coping with compassion fatigue. *Nursing.* 1992;22(4):116, 118–120.

44. Figley CR. *Compassion Fatigue: Coping with Secondary Traumatic Stress Disorder in Those Who Treat the Traumatized.* New York: Brunner/Mazel; 1995.

45. Klimecki OM, Singer T. Empathic distress fatigue rather than compassion fatigue? Integrating findings from empathy research in psychology and social neuroscience. In: Oakley B, Knafo A, Madhavan G, Wilson DS, eds. *Pathological Altruism.* New York: Oxford University Press; 2012:368–383.

46. Dasan S, Gohil P, Cornelius V, Taylor C. Prevalence, causes and consequences of compassion satisfaction and compassion fatigue in emergency care: A mixed-methods study of UK NHS Consultants. *Emerg Med J.* 2015;32(8):588–594.

47. Klimecki OM, Leiberg S, Ricard M, Singer T. Differential pattern of functional brain plasticity after compassion and empathy training. *Soc Cogn Affect Neurosci.* 2014;9(6):873–879.

48. Luks A. Doing good: Helper's high. *Psychol Today.* 1998;22(10):39–42.

49. Shamay-Tsoory S, Lamm C. The neuroscience of empathy: From past to present to future. *Neuropsychologia.* 2018;116:1–4.

50. Stellar JE, Cohen A, Oveis C, Keltner D. Affective and physiological responses to the suffering of others: Compassion and vagal activity. *J Personality Soc Psychol.* 2015;108(4):572–585.

51. Brown SL, Brown RM. Connecting prosocial behavior to improved physical health: Contributions from the neurobiology of parenting. *Neurosci Biobehav Rev.* 2015;55:1–17.

25

Treatment of Suffering in Patients with Advanced Cancer

Nathan I. Cherny and Anna K. L. Reyners

Despite the advances of modern oncology, most adult patients with metastatic cancer still die of their disease. Advanced cancer therefore remains a major cause of disability, distress, suffering, and, ultimately, death.[1] When cure is not possible, the relief of suffering is the cardinal goal of medicine. Recognition of this axiom is at the heart of the philosophy, science, and practice of palliative medicine.

Understanding Suffering

For the patient with incurable illnesses such as cancer, the goals of care may be stated as the alleviation of suffering, the optimization of quality of life until death ensues, and the provision of comfort in death. Persistent suffering that is inadequately relieved (or the anticipation of this situation) undermines, for the sufferer, the value of life. Without hope that this situation will be relieved, patients, their families and loved ones, and professional healthcare providers may see elective death as their best alternative.

The alleviation of suffering is universally acknowledged as a cardinal goal of medical care. The ability to formulate a response to the challenge of suffering requires a clinically relevant understanding of the nature of the problem.

A Conceptual Framework for Suffering

Suffering can be defined as an aversive experience characterized by the perception of personal distress that is generated by adverse factors that undermine quality of life.[2] The

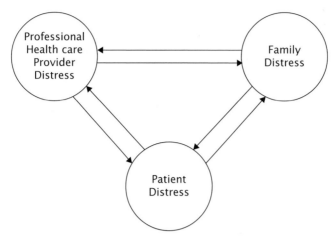

FIGURE 25.1 The interrelationship between the distress of the patient, the familiy, and healthcare providers.

defining characteristics of suffering include the presence of perceptual capacity (sentience), that the factors undermining quality of life are appraised as distressing, and that the experience is aversive.

According to this definition, suffering is a phenomenon of conscious human existence, the intensity of which is determined by the number and severity of the factors diminishing quality of life, the processes of appraisal, and perception. Each of these variables is amenable to therapeutic interventions.

The encounter with advanced cancer is a potential cause of great distress to patients, their families, and the professional caregivers attending them.[2] Many patients endure significant pain and numerous other physical symptoms, psychological distress, and, in some cases, from an existential perspective that continued life may be without meaning, even without the presence of pain or other physical symptoms.

For the families and loved ones of patients there is, likewise, great distress in this process: anticipated loss, changing relationships, standing witness to the physical and emotional distress of the patient, and bearing the burdens of care. Finally, professional caregivers may potentially be stressed by the suffering which they witness and which challenges their clinical and emotional resources. According to this model,[2] the suffering of each of these three groups is inextricably interrelated, such that the perceived distress of any one of these three groups may amplify the distress of the others (Figure 25.1) in a pattern than can be described as *reciprocal suffering*.[3]

Suffering, Personal Growth, and Resilience

The potential for personal development and net positive gain in overcoming situations of adversity and suffering is widely recognized, and it is often referred to as *posttraumatic growth*.[4] This potential, however, is predicated on the ability to cope with the prevailing problems and challenges. It is the phenomenon of coping that generates the potential for growth and reward.[5]

Coping does not occur if the demands of the situation are overwhelming (as distinct from merely being appraised as overwhelming). For example, the patient with inadequately relieved pain, shortness of breath, or vomiting may be absolutely unable to address issues related to his offspring and spouse. Nonprofessional caregivers, who are family or friends, may be overwhelmed by daily care requirements and, consequently, may be absolutely unable to appreciate time with the patient.

Suffering in the setting of progressive debilitating illness cannot be eliminated, but if adequate relief is achieved, then coping and growth can occur. By understanding and addressing the factors that may potentially overwhelm the patient, family, and healthcare providers, the necessary preconditions for coping and growth are established.

The potential for growth and adaptation are related to the quality and process of resilience.[6] *Resilience* is the capacity of an individual person or a social system to grow and to develop in the face of very difficult circumstances. Situational challenges, therefore, may trigger the development of hitherto occult personal resources, generating a process of personal development and growth.

Resilience has several important attributes: resilience is not absolute; rather it is a relative personal attribute which may vary in strength over time. It consists of two dimensions: resistance to adversity and the ability to make constructive adaptations. This latter characteristic implies the capacity to transform a negative event into an element of growth. It is important to emphasize that resilience does not invoke denial; it involves negative emotions such as sadness, fear, and loss, but also looking for positive elements to (re) build life incorporating a realistic appraisal which also recognizes and identifies positive opportunities.

Relieving Suffering: A Right

It is widely held that terminally ill patients have a right to adequate relief of uncontrolled suffering.[7] Indeed, the World Health Organization asserts that the relief of pain and other symptoms is a right of the patient with life-threatening diseases such as advanced and incurable cancer,[8] and the right to the adequate provision of palliative care for the terminally ill has been widely ratified by medical societies and professional organizations. This right has legal status recognized by the Supreme Court of the United States[9] and in Israeli statute law defining the rights of the dying.[10]

The corollary of this right is the responsibility of caregivers to ensure that adequate provisions are made for relief. The formulation of a therapeutic response to suffering, however, requires an understanding of the phenomenology of suffering and the factors contributing to it. Indeed, the failure to appreciate or effectively address the full diversity of contributing factors may confound effective therapeutic strategies.[11]

Patient Distress

Physical Symptoms

Among patients with advanced incurable illness physical symptoms are common, they are often multiple, and they cause a variable degree of distress. Among patients with advanced cancer, 70–90% will have significant pain that requires the use of opioid drugs.[12] Persistent pain interferes with the ability to eat, sleep, think, or interact with others, and it is correlated with fatigue, depression, and anxiety. The prevalence of symptoms other than pain in the advanced cancer patient has been well documented in the hospice and palliative care literature.[13]

Symptoms often appear to cluster and indeed several common patterns of symptom clusters have been recognized including one cluster of nausea-vomiting, anxiety-depression, fatigue-drowsiness, and pain-constipation and another of nausea-vomiting, anxiety-depression, and dyspnea-cough. Multiple concurrent physical symptoms are common during the last weeks of life, with a particularly high prevalence of fatigue and generalized weakness.[14] In the last few days of life, dyspnea, delirium, nausea, and vomiting are most common.[14]

Psychological Symptoms

Among cancer patients, the prevalence of psychological distress is high.[15] Whatever the prevalence, there is agreement that the most common problems are adjustment disorders, depression, and anxiety. All three may contribute to the development of substantial distress and, for some patients, a desire for death. Factors that adversely influence the prevalence and severity of psychological distress are listed in Box 25.1.

Anxiety is endemic among patients with advanced cancer. Among patients it commonly coexists with depression. Anxiety has many expressions. Common ones include

1. *Fearfulness* characterized by apprehension and dread. These symptoms may become even more exaggerated and manifest as panic or alarm.
2. *Physical reactions not attributable to organic disease or drug reactions* which may present as hyperventilation, a sensation of lump in throat, palpitations, tightness in chest or stomach, and nausea.
3. *Cognitive impairment* which may manifest as difficulty in concentrating, difficulty assimilating or recalling information or altered perceptions such as seeing the environment, procedures, or treatments as threatening.
4. *Restlessness.* This may find expression in hypervigilance about new treatments or symptoms, phobic avoidance of feared procedures or situations, paralysis of effective coping, indecision, and poor sleeping.

Among patients with cancer, anxieties are often associated with specific identifiable themes that are related to their cancer experience. *Uncertainty* may relate to the outcome of treatments, likelihood of cure, or relapse or duration of survival. Uncertainty may also relate to the potential trauma of unfamiliar treatments and procedures. Some patients have feelings that their lives have been surrounded and overtaken by forces which threaten and dominate the present and possibly the future, too—a *life under siege*. Finally, many patients experience *fear of progression*, which refers to the range of biopsychosocial fears experienced by patients with respect to the progression of their illness and its possible dire consequences.[16]

BOX 25.1 Factors contributing to psychological distress

Disease-related
   The presence of advanced disease
   Distressing physical symptoms (especially pain)
   Disability
Past personal history
   Previous experiences of loss or separation
   Feelings of frustration and hopelessness
Social
   A lack of perceived support from at least one loved person
   Strained interpersonal relationships
   Economic concerns
Comorbidities and premorbid personality
   Controlling personality trait
   Impaired cognitive abilities
   Limited adaptive capacities
   Catastrophization
Clinician-related
   Unsatisfactory communication regarding illness or treatment
   Precipitous disclosure of poor prognosis
   Unempathic care

Depression is less common than anxiety, but it is also common. It is more common among patients with a family history of depression and history of previous depressive episodes. In some cases depression may be iatrogenic: corticosteroids, hormonal therapies, and whole-brain radiation have all been implicated as potential causes.

Spiritual and Existential Distress

Existential issues are also common among patients with cancer. These issues are universal and independent of religion and religious practice although their content is often influenced by one's culture.[17] For patients with advanced cancer these include concerns related to hopelessness, futility, meaninglessness, disappointment, remorse, death anxiety, and disruption of personal identity.

Existential distresses may be related to past, present, and/or future concerns.

- *Present*: Current personal integrity, the sense of who one is as a person, can be disrupted by changes in body image; somatic, intellectual, social, and professional function; and in perceived attractiveness as a person and as a sexual partner.

- *Past*: For some patients retrospection can trigger profound disappointment from unfulfilled aspirations or remorse from unresolved guilt or unsolved matters.
- *Future*: If life is perceived to offer, at best, comfort in the setting of fading potency or, at worst, ongoing physical and emotional distress, anticipation of the future may be associated with feelings of hopelessness, futility, or meaninglessness such that the patient sees no value in continuing to live.

Death anxiety is common among cancer patients; surveys have shown that 50–80% of terminally ill patients have concerns or troubling thoughts about death and that only a minority achieve an untroubled acceptance of death.

A 2017 integrative review[18] identified eight central spiritual needs of patients with advanced cancer: finding the meaning and purpose of life; finding the meaning in the experience of being ill; being connected to other people, God and nature; having access to religious/spiritual practices; physical, psychological, social, and spiritual well-being; talking about death and the experience of dying; making the best out of their time; being independent and being treated like a normal person.

Family/Social Distress

The perception by the patient of the distress of family, friends, and caregivers can further amplify the patient's distress[11] and thus contribute to the nihilistic conclusion that ongoing existence only constitutes a perpetuation of the burden to self and others.

Family Distress

The development of incurable cancer in a family member impacts the entire family. Very common issues include emotional strain, physical demands, uncertainty, fear that the patient will die, alteration in roles and lifestyles, financial concerns, ways to comfort the patient, perceived inadequacy of care services, existential concerns, sexuality, and nonconvergent needs among family members.

These issues can be profoundly influenced by the illness trajectory. For example, a long illness characterized by a remitting and relapsing course may produce persistent anxiety and uncertainty and severe physical and emotional fatigue. Indeed, in some circumstances, family members may hope for and even request the patient's rapid demise. In contrast, when the time from diagnosis to impending death has been short, there may have been little opportunity for family members to come to terms with the presence of the life-threatening illness let alone impending death.

The challenges confronting the family are to deal with impending losses, altered relationships and family dynamics, new care responsibilities, acknowledging the ending of life as they have known it, and defining a new way of constructively living out remaining time together as best possible. These engenders great stresses.

Furthermore, the family caregivers of adult persons with advanced chronic illness have been shown to constitute a vulnerable population.[19] Many family caregivers for the

---

BOX 25.2 Needs of family members

The prompt and effective relief of patient symptoms

Education in the comfort care of the patient

Adequate physician and nursing availability

Communication from healthcare providers

Around the clock accessibility

Honesty

Information regarding of the patient's condition

Compassion and empathy

Receptiveness and responsiveness to concerns and opinions of family members

Conveys information that can help in patient care

Allows ventilation of emotions

Material supports

Hospital bed

Assistive devices

Financial support

Home help

Personal care assistance

Sensitivity to the limits of family resources

Emotional

Physical

Financial

Psychological

Disrupted families (divorce, death, disrupted relationships)

Traumatized families

---

terminally ill have chronic health problems themselves, and often during the course of the illness family caregivers incur further detriment to their health. A very high prevalence of anxiety and adjustment difficulties have also been identified among family members, the severity of which is often as great as that of the patients themselves.[20]

The needs of the families of patients with advanced cancer are summarized in Box 25.2.

Psychosocial Distress Among Family Members

Psychological distress among family caregivers, expressed as anxiety, depression, and adjustment disorder, is very common, occurring in 40–60% of family caregivers who care for a loved one with advanced cancer, especially as the patient's dependency increases.[21]

Family characteristics and especially families with poor cohesiveness and low expressiveness of needs and feelings often have higher levels of psychological distress. In contrast, good communication within the family mitigates against psychological distress in general[22] and anxiety in particular.

Often, the pre-terminal phase is associated with a period of anticipatory grieving in which the family undergoes a transition associated with the patient's "fading away." Its onset is often triggered by deterioration in the patient's condition such as unrecoverable weakness, loss of independence in ambulation and personal care, or loss of mental clarity that challenge and undermine ongoing denial. These events are distressing in that they constitute losses, diminish hope for recovery, and focus attention on the inevitability of the patient's demise.

Caregiver Burden

Although most patients die in the hospital setting, most of the care prior to dying is carried out at home by the family members, with a variable and often low level of support by friends and healthcare professionals. The care of a terminally ill family member greatly strains the physical, emotional, and psychological resources of the family unit and its individual members.[23]

Family-administered care often involves participation in personal hygiene needs, administration of medication by noninvasive or invasive routes, attention to nutritional needs, psychological support, and emergency management of such problems as pain, dyspnea, or bleeding. The heavy physical work of transferring a weak or immobile patient and attending to other needs (such as laundering or cleaning), is often further compounded by exhaustion due to sleep deprivation due to intrusive worries or patient care needs. For many, this is a new experience, and the uncertainties about the dying process and the ability to cope with the problems that lie ahead may become a focus for anxiety or ruminative thoughts.

Family caregivers may be ill-prepared to assume these tasks, requiring information on the disease and treatment, as well as instruction in technical and care skills. Moreover, caregiving must be balanced against already established roles and role responsibilities.

Financial Distress

Financial distress has been underappreciated and is often neglected in routine care. Studies comparing the relative costs of home- and hospital-based terminal care have generally neglected the financial and social costs to the family. Many family caregivers need to take time off work, some lose their jobs, and most families endure a significant reduction in income due to either absenteeism or a change in work arrangements. Permanent loss of employment, even after the disease, is not infrequent, and it occurs most frequently among those who could least afford it: older women and low-income families. The costs of caring for a family member can leave the surviving family with severely compromised resources.

Caregiver Conflicts

Family caregivers sometimes have nontrivial conflicts in this situation: conflict between the desire to provide adequate relief of distressing symptoms while, at the same time, wanting to preserve their loved one's alertness and to avoid possibly hastening death; and conflict between the duty to care for a loved-one and to care for oneself and one's other responsibilities.

Additionally, within the family conflicts, symptoms arise between family members regarding goals of care, limits of care, and aggressiveness of care. Guilt, anger, denial, and other emotions sometimes contribute to conflicted opinions between family members whether to treat a devastating illness aggressively or discontinue life-sustaining measures. These conflicts may reflect low levels of preexisting cohesiveness, or they may threaten family closeness and collaboration in previously cohesive families.

Identifying Families at Risk

The endurability of the burdens of care is an important consideration in long-term care planning. The family members' current and future welfare is an important consideration, especially when care demands are great and supportive resources for home care are limited. The ability and willingness of family members to participate in care are very variable. In one retrospective survey, 22% of families of terminally ill patients were unable or unwilling to provide personal or medical care.[24]

The identification of populations at particularly high risk for early intervention is facilitated by an assessment of stressors, particular family needs, and the resources available to the family. A survey of bereavement councilors highlighted several different risk factors: perceived lack of caregiver social support (70%), caregiver history of drug/alcohol abuse (68%), poor caregiver coping skills (68%), caregiver history of mental illness (67%), and when the patient is a child (63%).[25]

Global family functioning is a predictor of coping. In a large longitudinal study, Kissane and colleagues identified characteristics of families with high prevalence of distress and poor coping.[26] "Hostile" families ware characterized by low cohesiveness, low expressiveness, and high conflict. These families cope poorly because family life is fraught with frequent arguing, little teamwork or felt closeness among members, and minimal communication. Families classified as "Sullen" were characterized by reduced cohesiveness and expressiveness, but with much less overt conflict. Outright hostility is less common in these families, suggesting that anger is muted, with depression gaining more prominence as the anger is directed inward.

Healthcare Professional Distress

Stressors

Work in palliative care and, in particular end-of-life care, is associated with inherent stressors that may negatively impact the well-being of clinicians working in the field. Among the stressors experienced by professionals working in this field are patients who experience high morbidity and mortality; high work pressure; frequent life-and-death decisions (which sometimes occur in ambiguous circumstances); high consumer expectations; interstaff conflict; severe patient dependency, debilitation, or disfigurement; severe emotional distress among patients and their families; and issues relating to suffering and distress caused by the treatments themselves.[27]

It is not unusual for clinicians to bond strongly with patients who remind them of someone special in their lives or identify with patients who are similar to themselves in age, appearance, or background. Identification with patients can revive personal pain and heighten feelings of guilt or a lack of control, resulting in burnout. Among nurses, the major sources of stress include perceived deficiencies in symptom control, deep emotional involvement in work, dealing with young patients, dealing with the emotional needs of distressed relatives, and conflict with the participating physicians over the goals of care.

The stressors generated by providing care may have diverse impacts on the emotional and professional lives of every member of the clinical team and may lead to burnout and compassion fatigue, both of which can negatively affect professional function, adversely influence the care given to patients and to the family.

Burnout

The burnout syndrome is characterized by losing enthusiasm for work (emotional exhaustion), treating people as if they were objects (depersonalization), and having a sense that work is no longer meaningful (low personal accomplishment). *Emotional exhaustion*— feelings of being overextended and depleted of one's emotional and physical resources— prompts efforts to cope by distancing oneself emotionally and cognitively from work. *Depersonalization* is another form of distancing characterized by negative, callous, cynical, or excessively detached responses to various aspects of the job. *Lack of personal accomplishment* refers to feelings of being ineffectual and underachieving at work.

Compassion Fatigue

Some researchers have asserted that repeated intense involvement with the distress of patients and their families in the time leading up to and after the death can traumatize healthcare providers and contribute to "the compassion fatigue syndrome"[28] characterized by avoidance of contact with the patient, a negative self-assessment of performance, and a host of other responses that may adversely impact on personal and professional well-being and function. Compassion fatigue is one of the factors contributing to burnout, but it may occur without signs of burnout when it occurs despite maintaining engagement and enthusiasm for work.[28]

Compassion fatigue may be expressed across psychological, cognitive, or interpersonal domains. Sometimes symptoms are similar to the classic features of posttraumatic stress disorder (PTSD): hyperarousal, disturbed sleep, outbursts of anger or hypervigilance, or, alternatively, avoidance, "not wanting to go there again," or the desire to avoid thoughts, feelings, and conversations associated with the patient's pain and suffering. Clinicians may become either overinvolved or detached.

Compassion fatigue can express itself in several behavior patterns. *Splitting* is a form of good–bad polarization. It involves perceiving oneself or other members of the care team as entirely good and helpful and others as entirely bad and extremely unhelpful. It produces intra-team conflicts and tensions that compromise teamwork and the cohesiveness of the care team. Additionally, caregivers may demonstrate splitting between their "good patients" and their "bad patients." Taking on the role of "the savior" can be a manifestation of compassion fatigue. Among oncologists with compassion fatigue, the savior syndrome is often manifested as a "counterphobic determination to treat," whereby oncologists caring for dying patients focus their energies on trying new treatments rather than addressing the more challenging issues of end-of-life care. Clinicians with compassion fatigue may gradually or abruptly became *detached* as the emotional intensity increases.

Compassion fatigue is not universally considered distinct from burnout, and this view is argued in Chapter 24.

Factors Exacerbating the Risk of Burnout and Compassion Fatigue

Workload: Dealing with dying patients and their families, excessive caseload of challenging patients and families, inadequate supports, excessive bureaucracy, and lack of time to talk to patients have all been identified as workload stressors. The greater the mismatch between the person's capacity and the demands of the work environment, the greater is the likelihood of burnout.

Control (and training): When clinicians are expected to take responsibility without adequate training, they may experience extreme lack of control. Among palliative care clinicians, this may occur if they lack communication skills or specific management skills in palliative care. Clinicians with inadequate communication training in stress management, recognition and management of compassion fatigue, conflict resolution, and symptom control have a higher risk of burnout.

Inter-professional and team issues: Team conflict between doctors and nurses, among nurses, or between other members of the care team all contribute to burnout. Characteristics commonly seen in poorly functioning interdisciplinary care teams include lack of collaborative practice among professionals, strong hierarchical characteristics, lack of a shared philosophy of care, stifled expression of concerns, and strong professional territoriality. Often, conflicts are generated by lack of common understandings of the prevailing goals of care, role diffusion issues, or differences of opinion regarding the appropriate clinical management or issues related to management style.

Values: Moral distress arising from situations in which clinicians are expected to perform duties that run contrary to their moral compass may be a major stressor contributing to distress and burnout.[29] Moral distress, in turn, may be precipitated by the perceived inability to live up to one's own standards or provide an idealized, and often unattainable, vision of the "good death."

Reward: Limited or inadequate financial rewards for the extremely challenging work of palliative care can contribute to burnout.

Emotion-work variables: When patients die, professional caregivers may experience grief, loss, or chronic grief, particularly if the relationships was long. These reactions may be especially difficult when patients or their children are young, or in situations where the patient's distress was poorly uncontrolled and the staff feel that they were unable to deliver the best possible care. Professionals must continually balance support for those facing death with the need to avoid being overwhelmed by the patient's suffering.

Extrinsic factors: Palliative care staff may also have personal sources of pressure outside of the work environment. These include family, financial health, societal pressures, limited supports, and problems with interpersonal relationships unrelated to their roles as caregivers.

Personality factors: Clinicians with an exaggerated sense of responsibility, doubt, and guilt can have an enormous impact on clinicians' professional, personal, and family lives.

An Approach to Suffering Assessment and Therapeutic Planning

An effective approach to the alleviation of suffering for patients with incurable or terminal illness is predicated on careful case assessment, identification of care needs, formulation of a multidisciplinary therapeutic interventions to address those needs, and the provision of ongoing monitoring with readiness to re-evaluate the care plan as problems arise or needs change.

Assessment: Looking at the Full Triad

An appreciation of the full diversity of factors that may contribute to suffering underscores the need for a methodical approach to the assessment of each individual patient, those close to him, and the professionals involved in the care. The objectives of the assessment are to identify current problems that are a source of distress to each of the parties, assess their care needs, and evaluate the adequacy of the available resources.

This evaluation must include medical variables in the patient, family, and available community medical and nursing supports; psychological variables in the patient and family; the well-being and coping of the professional caregivers; and social and financial variables in the patient and family. Since both the patient and family are part of the unit of care, assessment requires discussion with both. The clinician must maintain a clinical posture that affirms relief of suffering as the central goal of therapy, which encourages open and effective communication about perceived problems.

Formulating a Care Plan to Mitigate Suffering

Based on this assessment, one can formulate a care plan that addresses all aspects of the care triad: patient, family, and healthcare providers. The formulation can be summarized in a document or report that describes

1. The medical condition of the patient and the goals of care
2. Description of the involved family and professional caregivers
3. Patient issues: Physical, psychological, existential, social, communication, understanding
4. Family issues: Physical, psychological, existential, social, communication, understanding
5. Professional caregiver issues: Staffing, training, resources, resource/need match, emotional coping

6. Coping assessment: Patient, family, and professional staff
7. Contingency planning: Anticipated contingencies, planned interventions

The multidimensional nature of suffering demands an approach to care that is interdisciplinary, bringing together the skills of healthcare professionals to address the full range of physical, psychological, existential, and social sources of distress confronting the patient and their family caregivers. This underscores the need for multidisciplinary care teams including cancer experts, nurse and physician palliative care experts, social workers, psychologists, and spiritual caregivers to address these challenges in a coordinated manner. Depending on the prevailing problems of the patient and family, different parts of the interdisciplinary team may have greater or lesser roles in the provision of care, and the roles may change over time. In each case there is a need for individualization of the care plan developed, based on the specific needs that are identified in the assessment process and which are continually re-evaluated.

Implementation of Ongoing Assessment

Advanced incurable cancer leading toward death is characterized by the potential for rapid and dramatic change. The overall tendency is for increasing dependency and an increasingly complex confluence of physical, psychological, existential, ethical, and social concerns. Just as care for the palliative care patient is a longitudinal commitment, so is assessment. Consequently, this assessment must be repeated at appropriate intervals which will be determined by the rate of change in the patient's clinical condition or at points of major change in goals, care plan, or the patient's condition.

Coordination of the many participants in this sort of multidisciplinary care requires an identified leader for each case. This role is usually filled by either a physician or nurse, and the specific person may change during the course of an illness as the predominant care needs change. For example, with the progression of the cancer from a diagnostic stage to a palliative stage, the responsibility may shift sequentially from a surgeon, to a medical oncologist, and, finally, to a palliative care nurse. The coordinator, or case manager, is responsible for monitoring the degree to which care needs are being met and for facilitating change when necessary.

Similarly the well-being and function of the healthcare professionals must be monitored, ensuring the availability of appropriate manpower and expertise to effectively manage the prevailing problems. For security and safety in the event of a clinical crisis, it is essential that the patient and family have access to a contact person with 24-hour availability. This model represents a family-centered, multidisciplinary, collaborative approach among physicians, nurses, social workers, other therapists, and community supports.

Future Directions

Continual electronic patient-reported outcomes (ePRO) monitoring systems have already established themselves as an approach to the early identification and treatment of patient distress.[30] Widening this model to monitor for distress in the full triad of patient, family, and healthcare providers needs to be evaluated as a more comprehensive approach to the relief of suffering in its wider context, in the management of patients with advanced cancer.

Key Points

- An understanding of the nature of suffering and of the factors that contribute to it are essential to the task of palliative medicine.
- Suffering is a complex human experience which requires evaluation in order to construct an effective therapeutic response that is appropriate to presenting problems.
- An appreciation of the full diversity of factors that may contribute to suffering underscores the need for a methodical approach to the assessment of each individual patient, those close to him, and the professionals involved in his care.
- The objectives of the assessment are to identify current problems that are a source of distress to each of the parties, assess their care needs, and evaluate the adequacy of the available resources.
- This broad approach to suffering can assist in the formulation of a multidisciplinary therapeutic intervention to address critical needs.
- All patients need provision of ongoing monitoring with readiness to re-evaluate the care plan as problems arise.

References

1. Knaul FM, Bhadelia A, Rodriguez NM, Arreola-Ornelas H, Zimmermann C. The Lancet Commission on Palliative Care and Pain Relief: Findings, recommendations, and future directions. *Lancet Global Health.* 2018;6:S5–S6.
2. Cherny NI, Coyle N, Foley KM. Suffering in the advanced cancer patient: A definition and taxonomy. *J Palliat Care.* 1994;10(2):57–70.
3. McCauley R, McQuillan R, Ryan K, Foley G. Mutual support between patients and family caregivers in palliative care: A systematic review and narrative synthesis. *Palliat Med.* 2021:0269216321999962.
4. Gori A, Topino E, Sette A, Cramer H. Pathways to post-traumatic growth in cancer patients: Moderated mediation and single mediation analyses with resilience, personality, and coping strategies. *J Affect Disord.* Jan 15 2021;279:692–700.
5. Fujimoto T, Okamura H. The influence of coping types on post-traumatic growth in patients with primary breast cancer. *Jap J Clin Oncol.* Jan 1 2021;51(1):85–91.
6. Li L, Hou Y, Kang F, Wei X. The mediating and moderating roles of resilience in the relationship between anxiety, depression, and post-traumatic growth among breast cancer patients based on structural equation modeling: An observational study. *Medicine (Baltimore).* Dec 11 2020;99(50):e23273.
7. Radbruch L, Payne S, de Lima L, Lohmann D. The Lisbon Challenge: Acknowledging palliative care as a human right. *J Palliat Med.* Mar 2013;16(3):301–304.
8. World Health Assembly S-S. Strengthening of palliative care as a component of comprehensive care throughout the life course. 2014. http://apps.who.int/gb/ebwha/pdf_files/wha67/a67_r19-en.pdf2014
9. Burt RA. The Supreme Court speaks: Not assisted suicide but a constitutional right to palliative care. *N Engl J Med.* 1997;337(17):1234–1236.

10. Steinberg A, Sprung CL. The dying patient: New Israeli legislation. *Intensive Care Med.* Aug 2006;32(8):1234–1237.

11. Krikorian A, Limonero JT, Mate J. Suffering and distress at the end-of-life. *Psycho-oncology.* 2012;21(8):799–808.

12. Knaul FM, Farmer PE, Krakauer EL, De Lima L, Bhadelia A, Jiang Kwete X, et al. Alleviating the access abyss in palliative care and pain relief: An imperative of universal health coverage: The Lancet Commission report. *The Lancet.* 2018;391(10128):1391–1454.

13. Reilly CM, Bruner DW, Mitchell SA, Minasian LM, Basch E, Dueck A, et al. A literature synthesis of symptom prevalence and severity in persons receiving active cancer treatment. *Support Care Cancer.* Jun 2013;21(6):1525–1550.

14. Kehl KA, Kowalkowski JA. A systematic review of the prevalence of signs of impending death and symptoms in the last 2 weeks of life. *Am J Hospice Palliat Care.* 2013;30(6):601–616.

15. Carlson LE, Zelinski EL, Toivonen KI, Sundstrom L, Jobin CT, Damaskos P, et al. Prevalence of psychosocial distress in cancer patients across 55 North American cancer centers. *J Psychosoc Oncol.* 2019;37(1):5–21.

16. Dinkel A, Herschbach P. Fear of progression in cancer patients and survivors. *Psycho-Oncology.* 2018:13–33.

17. Puchalski CM, King SDW, Ferrell BR. Spiritual Considerations. *Hemonc Clin N Am.* Jun 2018;32(3):505–517.

18. Mesquita AC, Chaves ECL, Barros GAM. Spiritual needs of patients with cancer in palliative care: An integrative review. *Curr Opin Support Palliat Care.* Dec 2017;11(4):334–340.

19. Janssen DJ, Spruit MA, Wouters EF, Schols JM. Family caregiving in advanced chronic organ failure. *J Am Med Dir Assoc.* 2012;13(4):394–399.

20. Teixeira RJ, Remondes-Costa S, Graça Pereira M, Brandão T. The impact of informal cancer caregiving: A literature review on psychophysiological studies. *Eur J Cancer Care.* 2019;28(4):e13042.

21. Northouse LL, Katapodi MC, Schafenacker AM, Weiss D. The impact of caregiving on the psychological well-being of family caregivers and cancer patients. *Semin Oncol Nurs.* 2012;28(4):236–245.

22. Ozono S, Saeki T, Inoue S, Mantani T, Okamura H, Yamawaki S. Family functioning and psychological distress among Japanese breast cancer patients and families. *Support Care Cancer.* Dec 2005;13(12):1044–1050.

23. Johansen S, Cvancarova M, Ruland C. The effect of cancer patients' and their family caregivers' physical and emotional symptoms on caregiver burden. *Cancer Nurs.* 2018;41(2):91–99.

24. Wellisch D, Fawzy F, Landsverk J, Pasnau R, Wolcot D. An evaluation of psychosocial problems of the homebound cancer patient: Relationship of patient adjustment to family problems. *J Psychosoc Onc.* 1989;7:55–76.

25. Ellifritt J, Nelson KA, Walsh D. Complicated bereavement: A national survey of potential risk factors. *Am J Hospice Palliat Care.* Mar-Apr 2003;20(2):114–120.

26. Kissane DW, McKenzie M, McKenzie DP, Forbes A, O'Neill I, Bloch S. Psychosocial morbidity associated with patterns of family functioning in palliative care: Baseline data from the Family Focused Grief Therapy controlled trial. *Palliat Med.* Sep 2003;17(6):527–537.

27. Vachon M. Occupational stress in palliative care. In: O'Connor M, Aranda S, Wilkinson S, eds. *Palliative Care Nursing.* New York: Routledge; 2018:41–51.

28. Slocum-Gori S, Hemsworth D, Chan WW, Carson A, Kazanjian A. Understanding compassion satisfaction, compassion fatigue and burnout: A survey of the hospice palliative care workforce. *Palliat Med.* 2013;27(2):172–178.

29. Sundin-Huard D, Fahy K. Moral distress, advocacy and burnout: Theorizing the relationships. *Int J Nurs Pract.* Mar 1999;5(1):8–13.

30. Basch E, Barbera L, Kerrigan CL, Velikova G. Implementation of patient-reported outcomes in routine medical care. *Am Soc Clin Oncol Educ Book.* 2018;38:122–134.

26

Demoralization in Palliative Care

David W. Kissane, Irene Bobevski, and Luigi Grassi

Introduction

Nearly 70 years ago, clinicians such as G. Engel, V. Frankl, and J. Frank observed given-up and defeated states of mind.[1] Although some tools were developed to assess some psychosocial dimensions, including an interview to assess demoralization in the medically ill,[2] it was not until systematic measurement was undertaken 20 years ago with a psychometrically validated scale, the Demoralization Scale (DS), that more rapid progress in recognition and treatment began to occur.[3] Demoralization is a disorder of adjustment or failure to cope in which morale is severely lowered by a stressor event, with resultant discouragement, hopelessness, worthlessness, and meaninglessness about life able to mediate suicidal thoughts. Systematic reviews of demoralization in palliative care have identified a prevalence of 15% toward the end of life, highlighting how it spoils the quality and value of life.[4] Much can be done to alleviate the inherent suffering found among demoralized patients and their families.[5]

The Clinical and Historical Landscape of Demoralization

The demoralized patient can be heard to say, "I don't see the point to life anymore. It has become too hard! Pain, nausea, and fatigue spoil my days. I feel trapped by this illness. Hope has flown out the window! My doctor seems to have given up on me. My family want me to fight but I cannot keep trying to go on like this. My life has lost its meaning. If I had a gun, I think I'd end it!"

Demoralization is an old construct, found in early church literature as the state of *acedia*, where the development of a tedious meaninglessness about life was considered sinful.[1] Victor Frankl (1963) recognized it as a form of suffering in the concentration camps, George Engel (1967) as a giving up/given-up syndrome in the medically ill, Ernest Gruenberg (1967) as social breakdown among asylum patients, and Jerome Frank (1968) as central to effective psychotherapy.[6] Whenever a stressor event occurs, the appraisal of threat is responded to with emotion-based, solution-focused, or meaning-centered coping. Should these coping responses prove inadequate, the stressful predicament can result in a failure to adapt, with the phenomenology of demoralization emerging clinically.

John de Figueiredo in Boston advanced the early understanding of the concept of demoralization with Frankl in the 1980s by pointing out that any distress is accompanied by what they termed "subjective incompetence,"[7] in which there was an inability to plan or initiate action to overcome the sense of entrapment which the stressor had brought on.[8] Working in Bologna, Giuseppe Fava's group, in the 1990s, took the concept further by recognizing that expectations of the patient or those around them were not fulfilled, with the hopeless-helpless stance breaking continuity between the person's past and their perception of the future.[8] Then, around 2000, the Melbourne group involving Kissane and Clarke saw the strongest link to existential distress, with meaninglessness, purposelessness, and pointlessness being added to the phenomena of hopelessness, entrapment, and isolation and their proposal that a diagnostic syndrome be recognized.[8]

Many dimensions of an illness experience can precipitate demoralization, especially so when the prognosis is poor, the disease state progressive, and life itself is threatened. Thus, clinical conditions where it is prevalent include cancer, incipient organ failure associated with chronic progressive disorders, severe neurological states, substance dependence, treatment-resistant mental illness, and poor symptom control, but it is also found in settings of poverty and social alienation, refugee status, adolescent disillusionment, and the mid-life crisis.

As a disorder of coping, demoralization can be found comorbidly with a range of other mental disorders, especially states of psychopathology that include depression, anxiety, cognitive impairment, and psychosis. Nosological systems of disease classification could employ demoralization as a "specifier" to more fully describe a clinical presentation and especially to guide treatment choices. Using a field survey where clinicians were asked to compare comparative clinical vignettes, strong sensitivity and specific ratings were found for diagnoses of adjustment disorder with demoralization and major depression with demoralization.[9] The specifier "with demoralization" was shown to deepen diagnostic understanding, enhance treatment choices, and optimize the ability to communicate with clinicians and patients.

Among several systematic reviews, one identified 25 studies of 4,545 patients from 10 countries.[3] Among these, 10 studies used the DS to reveal a prevalence of clinically significant demoralization in palliative care patients in the range of 13% to 18%.[3]

Demoralization is a contagious state of mind, readily transmitted to family and friends, clinicians, caregivers, and, at times, whole services or communities. Across this landscape, demoralization is recognized as a major expression of human suffering.

Presenting Symptoms

In the medically ill, disease progression, discussion of a limited prognosis, treatment side effects, or difficult symptom control can quickly precipitate the development of demoralization. Key symptoms include

- Low morale, discouragement, and grief at loss or change
- Sense of poor coping, with thoughts like "I'm struggling badly!"
- Feeling trapped by the illness, with deepening helplessness
- Pessimism about the illness and the future
- Hopelessness
- Loss of the value and meaning of life
- Pointlessness
- Purposelessness
- Feeling alone, isolated, or alienated from others
- Feeling a failure
- Worthlessness
- Readiness to give up on life, desire death, or wish to hasten death
- Active suicidal plans

Because of the chronicity and journey of illness, many patients will not conceptualize the illness as a stressor event, but their distress grows and impairs functioning in their adaptation, social and relational world, everyday roles and activities; it is an impairment that thus interferes with their quality of life. A cluster of nonspecific emotions can accompany this, including worry, irritability, anger, sadness, low mood, or distress. There may be social withdrawal, an urge to retreat or hide, and avoid contact and discussion of their predicament. These presenting symptoms may fluctuate in intensity or come in waves, but they tend to become established and persist, although retention of a sense of humor, absence of anhedonia, and reactivity to their social world differentiates them from a clinical depression.

Suicidal Thinking

One feature of the demoralized state is its propensity to induce suicidal thinking. Several studies have now confirmed this association. The exemplar study assessed mood, anxiety, adjustment, and suicidal states among 430 patients with mixed cancers using the Composite International Diagnostic Interview–Oncology (CIDI-O), as well as validated measures of demoralization (DS) and depression (the Patient Health Questionnaire [PHQ-9]).[10] While 21% of patients carried clinically relevant levels of demoralization, 14% did so without any mood or anxiety disorder. When the risk of suicidal thinking was assessed by controlling for mood and anxiety disorders, demoralization was also associated with a significantly increased risk for suicidal ideation (RR, 2.8; 95% confidence interval [CI], 1.2–6.7). When demoralization and depression were examined as simultaneous predictors of suicidal ideation, demoralization was a significant predictor, whereas depression was not. Demoralization explained a significant variance in suicidal ideation not explained by mental disorders. Failure to assess for demoralization may miss a key group of patients at risk because of suicidal thinking.

Recent Empirical Studies

A latent class analysis of 1,527 cancer patients assessed for demoralization, anxiety, depression, physical symptoms, and functional impairment identified four symptom clusters.[11] The largest class (54%) was defined by the absence of distress, while the next (22%) had functional impairment with somatic symptoms (insomnia, fatigue, and anorexia). A third class (13%) carried moderate demoralization with functional impairment, poorly controlled physical symptoms, and moderate suicidal ideation—a class that reflected poor adjustment to the cancer illness and its treatment. The fourth class (11%) displayed severe psychopathology, with anhedonia, anxiety, demoralization, suicidal ideation, and poor physical symptom control. However, there was an 81% probability of the poor adjustment with demoralization class endorsing suicidal thoughts and a 76% probability of the severe psychopathology class with anhedonia/anxiety/demoralization reporting suicidality. The adjustment disorder class had more patients with very advanced disease and a single status. This latent class analysis[11] supported the unidimensional model of adjustment disorder in the International Classification of Disease (ICD-11) and supported adjustment disorder being classified as an axis 1 disorder, rather than only being hierarchically diagnosed (as in the *Diagnostic and Statistical Manual of Mental Disorders* [DSM]) if a major depression or anxiety disorder diagnosis cannot be made.

An Italian study of 473 medically ill patients were assessed with the DS, PHQ-9, and the Diagnostic Criteria for Psychosomatic Research-Demoralization (DCPR-D) module interview to make a clinical diagnosis of demoralization.[12] Confirmatory factor analysis supported the four-factor structure previously confirmed in validation studies of the Italian version of the DS. However, item response theory was employed to examine briefer versions of the DS compared to the original 24 item scale. Using area under the curve (AUC) analyses to assess a six-item version against the interview diagnosis of demoralization using the DCPR-D, similar AUC values and satisfactory sensitivity and specificity were found.[12] These six items were loss of purpose, loss of role, loss of control, hopeless, angry, and feeling trapped, which can be considered as a screening tool to better recognize demoralization in palliative care.

A third body of work made further use of the Italian cohort of medically ill patients with network analysis, in which partial correlations are examined between every symptom in the dataset to display which symptoms are highly associated and belong to distinct communities, compared to other symptoms, in a Gaussian graphical model.[13] A case-dropping bootstrap procedure using 10,000 iterations ensured stability of the resultant symptom communities using the R program (see, e.g., Figure 26.1). Symptoms that are most central in any community make logical targets for therapeutic interventions. Using this analytic method,

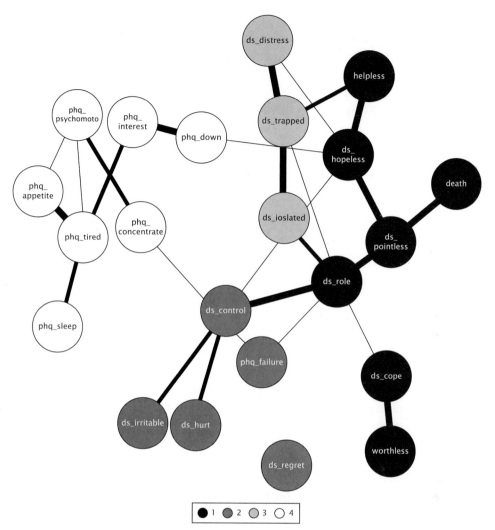

FIGURE 26.1 Exploratory graph analysis using 10,000 bootstrap iterations of the R program to display the median network of demoralization and depression symptoms clustering into four communities. There are 22 symptoms displayed here, derived from 1,527 patients with cancer. Each symptom is located in the community it is strongly associated with, where the strength of association between symptoms is represented by the thickness of the line joining it to other symptoms. Where symptoms only have a weak association, the linking line has been deleted for ease of representation. The notation of phq ahead of any symptom indicates its origin from the Patient Health Questionnaire-9 (PHQ-9) measure for depression, while the notation of ds ahead of a symptom indicates its origin from the Demoralization Scale-II. A latent symptom derived from one or more overlapping symptoms lacks either phq or ds preceding the symptom name (e.g., death, helpless, or worthless). Community 1 = pointlessness and hopelessness; Community 2 = loss of control; Community 3 = entrapment and isolation; Community 4 = anhedonic depression.

four communities emerged. First, anhedonic and depressive symptoms, as found in the PHQ-9 measure, formed a discrete community, confirming a distinct separation of depression from demoralization. Demoralization symptoms formed three communities, reflecting (1) loss of purpose/point and hope, (2) entrapment and distress, and (3) loss of control.[13]

The location of death wishes/suicidal ideation in the symptom map was very revealing. It was closely aligned in a cluster with pointlessness, purposelessness, and hopelessness and quite remotely located away from the depression symptoms.[13] Second, entrapment is closely associated with distress and is a very central symptom, suggesting its importance as a therapeutic target. Third, the most central symptoms in this overall network analysis were pointlessness, discouragement, hopelessness, and entrapment—key targets for interventions to address.

Given the strength of findings identified in the network analysis, we replicated the approach on the German cancer dataset of more than 1,500 patients. Findings were effectively identical (see Figure 26.1). Again, depressive symptoms sit in a very separate community, confirming their distinctness from demoralization symptoms. Second, suicidal thoughts are strongly associated with pointlessness and hopelessness. Third, the central symptoms in the demoralization communities are hopelessness, pointlessness, loss of role, and entrapment.

Differential Diagnoses

The key differential diagnoses include

- *Major depressive episode*, where persistent and pervasive anhedonia occurs over 2 or more weeks, with loss of interest and pleasure associated with low mood, reduced motivation, poor concentration, insomnia, lethargy, anorexia, weight loss, loss of libido, diurnal variation, guilt, and slowness of thoughts or activity, potentially culminating in suicidal thoughts
- *Agitated depression*, where noteworthy agitation and restlessness accompanies the major depressive episode
- *Major depression with melancholia*, where profound sleep disturbance with early awakening, mental slowing, marked diurnal variation, and very severe anhedonia lead to deep feelings of despair; The DSM thus uses melancholia as a specifier for the severity of the depressive episode.
- *Psychotic depression,* where thoughts of nihilism, a belief that one's body is dead, conviction that it is all over, or delusional beliefs of a paranoid nature develop in association with the clinical depression. The DSM again uses "with psychotic features" as a specifier.
- *Dysthymia*, where chronic unhappiness prevails across 2 or more years, spoiling quality of life, relationships, work, and life in general. It is hard to experience joy because pessimism, gloominess, and complaints prevail.
- *Anxiety disorders*, where generalized worry, panic attacks, agoraphobia, specific phobias (e.g., needle or magnetic resonance imaging tunnel phobia) or social anxiety develop.
- *Acute stress disorder* or *posttraumatic stress disorder* develop where the illness has been experienced as a trauma, and flashbacks, nightmares, and avoidance of cues start to dominate the clinical picture.
- *Organic affective disorders* and depression due to medical illness develop when thyroid disorders, parathyroid tumors, cortisol dysfunction, cytokine cascades, medication effects (steroids, chemotherapy), and paraneoplastic syndromes complicate the medical illness.

- *Comorbid mental states*, with mixed anxiety-depressive disorders or major depression with demoralization, complicate the clarity of presentations. The overlap of symptoms may make a clear-cut diagnosis difficult. Studies have shown that severe mental illness, such as a major depression, may lead to loss of morale and poor coping, so that demoralization develops on top of the depressive disorder. Alternatively, an initial mental state of moderate demoralization may persist and act as a harbinger for the development of major depression. Thus, whenever severe depression develops, symptoms of severe demoralization are likely to coexist in such patients.

This list of differentials is not exhaustive, but only captures the more common mental states—see other chapters in this book for further information. Because in this chapter we have defined demoralization as a form of adjustment disorder, including where a specifier "with demoralization" might be used, we have not added adjustment disorder to the list of differentials. If clinicians stuck to a strict DSM definition of adjustment disorder, then it could form yet another differential diagnosis of demoralization.[14]

Nonetheless, attention is needed to the health literacy and ethnic background of each patient if we are to understand the meaning of the illness, its treatment, and related perceptions of prognosis. How wounded or damaged is the body? How dire is the predicament? What illness expectations come from the family and its traditions? How is such an illness dealt with according to the customs of each culture? In this sense, a comprehensive understanding of each patient, their developmental journey, and their family of origin is desirable to make sense of where they are at in the illness trajectory and what this means personally to them.

Instruments to Measure Demoralization

Instruments to measure demoralization are set out in Table 26.1. From the early insight that Dohrenwend and colleagues had in 1980, in measuring nonspecific distress in the community, to the sterling work of Fava's group from 1995 in studying psychosomatic conditions affecting the medically ill, the systematic measurement of demoralization established its prominence and significance as a diagnostic condition. The DS was translated into more than 15 languages and saw a burgeoning of empirical studies highlighting its prominence. In the process, refinement and validation of this measure across cultures revealed the striking prevalence of this clinical syndrome and its association with wellness, quality of life, social support, and the will to live.[7] There have been repeated calls to incorporate the construct into the phenomenology of adjustment disorder within the ICD of the World Health Organization or as a specifier for both adjustment disorder and major depression with the DSM of the American Psychiatric Association.[1,5,8]

This work is now maturing into two directions. First, within psycho-oncology research, collaborative studies are under way in Germany and Australia to validate a diagnostic interview for adjustment disorder with demoralization. Second, in Australia, studies of screening for existential distress using the Psycho-existential Symptom Assessment Scale (PeSAS) are examining the contribution that better recognition of existential distress makes to clinical outcomes and the amelioration of suffering in the palliative care setting.[15]

TABLE 26.1 Instruments to measure demoralization

Instrument		Nature and role of measure
Psychiatric Epidemiological Research Interview, Demoralization. (Dohrenwend et al., 1980)[19]	PERI-D	27-item self-report, 5-point response format, 8 dimensions, concurrent validity with Center for Epidemiologic Studies Depression Scale (CES-D), high reliability coefficients, assesses symptoms across prior year.
Diagnostic Criteria for Psychosomatic Research, Demoralization module (Fava et al., 1995)[2]	DCPR	Structured interview with 5 items, yes-no response format, part of longer 58 item interview for 12 psychosomatic syndromes. Emphasis on failed expectations and inability to cope. Assesses symptoms over 1 month. Shows level of coping with illness stress of a chronic nature.
Minnesota Multiphasic Personality Inventory-II, Demoralization Scale (Tellegen et al., 2003)[20]	MMPI-II-D	Overarching latent factor of demoralization was extracted from earlier versions; general distress measure linked to hopeless-helpless, low self-esteem, and inefficacy. Affects of poor coping distinct from personality traits and responsive to treatments of depression.
Demoralization Scale (Kissane et al., 2004)[3]	DS	24-item, self-report, quantitative scale, 5-point Likert response, 5 factors, Cronbach's $\alpha = 0.94$, sound concurrent and divergent validity, translated into 15+ languages. Assesses symptoms over past 2 weeks. Contains existential component of loss of meaning and purpose.
Subjective Incompetence Scale (Cockram et al., 2009)[21]	SCS	12-item, self-report, unidimensional scale, Cronbach's $\alpha = 0.90$, measures incompetence.
Demoralization Scale-II (Robinson et al., 2016)[22]	DS-II	16-item, 3-point response scale, 2x8-item factors, refined validation using item response analysis. Strong convergent and discriminant validity. Sound test-retest and Cronbach's $\alpha = 0.89$. Measure of change in intervention studies.
Demoralization Scale-Short version (Belvederi Murri et al., 2020)[11]	DS-6	6-item short version with comparable Area-under-the Curve (0.81), Sensitivity (75.7%) and Specificity (71.7%) to the 24-item original DS in achieving a DCPR diagnosis of demoralization.
Psycho-existential Symptom Assessment Scale (Kissane, 2020)[13]	PeSAS	10-item Visual Analogue Scale, symptom rating measure modeled on the Edmonton Symptom Assessment Scale, used for screening and monitoring change in psycho-existential symptoms during palliative care.

Management

Recognizing the presence of a core set of symptoms in the demoralized patient is the starting point in management. Routine screening with the PeSAS ensures that this mental state is not overlooked.[13] Empathic responsiveness is a basic skill as the presence of such symptoms is acknowledged.

When mild levels of discouragement and hopelessness are present, brief interventions have long been used to counter negative existential postures and restore hope. In settings where some bad news has been heard, prognosis may have been misunderstood, or physical symptom control has temporarily lapsed but can be restored, encouragement and support using supportive counselling will prove helpful. The clinician reinterprets any misunderstanding and functions as the source of hope, promoting optimism, determination, and courage as sources of resilient strength.

More moderate levels of demoralization are commonly precipitated by cumulative bad news and disease progression and less supportive communication, and they are accompanied by greater grief. The patient may be predisposed to this response by limited social support and more isolation, with symptoms perpetuated by pessimism that may derive from habitual negative automatic thoughts. Coping styles that are avoidant, passive, insecure and anxious, indecisive, involve ruminating worry, and leave the person feeling stuck in a predicament they cannot solve contribute to this demoralization. Therefore, the clinician's therapeutic stance may name the grief, empathically acknowledge the struggle, rally a sense of support, and point to more constructive cognitions that can displace catastrophizing attention to worst-case scenarios. Patients will vary in the themes that predominate, with the clinician flexibly responding to uncertainty, anticipatory grief, fear of the future, sense of unfairness, feeling a burden, aloneness, spiritual anguish, or loss of self-worth. Rather than being helped by a brief intervention, continuity of care is called for as some three to four sessions of counseling will be needed.

Severe demoralization warrants careful assessment for comorbid states of anxiety and depression, as psychotropic medication will be indicated when they coexist with demoralization (see Chapters 4 and 5 for the management of depression and anxiety, respectively). Severe demoralization can also present as an adjustment disorder, where poor coping with a stressor event is central, without anhedonia or anxiety coexisting. Here the management is essentially psychotherapeutic. Meaning-centered psychotherapies represent a group of existentially oriented interventions that respond to the loss of hope, meaning, and purpose present in severe demoralization. For example, as a secondary outcome assessed in the randomized controlled trial of CALM therapy (Managing Cancer and Living Meaningfully), for those CALM participants who presented with moderate death anxiety at baseline on the Death and Dying Distress Scale, their DS scores fell significantly by 6 months (DS change score 6.24 [95% CI 1.54 to 10.93, d = 0. 50, p = 0.01]).[16]

A core symptom that needs to be targeted in the treatment of demoralization is entrapment. Here a sense of "stuckness" typically arises from an illness rather than whole-of-life orientation, where the illness has been designated incurable, nonresponsive to anti-cancer treatments, and likely to progress to organ failure. The clinical predicament appears dire and unsolvable in terms of problem-based coping. Yet if death is an inevitable human outcome for all, a sole focus on the illness creates grief, despair, and suffering. As Yalom taught, the only reason to look death in the face is to embrace life more fully.[17] Hence, despite the illness predicament, there are still relationships to engage with, celebrations to join, life to feel fulfilled by, and meaningful activities to be pursued. The living remains meaningful until death intervenes. The therapeutic stance of the clinician is a metacognitive one as she invites the patient to revise this orientation from one of entrapment to a freedom to choose, be, and live in the present—to sustain Frankl's "will to meaning" until the end.

Another cluster of core symptoms includes hopelessness, pointlessness, and a desire to die. When loss of the meaning or purpose of life develops, life's value diminishes and culminates in suicidal thinking unless a more generalized philosophy of life can be called upon to sustain this sense of purpose. Similarly, when hopelessness worsens, it is a background sense of generalized hope that empowers a person to hope in the here-and-now, with short-term agendas becoming the focus. Attention to the coherent narrative of where an individual's sense of fulfilment and meaning lies, what role has been most precious, what relationships most beautiful, and what beliefs and philosophy most enduring offer a therapeutic pathway to recapture hope and meaning. These need to be the target to address these core symptoms.

A third cluster of core symptoms include social isolation, loss of control, and sense of failure. Levels of interpersonal sensitivity and emotional dysregulation may contribute to this cluster and be more amenable to approaches found in cognitively oriented and emotionally focused therapies. At a practical level, social connectedness may be enhanced with volunteers and helplessness with services and community resources, while affirmation of the dignity and worth of each person is always crucial. The general factors common to all psychotherapies remain important.

In the spirit of Jerome Frank's emphasis on restoring morale, Griffith and Gaby pointed to the method of countering negative existential postures of vulnerability by redirecting the patient toward more constructive coping strategies.[18] An expanded list of these postures are displayed in Table 26.2. The clinician adopts a supportive stance and employs gentle education, listening, empathic acknowledgment, and some reassurance and encouragement as explanation is offered about the clinical journey, with reality testing about

TABLE 26.2 Existential postures of vulnerability and constructive stances that enhance coping[a]

Vulnerability	Resilience
Low morale and discouragement	Fight and confidence
Uncertainty and bewilderment	Coherent direction across lifespan
Isolation and aloneness	Connected and supported
Despair and hopelessness	Optimism and hope
Helplessness, feeling trapped	Agency and mastery
Pointlessness and meaninglessness	Purpose and meaning
Cowardice and fear	Courage and determination
Resentment and anger	Gratitude and acceptance
Loss of control	Planning and action
Loss of roles	Directedness to the other
Spiritual angst, guilt, and regret	Valuing the sacred and acceptance
Desire to die and suicidal thoughts	Engagement with living

[a] This list is modeled on Griffith and Gaby,[18] who originally listed the following seven vulnerable postures: confusion, isolation, despair, helplessness, meaninglessness, cowardice, and resentment.

what is happening and what the future will hold. Adaptive responses need to be affirmed, drawing on the strengths of each individual as they are invited to adopt a more resilient stance. When pessimistic or catastrophizing attitudes prevail, the person can be invited to consider their impact on coping. Might a more balanced response be possible? This direction needs to be realistic, and so the evaluation of any attitude is less about rationality and more about what would be helpful. The clinician searches for a resilient attitude that can lead to courage and peace, and contentment with a wholesome life, albeit one that is never perfect.

Future Directions

The routine assessment and management of existential distress has long been neglected in palliative care. Demoralization provides a strong framework to redress this. Routine screening would identify patients of concern. More intervention studies are needed to better define therapeutic techniques, necessary dose of therapy, and key symptoms to be targeted so that services may confidently address the substantial suffering that occurs among patients who struggle to cope with existential realities at the end of life.

Key Points

- The phenomenology of demoralization offers a strong set of diagnostic criteria for adjustment disorders, wherein low morale and poor coping are associated with a sense of entrapment, hopelessness and helplessness, loss of role, and pointlessness, culminating in a desire to die.
- Demoralization forms an apt "specifier" for adjustment disorder in diagnostic classifications such as the DSM; thus, adjustment disorder with demoralization.
- Conceptualized as maladaptive coping which can be comorbid with a range of mental states including affective and psychotic disorders, the phenomena of demoralization can be commonly found in psychiatrically ill patients.
- Suicidal ideation and desire for death are located among the demoralization symptom communities, with desire for death being strongly associated with symptoms of pointlessness and hopelessness and remote from the neurovegetative symptoms of anhedonia.
- Symptom network analyses of the symptoms of depression and demoralization reveal a clear differentiation wherein the symptoms of depression form a distinct community quite separate from the symptoms of low morale, poor coping, and demoralization.
- Centrally located symptoms in the hub of a network community are key therapeutic targets. Entrapment is one target as it induces the loss of control, helplessness, and defeat that powerfully lower morale. Hopelessness, pointlessness, and loss of roles make up another set of core symptoms appropriately targeted to counter demoralization.
- Meaning-centered psychotherapies appear central to counter the existential angst present among demoralized patients. For instance, CALM therapy delivered to patients with

high death anxiety at baseline achieved a significant amelioration of demoralization at 6 months (effect size = 0.5, p = 0.01).

References

1. Kissane DW, Clarke DM, Street AF. Demoralization syndrome: A relevant psychiatric diagnosis for palliative care. *J Palliat Care*. 2001;17(1):12–21.
2. Fava GA, Freyberger HJ, Bech P, Christodoulou G, Sensky T, Theorell T, et al. Diagnostic criteria for use in psychosomatic research. *Psychother Psychosom*. 1995;63(1):1–8.
3. Kissane DW, Wein S, Love A, Lee XQ, Kee PL, Clarke DM. The Demoralization Scale: A preliminary report of its development and preliminary validation. *J Palliat Care*. 2004;20(4):269–276.
4. Robinson S, Kissane DW, Brooker J, Burney S. A systematic review of the Demoralization syndrome in individuals with progressive disease and cancer: A decade of research. *J Pain Sympt Manage*. 2015;49(3):595–610.
5. Kissane DW. Demoralization: A life-preserving diagnosis to make in the severely medically ill. *J Palliat Care*. 2014;30(4):255–258.
6. Robinson S, Kissane DW, Brooker J, Burney S. A review of the construct of demoralization: History, definitions, and future directions for palliative care. *Am J Hospice Palliat Med*. 2016;33(1):93–101.
7. de Figueiredo JM, Frank JD. Subjective incompetence, the clinical hallmark of demoralization. *Comprehens Psychiatry*. 1982;23:53–63.
8. Grassi L, Nanni MG. Demoralization syndrome: New insights in psychosocial cancer care. *Cancer*. 2016;122(14):2130–133.
9. Kissane DW, Bobevski I, Gaitanis P, Brooker J, Michael N, Lethborg C, et al. Exploratory examination of the utility of demoralization as a diagnostic specifier for adjustment disorder and major depression. *Gen Hosp Psychiatry*. 2017;46(5):20–24.
10. Vehling S, Kissane DW, Lo C, Glaesmer H, Hartung TJ, Rodin G, et al. The association of demoralization with mental disorders and suicidal ideation in patients with cancer. *Cancer*. 2017;123(17):3394–401.
11. Bobevski I, Kissane DW, Vehling S, McKenzie D, Glaesmer H, Mehnert A. Latent class analysis differentiation of adjustment disorder and demoralization, more severe depressive-anxiety disorders, and somatic symptoms in a cohort of patients with cancer. *Psycho-Oncology*. 2018;27(11):2623–30.
12. Belvederi Murri M, Zerbinati L, Ounalli H, Kissane D, Casoni B, Leoni M, et al. Assessing demoralization in medically ill patients: Factor structure of the Italian version of the demoralization scale and development of short versions with the item response theory framework. *J Psychosom Res*. 2020;128(1):109889
13. Belvederi Murri M, Caruso R, Ounalli H, Zerbinati L, Berretti E, Costa S, et al. The relationship between demoralization and depressive symptoms among patients from the general hospital: Network and exploratory graph analysis. *J Affect Dis*. 2020;276:137–146.
14. de Figueiredo JM. Distress, demoralization and psychopathology: Diagnostic boundaries. *Eur J Psychiatry*. 2013;27:61–73.
15. Kissane DW. Education and assessment of psycho-existential symptoms to prevent suicidality in cancer care. *Psycho-Oncology* 2020;29(9): PMID: 33463852
16. Rodin G, Lo C, Rydall A, Shnall J, Malfitano C, Chiu A, et al. Managing Cancer and Living Meaningfully (CALM): A randomized controlled trial of a psychological intervention for patients with advanced cancer. *J Clin Oncol*. 2018;36(23):2422–2432.
17. Yalom ID. *Existential Psychotherapy*. New York: Basic Books, 1980.
18. Griffith JL, Gaby L. Brief psychotherapy at the bedside: Countering demoralization from medical illness. *Psychosomatics*. 2005;46(2):109–116.
19. Dohrenwend BP, Shrout PE, Egri G, Mendelsohn FS. Non-specific psychological distress and other measures for use in the general population. *Arch Gen Psychiatry* 1980;37:1229–1236.

20. Tellegen A, Ben-Porath YS, Sellbom M, Arbisi PA, McNulty JL, Graham JR. *The MMPI-2 Restructured Clinical (RC) Scales*. Minneapolis: University of Minnesota Press; 2003.

21. Cockram CA, Doros G, de Figueiredo JM. Diagnosis and measurement of subjective incompetence: The clinical hallmark of demoralization. *Psychother Psychosom* 2009;78:342–345.

22. Robinson S, Kissane DW, Brooker J, Michael N, Fischer J, Franco M, et al. Refinement and revalidation of the Demoralization Scale: The DS-II, internal validity. *Cancer*, 2016;122:2251–2259; and external validity, 2260–2267.

27

Interprofessional Spiritual Care in Palliative Care

Christina Puchalski, Betty R. Ferrell, Vanessa Battista, Elisha Waldman, and Richard W. Bauer

Spiritual Care as a Key Aspect of Palliative Care

Palliative care is often referred to as "whole-person care," with the aim of relieving pain and suffering across the physical, emotional, psychosocial, and spiritual continuum.[1] The World Health Organization (WHO) was one of the first entities to define palliative care as "an approach that improves the quality of life of patients and their families facing the problems associated with life-threatening illness through the prevention and relief of suffering by means of early identification and impeccable assessment and treatment of pain and other problems, physical, psychosocial, and spiritual."[2] "From its inception, spirituality has been at the core of the definition of whole-person palliative care."[3 (p. 428)]

An increasing amount of evidence supports that individuals living with serious and/or life-threatening illness or facing the end of life, and their families, may discover "an intensified desire to access and enrich the spiritual aspect of their lives."[3] The National Consensus Project (NCP) for Quality of Palliative Care has identified spiritual, religious, and existential care as one of the eight essential domains of quality care. The NCP guidelines define spirituality as "the aspect of humanity that refers to the way individuals seek and express meaning and purpose and the way they experience their connectedness to the moment, to self, to others, to nature and to the significant or sacred."[4] The National Comprehensive Cancer Network has shown an increase in patient satisfaction with medical care related to "religiousness and spiritual support."[5 (p. 724)] Also, spiritual distress has been associated with "poor physical outcomes and higher rates of morbidity,"[5 (p. 724)] with a lack of spirituality leading to "greater emotional distress, higher indices of pain and fatigue, increased burden of illness, and a lower quality of life"[5 (p. 725)] in patients living with serious illness.

Palliative care is intended to be delivered by an interdisciplinary team (IDT) and involves the use of "comprehensive and thoroughly researched assessments and treatments for spiritual, physical, and psychosocial symptoms."[5] Currently, there is increased recognition that spirituality or spiritual care has evolved to encompass participation by all members of the IDT. Given the well-documented positive effects of spiritual health on overall health outcomes, the clinical relevance of providing spiritual care by all members of the interdisciplinary palliative care team, and providing them with the proper training to do so, is becoming more widely accepted and embraced. Many palliative care teams include chaplains; it is essential that members of the IDT work collaboratively to ensure that thorough spiritual assessment and adequate spiritual care are a part of routine evaluation and comprehensive care. Referral to or involvement of community spiritual resources should also be an important component of spiritual assessment and care.

Comprehensive palliative care, including a spiritual assessment, should be offered to all individuals living with life-threatening disease, and their families, and it should be tailored to the individual's chronologic and developmental age and ability. The American Academy of Pediatrics (AAP) has deemed that palliative care should be made available to all children who could benefit from it,[6] and it should include spiritual care as a core component, and "addresses the practices, beliefs, objects, and relationships that families turn to for help in times of crisis or concern."[7]

Addressing Spirituality at the End of Life

Spiritual care becomes especially important when an individual is nearing the end of life, as spirituality is "closely related to culture and encompasses religious beliefs as well as a broad array of dimensions including meaning, a sense of purpose, hope, and connection."[8] Spiritual distress is significant in advanced illness and is an important component of the dying process; therefore, there is a need for individuals receiving palliative care to experience "meaning-oriented and spiritual care interventions."[9] Spiritual well-being and identifying meaning in life seem to be "protective factors" against this distress.[9]

Comprehensive spiritual assessments should be included as part of palliative care, with a focus on "skilled expert therapeutic communication" between patients and members of the healthcare team so that therapeutic relationships can be maintained, and patients may experience a sense of control and meaning-making in the "complete dying process."[10] In the words of Dame Cicely Saunders, founder of the modern hospice movement, "Where a desolate sense of meaninglessness is encountered by the person at the end of life, one finds the essence of 'spiritual pain.'"[11] The recognition of the importance of addressing spiritual care as an essential component of palliative care has never been more important than it is now. The coronavirus pandemic has highlighted the urgent need for palliative care not only for individuals dying from the disease, but also for their families and community members and the providers caring for them.[11] Now, more than ever, there is a "need to recommit to spiritual care as an essential component of whole-person palliative care."[12 (p. e7)]

Interdisciplinary Palliative Care: The Roles of Spiritual Care Specialists and Generalists

The field of palliative care began as an extension of hospice care devoted to the end of life as both the public and healthcare professionals recognized the need for earlier integration of the core principles of hospice in serious illness. One of the core precepts of hospice was interdisciplinary care, creating a model for various disciplines to contribute separately but also collaboratively to provide patient- and family-focused care. As palliative care has evolved, new models of care have emerged demonstrating the value of care which incorporates the complex needs of patients and families across dimensions of psychological, social, and spiritual needs.

Role of the Spiritual Care Specialist

Concurrent with the evolution of the field of palliative care, healthcare professionals have recognized the importance of the role of chaplains and other spiritual care providers. Chaplains are increasingly included as core members of the IDT with increased recognition of their role in patient care, family support, and staff support. From time of diagnosis of serious illness through bereavement care for families, quality care is enhanced by inclusion of and leadership by chaplains.

The role of chaplains has not previously been well understood. Recent advances have helped to increase understanding of the role of chaplaincy at a time when there has been a recognition of the need for palliative care to serve diverse communities, including those with no religious affiliations. There has also been increased recognition of the relationship between spiritual care needs and psychosocial needs.[13] For example, patient symptoms such as depression or anxiety are often associated with sources of spiritual distress, yet without spiritual assessment they may be ignored. Also, there is growing recognition of the need for chaplains to train other team members in spiritual assessment and care.[14]

There is an increasing awareness of the role of chaplains in supporting and providing spiritual care for the often overwhelmed clinician members of the team. The COVID pandemic made evident the need for frontline clinicians to be knowledgeable in spiritual care as they faced overwhelming numbers of severely ill patients, deaths, and personal risk of illness or death. The role of chaplains at the time of death, in communicating with families and in the monumental support of beleaguered staff, was evident.

Role of the Spiritual Care Generalist

The concept of "generalist versus specialist" is a standard in most clinical practice. A primary care clinician may treat depression but recognizes when she needs the expertise of psychiatrists, for example. Similarly, in palliative care, clinicians whose practice focuses on serious illness populations should also have a basic palliative care knowledge base and skill set to integrate spiritual care into patient care.[15] All clinicians should therefore address spiritual needs with patients. Some clinicians may feel hesitant to explore spiritual needs, worried that they lack the language or ability to engage around these issues. While non-specialists should be thoughtful about limitations and boundaries, there are incredibly valuable contributions to be made by non-specialists, especially in attending to the suffering of another. Educating clinicians in generalist spiritual care is a necessary step in operationalizing spiritual care. Any clinician caring for patients and families facing serious illness should have a basic comfort with and knowledge of spiritual care issues and how to refer to a chaplain or other spiritual care specialist for complex cases. Without that comfort level, the number of multidisciplinary providers available to help integrate spiritual care into whole-patient and family care shrinks, leaving patients unable to have their spiritual needs addressed within their clinical care. The intention of the specialist–generalist approach is to extend spiritual care to all patients, referring to the spiritual care specialist to provide a deeper level of spiritual counseling and care which might also include rituals and practices.

Case Example

The following case example illustrates the need for spiritual care in palliative care and the roles of all IDT members.

Spiritual Care

Pedro Garcia was a 74-year-old man from Guatemala living alone in low-income housing in an urban area. He was diagnosed with advanced pancreatic cancer and had severe pain and GI symptoms upon his first visit to the county hospital oncology clinic. Pedro and the medical oncologist agreed that chemotherapy was not recommended due to his numerous other medical problems and very advanced disease. Pedro was referred to palliative care, where he was evaluated by a physician, nurse, and social worker, and several interventions were implemented to control his severe pain and nausea. A week later, the palliative care clinic nurse confirmed his symptoms were controlled and the team had prioritized his visit to be with a social worker who could begin to better understand his psychosocial needs, assess for strengths and supports, and explore end-of-life care options since his death was imminent and he lived alone. The social worker's assessment included spirituality, and Pedro reported that he "used to be Catholic"; he strongly asserted that he did not want to see a chaplain.

Over the next 3 weeks, Pedro was seen in the outpatient palliative care clinic, and each team member including the social worker, nurse, and physician, addressed his numerous concerns, including escalating pain, weight loss, depression, and nausea. He often mentioned God ("God, help this pain," "God, take me soon"), and, as he became closer to and more trusting of the palliative care team, he also spoke of his fear of death, estrangement from family, and the belief his pain was punishment for "many bad decisions." The palliative care team began the process of arranging placement in an inpatient hospice setting, but a bed was not yet available.

The palliative care nurse was called to the emergency department (ED) one day because Pedro had arrived by ambulance after being found by a neighbor who realized Pedro had not left his home for several days. Severely dehydrated and weak, Pedro told the nurse he knew he would die soon. The nurse told Pedro that the social worker was arranging for transfer to inpatient hospice, and she also told Pedro that often, as patients face approaching death, they may decide they would like to see a chaplain. Pedro said he had "been praying a lot lately" and yes, he would like to see a chaplain now.

The chaplain met with Pedro in the ED and again for the next 2 days before a bed was available at the hospice facility. The palliative care team communicated with the hospice about their care for Pedro, and the hospice chaplain agreed to visit him on admission. Pedro was discharged to hospice and died 1 week later.

Integrating Spiritual Care into Clinical Care

There are two main pillars to the operationalization of spiritual care. One is creating space for the work of a spiritual care specialist. This requires deliberately and thoughtfully creating opportunities for early and ongoing engagement with a spiritual specialist. If available, a spiritual specialist should engage with every patient and family facing serious illness early on, at least once.

The second pillar to the operationalization of spiritual care is to routinely integrate spiritual care by generalists and specialists into regular assessment and the formulation of care plans as well as rounds. Integrating spiritual care into the routine care of patients and families must be a joint effort between the clinicians, as spiritual care generalists, and the spiritual care specialists. Follow-up by both generalists and specialists on spiritual distress should be dictated in part by need, but should also include regular check-ins to see if new needs arise.

In addressing spiritual needs in both adult and pediatric palliative care, having an actual plan is critical. While providers should be prepared for and open to spontaneous discussions with patients and families, ready to follow where those discussions might lead, using a structured assessment and treatment/care plan model is critical so that spirituality is not completely overlooked. If spiritual distress is identified, it must be addressed as urgently as physical pain or depression.

Three major consensus conferences on improving the spiritual domains of palliative care[16] and whole-person care[17] developed process models for implementing interprofessional spiritual care in both the inpatient and outpatient settings through national and global consensus models. The model is based on the generalist-specialist model and on the biopsychosocial and spiritual model which serves as the foundation for palliative care. The process model for inpatient spiritual care, with modifications to include the role of multiple clinicians from the beginning, is portrayed in Figure 27.1.

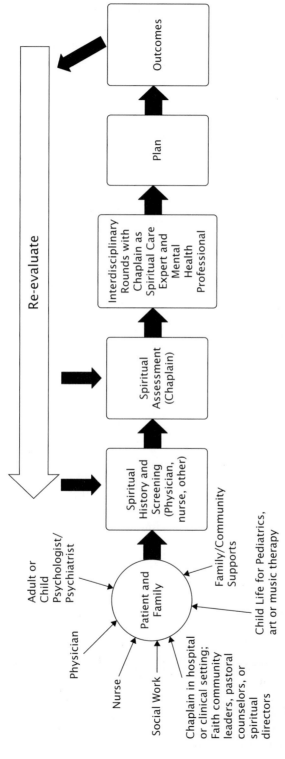

FIGURE 27.1 Integration of spiritual care into whole-patient care across settings. Adapted from Puchalski C, Ferrell B, Virani R, et al. Improving the quality of spiritual care as a dimension of palliative care: the report of the Consensus Conference. *J Palliat Med.* 2009;12(10):885–904.

It is important to note in this model that spiritual care is an iterative process and not a one-time intervention. The process is dependent on multidisciplinary participation, with providers alternately exploring spiritual health, including spiritual needs on their own with their patients as well as in collaboration with one another, to share insights and formulate plans. This also highlights the importance of including all members of the clinical care team, including psychosocial clinicians such as social workers and psychologists/psychiatrists.

Spiritual Screening, History-Taking, and Assessment

There are three main types of spiritual assessments: spiritual screening, history-taking, and assessment. Spiritual screening provides initial information about a patient in spiritual emergencies (i.e., spiritual distress which needs attention by a trained chaplain) or for referral to an in-depth spiritual assessment. The spiritual history is a more in-depth inquiry which clinicians who do the clinical assessment and plan use. Spiritual assessment done by chaplains is an in-depth, ongoing process of evaluating the spiritual needs and resources of patients. A professional chaplain listens to a patient's story to understand the patient's needs and resources. Various models of spiritual assessment are continually being developed. The first such model was the 7×7 model, which is an important model for spiritual assessment used by chaplains and that was developed by a team of Rush chaplains and nursing faculty. This model explicitly places spiritual assessment in the context of a holistic assessment and employs a multidimensional, contextual approach to a spiritual assessment including medical, psychological, and spiritual domains. [18]

The Spiritual History

The spiritual history is used as part of the clinical history to assess for spiritual health, including spiritual wellness and spiritual distress as part of the patient's total health. It affords the patient the space and opportunity to share what matters most to them, as well as their suffering, despair, or hopelessness. It enables the clinician to connect with the patient on a deeply caring level while helping identify spiritual distress. The clinician can then begin to treat the patient's spiritual distress through compassionate presence and reflective listening and by referral to spiritual care professionals for more in-depth assessment and treatment. The spiritual history is taken during the history of present illness or social history depending on the context of the visit. A review of symptoms should also include questions about spiritual or existential distress such as meaninglessness, despair, hopelessness, or religious or spiritual struggle.

Regardless of the results of the spiritual screening, clinicians should take a spiritual history to understand the patient's spiritual needs and resources . There are several spiritual history tools that have been developed. One of these tools, the FICA[19] (see Table 27.1), a validated tool in clinical practice, is primarily a communication aid inviting the patient to share their spiritual beliefs and values with their clinician but also affording the clinician the opportunity to assess for spiritual health including spiritual distress.

TABLE 27.1 FICA Spiritual History Tool

F - Faith, Belief, Meaning	"Do you consider yourself to be spiritual?" or "Is spirituality something important to you?" "Do you have spiritual beliefs, practices, or values that help you to cope with stress, difficult times?" or "What you are going through right now?" "What gives your life meaning?"
I - Importance and Influence	"What importance does spirituality have in your life?" "Has your spirituality influenced how you take care of yourself, particularly regarding your health?" "Does your spirituality affect your healthcare decision-making?"
C - Community	"Are you part of a spiritual community?" "Is your community of support to you and how?" For people who don't identify with a community consider asking "Is there a group of people you really love or who are important to you?" (Communities such as churches, temples, mosques, family, groups of like-minded friends, or yoga or similar groups can serve as strong support systems for some patients)
A - Address/Action in Care	"How would you like me, as your healthcare provider, to address spiritual issues in your healthcare?" *(With newer models, including the diagnosis of spiritual distress, "A" also refers to the "Assessment and Plan" for patient spiritual distress, needs, and/or resources within a treatment or care plan.)*

© Copyright Christina Puchalski, MD, 1996 (updated 2021).

The FICA tool is based on four domains of spiritual assessment: the presence of *Faith*, belief, or meaning; the *Importance* of spirituality in an individual's life and the influence that a belief system or values has on the person's healthcare decision-making; the individual's spiritual *Community*; and interventions to *Address* spiritual needs.[18] The spiritual history is performed as part of the social or personal history of the patient and should be done routinely as part of the initial intake evaluation.

For children, especially younger children, and adolescents, comprehensive assessment of spiritual beliefs, values, and practices may include assessment of parents and/or siblings as well. FICA can be used for parents and for adolescents.

Whole-Person Assessment and Treatment Plan

Once a clinician takes a spiritual history and identifies spiritual distress and spiritual resources of strength, this information is integrated into a bio-psychosocial-spiritual treatment plan. The clinician must attend to spiritual distress with the same urgency as any other distress. Patients with moderate or severe spiritual distress or with religious-specific needs should be referred to the trained chaplain. Minimal or mild spiritual distress may be attended to by the clinicians on the team or referral to other modalities, including art therapy, meaning-oriented therapy, or meditation. If the patient identifies specific spiritual or religious practices that are important to them, then encouraging those practices might be appropriate. These may include reconnecting with nature, prayer, meditation, community support, or rituals. All issues, whether simple or complex, should be documented in the patient's chart and shared with the patient's healthcare team.

Case Example

Katie was a 30-year-old woman with a history of childhood abuse and depression. In college, she was not able to function well because she drank too much alcohol. She sought therapy and attended a residential treatment center. After completing treatment, she returned to college and graduated with a degree in art therapy. She was recently diagnosed with breast cancer and is planning to see the surgeon and oncologist next week. She told her physician that she was "down," wondering why this was happening to her. She had overcome so much suffering in her childhood and chose art therapy as a profession because she wanted to help people. She had insomnia and decreased appetite. She denied suicidal ideation but felt so down sometimes that it was hard for her to get out of bed in the morning. She reported having "pain in the soul."

Her FICA spiritual history:

- F: Her parents were Christian, and, as a young child, she went to church regularly with them. Once her mother found out that an uncle abused Katie and her younger sister, the parents stopped going to church. Meditation and other practices have been very important to her. She attends 12-step meetings regularly. "I am searching right now for meaning in my life, I don't see a way out of this pain inside my soul. Why is this happening?"
- I: Her 12-step program is important and central to her life. "I don't want to go back to the place I was when I was drinking." She thinks about God because that was important to her as a child and wonders how she might begin to "understand God again."
- C: She has a strong spiritual community in AA and in a woman's support group.
- A: She asks her physician if there is a connection with how depressed she is feeling and her spirituality, but she does not know how to make the connection work for her right now.

Katie and her doctor formulated a plan of attending to her physical, emotional, social and spiritual issues.

Katie was a 30-yo-female with newly diagnosed breast cancer stage, depression, abuse, hypertension and alcoholism. She was currently sober and active in AA. Now presented with elevated hypertension. depression, and spiritual distress. Her elevated blood pressure was maybe secondary to anxiety and stress. She will be monitored at home, and we will adjust medications as needed. We discussed meditation practices, healthy nutrition, and exercise as tolerated. Her depression was likely situational but complicated by spiritual distress and significant past history of depression. Referral to psychiatry suggested. Socially, Katie had a good relationship with her mother and agreed to bring her mother to the next visit. She had significant spiritual distress, including existential distress, despair, questioning her understanding of God, and searching for meaning. Suggested referral to the chaplain, and meaning-oriented therapy as well as integrating her meditation practices into her daily activities.

Katie appreciated the time her physician took in listening to all her concerns and agreed with the recommendations. She expressed feeling supported by her physician and team. She planned to share more with her mother about her feelings and looked forward to the family meeting at the next visit. She agreed to set up appointments with the chaplain and psychiatrist and pursue meaning-oriented therapy.

Katie's case illustrates the essential role spirituality plays in the care of patients. She exhibited various aspects of spiritual distress, including despair, loss of meaning, desire for a search for meaning, and questions about her understanding of God in the setting of a traumatic childhood. Katie's care demonstrated the potential benefit of spiritual care, including an individual's ability to come to an understanding of their suffering at a deeper level, finding a source or sources of meaning and purpose, and perhaps reconnecting with a sense of transcendence or that which is sacred or significant in their life.

Addressing spiritual needs in both adult and pediatric palliative care and having an actual plan is critical. Using a communication tool such as the FICA spiritual history tool is a way to operationalize spiritual assessment so that spiritual issues are addressed routinely.

Spiritual Care for the Interprofessional Team

A growing body of literature highlights the role and impact of chaplains providing spiritual care and support to members of the interprofessional team. The professional board-certified chaplain is the member of the interprofessional palliative care team who highlights and focuses the team on the domain of spiritual care for both the patient and family and the team itself. This is more than religious care and may include moments of reflection, pause, ritual, and renewal to support the team in their shared values and vision of providing optimal palliative care.

The chaplain has been trained to deeply respect individual spiritual beliefs, practices, and experiences to provide spiritual care and support. When providing care for the interprofessional team, the chaplain must include respect for the spirituality of each individual as well as of the collective team. The chaplain can assist team members in reflecting on their own spirituality as well as that of the IDT's spirituality, or "collective soul."[19,20] It is the chaplain who often tries to give voice to the sacred and transcendent aspects of providing hospice and palliative care. Most certified chaplains report that, in addition to patient care, they also provide support to the IDT. Just as patients and families experience spiritual and existential distress in the midst of hospice and palliative care, so, too, may staff members experience distress or even compassion fatigue in the midst of their calling and vocation to serve and care for those with life-limiting illnesses.

Healthcare systems increasingly acknowledge the importance of clinical staff well-being for both optimal patient care and outcomes, as well as to reduce staff turnover and increase job satisfaction. This staff care and support often focuses only on physical and psychosocial distress and suffering. However, caring for the whole person means addressing the *spiritual* needs in both patient care and staff support.

King and colleagues[21] articulate four key areas that are essential for staff care. These include finding meaning and joy in work, addressing the accumulated grief from multiple patient deaths, providing closure with patients and families after leaving the palliative care service, and addressing stress for both emotional and spiritual well-being. If we understand spirituality and spiritual care as meaning, purpose, and connectedness, then each of these four areas has a spiritual dimension that can be addressed by the staff chaplain for the well-being of the entire team.

While the multiple roles, functions, and interventions of chaplains are well documented, Chaplain Rhonda Cooper stated, "the chaplain also has a peculiar role on the team, in that her most fundamental task is her intentional listening-and-hearing of the other person's story."[22] The palliative care clinician focuses so much of her time on really listening and hearing and being present to the patient, one must then ask, "who then, will listen to the clinician's story of providing care?" While this may involve any member of the interprofessional team, it is the expertise, vocation, and role of the professional chaplain to hear and honor each team member's story.

Many healthcare systems have integrated "the pause"[23] as an intervention following a patient death. This provides a solemn moment for staff who have cared for the patient to remember, honor, and acknowledge their work and compassion with this human being. "Chi time" or "tea for the soul" is an example of a chaplain-led intervention that provides an expanded "pause" for staff to be supported and silently reflect on the power and wonder of their vocation to care for others and to experience being served and cared for, often by the staff chaplain.

Daily spiritual experiences can mitigate the physical, emotional, and existential stress of working with death and dying on a continual basis. Chaplains integrated into the interprofessional palliative care team can provide not only moments of pause and reflection, but also ritual or readings of sacred texts or poetry that confirm and support the holy work of palliative care. The chaplain, knowing the individual members of the team, can incorporate rites and rituals from each member's spiritual or religious traditions that would be appropriate for group reflection, process, and grieving.

Many palliative care clinicians describe the sacred relationship between clinician and patient. Caring for patients and their families at the end of life is stressful. The chaplain acknowledges this aspect of care and serves as a beacon to remind and call staff members to care and support themselves and each member of the team, especially in the spiritual aspects of this work.

The chaplain is the one who can call each team member to recognize their deepest selves and the sacred, holy, and spiritual nature of caring for those with life-limiting illnesses and at the time of death. The spiritual aspect of our lives and work can serve as an energy to renew our vocation to service in healthcare and mitigate against the negative aspects of the daily stress of this work.

Conclusion

Spiritual care is an essential domain of palliative care. The essential way to operationalize spiritual care is for clinicians to routinely assess for and treat spiritual distress, working collaboratively with chaplains. While the evidence supports the integration of spiritual health in clinical care, models are needed to further create an evidence base for this field. Educating clinicians in generalist spiritual care is a necessary step in operationalizing spiritual care. One program, Interprofessional Spiritual Care Education Curriculum (ISPEC), serves as a standard curriculum that can educate clinicians across disciplines to provide quality spiritual care.[24]

Future Directions

Future directions include quality improvement and other research in spiritual care to develop models of interprofessional and collaborative generalist-specialist spiritual care and expansion and evaluation of current training programs.

Key Points

- Patients with serious, chronic illness or at the end of life often have significant spiritual or transcendent experiences. They may also experience severe spiritual distress that impacts their quality of life.
- Spiritual distress should be assessed and treated as any other palliative care symptom.
- Models and recommendations based on generalist-specialist spiritual care support the full integration of spirituality in clinical palliative care.
- Training programs such as ISPEC are needed to advance the field and ensure that patients' spiritual needs are fully addressed.

References

1. Ellis J, Lloyd- Williams M. Palliative care. In: Cobb M, Puchalski CM, Rumbold B, eds., *Oxford Textbook of Spirituality in Healthcare*. New York: Oxford University Press; 2012:257–264.
2. World Health Organization. Palliative care. Health topics. 2021. http://www.who.int/cancer/palliative/definition/en

3. Steinhauser KE, Fitchett G, Handzo GF, Johnson KS, Koenig HG, Pargament KI, et al. State of the science of spirituality and palliative care research Part I: Definitions, measurement, and outcomes. *J Pain Symptom Manage.* 2017;54(3):428–440. doi:10.1016/j.jpainsymman.2017.07.028

4. National Consensus Project for Quality Palliative Care. *Clinical Practice Guidelines for Quality Palliative Care.* 4th ed. Richmond, VA: National Hospice and Palliative Care Coalition; 2018. https://www.natio nalcoalitionhpc.org/ncp/.

5. Gomez-Castillo BJ, Hirsch R, Groninger H, Baker K, Cheng MJ, Phillips J, et al. Increasing the number of outpatients receiving spiritual assessment: A pain and palliative care service quality improvement project. *J Pain Symptom Manage.* 2015; 50(5):724–729. doi:10.1016/j.jpain symman.2015.05.012

6. American Academy of Pediatrics. Committee on Bioethics and Committee on Hospital Care: Palliative care for children. *Pediatrics.* 2000;106(2 Pt 1):351–357.

7. Sreedhar SS, Kraft C, Friebert S. Primary palliative care: Skills for all clinicians. *Curr Probl Pediatr Adolesc Healthcare.* 2020;50(6):100814. doi:10.1016/j.cppeds.2020.100814

8. Ferrell B. The role of the advanced practice registered nurse in spiritual care. In: Dahlin C, Coyne PJ, Ferrell BR, eds., *Advanced Practice Palliative Nursing.* New York: Oxford University Press; 2016:427–434.

9. Bernard M, Strasser F, Gamondi C, Braunschweig G, Forster M, Kaspers-Elekes K, et al. Relationship between spirituality, meaning in life, psychological distress, wish for hastened death, and their influence on quality of life in palliative care patients. *J Pain Symptom Manage.* 2017;54(4):514–522. doi:10.1016/j.jpainsymman.2017.07.019

10. Rome RB, Luminais HH, Bourgeois DA, Blais CM. The role of palliative care at the end of life. *Ochsner J.* 2011;11(4):348–352.

11. Saunders C. Spiritual pain. *J Palliat Care.* 1988;4(3):29–32.

12. Ferrell BR, Handzo G, Picchi T, Puchalski C, Rosa WE. The urgency of spiritual care: COVID-19 and the critical need for whole-person palliation. *J Pain Symptom Manage.* 2020;60(3):e7–e11. doi:10.1016/j.jpainsymman.2020.06.034

13. Handzo G, Bowden JM, King S. The evolution of spiritual care in the NCCN Distress Management Guidelines. *J Natl Comprehensive Cancer Network.* 2019;17(10):1257–1261.

14. Rosa W. Spiritual care intervention. In: Ferrell BR, Paice JA, eds., *Oxford Textbook of Palliative Nursing.* 5th ed. New York: Oxford University Press; 2019.

15. Zollfrank A, Trevino KM, Cadge W, Balboni MJ, Thiel MM, Fitchett G, et al. Teaching healthcare providers to provide spiritual care: A pilot study. *J Palliat Med.* 2015;18(5):408–414. doi:10.1089/jpm.2014.0306

16. Puchalski C, Ferrell B, Virani R, Otis-Green S, Baird P, Bull J, et al. Improving the quality of spiritual care as a dimension of palliative care: The report of the consensus conference. *J Palliat Med.* 2009;12:885–904.

17. Puchalski CM, Vitillo R, Hull SK, Reller N. Improving the spiritual dimension of whole-person care: Reaching national and international consensus. *J Palliat Med.* 2014:17(6);642–656.

18. Farran CJ, Fitchett G, Quiring-Emblen JD, Burck JR. Development of a model for spiritual assessment and intervention. *J Relig Health.* 1989;28:185–194.

19. Puchalski C, Romer AL. Taking a spiritual history allows clinicians to understand patients more fully. *J Palliat Med.* 2000;3:129–137.

20. Sinclair S, Raffin S, Pereira J, Guebert N. Collective soul: The spirituality of an interdisciplinary palliative care team. *Pall Supp Care.* 2006;4(1):13–24. doi:10.1017/S1478951506060032

21. King SD, Jarvis D, Cornwell M. Programmatic staff care in an outpatient setting. *J Pastoral Care Counsel.* 2005;59(3):263–273. doi:10.1177/154230500505900309

22. Cooper RS. The palliative care chaplain as story catcher. *J Pain Symptom Manage.* 2018;55(1):155–158 doi:10.1016/j.jpainsymman.2017.03.035

23. Kapoor S, Morgan C, Siddique MA, Guntupalli K. "Sacred pause" in the ICU: Evaluation of a ritual and interventions to lower distress and burnout. *Am J Hosp Palliat Care.* 2018 Oct;35(10):1337–1341. doi:10.1177/1049909118768247. Epub 2018 Apr 4.

24. Puchalski C, Jafari N, Buller H, Haythorn T, Jacobs C, Ferrell B. Interprofessional spiritual care education curriculum: A milestone toward the provision of spiritual care. *J Palliat Med.* 2020;23(6):777–784. doi:10.1089/jpm.2019.0375

PART V

Understanding and Managing Symptoms

28

Physical Symptom Management in the Terminally Ill

Russell K. Portenoy and Eduardo Bruera

Introduction

Pain, breathlessness, fatigue, and other physical symptoms are experienced by most patients with advanced illness.[1] If uncontrolled, physical symptoms may compromise mood, impair function, and prevent adaptation to advanced illness. All clinicians can contribute to symptom control by recognizing symptom-related distress and participating in assessment and management. This chapter describes these contributions as they pertain to several common physical symptoms—pain, breathlessness, and fatigue.

Pain

Effective pain management minimizes pain-related distress and mitigates the adverse impact of pain on function and quality of life. Pain management exemplifies best practices that may be applied to many other symptoms.

Assessment

The assessment of pain and other symptoms begins with a history, examination, and review of test results (Box 28.1). This information clarifies the relationship of the symptom to the primary disease, identifies specific etiologies related to the onset or persistence of the symptom, and allows inferences about pathophysiology. A treatment plan based on this assessment may include etiology-focused and/or symptom-focused interventions.

In pain management, etiology-focused treatment may address the disease itself (e.g., radiation therapy for a bone metastasis) or a comorbid process (e.g., antibiotic for infection),

---

BOX 28.1 Elements of a symptom-related history

Symptom Characteristics

Severity

- Verbal ("none," "mild," "moderate," "severe"); numeric ("0–10" where "0" is none and "10" is the worst imaginable"); analog (10 cm line anchored by none and worst imaginable), or pictorial (e.g., faces)
- Distinguish "right now," "on average during the past week," and "worst during the past week";

Temporal features

- Onset, duration. course (stable, improving, worsening, fluctuating, recurrent, or recurrent with episodes)

Location, if appropriate

Quality

- For pain, examples include "aching," "throbbing," or "burning"

Exacerbating or relieving factors

- Examples include coughing, eating, specific positions

Essential Historical Information

- Status of the primary illness
- Premorbid medical and psychiatric conditions
- Comorbid medical and psychiatric conditions
- Prior symptom evaluation
- Prior symptom treatments

Symptom Impact

Physical functioning

- Effect on walking or other physical activities
- Effect on sleep

Psychological functioning

- Mood
- Symptom-associated distress or catastrophization
- Coping, adaptation, resilience, and role of self-management

Social function

- Role integrity and functioning
- Effect on school, work recreation

---

and inferences about pathophysiology may rationalize specific symptom-focused treatments. The pathophysiology may be "nociceptive" (related to activation of pain sensitive structures by injury or inflammation) and/or "neuropathic" (related to abnormal somatosensory activity from a condition affecting the nervous system). Psychological processes that amplify or modify pain expression also may be evident.

TABLE 28.1 Analgesic approaches

Approach	Type	Example
Pharmacotherapy	Nonopioids	Acetaminophen, nonsteroidal anti-inflammatory drugs
	Adjuvant analgesics	analgesic antidepressants, gabapentinoids and other anticonvulsants, α-2 adrenergic agonists, topical therapies
	Opioids	Agonist-antagonists, partial agonists, full agonists
Psychological therapies	Psychoeducation	Managing expectations
	Cognitive behavioral therapy	Relaxation therapy, mindfulness, pacing
	Other psychotherapies	Individual, group
Integrative medicine therapies	Movement therapies	Pilates, tai chi
	Mind-body therapies	Music therapy, relaxation therapy, hypnosis
	Energy therapies	Reichi, therapeutic touch
	Other selected therapies	Acupuncture, massage,
Rehabilitative therapies	Physical therapy, occupational therapy, modalities	Heat, cold, ultrasound, transcutaneous electricity
Noninvasive neuromodulatory therapies	Transcutaneous or transcranial stimulation	Transcranial direct current stimulation, transcranial magnetic stimulation
Interventional therapies	Myofascial injections, neural blockade, implanted neurostimulation or infusion devices	Trigger point injection, temporary nerve blocks, spinal cord stimulation, subarachnoid infusion

Among the many symptom-focused interventions available for pain (Table 28.1), opioid-based pharmacotherapy is widely accepted as the mainstay approach in populations with advanced illness. Alternative nonpharmacological treatments always should be considered, however. These therapies are combined with drugs, potentially reducing the risks associated with higher doses or polypharmacy.

Management

Nonpharmacological Therapies

Noninvasive nonpharmacological therapies have broad applications for the management of pain and other symptoms. The simplest intervention is psychoeducational—supportive information that promotes self-management. Discussions with the patient or family may focus on modification of diet, activity, or sleep; use of simple cognitive strategies to reduce anxiety or catastrophization; or specific planning about the use of as-needed medications. These discussions support autonomy and self-efficacy.

Psychotherapeutic approaches, such as mindfulness training or cognitive behavioral therapy, may also be considered for symptom-focused care, particularly when symptoms are accompanied by distress and disability. Unfortunately, information about the use of these approaches in the context of advanced illness is very limited, and many patients decline participation or lack access to trained professionals.[2] To integrate psychotherapeutic approaches into the plan of care, clinicians should appreciate the professional resources in the community and be able to encourage participation by setting expectations about specific treatments.

Other types of noninvasive nonpharmacological therapies may be categorized as rehabilitative, integrative medicine, and neuromodulation (Table 28.1). Although the many therapies categorized in this way have a limited evidence base, they are generally safe and supported by positive observations in diverse populations. Clinicians providing care to those with pain due to serious chronic illness should know the capabilities of local providers and integrate referrals for one or more treatments into a plan of care.

Invasive therapies for pain management are usually considered when pain is refractory to pharmacotherapy and referral to appropriate professionals is possible. Therapies include injection therapies, neural blockade (such as celiac plexus block for pain related to pancreas cancer), and implanted devices for neurostimulation or neuraxial infusion.

Analgesic Pharmacotherapy

Competency in analgesic pharmacotherapy—the safe and effective use of opioids, nonopioids, and adjuvant analgesics—is the foundation for pain management in palliative care.[3]

Opioid Drugs

Opioids are usually the first-line treatment for patients with moderate or severe chronic pain in the context of advanced illness. These drugs can be divided into pure μ-receptor agonists, partial agonists, agonist-antagonists, and "mixed mechanism" drugs that combine pure μ-receptor agonism with other mechanisms (Table 28.2).

Given the absence of comparative trials, opioid selection is usually determined by the experience of the clinician, the patient's prior experience (if any), availability, and several properties of specific drugs. The pure μ-agonists, such as morphine, oxycodone, hydromorphone, fentanyl and others, are available in multiple formulations, have no clinically relevant ceiling dose for analgesia, and are usually preferred for the long-term management of pain. Codeine and meperidine (pethidine) should not be used, however; codeine has an unpredictable dose-response due to genetically determined variation in metabolism and meperidine (pethidine) has a toxic metabolite. Morphine should be used cautiously in those with renal impairment due to its active renally excreted metabolites, and methadone should not be used unless the clinician is familiar with its unique pharmacology—a long and variable half-life, potential for drug-drug interactions, possibility of QTc prolongation, and greater than expected potency when switching from other opioids.[4]

Buprenorphine, a partial μ-receptor agonist available in a long-acting transdermal delivery system, is favored by some experts for initiating long-term therapy in those with limited or no prior opioid exposure. This drug, like methadone, also is used for the treatment of opioid addiction and, for this reason, may be preferred when patients have a history of substance abuse. Buprenorphine's pharmacology includes a ceiling effect for respiratory

TABLE 28.2 Opioid analgesics

DRUG	Approximate equianalgesic doses (mg)		Elimination half–life (hr)	Comment
	Oral	IV		
Morphine	30	10	2–4	Available in extended-release oral formulations.
Codeine	200	100	2–4	Not recommended due to variation in metabolism.
Oxycodone	20	–	2–4	Available in an extended-release oral formulation.
Hydromorphone	7.5	1.5	2–4	Available in an extended-release oral formulation.
Oxymorphone	10	1	2–4	Available in an extended-release oral formulation.
Fentanyl transdermal system	–	–	–	Consult prescribing information when changing from another opioid to transdermal fentanyl. Dosing interval is 48–72 hours. Cachexia changes pharmacokinetics, and fever or external heat can result in unintended overdose.
Transmucosal immediate-release fentanyl	–	–	–	For selected patients with breakthrough pain. Multiple formulations with more rapid onset than oral drugs. Consult prescribing information for safe dosing.
Methadone	20	10	8– >100	Use only if familiar with pharmacology, including long and variable half-life, potential for drug-drug interactions, possibility of QTc prolongation, and greater than expected potency when switching from other opioids.
Levorphanol	4	2	12–15	Relatively long half-life.
Hydrocodone	30	–	2–4	Available combined with a non-opioid analgesic in immediate-release formulations and as single-entity extended-release formulation.
Tramadol	–	120	5–6	Mixed mechanism, partly opioid and partly due to monoamine effects. Available in extended-release formulation.
Tapentadol	–	–	4–5	Mixed mechanism, partly opioid and partly due to monoamine effects. Available in extended-release formulation.
Buprenorphine transdermal	–	–	–	Low-dose patches, changed weekly, can be used to initiate opioid therapy.

depression, and possibly analgesia, and the ability to induce abstinence when administered to a patient who is physically dependent on a pure μ-receptor agonist.

The mixed mechanism drugs—tramadol and tapentadol—are μ-receptor agonists and reuptake inhibitors at monoamine receptors (serotonin, norepinephrine, or dopamine). These drugs may be used for acute or chronic pain but evidence of comparative benefit relative to the pure μ-receptor agonists is lacking. They have a ceiling effect imposed by the potential for monoaminergic toxicity.

Opioid administration. A relatively safe approach to the initiation of therapy in an opioid-naïve patient employs "as-needed" dosing of a short-acting formulation (a combination product, e.g., hydrocodone plus acetaminophen [paracetamol] or a single-entity

opioid). If long-term pain management is anticipated, however, some experts prefer to initiate treatment with a low dose of a long-acting oral or transdermal (buprenorphine or
fentanyl) formulation.

An established need for around-the-clock treatment suggests the utility of fixed
schedule dosing with a long-acting formulation, which may improve adherence and convenience. Most patients are offered one of the extended-release oral formulations (e.g.,
long-acting morphine, oxycodone or others), a transdermal formulation, or methadone
(Table 28.2). In the absence of comparative data, drug selection again is based on experience and availability. There is some evidence that transdermal fentanyl therapy is associated
with relatively less constipation than oral therapy, but transdermal systems must be used
cautiously in cachectic patients due to variable drug absorption and in febrile patients due
to the potential for increased drug absorption.

In populations with serious chronic illness, particularly the cancer population, patients with chronic pain also have breakthrough pain—episodes that "break through" the
regularly scheduled opioid regimen and contribute to the adverse consequences of chronic
pain. When breakthrough pain is evident, conventional practice supports the administration of both a regularly scheduled opioid and a short-acting "as-needed" opioid.

Occasional patients require alternative routes of opioid delivery. The sublingual and
rectal routes are usually considered for short-term treatment when the oral route is unavailable. Sublingual administration may be accomplished using an injectable formulation or an
opioid compounded for this purpose, and some rectal formulations are commercially available. There is anecdotal experience with rectal administration of extended-release opioids.

The sublingual, transnasal, and buccal routes have been used for the delivery of fentanyl in a group of products collectively termed the "transmucosal immediate-release fentanyl" (TIRF) formulations.[5] TIRFs have been developed for the treatment of cancer-related
breakthrough pain. They have a more rapid onset of effect than the short-acting oral drugs
conventionally used to manage breakthrough pain and, where available, are typically considered when oral therapy for breakthrough pain is ineffective.

Parenteral subcutaneous dosing through a "butterfly" needle or a catheter placed
under the skin can be accomplished via repetitive injections or via infusion maintained by
portable pump. Intravenous infusion typically requires a central venous port. Techniques
for long-term intraspinal (neuraxial) infusion through an epidural or subarachnoid catheter are well accepted and are considered for patients whose pain has not responded to
systemic drug administration.

Effective opioid therapy requires individualization of the dose through an iterative
process of dose titration, the objective of which is to identify the dose associated with a
favorable balance between analgesia and side effects. Although a favorable dose is usually
identified and maintained for prolonged periods, most patients with progressive illness require periodic dose escalation to address worsening pain. When this happens, an opioid
dose increase of 30–50% is usually safe and effective. If the patient has access to an as-
needed opioid for breakthrough pain, the increase can be guided by the amount required
during the past several days. Typically, dose escalation involves both the regularly scheduled opioid and the opioid for breakthrough pain.

Opioid-poor responsiveness. If opioid titration results in treatment-limiting side effects instead of a favorable outcome, the patient should be designated "poorly responsive" to the therapy. Poorly responsive pain may be addressed by adding a pharmacologic treatment (such as a nonopioid analgesic) or a nonpharmacologic treatment (such as a psychological approach), or by switching opioids—a technique known as *opioid rotation.* Guidelines for opioid rotation are based on calculation of the equianalgesic dose based on published tables (Table 28.2), followed by dose reduction to ensure safety.[6]

Management of side effects and drug abuse risk. The prevention and treatment of side effects is an essential component of effective opioid therapy. The management of common physical symptoms subsumes this attention to opioid-related side effects. During long-term opioid therapy, the most salient side effects are constipation, somnolence or impaired cognition, neuroendocrine effects, and sleep-disordered breathing (Table 28.3).

Opioid abuse and addiction are serious adverse outcomes, and clinicians assume responsibility for risk assessment and management whenever they are prescribed. A systematic "universal precautions" approach is the safest strategy (Table 28.4).

TABLE 28.3 Common opioid side effects

Side effect	Principles of management

Constipation	• Reduce/eliminate nonessential drugs with constipatory effects
	• If appropriate, increase fluid intake
	• In nondebilitated patients, consider increasing fiber in diet or with supplements
	• Consider daily probiotic consumption
	• Consider switch to non-oral route for opioid administration
	• Consider conventional first-line therapy, prophylactically and during opioid treatment, including:
	  o Contact (stimulant) laxative (e.g., senna, bisacodyl) and/or
	  o Stool softener (e.g., docusate) and/or
	  o Osmotic laxative (e.g., polyethylene glycol, lactulose, or magnesium sulfate or sodium phosphate)
	• Consider treatments for refractory symptom
	  o Peripherally acting mu opioid receptor antagonists (PAMORAs), e.g., methylnaltrexone, naloxegol, naldemidine
	  o Chloride channel activator, e.g., lupiprostone
	  o Guanylate cyclase C activator, e.g., linaclotide, plecanatide
	  o 5-HT4 agonist, e.g., prucalopride phosphate)
	• Consider prokinetic treatment, e.g., metoclopramide

Somnolence/impaired cognition	• Reduce/eliminate nonessential drugs with sedating effects • Consider opioid rotation • Consider use of a psychostimulant, e.g., methylphenidate, modafinil, others
Neuroendocrine effects	• Suspect hypogonadism in patients with depressed mood, fatigue, sexual dysfunction, infertility; be aware that opioids can be associated with hypocortisolism and hypoglycemia • If appropriate, evaluate and consider hormone replacement therapy
Sleep-disordered breathing	• Be aware that opioids can worsen sleep apnea syndrome or produce a de novo central/obstructive sleep apnea syndrome. • If suspected, reduce/eliminate nonessential centrally acting drugs • If appropriate, consider sleep study and conventional treatment of sleep apnea

TABLE 28.4 Universal precautions when prescribing opioids

Steps	Considerations
1. Assess and stratify risk in all patients	Assess risk of opioid misuse/abuse based on history, examination, record review, and check of prescription drug monitoring program; consider obtaining a drug screen. Stratify risk into very low vs. moderate or high.
	Higher risk of misuse/abuse is associated with (1) past or present history of alcohol or drug abuse, (2) family history of alcohol or drug abuse, and (3) any type of major psychiatric disorder. Younger age and history of physical/sexual abuse are also associated. Validated measures are available.
2. Decision: Prescribe or not	Do not prescribe if diversion to the illicit market is suspected.
	If drug abuse is occurring, prescribing requires control of the behavior and adherence monitoring.
3. Structure prescribing to minimize risk	Implement adherence monitoring matched to risk. Consider prescribing quantities, pill counts, no short-acting drugs, biofluid drug testing, required consultation with psychiatry or addiction medicine.
4. Monitor drug-related behaviors	Continually monitor drug-related behaviors as one of the "Four A's": Analgesia (effectiveness); Adverse Effects (side effects), Activity (function), and Aberrant Drug-Related Behavior.
5. Respond to aberrant behaviors	If aberrant drug-related behavior occurs, re-assess to determine diagnosis. Consider recreational abuse, addiction, so-called "pseudoaddiction," psychiatric disorders associated with impulsive drug-taking, patient confusion about instructions for dosing, organic brain syndrome associated with confusion or impulsivity, family or caregiver issues, or criminal activity.
	Management is guided by diagnosis and may include discontinuation of therapy or increased adherence monitoring. Always document behaviors, their assessment and management.

Non-Opioid Analgesics

The nonopioid analgesics include acetaminophen (paracetamol) and the nonsteroidal anti-inflammatory drugs (NSAIDs). Anecdotal experience suggests that these drugs potentially benefit any type of pain but are more likely to yield analgesia when pain is related to injury to somatic tissue and inflammation. Clinical trials have confirmed the analgesic efficacy of NSAIDs in cancer pain;[7] the evidence base in other populations is lacking.

Acetaminophen (paracetamol) is not significantly anti-inflammatory but has a favorable toxicity profile. Hepatotoxicity is the major concern and is minimized by avoiding the drug in those with significant liver disease and those who imbibe three or more alcoholic drinks per day and by taking no more than 1.0 g as a single dose and 3.2 g per day. These limits are lowered by 25–50% if liver dysfunction exists.

NSAIDs include numerous prescription and over-the-counter oral drugs and parenteral formulations of ketorolac, ibuprofen, and diclofenac (Table 28.5). Among the potential serious toxicities are peptic ulcer disease and hemorrhage from the upper and lower gastrointestinal tracts; acute or chronic kidney injury; a bleeding diathesis due to inhibited platelet aggregation; prothrombotic effects leading to a risk of cardiac, cerebrovascular, and peripheral vascular events; and acute and chronic liver disease. Patients at high risk of

TABLE 28.5 Nonsteroidal anti-inflammatory drugs (NSAIDs)

	Adult starting dose	Comment
COX-2 INHIBITORS		
Celecoxib	100–200 mg q12h	Fewer GI side effects; no effect on platelet function.
NAPTHYLALKANONES		
Nabumetone	500–1,000 mg q12h	Relatively COX-2 selective; lesser GI effects.
SALICYLATES		
Aspirin	650 mg q4h (5 daily)	May not be tolerated as well as some of the newer NSAIDs. Not recommended in children.
Diflunisal	1,000 mg × 1, then 500 mg q12h	—
Choline magnesium trisalicylate	500–1,000 mg q12h	Relatively low GI toxicity and no effect on platelet aggregation
Salsalate	500–1,000 mg q12h	
PROPRIONIC ACIDS		
Ibuprofen[c]	400–600 mg q8h	Available over-the-counter. First-line therapy for children. Relatively low risk of cardiovascular events.
Naproxen[c]	250–500 mg q12h	Available over-the-counter and as a suspension. Relatively low risk of cardiovascular events
Naproxen sodium[c]	275–550 mg q12h	Relatively low risk of cardiovascular events
Fenoprofen	200 mg q6h	—
Ketoprofen	25–50 mg q8h	—
Flurbiprofen[c]	100 mg q12h	—
Oxaprozin	600 mg q24h	Once-daily dosing may be useful.
ACETIC ACIDS		
Indomethacin	25 mg q8h	Available in sustained-release and rectal formulations. Higher incidence of side effects, particularly GI and CNS, than proprionic acids.
Tolmetin	200 mg q8h	
Sulindac	150 mg q12h	
Etodolac	200–400 mg q6–8h	Relatively COX-2 selective; lesser GI effects
Diclofenac	25 mg q8h	Topical formulation available
Ketorolac[c]	30–60 mg load, then 15–30 mg q6h (parenteral); 10 mg q6h (oral)	Parenteral formulation available.
Oxicams	7.5 mg daily	Relatively COX-2 selective; lesser GI effects
Meloxicam		Relatively COX-2 selective; lesser GI effects
Piroxicam	20 mg q24h	Administration of 40 mg for over 3 weeks is associated with a high incidence of peptic ulcer, particularly in the elderly.

[a]Starting dose should be one-half to two-thirds of the recommended starting dose for the medically frail, those with mild nephropathy or hepatopathy, and those taking multiple drugs. Toxicity of all drugs is related to dose and duration of therapy; the minimal effective dose should be used.

ulcer disease, vascular events, or bleeding, and those with renal or liver disease, have relative contraindications to NSAID therapy. A careful assessment of benefit versus risk and a monitoring plan is needed for long-term therapy.

In those with advanced illness, NSAID selection should minimize risk. Selective COX-2 inhibitors have a lower risk of upper gastrointestinal adverse effects. They include celecoxib, nabumetone, meloxicam, etodolac, and others; the non-acetylated salicylates, choline magnesium trisalicylate and salsalate, also have low gastrointestinal toxicity. Risk of upper gastrointestinal toxicity is further reduced by co-administration of a proton pump inhibitor, such as omeprazole. There is some evidence that naproxen and ibuprofen have relatively low cardiovascular risk, and the non-acetylated salicylates lack effect on platelet aggregation.

Adjuvant Analgesics

The term "adjuvant analgesic" describes drugs that were developed for indications other than pain but are currently used for the management of chronic pain. Based on conventional practice, the adjuvant analgesics can be divided into multipurpose analgesics, drugs used for neuropathic pain, and drugs used for musculoskeletal disorders (Table 28.6). Some drugs used for specific types of cancer pain also may be described as adjuvant analgesics.

The most important multipurpose adjuvant analgesics are the glucocorticoids, the analgesic antidepressants, and topical analgesics. The glucocorticoids, such as dexamethasone, are widely used in the setting of advanced illness, notwithstanding limited evidence of analgesic efficacy. The antidepressants, specifically the serotonin-norepinephrine reuptake inhibitors (SNRIs) and the tricyclic antidepressants (TCAs), have strong evidence of efficacy and may be used for all types of pain, singly or in combination with opioids. Topical therapies should be considered for pains that have a focal or regional distribution (Table 28.6). Other multipurpose drugs include the α-2 adrenergic agonists (e.g., clonidine and tizanidine), the cannabinoids (e.g., nabiximols), and botulinum toxin.

Neuropathic pain may be treated with the multipurpose analgesics or with other adjuvant analgesics used selectively for pain of this type. The most important of the latter group are gabapentin and pregabalin. Evidence-based guidelines suggest that these gabapentinoids, the analgesic antidepressants, and the topical local anesthetics are the preferred therapies for neuropathic pain.[8] When neuropathic pain is refractory to standard treatment, other drugs, such as selected anticonvulsants (e.g., oxcarbazepine) and NMDA receptor antagonists (e.g., ketamine) may be tried (Table 28.6).

Dyspnea

Dyspnea is defined as an uncomfortable awareness of breathing. It is a frequent and distressing symptom in diverse populations with chronic illness. Most patients experience significant episodes before death. Like pain, the etiologies and mechanisms of dyspnea are multiple and protean. In the cancer population, for example, dyspnea may be due to primary or metastatic lung involvement, often complicated by pleural effusion or

TABLE 28.6 Adjuvant analgesics

Category	Class	Types	Examples	Comment
Multipurpose analgesics	Glucocorticoids	–	Dexamethasone, prednisone	Limited evidence but extensive anecdotal experience suggests potential benefit for pain, nausea, and fatigue associated with advanced illness.
	Antidepressants	SNRIs	duloxetine, milnacipran	Duloxetine often selected first for chronic pain.
		Secondary amine TCAs	desipramine, nortriptyline	Better tolerated than the tertiary amine TCAs.
		Tertiary amine TCAs	amitriptyline, imipramine	Established analgesics, but high side effect potential.
		SSRIs	paroxetine, citalopram	Poor evidence of analgesia.
	Alpha-2 adrenergic agonists	–	tizanidine, clonidine, dexmedetomidine	Oral tizanidine is a second-line analgesic.
	Cannabinoids	–	nabilone, dronabinol medical cannabis	Limited evidence.
	NMDA receptor antagonists	–	ketamine, memantine, amantadine, dextromethorphan	Ketamine used in palliative care for severe opioid-refractory pain.
	Neuroleptics	First/second generation	haloperidol/ olanzapine, risperidone	Poor evidence of efficacy.
	Topical agents	Local anesthetics	5% patch, lower concentration creams, gels and patches	5% patch used for neuropathic and musculoskeletal pains.
		NSAIDs	Diclofenac, ketoprofen	Approved for acute musculoskeletal pains.
		Capsaicin	0.075% patch or cream, 8% patch,	0.075% used for diverse pains and 8% patch approved for postherpetic neuralgia.
		Compounds	ketamine, amitriptyline, menthol, others	Limited evidence.
	Botulinum toxin	Botulinum A, B	–	Evidence for use in many focal and regional neuropathic and musculoskeletal pains.

(continued)

TABLE 28.6 Continued

Category	Class	Types	Examples	Comment
Drugs used for neuropathic pain	Multipurpose adjuvant analgesics	See above	–	Guidelines state that antidepressants and topical drugs—along with the gabapentinoids—are first-line for neuropathic pain
	Gabapentinoids	–	Pregabalin, gabapentin	Evidence in acute pain and chronic neuropathic pain; used first for neuropathic pain, unless comorbid depression supports antidepressant.
	Other anticonvulsants	–	oxcarbazepine, lacosamide	Limited evidence overall.
	GABA agonist	GABA$_A$ GABA$_B$	Baclofen (GABA$_A$) Clonazepam (GABA$_B$)	Limited evidence of analgesia for baclofen. Clonazepam is sometimes used, but the risks suggest a very limited role.
	Sodium channel blockers	–	IV lidocaine, mexiletine	IV lidocaine used for pain in monitored settings; oral drugs rarely used pain due to side effects.
Drugs used for musculoskeletal pains	Multipurpose adjuvant analgesics	see above	–	–
	"Muscle relaxants"	–	methocarbamol, carisoprodol, chlorzoxazone, metaxalone, cyclobenzaprine	No evidence in chronic pain; not generally used for chronic pain
Drugs used in cancer pain management	For bone pain	Bisphos-phonates Monoclonal antibodies Radiopharmaceuticals	Zolendronate, ibandronate Denosumab Strontium[89], samarium[153]	Bisphosphonates used to prevent skeletal-related events and treat pain specifically; denosumab equieffective with bisphosphonates.
	For pain due to bowel obstruction	Somatostatin analogues	Octreotide, lanreotide	Evidence of efficacy of somatostatin analogues is mixed. Octreotide may be added to other drugs, including an opioid, an anticholinergic, and a glucocorticoid, to manage severe obstructive symptoms.

SNRIs, serotonin norepinephrine reuptake inhibitors; TCAs, tricyclic antidepressants; SSRIs, serotonin selective reuptake inhibitors; NSAIDs, non-steroidal anti-inflammatory drugs; GABA, gamma aminobutyric acid; NMDA, N-methyl-D-aspartate.

lymphangitis; treatment-related pneumonitis; or comorbid infections, embolism, congestive heart failure, chronic obstructive pulmonary disease (COPD), or anemia (Figure 28.1). Among those with advanced illness, respiratory muscle dysfunction related to cachexia and neuromyopathy may be prominent.

Assessment

Dyspnea is subjective and is only moderately correlated with objective findings, such as tachypnea, pulmonary function tests, blood gases, or imaging studies. The patient's subjective estimation of severity and other characteristics is the gold standard for assessment.

The principles of pain assessment are applicable to dyspnea. To measure severity, for example, a simple numerical scale from 0 to 10, a verbal rating scale, or a visual analogue scale can be used. Given the frequency with which dyspnea associates with other symptoms, however, measurement using a multisymptom tool, such as the Edmonton Symptom Assessment Scale (ESAS),[9] is particularly useful, allowing patients to rate the severity of 10 symptoms on 0–10 scales in less than 1 minute. Tools such as the ESAS complement the clinical assessment and may reveal symptoms that amplify or change the experience of dyspnea, or require concurrent treatment.

Management

Whenever possible, etiology-focused treatment should be offered. This may require complex interventions, such as pleural drainage, bronchial stents, anticoagulation, or transfusions. If dyspnea is severe, initial management should take place in settings where these interventions are readily accessible if needed.

Other etiology-focused treatments include bronchodilators and oxygen therapy. Bronchodilators are often administered by nebulization and are most likely to help when bronchospasm is indicated by examination or pulmonary function tests. Oxygen can

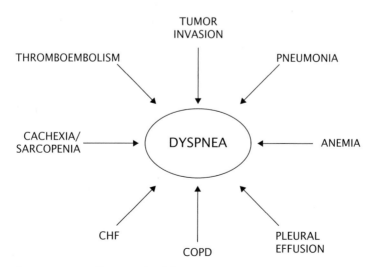

FIGURE 28.1 Frequent causes of cancer-related dyspnea.

mitigate dyspnea when hypoxemia exists; it is not effective when the pO_2 is normal. Recent research shows that high-flow oxygen is also capable of reducing dyspnea.

When no reversible causes are identified or when dyspnea is refractory to such interventions, symptom-focused management is frequently capable of reducing the severity (Box 28.2).[10,11] For some patients, treatment focuses on mitigation of episodic dyspnea, which occurs only with activity; other patients have continuous dyspnea, which worsens with exertion.

Pharmacological Management

In advanced illness, opioid drugs are preferred for the management of dyspnea, notwithstanding a limited evidence base. Conventionally, the drugs, initial doses, and titration approach used for dyspnea are similar to those used in pain management. Due to the episodic nature of dyspnea, short acting opioids are useful, ideally administered orally 30–45 minutes before a walk, shower, or other activities. When dyspnea is continuous, long-acting formulations or parenteral infusions can be useful. The best type and dose of opioids have not been well characterized.[10,11]

Glucocorticoids may be useful to manage dyspnea related to bronchospasm, bronchial or tracheal obstruction, or metastatic deposits or lymphangitic spread. A relatively high dose of one of the commercially available drugs is used for the first 2 days and then rapidly decreased to the lowest effective dose, which is maintained.

Benzodiazepines are used for the management of refractory dyspnea. They may be helpful to reduce anxiety, which may be both a cause and an effect of worsening dyspnea. Whenever opioids and benzodiazepines are co-prescribed, access to intranasal naloxone should be provided since the frequency of severe sedation and respiratory depression increases when these drugs are combined.[10,11]

In end-of-life care, palliative sedation using a benzodiazepine may be needed to address refractory distress associated with dyspnea. Palliative sedation should be provided according to guidelines that ensure an ethical and medically effective intervention.

BOX 28.2 Management of dyspnea

- Diagnose and treat reversible causes
- Symptomatic treatment
  - Opioids
  - Oxygen (low-high flow)
  - Respiratory rehabilitation
  - Corticosteroids
  - Psychosocial support
  - Fan
  - Integrative therapies

Nonpharmacological Management

Non-drug therapies may ameliorate dyspnea and should always be considered in the context of advanced illness. High-flow air directed to the face is a simple approach and cognitive approaches, such as relaxation training, may acutely reduce anxiety and be particularly helpful with episodic symptoms.[12,13] Psychosocial support for the patient and dyadic interventions with the spouse or caregiver have been reported to help relieve dyspnea and associated distress. Respiratory physiotherapy and exercise including incentive spirometry has been used in patients with COPD; the latter approaches may be helpful when dyspnea has a major component of sarcopenia and cachexia.[13]

Fatigue

Fatigue is a very prevalent symptom—the most common symptom reported by cancer patients. It is an experience fundamentally different from the exhaustion experienced by a healthy person, which is resolved with rest or sleep. When associated with serious chronic illness, fatigue is synonymous with asthenia; refers to a perceived lack of physical and mental energy as well as tiredness and weakness, and it is not reliably relieved by rest or sleep. It may vary over time, progress, and result in major impairments in function and socialization, leading to reduced physical activity. The deconditioning that occurs as the fatigued person reduces activity may worsen the symptom.

Fatigue is a multicausal syndrome and the pathophysiology is yet poorly understood.[14] In the cancer population, tumor-related byproducts and cytokines are known to affect brain function, resulting in fatigue and other symptoms, such as anorexia and mood changes (Figure 28.2). The mechanisms of disease-related fatigue in those with other conditions, such as heart failure, COPD, cirrhosis, and chronic kidney disease, are not known. Disease-modifying treatments for cancer and other conditions may cause fatigue through

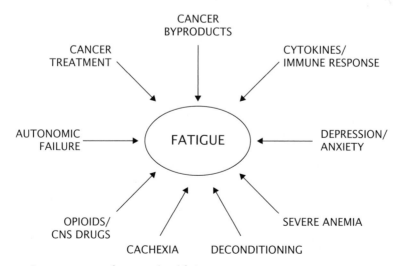

FIGURE 28.2 Frequent causes of cancer-related fatigue.

central nervous system interactions or effects on peripheral nerves or muscles, and varied drugs used to treat symptoms can increase fatigue, including opioids, sedative-hypnotics, antihistamines, and drugs with anticholinergic effects. Severe anemia, electrolyte abnormalities, and metabolic disturbances associated with organ dysfunction, poor nutrition, or other factors also may be important causes of fatigue. Other contributing factors include anxiety and depression and early stages of delirium.

Assessment

Like pain and dyspnea, fatigue is subjective and the patient's perception is the gold standard for assessment. The approach to pain assessment applies to fatigue and may be complemented by tools developed to clarify fatigue characteristics and measure severity. Examples include the Functional Assessment of Cancer Therapy-Fatigue and the Brief Fatigue Inventory. Multisymptom severity or distress measures, like the ESAS, also may be used to evaluate fatigue and concurrent symptoms.

Management

Due the multiple contributors, most patients require multidimensional management of fatigue.[15] Etiology-focused treatments should be considered as a first step. A medication review may identify centrally acting drugs that might be discontinued or reduced. If a mood disorder is diagnosed, an antidepressant may produce a secondary increase in energy. In cancer patients with cachexia, progestational drugs have found to improve both appetite and fatigue; the main limitation of these drugs is their prothrombotic effect.

Pharmacological Management

If fatigue cannot be ameliorated through management of contributing factors, drug therapy should be considered (Box 28.3). In the cancer population, glucocorticoids improve fatigue in most patients with advanced illness.[16] It is useful to start at a relatively high dose (i.e., dexamethasone 10 mg twice daily) and reduce the dose after 2–3 days if there is a positive effect; the lowest effective dose is continued. If there is no improvement after a few days, the drug should be discontinued.

BOX 28.3 Management of fatigue

- Diagnose and treat reversible causes
- Symptomatic treatment
  - Physical activity/exercise
  - Corticosteroids
  - Psychosocial support
  - Methylphenidate/stimulants
  - Integrative therapies

Methylphenidate and other psychostimulants can improve fatigue, especially in patients who report sedation or depressive symptoms. There is strong evidence supporting the use of methylphenidate to reduce opioid-induced sedation and fatigue.

Nonpharmacological Management

Physical activity is very effective in reducing fatigue. Patients who are capable of activity should be instructed to initiate exercise slowly, always aiming for activity at a level that does not acutely worsen symptoms. Walking is the simplest type of physical activity, and both activity trackers and support by a partner can be helpful.[17] A glucocorticoid and/or a psychostimulant might be considered to help patients initiate and adhere to increased activity. In some situations, referral for physical therapy can be used to develop a program of graduated activity. Patients with physical impairments should be considered for referral to a physiatrist, who may be able to identify safe physical activity enhancement.

Other nonpharmacological therapies also may be considered. Integrative therapies have been found to be promising for patients with persistent fatigue.[18] Some patients appear to benefit from exposure to natural light, yoga or other movement therapies, meditation, or acupuncture.

In the context of advanced illness, fatigue contributes to functional decline. Progressive adaptation to losses by counseling and the use of assistive devices such as ambulation aids or a bedside commode and shower stool may help patients accept some of the loss in function and improve the quality of the remaining life.

Future Directions

Although the evidence base available to guide the assessment and management of diverse physical symptoms is very limited, conventional best practices provide a roadmap to care that benefits many patients. Nonetheless, gaps in knowledge continue to constrain the ability to manage symptoms and relieve symptom distress in the context of serious illness. Little is known about the heterogeneous mechanisms responsible for symptoms, and there is a compelling need to investigate the common symptoms in terms of contributing mechanisms and the relationships between these mechanisms and phenomenology. In pain management, the process has begun with the development of guidelines for identifying neuropathic pain and some treatments specific for this type. Far more is needed to understand pain, and there should be parallel research initiatives that identify the mechanisms underlying various types of dyspnea, fatigue, and other symptoms. The goal of mechanism-based treatment will be pursued in this way.

Symptom-focused treatments reveal similarly challenging gaps in knowledge about therapeutics. The evidence base underlying the decision to select a pharmacologic or nonpharmacologic treatment for a specific symptom is limited in all cases and entirely absent in many. Clinical trials are difficult to do but are badly needed to improve treatment outcomes.

Palliative care is predicated on clinical competency in the management of common physical symptoms. All clinicians may contribute to effective symptom management.

Key Points

- Pain, dyspnea, and fatigue are among the most frequent and distressing symptoms in patients with cancer.
- Regular screening for the presence and severity of symptoms should be conducted in every clinical encounter with patients with cancer.
- Most symptoms are multidimensional, and it is important to determine the main contributors to symptom expression.
- Opioids remain the most important intervention for the management of pain and dyspnea.
- Patients with symptoms that persist after initial management by the oncologist or hospitalist should be referred to palliative care specialists.

References

1. Moens K, Higginson IJ, Harding R; EURO IMPACT. Are there differences in the prevalence of palliative care-related problems in people living with advanced cancer and eight non-cancer conditions? A systematic review. *J Pain Symptom Manage*. 2014 Oct;48(4):660–677. doi:10.1016/j.jpainsymman.2013.11.009. Epub 2014 May 5. PMID: 24801658

2. Brebach R, Sharpe L, Costa DS, Rhodes P, Butow P. Psychological intervention targeting distress for cancer patients: A meta-analytic study investigating uptake and adherence. *Psychooncology*. 2016 Aug;25(8):882–90. doi:10.e1002/pon.4099. Epub 2016 Feb 18. PMID: 26893285

3. Swarm RA, Paice JA, Anghelescu DL, Are M, Bruce JY, Buga S, et al. Adult cancer pain, version 3.2019, NCCN clinical practice guidelines in oncology. *J Natl Compr Canc Netw*. 2019 Aug 1;17(8):977–1007. doi:10.6004/jnccn.2019.0038. PMID: 31390582

4. McPherson ML, Walker KA, Davis MP, Bruera E, Reddy A, Paice J, et al. Safe and appropriate use of methadone in hospice and palliative care: Expert consensus white paper. *J Pain Symptom Manage*. 2019 Mar;57(3):635–645.e4.0

5. Brząkała J, Leppert W. The role of rapid onset fentanyl products in the management of breakthrough pain in cancer patients. *Pharmacol Rep*. 2019 Jun;71(3):438–442. doi:10.1016/j.pharep.2019.01.010. Epub 2019 Jan 31. PMID: 31003154

6. Schuster M, Bayer O, Heid F, Laufenberg-Feldmann R. Opioid rotation in cancer pain treatment. *Dtsch Arztebl Int*. 2018 Mar 2;115(9):135–142. doi:10.3238/arztebl.2018.0135. PMID: 29563006; PMCID: PMC5876542

7. Schüchen RH, Mücke M, Marinova M, Kravchenko D, Häuser W, Radbruch L, Conrad R. Systematic review and meta-analysis on non-opioid analgesics in palliative medicine. *J Cachexia Sarcopenia Muscle*. 2018 Dec;9(7):1235–1254. doi:10.1002/jcsm.12352. Epub 2018 Oct 29. PMID: 30375188; PMCID: PMC6351677

8. Deng Y, Luo L, Hu Y, Fang K, Liu J. Clinical practice guidelines for the management of neuropathic pain: A systematic review. *BMC Anesthesiol*. 2016 Feb 18;16:12. doi:10.1186/s12871-015-0150-5. PMID: 26892406; PMCID: PMC4759966

9. Hui D, Bruera E. The Edmonton symptom assessment system 25 years later: Past, present, and future developments. *J Pain Symptom Manage*. 2017 Mar;53(3):630–643. doi:10.1016/j.jpainsymman.2016.10.370. Epub 2016 Dec 29. PMID: 28042071; PMCID: PMC5337174

10. Clemens KE, Faust M, Bruera E. Update on combined modalities for the management of breathlessness. *Curr Opin Support Palliat Care.* 2012 Jun;6(2):163–167. doi:10.1097/SPC.0b013e3283530fee. PMID: 22469671

11. Del Fabbro E, Dalal S, Bruera E. Symptom control in palliative care Part III: Dyspnea and delirium. *J Palliat Med.* 2006 Apr;9(2):422–36. doi:10.1089/jpm.2006.9.422. PMID: 16629572

12. Qian Y, Wu Y, Rozman de Moraes A, Yi X, Geng Y, Dibaj S, Liu D, Naberhuis J, Bruera E. Fan therapy for the treatment of dyspnea in adults: A systematic review. *J Pain Symptom Manage.* 2019 Sep;58(3):481–486. doi:10.1016/j.jpainsymman.2019.04.011. Epub 2019 Apr 18. PMID: 31004769

13. Hui D, Maddocks M, Johnson MJ, Ekström M, Simon ST, Ogliari AC, Booth S, Ripamonti CI; ESMO Guidelines Committee. Management of breathlessness in patients with cancer: ESMO Clinical Practice Guidelines†. *ESMO Open.* 2020 Dec;5(6):e001038. doi:10.1136/esmoopen-2020-001038. PMID: 33303485

14. Thong MSY, van Noorden CJF, Steindorf K, Arndt V. Cancer-related fatigue: Causes and current treatment options. *Curr Treat Options Oncol.* 2020 Feb 5;21(2):17. doi:10.1007/s11864-020-0707-5. PMID: 32025928

15. Vannorsdall TD, Straub E, Saba C, Blackwood M, Zhang J, Stearns K, Smith KL. Interventions for multidimensional aspects of breast cancer-related fatigue: A meta-analytic review. *Support Care Cancer.* 2021;29(4):1753–1764. doi:10.1007/s00520-020-05752-y. Epub ahead of print. PMID: 33089371

16. Yennurajalingam S, Bruera E. Review of clinical trials of pharmacologic interventions for cancer-related fatigue: Focus on psychostimulants and steroids. *Cancer J.* 2014 Sep-Oct;20(5):319–24. doi:10.1097/PPO.0000000000000069. PMID: 25299141

17. Ng A, Gupta E, Bansal S, Fontillas RC, Amos CE Jr, Williams JL, Dibaj S, Bruera E et al. Cancer patients' perception of usefulness of wearable exercise trackers. *PM R.* 2020 Aug;13(8):845–851. doi:10.1002/pmrj.12475. Epub ahead of print. PMID: 32844592

18. Arring NM, Barton DL, Brooks T, Zick SM. Integrative therapies for cancer-related fatigue. *Cancer J.* 2019 Sep/Oct;25(5):349–356. doi:10.1097/PPO.0000000000000396. PMID: 31567463; PMCID: PMC7388739

29

Psychiatric Aspects of Pain Management in Palliative Care

R. Garrett Key and William Breitbart

Introduction

Pain is one of the most prevalent and distressing symptoms encountered in palliative care settings. Effective pain management requires clear knowledge of the physiologic etiology of pain and an understanding of the relationship between pain and psychiatric symptoms. There is a bidirectional relationship between pain and mental health: uncontrolled pain and physical symptoms can produce behaviors that manifest like psychiatric illness, and untreated psychiatric disorders and psychological distress will amplify the pain experience. Practitioners of all types can integrate elements of mental health treatment into the care plan to optimize pain control and overall well-being of their patients.[1] This chapter reviews the prevalence of pain in palliative populations, specific common pain syndromes, pain assessment strategies, and adjuvant pharmacologic interventions for pain in medically compromised patients. A brief overview of some psychotherapeutic approaches to pain in this population is included. Detailed review of psychotherapy approaches in palliative care can be found in Part VI.

Prevalence of Pain

Cancer

Although there has been increased attention on the importance of pain control in cancer, it remains a persistent and common problem. A recent meta-analysis reviewing the prevalence and severity of pain in cancer patients found that 39.3% of people who had curative treatment still reported pain, 55% of those being actively treated reported pain, and 66.4% of those with advanced, metastatic, or terminal disease reported problematic pain.

Moderate to severe pain was reported by 38% of cancer patients when the group was examined as a whole.[2] Evidence suggests that approximately one third of cancer patients are undertreated for pain.[3]

Human Immunodeficiency Virus/Acquired Immunodeficiency Syndrome (HIV/AIDS)

Between 54% and 83% of HIV-infected people report moderate to severe pain, with a moderate amount of interference in daily function from their pain. Pain in HIV/AIDS is typically present at multiple anatomical sites and often results from multiple ongoing processes. Despite the longitudinal focus on pain in HIV/AIDS, the overall prevalence rates for pain remain stable and high, as described above.[4]

Amyotrophic Lateral Sclerosis

People with amyotrophic lateral sclerosis (ALS) typically suffer from significant pain that may be refractory to treatment. Estimates of pain prevalence in ALS are around 60% with the most common site of pain being the shoulders and upper limbs. Pain may vary significantly in quality but is most commonly related to muscle cramps or spasms.[5]

Dementia

The prevalence of pain in dementing illnesses has presented challenges in assessment and is based on limited data, but what data does exist suggests a range of 45% to 56%. Despite the difficulties in the accurate assessment of pain in this population, it is clear that undertreatment of pain remains significant and clinically complex in this heterogenous group of patients.[6]

Sickle Cell Disease

Sickle cell disease (SCD) is a chronic, lifelong condition resulting in episodes of vaso-occlusive pain crisis and significant end organ morbidity. These patients are seen both by palliative medicine practitioners and in chronic pain treatment settings. Opioids are the central component of pain crisis management; however, in the context of the modern opioid crisis, there is evidence that accessing opioid analgesics has become more difficult. SCD typically affects Black people and the well-documented healthcare stigma against the Black population further increases barriers to accessing care and optimal pain control.[7]

End-Stage Renal Disease

Patients with end-stage renal disease have been found to have extremely high levels of pain, with estimates of acute and chronic pain in 27–93% and 33–82%, respectively. The range of estimates is quite large, but even the low end of the range is a significant proportion and worth carefully addressing. Specific pain complaints in these people are vascular access pain, headache, limb pain, chest pain, abdominal pain, and neuropathic pain.[8]

Congestive Heart Failure

Pain is common in congestive heart failure (CHF), estimated to occur in 23–75% of patients and closely associated with functional impairment, anxiety, and depression. Pain is a precipitant for hospital admission in CHF patients and typically worsens as death approaches. Pain disrupts self-management habits of CHF patients, thus it is critical to address so that these people can continue to successfully manage their care at home.[9]

End-Stage Liver Disease

Prevalence estimates for pain in people with end-stage liver disease (ESLD) range from 30% to 79%. Of those with pain, more than 50% were found to have daily pain and 75% of ESLD patients complained of some degree of pain related disability. Although the vast majority of patients with pain from ESLD reported that they were prescribed pain medications, only 33% indicated that their pain relief was effective.[10]

Multidimensional Concept of Pain

Pain is not a purely nociceptive phenomenon and involves a complex cascade of psychosocial inputs including personality, affect, cognition, behavior, and environmental context.[11] The Gate Control Theory advanced by Melzack and Wall has been perhaps the most influential model of the effect of psychosocial factors on how we experience pain. Gate Control Theory describes the modulation of pain based on physical damage, emotional context, and salience of the pain.[12] Study of the relationship between mental state and pain has led to the development and wide adoption of a biopsychosocial model of pain. It is now widely accepted that optimal pain management requires treatment of psychological distress.[13,14]

The bidirectional relationship between physiologically based pain and psychological distress demands intervention in both domains. Treatments targeting the physical sources of pain will benefit the psychological well-being of patients. Efforts focused on minimizing anxiety, depression, and psychosocial distress will diminish the overall impact of residual pain and diminish pain-related functional losses and disability.[15] Both physical and psychological components of pain must be untangled and addressed. It is common for fragmentation of care to create communication barriers between a patient's primary pain team, who are likely to manage opioids, and the psychosocial care clinicians managing adjuvant analgesics and psychotropics. Close collaboration between these two groups is essential for optimal pain control, minimizing polypharmacy, and presenting the patient with a clear and consistent pain management plan.

Pain Assessment in Complex Illness

The initial step in pain management is a comprehensive assessment of pain symptoms that includes measures of psychosocial distress. Clinicians must have a solid understanding of the etiology and treatment of pain in a wide variety of illness states and also take into account the life circumstances and context of the patient.

Pain can be categorized broadly into two categories based on pathophysiology: nociceptive or neuropathic.[16] Nociceptive pain arises from stimulation of pain receptors (nociceptors and can be subdivided into somatic pain (skin, soft tissue, muscle, and bone) or visceral pain (internal organs and viscera). Nociceptive pain may be localized (common in somatic pain) or diffuse (common in visceral pain) and may be sharp, dull, aching, gnawing, throbbing, constant, or spasmodic.

Neuropathic pain comes from stimulation of damaged or compromised nervous tissue. It can be burning, tingling, stabbing, shooting, or electrical. *Allodynia*, the sensation of pain produced by a typically non-noxious stimulus like light touch, is a type of neuropathic pain. The differentiation of pain into subtypes can help determine appropriate therapy. Tracking change in pain descriptors described in Box 29.1 can be helpful in charting the course of treatment.

BOX 29.1 Pain History and Descriptors

- When did it start?
- How long has it been present?
- Has it changed in any way?
- Is it intermittent or constant/continuous?
- Are there any other symptoms?
- Does the pain radiate or move anywhere?
- What makes the pain worse or better?
- What has been tried to treat the pain? Has it helped? Are there side effects? What are the scheduled doses?
- **Psychosocial issues**: Evaluate for patient distress, cultural beliefs toward pain, family/caregiver support, psychiatric/substance abuse history, and patients' goal for comfort and function.
- **Distress**: How much distress is the pain causing? Is the pain bearable or unbearable? Does the diffuseness of the distress suggest emotional suffering rather than nociception? What does the patient think that the pain means (e.g., tumor spread)? What are cultural, spiritual, or religious concerns about pain?
- **Support**: Who does the patient have for support? Are family members or others available? Is anyone reliably helping to manage the pain and medications at home? Evaluate for polypharmacy and possible medication interactions/side effects.
- **Psychiatric illness**:
  Anxiety: Conditioned anticipatory anxiety may begin before dressing changes or painful walking. Patients may seek analgesics to treat anxiety or insomnia rather than pain.
  Depression: Pain is amplified in depressed patients. Assess history of depression and current depressive symptoms (sleep disturbance; loss

of interest; guilt, hopelessness, helplessness; low energy; concentration difficulties; appetite changes; psychomotor retardation; suicidal ideation). Treat the depressive syndrome as appropriate.

Substance Use Disorders: Patients with psychiatric or opiate abuse histories may require higher doses due to tolerance. Addictive behavior: Use caution in patients with a history of drug dependence or alcoholism. Use initial screening with the Opioid Risk Tool (ORT): a higher risk score correlates with an increased likelihood of drug abuse.[17] Partnering with an addiction specialist and opioid contracts are recommended in such situations. Making sure that these patients never run out of their analgesics may work as a preventive strategy in avoiding pain crisis or aberrant drug-seeking behavior.

- **Goals and expectations**: Discuss patients' goals and expectations regarding pain management in the context of level of comfort and function. Include family/caregivers. Provide after- and off-hours backup support to manage severe pain over the phone.
- **Medical/Oncological history**: Pain should be evaluated in the context of the cancer and other significant medical illnesses.
- **Current medications**, including over-the-counter and complementary substances should be reviewed.
- **Physical examination** with review of appropriate laboratory and imaging studies.

A careful history and physical examination may identify a pain syndrome that can be treated in a standard fashion. The pain history will provide information about the nature of the underlying process and may reveal associated problems. There is a lack of consensus on which standardized pain assessment tool is best in palliative settings.[18] Several tools which balance brevity, ease of administration, and extraction of good information from the patient are listed in Box 29.2

Pain assessment is done continuously through the course of illness. There are essentially four aspects of pain experience that require ongoing evaluation: intensity, degree of relief, pain-related functional interference (e.g., mood state, general and specific activities), and monitoring for side effects and misuse.

Psychological Factors in the Pain Experience

Patients in a palliative setting may bear many stressors including loss of independence, disability, and fear of unmitigated suffering. Concerns about these threats are universal, but the level of psychological distress depends on medical factors, social support, coping skills, and can be significantly improved by the efforts of the treatment team. Uncontrolled pain amplifies psychological distress. Psychological factors such as anxiety, depression, and the meaning of pain can magnify the degree of pain experienced.

BOX 29.2 Pain Assessment Tools

- Brief Pain Inventory (eight-item questionnaire that assesses the presence, location, and severity of pain; interference caused by pain; and response pain treatment)[19]
- McGill Pain Questionnaire (20-item questionnaire that assesses sensory, affective, and qualitative aspects of pain)[20]
- Memorial Pain Assessment Card (visual analog scales that measure pain intensity, pain relief, and mood. Patients can complete the MPAC in less than 30 seconds)[21]
- The Pain Assessment in Advanced Dementia (PAINAD) scale (using observation of breathing, vocalization, facial expression, body language, and consolability)[22]

Psychological variables, such as the amount of control people believe they have over pain, emotional associations and memories of pain, fear of death, depression, anxiety, and hopelessness, contribute to the experience of pain.[23] Pain thought to be related to life-threatening causes such as cancer may be perceived to be worse than pain known to be from a benign source like osteoarthritis. Educating patients about the mechanisms of their pain can improve anxiety and pain reports. Although psychosocial factors can significantly influence pain, it is crucial to avoid overly attributing difficult to treat pain to psychological sources or blaming the patient for challenges in how they cope with pain.

Specific psychological factors appear related to functional outcomes and the overall impact of pain. Vulnerability to worse outcomes appears related to overall psychological distress, a history of trauma with particularly high risk with childhood trauma, fear of pain, and pain catastrophizing. Conversely, it has been seen that intact social support, active coping strategies, acceptance of injury and limitations, and self-efficacy are associated with better recovery and function in chronic pain conditions.[24] Identification of risk factors in a patient can guide interventions aimed at minimizing negative factors and working to emphasize and strengthen positive coping attributes.

Psychiatric Disorders and Pain

Psychiatric disorders, particularly anxiety and depressive disorders, are significantly more common in people living with pain. As mentioned above, anxiety and depression are known to amplify pain perception and are associated with refractory pain, pain-related disability, and an increased risk of substance use disorders. Comprehensive pain management requires that all patients be assessed and treated for psychiatric illness when it is present.

The most common disorders found in pain patients are major depression (31%), dysthymia (20%), posttraumatic stress disorder (PTSD; 9%), and adjustment disorder (9%). Notably, patients with higher negative affect (mood states such anger, guilt, and fear) have significantly less pain improvement, more intense opioid side effects, and increased risk for opioid misuse.[25]

Despite the clear association between anxiety, depression, and chronic pain there is a paucity of rigorous study on pharmacotherapy targeting depression and/or anxiety in the context of chronic pain. It is evident that co-treatment of anxiety and depression will have collateral benefit to pain treatment and that the analgesic effects of some psychotropics can be further leveraged to optimize pain control and functional improvement. A reasonable recommendation is for to use serotonin–noradrenaline reuptake inhibitors (SNRIs) as initial treatments for depression and anxiety in the setting of persistent pain because of their potential utility as adjuvant analgesics.[26] Tricyclic antidepressants (TCAs) have similar benefits and receptor binding profiles, but also come with a greater burden of anticholinergic side effects and CYP450 interactions. Typical approaches to mood and anxiety continue to be employed routinely in the context of chronic pain, including psychotherapeutic approaches discussed later in this chapter.

Suicidality in Chronic Pain

Thoughts of suicide, suicide attempts, and completed suicide are all more common in people living with pain. Chronic pain is estimated to increase the risk for suicidal thinking and behavior about four times the rate in the general population. Lifetime incidence of suicidal ideation in chronic pain patients is estimated around 23%, and 15% for suicide attempts. Typical risk factors for suicide in the general population include unemployed or disabled status, a history of childhood adverse events such as abuse or violence in the home, known psychiatric illness, and substance use problems. Factors related to pain which are associated with increased suicidality are the number of pain conditions, comorbid sleep problems, poorer perceived mental health, and pain catastrophizing.[27] A newer approach that examines traits found in patients with both psychiatric disorders and pain has identified so-called *transdiagnostic risk factors* that span both groups and can help identify people at elevated risk for self-harm. Current transdiagnostic risk factors associated with higher suicidality in people with pain are diminished future orientation, presence of vivid mental imagery around either pain or suicide, psychological inflexibility, perceived burdensomeness, isolation or lack of belonging, and a sense of mental defeat.[28]

Adjuvant Analgesics

Psychotropics are valuable tools in the treatment of pain through both direct analgesia and reduction in anxious and depressive symptoms. The current literature supports the use of psychotropics as adjuvant analgesics in a wide variety of pain syndromes.[29] Table 29.1 lists psychotropic medications with analgesic properties, their routes of administration, and their approximate daily doses.

Caution should be taken to monitor for development of serotonin syndrome whenever medications with serotonin reuptake inhibition are combined with opioids. SNRIs, selective serotonin reuptake inhibitors (SSRIs), TCAs, and trazodone all require vigilance, but the contraindication is relative and can be managed with close clinical observation and gentle titration. Opioids with known serotonin reuptake inhibition, and therefore

TABLE 29.1 Psychotropic adjuvant analgesic drugs

GENERIC NAME	Approximate daily dosage range (mg)	Route
TRICYCLIC ANTIDEPRESSANTS		
Amitriptyline	10–300	PO, IM
Nortriptyline	10–150	PO
Imipramine	10–300	PO, IM
Desipramine	10–150	PO
Clomipramine	10–150	PO
Doxepin	12–150	PO, IM
HETEROCYCLIC AND NON-CYCLIC ANTIDEPRESSANTS		
Trazodone	125–300	PO
Maprotiline	50–300	PO
SEROTONIN-REUPTAKE INHIBITORS		
Fluoxetine	20–80	PO
Paroxetine	10–60	PO
Sertraline	50–200	PO
Citalopram	10–40	PO
Escitalopram	10–20	PO
SEROTONIN-NOREPINEPHRINE REUPTAKE INHIBITORS		
Venlafaxine	75–375	PO
Desvenlafaxine	25–100	PO
Duloxetine	20–120	PO
H_1 HISTAMINE, $5HT_2$/ $5HT_3$ SEROTONIN ANTAGONIST		
Mirtazapine	7.5–60	PO
Psychostimulants		
Methylphenidate	2.5–20 BID	PO
Dextroamphetamine	2.5–20 BID	PO
Modafinil	100–400	PO
Armodafinil	50–150	PO
PHENOTHIAZINES		
Fluphenazine	1–3	PO, IM
Methotrimeprazine	10–20 q6h	IM, IV
BUTYROPHENONES		
Haloperidol	1–3	PO, IV
Pimozide	2–6 BID	PO
ANTIHISTAMINE		
Hydroxyzine	50 q4–6h	PO
ANTICONVULSANTS		
Carbamazepine	200–400 TID	PO
Phenytoin	300–400	PO
Valproate	250–1,000 BID	PO
Gabapentin	300–1,200 TID	PO
Oxcarbazepine	300–1200 BID	PO
Pregabalin	50–150 BID/TID	PO

PO, per oral; IM, intramuscular; IV, intravenous; Q6H, every 6 hrs; BID, twice a day; TID, three times a day; QID, four times a day.

increased risk of serotonin syndrome, include fentanyl, meperidine, tramadol, methadone, dextromethorphan, and propoxyphene. Conversely, codeine, morphine, oxycodone, and buprenorphine are not known to have serotonin reuptake inhibition.

In the palliative setting, care should be taken to monitor for decreased clearance of medications in the context of end organ failure. Liver dysfunction may reduce CYP450 enzyme function and result in altered rates of metabolism. Hypoalbuminemia is common in serious illness states where either liver function is impaired or nutritional status is compromised. The vast majority of the psychotropics are highly protein bound. Reduction in albumin can increase the amount of unbound, and therefore active, drug in the bloodstream.

Serum level monitoring is important for TCAs and valproic acid preparations, otherwise clinical observation for evidence of emerging side effects can be used to guide most medication dosing in progressive hepatic illness. Of note, the SNRI venlafaxine and the SSRI escitalopram are less protein bound and thus can be more easily dosed in patients with hypoalbuminemia.

Renal disease can require dose adjustment for some psychotropics due to the presence of potentially toxic renally excreted metabolites. Due the highly protein bound nature mentioned above, these medications are not effectively removed by dialysis. Exceptions again are venlafaxine and escitalopram. Gabapentin and TCAs require adjusted dosing in renal impairment as well.

Tricyclic Antidepressants

TCAs can potentiate the effects of opioid analgesics and also work as a primary treatment for neuropathic pain. Amitriptyline is the TCA most studied and proved as an analgesic in a wide variety of chronic pain, and nortriptyline has also been found to be effective. Patients may respond variably to different to TCAs, so if one TCA is ineffective then others should be tried.

Treatment should be initiated with a low dose at bedtime and titrated slowly to effect. Maximal effect as an adjuvant analgesic may require 2–6 weeks of therapy, and serum levels can be checked to confirm therapeutic range or toxicity.

TCAs cause anticholinergic side effects like constipation, dry mouth, blurred vision, urinary retention, incoordination, worsened cognition, and tremor. These side effects are common and dose-dependent. Anticholinergic delirium can be precipitated at higher doses, particularly in elderly or medically compromised patients. Slow and careful titration is advised, particularly in the context of opioid treatment.

Selective Serotonin Reuptake Inhibitors

SSRIs have equivocal benefits in terms of direct anti-nociceptive properties. Their benefits to mood and anxiety can have indirect effects on the total pain experience of patients. Their efficacy as adjuvant analgesics in pain patients without anxiety or depression is not established.

Serotonin and Norepinephrine Reuptake Inhibitors

SNRIs have good analgesic properties which arise from the mechanism of norepinephrine reuptake inhibition, similar to TCAs. In most situations SNRIs are preferred over TCAs because of the lower burden of anticholinergic side effects seen with SNRIs.

Mirtazapine, Bupropion, and Trazodone

These mechanistically distinct medicines are effective for treating depressive symptoms and have side effect profiles that can be leveraged advantageously.

Mirtazapine can be helpful for pain, poor sleep quality, and irritability. It has potent antiemetic effects related to $5HT_3$ antagonism and promotes appetite which can benefit patients with nausea or poor appetite.

Bupropion is effective for treatment of depression, may offer some benefit to fatigue, and has an independent FDA indication for use in smoking cessation. Unlike most antidepressants, bupropion does not typically cause sexual dysfunction. Bupropion is usually less effective for anxiety and may worsen anxiety in some patients.

Trazodone is often prescribed as a sleep aid with less risk of delirium than the stronger sedative-hypnotics such as zolpidem, zaleplon, and eszopiclone. Trazodone shares some similarity in receptor binding with TCAs and SNRIs but has not been proved to have the same level of benefit for pain.

Monoamine Oxidase Inhibitors

Monoamine oxidase inhibitors (MAOIs) are less useful because of dietary restrictions on tyramine-containing foods and potentially dangerous interactions between MAOIs and opioids which can result in serotonin syndrome. Their use as adjuvant analgesics in most palliative settings is not advised.

Anticonvulsants

Many anticonvulsant drugs are effective treatments of neuropathic pain.[30] These drugs include gabapentin, pregabalin, oxcarbazepine, lamotrigine, and felbamate. Of these anticonvulsants, anecdotal experience has been most favorable with gabapentin, which has a relatively high degree of safety, including no known drug–drug interactions and a lack of hepatic metabolism. Pregabalin is approved by the US Food and Drug Administration (FDA) for neuropathic pain associated with diabetic neuropathy, as well as for post-herpetic neuralgia and is used broadly for all types of neuropathic pain.

Psychostimulants

Psychostimulants can be useful in treating depressed mood, potentiating analgesia, and reducing sedation from opioid analgesics, and they may potentiate opioid analgesia. Psychostimulants can encourage appetite, promote a sense of well-being, and improve weakness and fatigue. Tolerance may develop, and adjustment of dose may be necessary. Side effects include a sense of overstimulation, anxiety, paranoia, and insomnia. Caution to avoid misuse is advised.

Treatment with dextroamphetamine or methylphenidate begins with a low dose at morning and midday with titration over several days to desired effect.

Modafinil and armodafinil are non-amphetamine wakefulness-promoting agents approved by the FDA for the treatment of excessive daytime sedation secondary to sleep disorders (e.g., narcolepsy, sleep apnea); they are used in palliative settings to combat sedation and daytime fatigue and diminished attention and concentration. Modafinil/armodafinil are not sympathomimetic agents and may have lower abuse potential in general although caution is advised in patients with known substance misuse.

Antipsychotics

Neuroleptic medications, typically used for psychotic symptoms, have a critical role in the treatment of a variety of symptoms including nausea, vomiting, insomnia, and anxiety. There is little evidence to support their use as direct analgesics. Of note, it can help allay patient concerns about taking a medicine with labeled use in psychotic illness to explain that these drugs work through the modulation of dopamine and serotonin, which have many functions in the body unrelated to psychosis.

Phenothiazine neuroleptics treat anxiety, nausea, and vomiting primarily through dopamine blockade. Chlorpromazine and prochlorperazine are useful as antiemetics but have limited use as analgesics.

Atypical antipsychotics such as olanzapine, risperidone, quetiapine, aripiprazole, and ziprasidone are primarily used to treat symptoms of delirium in the palliative care setting but also are useful in reducing anxiety and augmenting depression treatment and thereby helping to reduce the pain amplification that can come from those states.

Benzodiazepines and Hydroxyzine

Benzodiazepines and the antihistamine hydroxyzine can be used in the treatment of pain through their anxiolytic effect. Benzodiazepines are not thought to have direct analgesic properties. The synergistic sedative effects of benzodiazepines when combined with opioids require caution and judicious use of both drugs to avoid oversedation and potentially lethal apnea.

Hydroxyzine is an antihistamine useful as a mild anxiolytic with mild sedative and analgesic properties.

Ketamine

Ketamine is an anesthetic agent and analgesic that is thought to exert its effects via antagonism of N-methyl-D-aspartate (NMDA) receptors. It has shown some promise in the treatment of pain but the quality of evidence remains modest as described in recent reviews.[31,32] In addition to the lack of a solid evidence base currently, issues in administration arise due to the best evidence for use with intravenous preparations and less reliable information available about the utility of oral ketamine in outpatient treatment of chronic pain. Ketamine may have a place in the standard treatment of chronic pain in the future, but, at the time of writing, a need for more robust investigation precludes recommendation of its use in routine practice.

Cannabis and Derivative Compounds

Decriminalization and a more permissive environment for formal research has moved cannabis into the realm of legally available medical treatments. Many states have it available as prescription medication, others have opened the doors for recreational use, and specifical legal channels have been made in other states for "compassionate use" in people with life-limiting conditions. A wide variety of preparations of whole leaf cannabis extracts, cannabidiol (CBD), and tetrahydrocannabinol (THC) are readily available and marketed to lay people for treatment of psychiatric illness, pain, seizures, nausea, cachexia, and other neurological conditions. In chronic pain the number needed to treat is high, around 24, while the number needed to harm is estimated at 6 individuals. The utility of these compounds in the treatment of both pain conditions and most psychiatric conditions including anxiety, depression, and PTSD is not well supported by current literature.[33,34]

Psychological Management of Pain

Psychological approaches to pain management have been the subject of a significant amount of study and are a common part of comprehensive pain management in palliative care settings. Pain can lead to depression, anxiety, disability, loss of social contact. Some people may feel that life has been irreversibly damaged by pain or see pain as an uncontrollable catastrophe. The goals of psychological treatment specifically related to pain can be collapsed into four broad categories: pain, mood, catastrophizing, and pain-related disability. In a palliative setting, there are also a number of focused techniques around death and dying which are reviewed in Part VI of this text.

The variety of psychological techniques that have been studied specifically around pain is wide and includes cognitive behavioral therapy (CBT) and a number of other techniques that can be grouped into behavior therapies. The behavior therapies include but are not limited to acceptance and commitment therapy (ACT), mindfulness-based stress reduction (MBSR), biofeedback, mindfulness meditation, hypnosis, progressive relaxation, and music/art/aromatherapy. CBT and behavioral therapies both attempt to change behavior that reinforces or maintains pain, psychological distress, catastrophic thinking, or disability. CBT adds a focus on the maladaptive thoughts and feelings associated with pain.

The evidence base supporting effectiveness of CBT is good and indicates a small benefit for catastrophizing and pain-related disability but without clear evidence of improvement in mood or pain. Behaviorally based therapies, taken as a whole, have a weaker evidence base and show only transient benefit for catastrophizing and no benefit for other domains. It is notable that the lack of effect seen in behavior therapies at the meta-analysis level may be related to limitations in our understanding of optimal patient selection and treatment application within chronic pain subgroups.[35] It is likely that proper patient selection; consistent, capable application of the psychologically based techniques; and improved study methodologies will improve the large scale outcome data.

Cognitive Behavioral Therapy

The goal of CBT is to develop the ability to observe and assess thoughts (cognitions) associated with pain and minimize maladaptive behaviors that exist around avoiding unpleasant thoughts and the pain itself. A core tenet of CBT is that strongly held negative beliefs about pain lead to behaviors that worsen disability, mood, and the overall impact of chronic pain. The cognitive work focuses on identifying and improving the negative beliefs about pain. The behavioral aspect centers on identifying behaviors that are contingent on pain or focused on avoiding and relieving pain and then developing new behaviors contingent on a person's goals and values. Instead of yielding to pain and focusing on comfort and avoidance, the patient will begin to set and achieve goals in the context of living with their chronic pain.

Notably, the benefit of CBT is best when delivered by experienced staff with formal training in CBT. Detailed instruction in the practice of these techniques is encouraged for anyone wishing to employ them in clinical practice; however, that information is beyond the scope of this work.

Behavioral Therapies

Behavioral techniques for pain control seek to modify physiologic pain reactions, respondent pain behaviors, and operant pain behaviors.

Acceptance and Commitment Therapy

ACT is based on the core concept that one can limit the impact of pain by accepting the pain as it is and learning to live with it. Elimination of pain is removed as a goal and replaced with finding ways to live as well as possible with whatever degree of residual pain exists with available treatment. Patients move away from efforts to control pain and instead attempt to accept the limits of pain control and work on ways to set and achieve goals for living in the presence of pain.

Mindfulness Meditation and Mindfulness-Based Stress Reduction

Mindfulness meditation approaches attempt to reduce the impact and experience of pain by experiencing physical feelings without judgment and associated negative emotions and cognitions. There is a focus on separating awareness from thinking that subsequently allows one to be aware of pain without also experiencing negative thoughts related to the pain. MBSR is a specific form of mindfulness meditation developed by Dr. Jon Kabat-Zinn which is manualized and has gained popularity since its introduction in 1979.[36]

Mindfulness meditation techniques include body scanning (focusing awareness on parts of your body to improve accuracy of sensation), breathing and/or progressive relaxation exercises to diminish anxiety and increase body awareness, and distraction techniques that shift the patient's attention away from their body and pain.

Biofeedback

Biofeedback uses sensors connected to the body to provide immediate information about its physical state; this allows the patient to try new ways of relaxing muscles or otherwise altering their body to improve how they feel. Sensors can return a variety of information including brain waves via electroencephalograph, breathing, heart rate, muscle contraction, sweat gland activity, and temperature.

Hypnosis

Hypnosis, which can also be called *hypnotherapy*, *hypnotic suggestion*, or more recently *hypno-algesia* when focused on pain relief, is a technique that encourages a patient to reach a deeply relaxed state where one becomes open to suggestions that are aligned with the goals of therapy. It has application in many areas, and in pain control the suggestions are set to encourage reduction in the patient's pain experience and pain interference. Studies of hypnosis suggests good efficacy for most people, with success depending on the suggestibility of the patient. The evidence is of low quality in terms of rigor and reproducibility, unfortunately.[37]

Music, Aroma, and Art Therapies

Pain treatment augmentation using music, aromatherapy, and artistic expression have been found to improve pain scores and psychological variables such as anxiety and depression in a variety of illness states including cancer, non-cancer terminal illnesses, and chronic pain. The quality of the evidence, however, is poor, and thus further study is recommended. These modalities can be easily employed in almost any setting and are minimally risky, noninvasive, and thus can be made available to essentially all patients who might benefit or express interest.

Future Directions

We know more now about the relationship between mental state and how pain is experienced than ever before. We have clear evidence for the entanglement of physical sources of pain and the modulating effect of mental state influences.[38] The opioid backbone of pain treatment can now be augmented with a variety of other medications, psychotherapeutic approaches, and behavioral methods. Yet the high prevalence and persistence of pain highlights how far we have to go and urges us onward.

Perhaps the most critical knowledge gap for both pharmacotherapies and psychologically based therapies is greater understanding of the molecular mechanisms of the pain experience. Rather than pursuing more trial-and-error approaches, we might seek to create more nuanced models of neurotransmitter effects, neural plasticity, and mechanistically based combination therapy trials.

In terms of specific agents, further study of endogenous and exogenous cannabinoids, MDMA, and psilocybin are potentially fruitful avenues of investigation. The controversial history of these pharmaceuticals makes it clear that their study and use should be pursued carefully and with respect for potential harms.

Improved rigor in the study of psychologically based therapies will yield more effective strategies for treatment. Improved trial design focused on identifying responsive subgroups of patients could help improve signal identification from the currently noisy data produced by trials with heterogenous patient populations studied under the non-specific banner of "chronic pain." Trials of psychological therapies tend toward heterogeneity in how treatments are delivered, further confounding the signal. Small subgroups of responders may disappear in large group analysis of larger, less sensitive aggregate datasets. Control group design is problematic. Many trials may compare an intervention to a waitlist or treatment as usual condition that lacks active engagement components of the treatment arm.

Outside of the realm of science, we must make our current treatments readily available and integrated into practice. Despite the widespread evidence supporting multimodal pain treatment, many patients must navigate the healthcare maze to find the various clinicians they need. We must improve the design of our system so that patients are not required to build their own treatment teams. Mental health access is particularly challenging, with a lack of clinicians and a marginal reimbursement climate that drives many clinicians to cash-only practice. Siloed medical disciplines are the norm outside of major medical centers, and this must change if meaningful integration of pain treatment and psychosocial care is to be achieved.

Key Points

- Pain is highly prevalent in palliative populations and has a large negative impact on functional status and quality of life.
- Psychosocial variables including depression, anxiety, and existential distress can amplify pain and reduce a person's ability to manage their pain effectively.
- Psychotropic medications are safe and effective for augmentation of other analgesic approaches.
- Psychologically based therapies, although less clearly supported by high-quality evidence, are an important component of a comprehensive pain management plan.
- The goals of pain management in palliative care focus on optimizing functional status and quality of life.

References

1. Foley KM. The treatment of cancer pain. *N Engl J Med.* Jul 11 1985;313(2):84–95. doi:10.1056/NEJM198507113130205
2. Van Den Beuken-Van MH, Hochstenbach LM, Joosten EA, Tjan-Heijnen VC, Janssen DJ. Update on prevalence of pain in patients with cancer: Systematic review and meta-analysis. *J Pain Sympt Manage.* 2016;51(6):1070–1090.

3. Greco MT, Roberto A, Corli O, Deandrea S, Bandieri E, Cavuto S, et al. Quality of cancer pain management: An update of a systematic review of undertreatment of patients with cancer. *J Clin Oncol.* 2014;32(36):4149–4154.

4. Parker R, Stein DJ, Jelsma J. Pain in people living with HIV/AIDS: A systematic review. *J Int AIDS Soc.* 2014;17(1):18719.

5. Hurwitz N, Radakovic R, Boyce E, Peryer G. Prevalence of pain in amyotrophic lateral sclerosis: A systematic review and meta-analysis. *ALS Frontotemp Degen.* 2021:1–10.

6. Zwakhalen SM, Hamers JP, Abu-Saad HH, Berger MP. Pain in elderly people with severe dementia: A systematic review of behavioural pain assessment tools. *BMC Geriatr.* 2006;6(1):1–15.

7. Sinha CB, Bakshi N, Ross D, Krishnamurti L. Management of chronic pain in adults living with sickle cell disease in the era of the opioid epidemic: A qualitative study. *JAMA Network Open.* 2019;2(5):e194410-e194410.

8. Brkovic T, Burilovic E, Puljak L. Prevalence and severity of pain in adult end-stage renal disease patients on chronic intermittent hemodialysis: A systematic review. *Patient Preference Adherence.* 2016;10:1131.

9. Godfrey C, Harrison MB, Medves J, Tranmer JE. The symptom of pain with heart failure: A systematic review. *J Cardiac Failure.* 2006;12(4):307–313.

10. Peng J-K, Hepgul N, Higginson IJ, Gao W. Symptom prevalence and quality of life of patients with end-stage liver disease: A systematic review and meta-analysis. *Palliat Med.* 2019;33(1):24–36.

11. Zaza C, Baine N. Cancer pain and psychosocial factors: A critical review of the literature. *J Pain Sympt Manage.* 2002;24(5):526–542.

12. Melzack R, Wall PD. Pain mechanisms: A new theory. *Science.* Nov 19 1965;150(3699):971–979.

13. Syrjala KL, Chapko ME. Evidence for a biopsychosocial model of cancer treatment-related pain. *Pain.* 1995;61(1):69–79.

14. Gatchel RJ, Peng YB, Peters ML, Fuchs PN, Turk DC. The biopsychosocial approach to chronic pain: Scientific advances and future directions. *Psychol Bull.* 2007;133(4):581.

15. Breitbart W. Psychiatric management of cancer pain. *Cancer.* Jun 1 1989;63(11 Suppl):2336–2342.

16. Doyle D, Hanks GWC, MacDonald N, eds. *Oxford Textbook of Palliative Medicine.* 2nd ed. New York: Oxford University Press; 1998.

17. Hjermstad MJ, Gibbins J, Haugen D, et al. Pain assessment tools in palliative care: An urgent need for consensus. *Palliat Med.* 2008;22(8):895–903.

18. Cleeland CS, Tearnan, BH. Behavioral control of cancer pain. In: Holzman AD, Turk DC, eds. *Pain Management: A Handbook of Psychological treatment approaches.* Oxford: Pergamon Press; 1986:93–212.

19. Edwards RR, Dworkin RH, Sullivan MD, Turk DC, Wasan AD. The role of psychosocial processes in the development and maintenance of chronic pain. *J Pain.* 2016;17(9):T70–T92.

20. Van Rijswijk S, van Beek M, Schoof G, Schene A, Steegers M, Schellekens A. Iatrogenic opioid use disorder, chronic pain and psychiatric comorbidity: A systematic review. *Gen Hosp Psychiatry.* 2019;59:37–50.

21. IsHak WW, Wen RY, Naghdechi L, et al. Pain and depression: A systematic review. *Harvard Rev Psychiatry.* 2018;26(6):352–363.

22. Racine M. Chronic pain and suicide risk: A comprehensive review. *Prog Neuro-Psychopharmacol Biol Psychiatry.* 2018;87:269–280.

23. Kirtley OJ, Rodham K, Crane C. Understanding suicidal ideation and behaviour in individuals with chronic pain: A review of the role of novel transdiagnostic psychological factors. *Lancet Psychiatry.* 2020;7(3):282–290.

24. Jacox A, Carr D, Payne R, Berde C, Breitbart W, Cain J. *Management of Cancer Pain. Clinical Practice Guideline No. 9.* AHCPR Publication No. 94-0592. Rockville, MD: Agency for Health Care Policy and Research, US Department of Health and Human Services, Public Health Service; 1994:257.

25. Swarm RA, Paice JA, Anghelescu DL, et al. Adult cancer pain, version 3.2019. *NCCN Clin Pract Guidelines Oncol.* 2019;17(8):977. doi:10.6004/jnccn.2019.0038

26. Michelet D, Brasher C, Horlin AL, et al. Ketamine for chronic non-cancer pain: A meta-analysis and trial sequential analysis of randomized controlled trials. *Eur J Pain.* 2018;22(4):632–646.

27. Orhurhu V, Orhurhu MS, Bhatia A, Cohen SP. Ketamine infusions for chronic pain: A systematic review and meta-analysis of randomized controlled trials. *Anesth Analg.* 2019;129(1):241–254.

28. Black N, Stockings E, Campbell G, et al. Cannabinoids for the treatment of mental disorders and symptoms of mental disorders: A systematic review and meta-analysis. *Lancet Psychiatry.* 2019;6(12):995–1010.

29. Fisher E, Moore RA, Fogarty AE, et al. Cannabinoids, cannabis, and cannabis-based medicine for pain management: A systematic review of randomised controlled trials. *Pain.* 2021;1(162 Suppl):S45–S66.

30. de C Williams AC, Fisher E, Hearn L, Eccleston C. Psychological therapies for the management of chronic pain (excluding headache) in adults. *Cochrane Database Syst Rev.* 2020 Aug 12;8(8):CD007407. pub4. PMID: 32794606; PMCID: PMC7437545

31. Kabat-Zinn J. Minfulness-Based Stress Reduction. *Constructivism in the Health Sciences.* 2003;8(2):73–107.

32. Thompson T, Terhune DB, Oram C, et al. The effectiveness of hypnosis for pain relief: A systematic review and meta-analysis of 85 controlled experimental trials. *Neurosci Biobehav Rev.* 2019;99:298–310.

33. Melzack R, Wall PD. Pain mechanisms: A new theory. *Science.* 1965;150(3699):971–979.

34. Cleeland C, Ryan K. Pain assessment: Global use of the Brief Pain Inventory. *Ann Acad Med Singapore.* 1994;23(2):129–138.

35. Melzack R. The McGill Pain Questionnaire: Major properties and scoring methods. *Pain.* Sep 1975;1(3):277–299.

36. Fishman B, Pasternak S, Wallenstein SL, Houde RW, Holland JC, Foley KM. The Memorial Pain Assessment Card: A valid instrument for the evaluation of cancer pain. *Cancer.* 1987;60(5):1151–1158.

37. Warden V, Hurley AC, Volicer L. Development and psychometric evaluation of the Pain Assessment in Advanced Dementia (PAINAD) scale. *J Am Med Dir Assoc.* Jan–Feb 2003;4(1):9–15. doi:10.1097/01.JAM.0000043422.31640.F7

38. Chou R, Fanciullo GJ, Fine PG, Miaskowski C, Passik SD, Portenoy RK. Opioids for chronic noncancer pain: Prediction and identification of aberrant drug-related behaviors: A Review of the evidence for an American Pain Society and American Academy of Pain Medicine clinical practice guideline. *J Pain.* Feb 2009;10(2):131–146. doi:10.1016/j.jpain.2008.10.009

30

Eating Issues in Palliative Cancer Patients

A Source of Cachexia-Related Distress

Jane B. Hopkinson, Koji Amano, and Vickie E. Baracos

Introduction

Cancer cachexia is the wasting syndrome experienced by many people with a cancer diagnosis.[1,2] It is a debilitating condition associated with muscle wasting, involuntary weight loss, physical decline, fatigue, and poor appetite. These symptoms have emotional and social impact that can adversely affect the quality of life of both patients and their family members.[3,4]

This chapter gives an overview of what is known about cancer cachexia and treatments, its emotional and social impact, and the measurement of associated distress. It concludes by considering the implications for clinical management.

Cancer Cachexia

Cancer cachexia is defined as a multifactorial syndrome of weight loss characterized by an ongoing loss of skeletal muscle mass (with or without loss of fat mass) that cannot be fully reversed by conventional nutritional support and leads to progressive functional impairment. The pathophysiology is characterized by a negative protein and energy balance driven by a variable combination of reduced food intake and abnormal metabolism.[5]

Cancer cachexia is a type of *sickness behavior*, which is defined as a coordinated set of changes during illness encompassing some or all of fever, lethargy, depression, anxiety, malaise, weight loss, loss of appetite, increased catabolism (increased proteolysis and lipolysis), sleepiness, hyperalgesia, reduction in grooming, difficulty concentrating, and reduced so-cial interaction. Sickness behavior is a hallmark of infection and is thought to have evolved as an adaptive response to facilitate recovery and decrease disease transmission among group mates.[6,7] The idea that the sickness behavior might be advantageous launched a new area of research aimed at understanding how the immune system communicates with the central nervous system (CNS). Sickness behaviors have been extensively studied in animal model systems, as well as in free-living animals of different species in their natural environ-ment. Pro-inflammatory cytokines are the main actors of this communication in infection, as well as other inflammatory states, including cancer.[8,9] These cytokines are secreted by leukocytes and include interleukin (IL)-1β, IL-6, and tumor necrosis factor-α (TNF-α). The cytokines are secreted by activated mononuclear phagocytic cells, and numerous studies show that both peripheral and central injection of IL-1β, IL-6, and TNF-α induce sickness behavior. Several labs have described a CNS-based mechanism of cancer cachexia in which cytokines generated in the periphery are amplified and modified within the hypothalamus, leading to aberrant activity of weight- and activity-modulating neurons.[10]

Sickness clearly invokes a catabolic state, with specific reduction of appetite along-side mobilization of body stores including activation of proteolysis in muscle and lipolysis in adipose tissue. Pro-inflammatory cytokines are again the actors of these responses via actions both in the CNS and directly at the tissue level via cytokine receptors. In addition to altered metabolism, sickness behavior also entails specific alterations in motivational state. Whereas motivation for feeding might be high in health, in sickness motivation this behavior is reduced and motivation to rest is increased. In what ways might this sacrifice of energy homeostasis enhance the chance of survival? It has been postulated that anorexia reduces motivation to engage in foraging, which would spare body energy for allocation to support the metabolic cost of inflammation. Likewise, increased somnolence/lethargy reinforces the urge to take shelter, reducing energy expenditure and body heat dissipation. In evolution, those responses would also reduce the likelihood of being killed by a predator while physically compromised.[6] Last, sickness can be a strong driver of behavioral inter-actions among individuals.[11] In the case of communicable illness, social isolation could be adaptive, in the sense of limiting potential for disease transmission to kin.[12]

Normally, infections are overcome by the immune system, the inflammatory response subsides, and, with it, the sickness behavior also subsides. In chronic disease, such as cancer, however, the persistent sickness behavior becomes pathological as it is naturally only ten-able until body stores of energy and protein are depleted or exhausted. The body condition of the individual worsens and energetic demands on the immune system (and of the tumor) increase. In animals, cancer progression also further reduces the connectivity of tumor-infected individuals within their social network.[13] In advanced stages of incurable cancer, anorexia and wasting progress relentlessly and may lead ultimately to emaciation and death.

The understanding of the pathophysiology of sickness behavior is relevant to un-derstanding several aspects of suffering experienced by patients with cancer and their im-mediate family and caregivers. Human relationships around food, eating, and caring are profoundly disturbed by the presence of sickness. Provision of food is a basic form of caring, but burdened with anorexia, anhedonia, and sensory alterations, patients all too often have little desire for and may even be actively repelled by certain foods. This is extremely frustrating on both sides and requires different strategies to alleviate the situation. Patients and their caregivers require information and education about the physiological and psychological changes generated by the cancer. This can help patients be aware of what to expect and ease their frustration about continued weight loss in spite of laborious efforts to eat. Family members can gain an appreciation of patient's loss of interest in food and redirect their care toward non–food related supports.

The Medical Management of Cancer Cachexia

Although science is building our understanding of the molecular basis of cancer cachexia and pathophysiology explaining its progression, the development of medical treatment has proved to be difficult. A variety of therapeutic targets (e.g., ghrelin receptor, type 4 melanocortin receptor, growth and differentiation factor GDF-15) for relief of cancer anorexia are in clinical development and new results are eagerly awaited. Anamorelin, a ghrelin receptor agonist that can be administered orally, has been developed and tested in cancer patient populations and shown to induce robust increases in lean and fat mass. It is the only pharmacological agent yet to be licensed to treat the syndrome and then only in Japan.[14] Loss of motivation to eat remains a significant problem. Corticosteroids or progesterone analogs can be of benefit to patients suffering from loss of appetite or weight loss with advanced progressing cancer, although possible benefit needs to be weighed against potential side effects in each case.[15] Recent research has also shown the possibilities of Chinese/Japanese herbal medicines (e.g., Yukgunja-Tang and Ninjinyoeito) for sickness behavior and cancer cachexia.[16–18] The effectiveness of Chinese/Japanese herbal medicines in combination with standard Western medicinal treatment needs to be investigated in the future.

Cachexia and anorexia can be in part alleviated through nutritional management. The reader is referred to recent clinical practice guidelines of international Medical Oncology Societies (ASCO[15], ESMO[19]) as well as those concerned with Clinical Nutrition and Metabolism (e.g., ESPEN[20,21]). Nutritional assessment and nutritional support of patients is exhaustively covered in the Guidelines. The low levels of clinical research in this area and the low quality of available evidence are a frequently cited concern; however, these guidelines provide valuable practical information. Medical management is possible for a variety of nutritional impact symptoms (e.g., pain, nausea, early satiety, constipation), and all Guidelines stress the need for impeccable symptom management and psychosocial support to enable dietary intake.

The Psychosocial Impact of Cancer Cachexia

Involuntary weight loss, poor appetite, weakness, and fatigue can be troubling, even distressing for patients.[22] The symptoms are challenging to manage and have negative emotional and social impact for patient and their family.[23] However, there is a growing community of clinicians who recognize the benefits of offering a supportive care plan to improve quality of life in people experiencing cachexia-related suffering.

The symptoms of cachexia can be experienced across the whole cancer pathway from diagnosis to death or survivorship. They are typically more pronounced in advanced disease with increased prevalence as end of life approaches and in some cancers, including lung cancer, esophageal cancer, pancreatic cancer, and gastric cancer. Cancer cachexia can be reversed if the cancer itself is treated successfully. When cancer is progressing and incurable, cachexia similarly becomes refractory.

Eating and Drinking with Refractory Cachexia

Eating problems can be caused by cancer treatments, their nutritional impact side effects, or the cancer itself obstructing the gastrointestinal tract or causing metabolic change that suppresses appetite. These obstacles to eating compromise nutritional intake. The resultant depletion of nutrients then contributes to muscle wasting, weight loss, and debilitation. Attention to both the pharmacological and nonpharmacological management of treatment side effects and nutritional impact symptoms is important to help the patient maintain an adequate nutritional status for as long as possible.

Problems with eating can be difficult for patients to understand, particularly if the cause is a hidden metabolic process rather than a symptom, such as a sore mouth. The problem may be even more difficult for a family member to understand, especially if they have no prior experience of disease-induced appetite loss. Fears expressed by patients include those of increasing physical dependency, loss of autonomy, and fear of death. Family members can similarly fear how they will cope with the patient's increasing physical dependency while fearing (in the absence of an obvious cause of the eating problem) that they are themselves to blame because they have been unable to provide sufficient nourishment. Emotional responses range from acceptance to extreme distress and conflict between family members. The emotional responses of the patient and family members can be interdependent[24] and influenced by culture or religious beliefs.[25,26]

Limitations on the ability to share meals can cause a decline in social activity. Some patients elect to eat alone to avoid the embarrassment of being able to eat too little or to avoid judgmental encouragement to eat. Thus, there is loss of enjoyment in social activities involving food and disruption to social life.[27] A sense of isolation evoked by cancer progression can be reinforced by difference in what can be eaten and drunk; difference that can also be experienced as isolating for a family member who witnesses a divergence between their own and the patient's eating habits. In a counterproductive effort to address such divergence, some family members even place themselves at nutritional risk by seeking to maintain congruence between the patient's oral intake and their own.

Living with Involuntary Weight Loss and Refractory Cachexia

Nutritional depletion and the impact of the cachectic process on muscle mass leads to involuntary weight loss. This effect might not be recognized if the patient was previously overweight as they may still appear adequately nourished despite losing muscle mass and experiencing progressive weakness. By not causing alarm to the patient or others, the progression of cachexia can thus be insidious. Weight loss among the previously overweight may even be welcomed by those who associate it with health improvement based on the healthy lifestyle messages promoted to the wider and well population. Opportunity is then lost for increasing protein and energy intake along with maintenance of activity to maintain muscle mass and physical function for as long as possible. However, once the realities of involuntary weight loss become visible, they can cause dismay,[28] even shock, as family and old friends come to interpret the change in physical appearance as being a portent of approaching death. This is a realistic interpretation as rapid weight loss and low body mass index (BMI) is associated with poor prognosis. Change in appearance is the most significant predictor of decrease in a sense of dignity—the sense of being valued and respected.[29] An approach that respects personhood by acknowledging interests, achievements, and past roles in life is important for supporting identity.

Relationships and Refractory Cachexia

The symptoms of refractory cachexia change roles and responsibilities. Food, eating, and the patterning of meals plays a part in negotiating a valued identity and role within the family and beyond. Change in what can be eaten disrupts the usual patterns of mealtime behavior and interaction that help maintain a sense of control and safety. An example of such disruption is physical frailty requiring meal preparation to be passed to another family member. Not only is this logistically disruptive, but it also disrupts long-standing family roles and their associated status. In this case, the patient would lose their important role of cook and the rewards of their family enjoying what is offered and giving praise. Family members may also experience loss. An example would be the loss of the reward from being able to feed someone they love, which may, in turn, disrupt their sense of self as the person who nourishes and nurtures in the home. The emotion evoked by such changing behavior patterns and roles can be well managed. However, when there is doubt about the cause or an assumption that it is volitional, misunderstandings and miscommunication can progress to conflict between family members. The effective management of change thus depends on the recognition that disease progression is causative. Education in the cachectic process is important.

Quality of Life and Refractory Cachexia

Health-related quality of life is, unsurprisingly, affected by refractory cachexia.[3] Cachexia-related factors with influence identified from a systematic review of literature[30] can be summarized as being physical function, oral intake, emotions, coping response, sense of control, identity, and relationships. It follows that clinical management may need to include intervention within each of these domains to improve quality of life (see Figure 30.1).

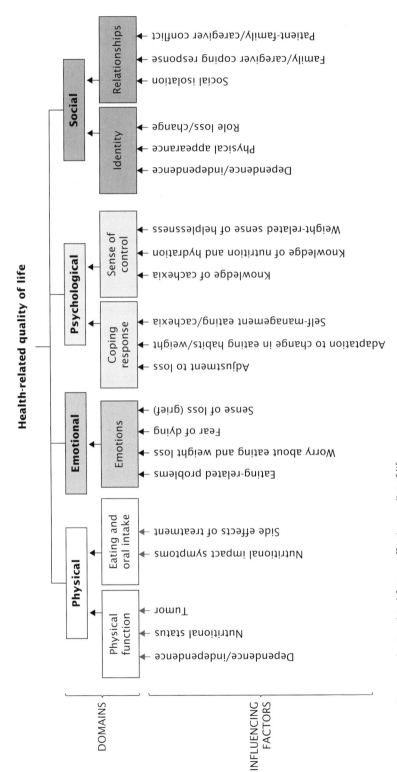

FIGURE 30.1 Cancer cachexia-related factors affecting quality of life.

Multimodal Intervention for Refractory Cachexia

Multimodal interventions that can address the physical, emotional, psychological, and social consequences of cancer cachexia are now thought to be the best approach to supporting affected patients. Multimodal interventions comprise components intended to work synergistically to treat cachexia and/or address cachexia-related problems. The selection of intervention components may be supported by an assessment of cachexia-related problems by members of a multidisciplinary team working together and aided by a cachexia-sensitive quality of life tool, such as the FACT-C[31] or EORTC QLQ CAX24,[32] or a measure of cachexia-related distress. High levels of distress are associated with poor quality of life.

Measurement of Cancer Cachexia-Related Distress

Few studies have investigated the prevalence, severity, and structure of cachexia-related distress, or eating-related distress, among patients with advanced cancer and their family members. However, recent studies have revealed that patients and family members often experience complicated eating-related distress due to tumors themselves, side effects of cancer treatments, and negative impacts of cancer cachexia.[33] Furthermore, there are currently no full-scale validated tools for measuring eating-related distress experienced by patients and family members. Thus, there is no structured method to help physicians and nurses to identify and target interventions for the problem in palliative care. It is also difficult for members of a multidisciplinary team to develop a new care strategy for alleviating eating-related distress in these patients and family members because information on the underlying factorial structure of their distress is very limited. We have therefore developed a preliminary version of a questionnaire for eating-related distress in cancer patients with cachexia receiving palliative care[34] (Figure 30.2). The study used for this development identified that eating-related distress in this population had three domains or factors: Factor 1, difficulties in coping with eating problems, Factor 2, eating-related distress, and Factor 3, conflict-related distress between patients and family members. (This is consistent with the findings of our systematic literature review[30] of psychological, emotional and social factors influencing quality of life, captured in Figure 30.1.) The underlying factorial structure elucidated can contribute to establishing fully validated tools for eating-related distress.

Development of multidisciplinary team approaches and improvement of cachexia-related quality of life in both patients and family members are key issues in cachexia care. Future tasks that we ought to perform to improve supportive care include the following:

- Elucidating the structures of cachexia-related distress in patients and family members, respectively
- Developing patient- and/or family member-reported questionnaires, respectively, as validated tools for measuring cachexia-related distress in daily clinical practices

Please circle the number that best describes how you feel now or during the past one week.

Distress originating from the feelings of patients themselves	No	Seldom	Sometimes	Frequently	Always
Although I know that I have to eat enough, I cannot do that.	1	2	3	4	5
I want attention to be paid to my eating-related distress.	1	2	3	4	5
I do not know why I cannot eat enough.	1	2	3	4	5
I feel that a lack of nutrition makes my condition worse.	1	2	3	4	5
Distress originating from concerns regarding information about the patient's diet	**No**	**Seldom**	**Sometimes**	**Frequently**	**Always**
I wonder what kinds of food I can eat.	1	2	3	4	5
I wonder which nutrients I should preferentially consume.	1	2	3	4	5
I wonder how I can eat more.	1	2	3	4	5
I feel that more medical support about my daily diet is needed.	1	2	3	4	5
Distress originating from the relationship between patients and their families	**No**	**Seldom**	**Sometimes**	**Frequently**	**Always**
I am burdened by the meals that my family serves me.	1	2	3	4	5
I have experienced conflict about my meals with my family.	1	2	3	4	5
I feel that I disregard the effort that my family shows by making my meals.	1	2	3	4	5
I feel sad because I cannot enjoy dinner with my family.	1	2	3	4	5

FIGURE 30.2 Questionnaire for Eating-Related Distress (QERD) among patients with advanced cancer. Source: Reproduced with permission from Amano K, Morita T, Mitsunori T. Potential measurement properties of a questionnaire for eating-related distress among advanced cancer patients with cachexia: Preliminary findings of reliability and validity analysis. *J Palliat Care.* 2020. doi.org/10.1177/0825859720951356.

- Educating clinicians who are responsible for patients with advanced cancer and family members in the structures of cachexia-related distress, how cachexia-related distress can be measured using the questionnaires, and how cachexia-related distress can be managed

Holistic Multimodal Management of Cancer Cachexia

Elucidating the factors influencing a patient's cachexia-related distress is a holistic, rather than purely medical, approach to cancer cachexia. It enables supportive care not only for physical health problems but also for those in the domains of emotional, psychological, and social well-being.[30] It is underpinned by a biopsychosocial understanding of health and illness, which attends not only to sustaining the physical body but also to health-related quality of life.

The psychosocial components of multimodal interventions for refractory cachexia can

- support adherence of multimodal therapies,
- support adaptation and coping, and
- treat comorbid mental health problems, such as anxiety and depression.[30]

Different methods can be embedded within a multimodal intervention to achieve these outcomes. Behavioral change techniques are important for the support of adherence to multimodal components, such as nutritional advice and prescribed exercise. Educational methods that support learning are important for adaptation and coping. The treatment of anxiety and depression can include therapies such as mindfulness meditation that support cognitive reframing and the management of emotion.

Future Directions

Cancer cachexia is a debilitating condition with physical, emotional, psychological, and social impact. It affects health-related quality of life in patients with advanced and progressing disease. It also affects the patient's family. To support quality of life we recommend the following Key Points.

Key Points

- A holistic approach is essential to supportive care in cachexia.
- Cachexia-sensitive measures of quality of life/distress must be used in clinical assessment.
- Cachexia-related factors affecting quality of life must be addressed through multimodal intervention.
- Multimodal intervention should include support for family members of patients with cancer cachexia.

- In the absence of treatment for cancer cachexia, attention to psychosocial factors affecting cachexia-related quality of life is key to improvement in cachexia care.

References

1. Vagnildhaug OM, Balstad TR, Almberg SS, Brunelli C, Knudsen KA, et al. A cross-sectional study examining the prevalence of cachexia and areas of unmet need in patients with cancer. *Support Care Cancer*. 2018;26:1871–1880. doi.org/10.1007/s00520-017-4022-z

2. Aapro M, Arends J, Bozzetti F, Fearon K, Grunberg SM, et al. Early recognition of malnutrition and cachexia in the cancer patient: A position paper of a European School of Oncology Task Force. *Ann Oncol*. 2014; 25(8):1492–1499. doi:10.1093/annonc/mdu085

3. Kasvis P, Vigano M, Vigano A. Health-related quality of life across cancer cachexia stages. *Ann Palliat Med*. 2019;8(1):33–42. doi:10.21037/apm.2018.08.04

4. Wheelwright S, Hopkinson J, Darlington A-S, Fitzsimmons D, Johnson C. A systematic review and thematic synthesis of quality of life in the informal carers of cancer patients with cachexia. *Palliat Med*. 2016;30(2):149–160.

5. Fearon K, Strasser F, Anker SD, Bosaeus I, Bruera E, Fainsinger RL, et al. Definition and classification of cancer cachexia: An international consensus. *Lancet Oncol*. 2011;12:489–495.

6. Hart BL. Biological basis of the behavior of sick animals. *Neurosci Biobehav Rev*. 1988;12:123–137. doi:10.1016/S0149-7634(88)80004-6

7. Hart BL, Hart LA. Sickness behavior in animals: Implications for health and wellness. In: Choe JC, ed. *Encyclopedia of Animal Behavior*. 2nd ed. Oxford: Academic Press; 2019:171–175.

8. Dantzer R. Cytokine-induced sickness behavior: Mechanisms and implications. *Ann NY Acad Sci*. 2001;933:222–234.

9. Bluthé RM, Layé S, Michaud B, Combe C, Dantzer R, Parnet P. Role of interleukin-1beta and tumor necrosis factor-alpha in lipopolysaccharide-induced sickness behavior: A study with interleukin-1 type I receptor-deficient mice. *Eur J Neurosci*. 2000;12(12):4447–4456.

10. Burfeind KG, Michaelis KA, Marks DL. The central role of hypothalamic inflammation in the acute illness response and cachexia. *Semin Cell Dev Biol*. 2016;54:42–52.

11. Kappeler PM, Cremer S, Nunn CL. Sociality and health: Impacts of sociality on disease susceptibility and transmission in animal and human societies. *Phil Trans R Soc B*. 2015;370:20140116. doi:10.1098/rstb.2014.0116

12. Johnson RW. The concept of sickness behavior: A brief chronological account of four key discoveries. *Veterin Immunol Immunopathol*. 2002;87:443–450. doi:10.1016/S0165-2427(02)00069-7

13. Hamilton DG, Jones ME, Cameron EZ, Kerlin DH, McCallum H, Storfer A, et al. Infectious disease and sickness behavior: Tumor progression affects interaction patterns and social network structure in wild Tasmanian devils. *Proc R Soc B: Biol Sci*. 2020;9:287(1940):20202454. doi:10.1098/rspb.2020.2454

14. Wakabayashi H, Arai H, Inui A. The regulatory approval of Anamorelin for treatment of cachexia in patients with non-small cell lung cancer, gastric cancer, pancreatic cancer, and colorectal cancer in Japan: Facts and numbers. *J Cachexia Sarcopenia Muscle*. 2021;12:14–16.

15. Roeland EJ, Bohlke K, Baracos VE, Bruera E, del Fabbro E, Dixon S, et al. Management of cancer cachexia: ASCO guideline. *J Clin Oncol*. 2020;38(21):2438–2453. doi:10.1200/JCO.20.00611.

16. Ko MH, Song SY, Ha SJ, Lee JY, Yoon SW, et al. Efficacy and safety of yukgunja-tang for patients with cancer-related anorexia: A randomized, controlled trial, pilot study. *Integr Cancer Ther*. 2021;20:15347354211019107. doi:10.1177/15347354211019107.PMID: 34032151

17. Miyano K, Ohshima K, Suzuki N, Furuya S, Yoshida Y, et al. Japanese herbal medicine ninjinyoeito mediates its orexigenic properties partially by activating orexin 1 receptors. *Front Nutrition*. 2020;7:5. doi:10.3389/fnut.2020.00005. eCollection 2020.PMID: 32175325

18. Takayama S, Arita R, Ohsawa M, Kikuchi A, Yasui H, et al. Perspectives on the use of ninjin'yoeito in modern medicine: A review of randomized controlled trials. *Evidence-Based Complem Altern Med.* Sep 2;2019:9590260. doi:10.1155/2019/9590260. eCollection 2019.PMID: 31565066

19. Arends J, Strasser F, Gonella S, Solheim TS, Madeddu P, et al. On behalf of the ESMO Guidelines Committee. Cancer cachexia in adult patients: ESMO clinical practice guidelines. 2021. https://www.esmo.org/guidelines/supportive-and-palliative-care/cancer-cachexia-in-adult-patients

20. Arends J, Bachmann P, Baracos V, Barthelemy N, Bertz H, et al. ESPEN guidelines on nutrition in cancer patients. *Clin Nutrition.* 2017;36(1):11–48. doi:10.1016/j.clnu.2016.07.015

21. Muscaritoli M, Arends J, Bachmann P, Baracos V, Barthelemy N, et al. ESPEN practical guideline. *Clin Nutrition.* 2021;40(5):2898–2913. doi:10.1016/j.clnu.2021.02.005

22. Amano K, Maeda I, Morita T, Okajima Y, Hama T, et al. Eating-related distress and need for nutritional support of families of advanced cancer patients: A nationwide survey of bereaved family members. *J Cachexia Sarcopenia Muscle.* 2016;7(5):527–534.

23. Hopkinson J. Psychosocial impact of cancer cachexia. *J Cachexia Sarcopenia Muscle.* 2014;5:89–94.

24. Hopkinson JB. Food connections: A qualitative exploratory study of weight- and eating-related distress in families affected by advanced cancer. *Eur J Oncol Nurs.* 2016;20:87–96.

25. Molassiotis A, Cheng HL, Byrnes A, Chan RJ, et al. The effects of a family-centered psychosocial-based nutrition intervention in patients with advanced cancer: The PiCNIC2 pilot randomised controlled trial. *Nutrition J.* 2021;20:2 https://doi.org/10.1186/s12937-020-00657-2

26. Pettifer A, Froggatt K, Hughes S. The experiences of family members witnessing the diminishing drinking of a dying relative: An adapted meta-narrative literature review *Palliat Med.* 2019;33(9):1146–1157.

27. Lize N, Raijmakers N, van Leishout R, et al. Psychosocial consequences of a reduced ability to eat for patients with cancer and their informal caregivers: A qualitative study. *Eur J Oncol Nurs.* 2020;49:101838.

28. Amano K, Morita T, Miyamoto J, et al. Perception of need for nutritional support in advanced cancer patients with cachexia: A survey in palliative care settings. *Support Care Cancer.* 2018;26:2793–2799.

29. McClement S. Cancer cachexia and its impact on patient dignity: What nurses need to know. *Asia Pac J Oncol Nurs* 2016;3:218–219.

30. Hopkinson JB. The psychosocial components of multimodal interventions offered to people with cancer cachexia: A scoping review. *Asian Pacific J Nurs.* 2021;8(5):450–461.

31. LeBlanc GP, Samsa SP, Wolf SC, et al. Validation and real-world assessment of the Functional Assessment of Anorexia-Cachexia Therapy (FAACT) scale in patients with advanced non-small cell lung cancer and the cancer anorexia-cachexia syndrome (CACS). *Support Care Cancer.* 2015;23:2341–2347.

32. Wheelwright SJ, Hopkinson JB, Darlington A-S, Fitzsimmons DF, Fayers P, et al. on behalf of the EORTC Quality of Life Group. Development of the EORTC QLQ-CAX24: A questionnaire for cancer patients with cachexia. *J Pain Sympt Manage.* 2017;53(2):232–242. doi:10.1016/j.jpainsymman.2016.09.010

33. Amano K, Baracos V, Hopkinson J. Integration of palliative, supportive, and nutritional care to alleviate eating-related distress among advanced cancer patients with cachexia and their family members. *Crit Rev Oncol/Hematol.* 2019;143:117–123. doi:10.1016/j.critrevonc.2019.08.006

34. Amano K, Morita T, Mitsunori T. Potential measurement properties of a questionnaire for eating-related distress among advanced cancer patients with cachexia: Preliminary findings of reliability and validity analysis. *J Palliat Care.* 2020. doi.org/10.1177/0825859720951356

31

Fatigue at End of Life

Meredith Hays, Han Le Santisi, and
Margaret M. Mahon

Introduction

Fatigue is a complex symptom that is often burdensome to patients and to their families. Incomplete understanding of the causes and effects of fatigue contributes to its underdiagnosis. Fatigue is qualitatively different from being tired and is not relieved by taking a nap. Providers' failure to recognize and treat fatigue leads to lack of understanding by patients and families. It is not uncommon for people living with a severe illness to be told to "try harder" or "power through." Family members may be frustrated or angry and perceive a lack of engagement or effort by the person with severe illness. In this chapter, the complexity of fatigue and means to manage it, with a goal of improving quality of life, are explored.

Definition

Fatigue is the most common symptom reported among people receiving palliative care and is perhaps one of the most underrecognized symptoms by providers.[1] While frequently documented in people with cancer, fatigue occurs frequently among people living with other chronic progressive diseases such as HIV/AIDS, or with chronic heart, lung, or kidney disease.[1] Fatigue is a decrement in physical or mental performance of tasks. It is a subjective sense of physical, emotional, or cognitive tiredness or exhaustion.[1,2] Especially at end of life, the symptom burden of fatigue can have a highly detrimental impact on quality of life.[1-3] Physical and mental fatigue often limit one's ability to participate in favorite activities, as well as in activities of daily living (ADLs).[1] Fatigue may be related to the disease process or to treatments and other interventions; fatigue is typically not improved with rest.[2,3]

Manifestations of fatigue vary, but typically include decreased activity tolerance, emotional lability, and impaired or slowed cognition.[3]

Fatigue at the end of life can be particularly burdensome; even then, it is often underrecognized and undertreated.[1,2] Most of what is known about fatigue is based on specific disease or pathology; few researchers have focused on people who are close to death.[1] Sandvick and colleagues found that increased fatigue was significantly associated with being able to determine the actual day of a person's death.[4] The burdens of fatigue, however, typically far predate the day of death. If end of life is understood as a time of weeks to months, many opportunities for assessment and intervention exist. Were it better recognized, interventions to decrease fatigue could lead to improved quality of life and thus, for many, dying better. Both the physical and cognitive aspects of fatigue should be addressed, and reversible causes should be considered.[2,4] At end of life, this can be more difficult as it may become a balancing act between the burdens of symptoms, treatments, and interventions.

Many researchers have explored fatigue in specific disease states such as cancer or end-stage kidney disease (ESKD).[4–7] For example, Artom and colleagues found fatigue in patients with ESKD, patients with higher C-reactive protein (CRP), and anorexic patients, as well as those receiving a range of types and duration of renal replacement therapy.[8] In a critical review, Picariello and colleagues looked at psychological factors of fatigue in people with ESKD. These included depression and anxiety, perceived lack of social support, poor sleep quality, and personal perception of illness and symptom burden.[5] The definition of fatigue is common across diseases, but the symptoms and impact of fatigue are highly variables between individuals, not only across diseases, but also with the same disease.[1,2,5]

Measurement

Despite the prevalence of fatigue at the end of life, there are many limitations to its quantification. Fatigue is a subjective experience; it cannot be measured objectively by an observer. Thus, patients' reports have been the mainstay for assessing fatigue and its impact on individuals.[9] Variations in the definition of fatigue have led to inconsistencies in detection and assessment between studies. Assessments of other variables that may affect the impact of disease and how it may affect fatigue are often incomplete.

Understanding of the experiences of fatigue and the end of life is further confounded because of the variability in accuracy of identifying when a person is at end of life. A person with fatigue, however, is likely to have the symptom weeks, months, or even years before the close proximity of death. Early assessment and intervention can improve quality of life for whatever time the person does have left.

Many assessment tools have been developed over the past four decades. More than 250 assessment tools for fatigue in cancer and other illnesses have been developed; the tools vary in structure, content, scoring, and psychometric properties assessed.[10] More than half of these assessment tools, however, were used only for a single study. To this day, no single standardized patient-reported instrument has been widely adopted in research or clinical practice.[10–13]

Current measures of fatigue include both unidimensional and multidimensional assessment tools. Unidimensional tools are used to screen for the presence and severity of fatigue; they are relatively quick to administer. Unidimensional tools include the National Comprehensive Cancer Network (NCCN) patient-reported fatigue intensity rating,[14] Brief Fatigue Inventory,[11] and the Fatigue Severity Scale.[15] Unidimensional tools can also be a validated subscale of larger quality-of-life measurement tools such as the Functional Assessment of Cancer Therapy[16] and the European Organization for Research and Treatment of Cancer Quality of Life questionnaire.[13]

Multidimensional tools are used to examine various dimensions of fatigue, including physical, cognitive, and emotional aspects. Multidimensional data can help practitioners not only diagnose fatigue but also determine its impact on function and quality of life and thus support the initiation of specific interventions.

The Fatigue Symptom Inventory[12] and Multidimensional Fatigue Inventory[17] are relatively short and simple multidimensional tools. The Memorial Symptom Assessment Scale (MSAS) is a frequently used, comprehensive symptom measure that allows the rater not only to record the prevalence of specific physical and psychological symptoms, but also to characterize symptoms' severity, frequency, and distress.[18] The MSAS, however, was developed for and validated in people with cancer. When used in the study of patients at end of life, the MSAS has often been modified so that proxies can assess for symptoms.[19]

Guidelines for screening, assessment, and intervention for cancer-related fatigue (CRF) have been developed, for example by the Canadian Association of Psychosocial Oncology (CAPO). Regardless, such guidelines are not consistently implemented in practice.[20–22] Jones and colleagues conducted a pilot study to determine whether a training session on the acceptability and feasibility of CAPO CRF guidelines would change the practice habits of providers. A one-time in-person training session was administered to 18 healthcare and community support providers. A knowledge translation tool was used to measure knowledge of CAPO CRF guidelines and intentions and the efficacy of applying guidelines in practice both before and after the training session. Mean comparisons for before-and-after comparisons revealed significant increases on the part of participants in perceived level of CRF-related knowledge ($t = -3.959(14)$; $p = 0.001$), self-efficacy in assessing CRF ($t = 2.621(13)$, $p = 0.021$), self-efficacy to intervene for CRF ($t = 2.924(13)$, $p = 0.012$), and intent to apply CAPO CRF guidelines in practice ($t = 4.786(13)$, $p = 0.000$). The researchers found that the training was both acceptable and feasible, with a high participation rate (88.89%) and high mean satisfaction scores for the study (52.27 ± 6.97 out of 60 points maximum).[23]

Prevalence

Fatigue is the most common symptom reported in patients with advanced life-threatening illnesses.[1] The complex nature of its presentation and lack of consistent guidelines for screening and diagnosis also make it one of the most underreported and undertreated symptoms.[24,25] Fatigue is addressed in fewer than half of outpatient palliative care consultations and typically is addressed only if the patient expresses concerns about being fatigued.[26] Furthermore, fatigue is often inappropriately conflated with "being tired" despite its different pathophysiology and greater complexity.

The prevalence of fatigue varies between diseases, the stage or severity of disease, type of treatments given, and years with disease process.[27] The prevalence of fatigue has been studied most often in patients with cancer at all stages. Two recent systematic reviews with meta-analyses reported the frequency of fatigue in patients with cancer to be 52% and 49%, respectively (95% confidence interval [CI]: 48–56%, 45–53%, respectively).[28,29] Though neither group of research reported a subgroup analysis of cancer patients at end of life, Ma and colleagues found lower performance status was the most prominent risk factor for CRF (odds ration [OR] = 6.58, 95% CI: 2.60–16.67, P < 0.0001), while Maqbali and colleagues found the highest frequency of CRF in patients with advanced disease (60.6%, 955 CI = 49.5–70.7).[29]

Kutner and colleagues used the MSAS to assess symptoms in 348 patients receiving hospice care. "Lack of energy" was the most common symptom (83%).[30] Fatigue may be underrecognized at the end of life if a proxy (e.g., physician, nurse, or family member) assesses symptoms.[19] More recently, researchers have found that fatigue is more distressing and associated with impaired quality of life in patients with 2–6 months left in life; this association disappeared during the last weeks and days of life.[31,32]

Ingham and colleagues undertook a large, prospective study using national data in Australia to assess patterns of distress from fatigue in patients with malignant and non-malignant diagnoses in the 60 days before death. The researchers found that distress from fatigue affected up to 80% of patients; the majority reported moderate to severe distress from fatigue. The researchers also found that reported distress from fatigue decreased in the 10 days before death across all disease cohorts. This may be correlated to the patient's performance status. Patients with Karnofsky performance status (AKPS) of 100 reported significantly less distress from fatigue than patients with lower AKPS scores until the patients become bedfast (AKPS 10–20) and level of distress decreases. Approximately 10% of bedfast patients reported distress from fatigue, compared with 80% of patients with Karnofsky performance status of greater than 30 reporting distress.[32]

The prevalence of fatigue is high in patients at the end of life across the disease processes. Tranmer and colleagues studied 135 patients hospitalized at end of life, comparing those with cancer to those with other diseases (congestive heart failure [CHF], chronic obstructive pulmonary disease [COPD], and cirrhosis). They found a significantly higher prevalence of most physical symptoms in people with cancer (e.g., pain [78% vs. 49%], nausea [61% vs. 28%], and constipation [48% vs. 38%]) (all p < 0.01); however, they found no significant difference in prevalence of fatigue (operationalized as lack of energy) between the cancer and non-cancer patients. Of note, lack of energy was also the most prevalent symptom, both physical and psychological, in both groups.[33]

People with advanced disease and concomitant depression have reported higher levels of fatigue than similar patients without depression.[34] Psychiatric disorders such as depression and anxiety are common in many end-stage disease processes, including AIDS,[35] lung disease,[36] and renal disease.[37] Depression is also independently associated with decreased survival and lower quality of life in heart failure[38] and end-stage liver disease.[39]

Pathophysiology

Consistent with the whole concept, the pathophysiology of fatigue is incompletely understood. Fatigue can caused by disease and by treatments. (Table 31.1 outlines, broadly, various disease processes that are commonly encountered and some of the known or suspected contributing physiological factors.) Factors such as proinflammatory cytokines, neuroendocrine and autonomic dysfunction, mitochondrial dysfunction, and decreased energy intake contribute to fatigue. Elevated serum concentration of inflammatory biomarkers, such as CRP and interleukin (IL)-1ra is associated with fatigue in cancer patients. Cytokines have

TABLE 31.1 Causes of fatigue at end of life by disease process

Disease process	Physiological causes
Cancer	Elevated inflammatory cytokines neuroendocrine dysfunction Autonomic dysfunction Mitochondrial dysfunction Deconditioning Depression Anxiety[1–3,41]
Delirium and cognitive dysfunction	Dehydration Opioid toxicity Infection Deconditioning Depression Anxiety[44]
End-stage renal disease	Metabolic dysfunction Anemia Medication interactions Subjective sleep quality Dialysis Illness perception Depression Lack of social support Anxiety[57]
Cardiac disease, including congestive heart failure (CHF)	Reduced cardiac output Changes to metabolism and blood flow to skeletal and cardiac muscle Deconditioning Depression Anxiety[6]
Pulmonary diseases, including chronic obstruction pulmonary disease (COPD)	Illness perception Deconditioning Depression Anxiety[43,45]
Liver disease	Metabolic dysfunction Deconditioning Depression Anxiety[45]

been found to be elevated in noncancer conditions associated with chronic fatigue such as myalgic encephalomyelitis/chronic fatigue syndrome, though these syndromes remain incompletely understood.[8,40] Fatigue is a common adverse effect of therapeutic cytokine administration, often used in cancer treatment.[3,41,42] In CRF, cytokines act as autocrine or paracrine growth factors in the neoplastic cells. Cytokines also cause secondary issues that contribute to fatigue such as anemia, fever, and night sweats.[42,43] Cachexia, a consequence of mitochondrial dysfunction leading to decreased ATP, leads to impaired energy production and increased fatigue.[42] Additional factors, such as medication interactions, uncontrolled pain, and metabolic derangements, among others, also play a role in the development and severity of fatigue.[1,2,5,6]

Treatment

Fatigue often results from the cumulative physiological, psychological, and situational dimensions of serious illness. Assessment should include a comprehensive history, including assessment of disease status and physical exam, as well as objective data, including laboratory and imaging results. It is not uncommon for people with fatigue to be incompletely aware of how significantly fatigue is affecting their lives. Asking specific questions about daily activities (e.g., walking the dog, getting the mail, shopping) and whether one has had to change how they accomplish these tasks or if they are less able to participate is a good place to start.

Patients benefit from an interdisciplinary team approach to develop individualized, multimodal interventions. It is unlikely that any single pharmacologic or nonpharmacologic intervention will completely mitigate fatigue at the end of life. The first step in treating fatigue is to optimize medical and nutritional status, review medications, and treat other distressing symptoms that may contribute to fatigue. Physiologic factors that contribute to fatigue are extensive and should be treated whenever possible[45-47] (see Box 31.1).

Again, fatigue is a subjective symptom and much more than a physical syndrome.[47] Fatigue at end of life often leads to psychological and psychosocial distress; evaluation, therefore, must be comprehensive. There is a strong correlation between fatigue and depression; this means that distinguishing fatigue from psychiatric conditions such as depression is not always possible.[48] Fatigue is a prominent symptom of many psychiatric disorders, including depression, anxiety, and substance/medication misuse.[48,49] Furthermore, the burden of fatigue from untreated physiologic or psychosocial contributors can lead to psychiatric disorders at the end of life. Curt and colleagues studied factors related to fatigue in people with cancer. Individuals with fatigue described several manifestations and effects, including needing to push themselves to do things (77%), decreased motivation or interest (62%), and feelings of sadness, frustration, or irritability (53%).[50]

Tchekmedyian and colleagues used a randomized, double-blind, placebo-controlled clinical trial of 250 patients to evaluate the effect of treating anemia with darbepoetin alfa, including the effects on reported fatigue, anxiety, and depression. The correlations of change in anxiety and depression with changes in fatigue scores had coefficients of −0.45

BOX 31.1 Physiologic contributors to fatigue

Undertreated symptoms, including pain, nausea, insomnia

Treatment-related symptoms, including cytotoxic therapy, radiotherapy, bio-immunotherapy

Medication-related symptoms, including opioids, benzodiazepines, anticholinergics, antihistamines, anticonvulsants, beta blockers, muscle relaxants, statins

Comorbidities (cardiac, hepatic, renal)

Infection/inflammation/cytokine dysregulation

Anemia

Hypoxia

Autonomic nervous system dysfunction

Metabolic/electrolyte disturbances

Neuroendocrine abnormalities (e.g., hypogonadism, hypothyroidism)

Cachexia

Dehydration

($p < 0.001$) and -0.44 ($p < 0.001$), respectively. That is, patients who had improved levels of fatigue were also more likely to have significant benefits in multiple mental and emotional symptoms, including reductions in anxiety and depression.[51]

Identifying underlying physiologic, psychiatric, and psychosocial factors that can contribute to fatigue is an important first step in the management of fatigue. (See Chapters 4, 5, and 6 for discussion of the diagnosis and management of depression, anxiety, and delirium in palliative care.) As with any symptom, identifying the cause whenever possible is essential. Symptomatic treatment should first consider treatment of reversible causes. Regardless, largely because of the multidimensional nature of the symptom, fatigue often persists. The National Comprehensive Cancer Network Clinical Practice Guidelines in Oncology recommends first using nonpharmacological interventions for the treatment of CRF.[52] There are, however, few standard interventions for the treatment of fatigue at the end of life.

Nonpharmacologic Treatment of Fatigue

Much of the evidence on therapies for management of fatigue is based on studies of people with cancer. Subjects have included those undergoing treatment, as well as those post-treatment. Nonpharmacological management includes exercise, energy conservation, nutritional interventions, complementary therapies (e.g., aromatherapy, meditation, and massage), and cognitive behavioral therapy.[1,2,45,53] A systematic review done in 2019 by Lee and colleagues described the increasing interest in the use of complementary therapies used to aid in the improvement of quality of life for cancer patients, including fatigue. Interventions were diverse and include modalities such as art therapy, yoga, acupuncture, psychosocial interventions, and massage.[53] The methodology of many of these studies, however, limits generalizability. In a systematic review of 120 studies examining complementary therapies including acupuncture, massage, yoga, and relaxation training, researchers found insufficient evidence to conclude the effectiveness of any of the modalities in reducing CRF.[54]

Exercise

Fatigue typically includes reduced energy and decreased physical activity, which makes exercise therapy seem almost counterintuitive. One of the most extensively evaluated nonpharmacologic interventions for fatigue has been aerobic exercise.[55–57] Though the majority of research has been on people with cancer, other conditions have also been studied.[1,5,6,55–57] Resistance training can also be effective.[58] Many researchers have found that exercise and psychological interventions have small to moderate effects on fatigue[48,59] and improved capacity for performing activities of daily life, for both people currently receiving treatment for cancer and those who are post-treatment.[60,61]

In a systematic review of 245 studies comparing the effectiveness of different types of exercise (e.g. aerobic vs. resistance training vs. combined training vs. dance vs. yoga, etc.) on CRF in patients during and after cancer treatments, Hilfiker and colleagues found that all types of exercise showed small to moderate benefits in decreasing fatigue when compared to usual care.[62] Yoga[63,64] and qigong/tai chi[65] significantly improved CRF in patients receiving cancer treatment, as well as for those who had completed treatments.

Wu and colleagues conducted a systematic review and Bayesian network meta-analysis of all major nonpharmacological interventions for CRF.[66] The researchers concluded that multimodal therapy (a combination of at least two therapies) including qigong, aerobic exercise, resistance exercise, mindfulness-based stress reduction, combined psychosocial therapies, cognitive behavioral therapy (CBT), and/or acupuncture were most effective interventions for CRF. The researchers did find variability between tools used and research methodologies. They concluded that multimodal therapy, CBT, and qigong were most frequently beneficial and thus may be optimal first selections for mitigating CRF.[66] Though these researchers focused on patients with cancer, these therapies are frequently recommended for patients with non-cancer diagnoses, with benefit.

Oldervoll and colleagues conducted a randomized controlled trial with 231 cancer patients with life expectancy of 3 months to 2 years where participants were assigned to either a physical exercise group (60 minutes twice a week for 8 weeks) or control group (usual care). The primary outcome was physical fatigue; the secondary outcome was physical performance as measured by Shuttle Walk Test and hand grip strength test. The investigators found that physical fatigue was not reduced; however, participants in the physical exercise group had significant improvement in physical performance.[67]

Exercise programs should be tailored for the individual; such programs may not be appropriate for people with bone metastases, active infection, or other limitations.[1,2,45] Exercise programs are likely to be of more limited benefit in inpatients with extremely advanced disease, including those for whom death is a more proximal reality. Consultation with physical therapists and recreational therapists can be very helpful in identifying regimens that benefit specific individuals, considering the patient's abilities and disabilities.

Energy Conservation

In addition to exercise, energy conservation management (ECM) may reduce fatigue, including for those who are at the end of life. Barsevick and colleagues defined energy conservation as "the deliberate, planned management of an individual's personal energy resources to prevent their depletion."[68 (p. 1303)] Blikman and colleagues completed a systematic review of six studies in which they compared ECM to no fatigue-related treatment in patients with multiple sclerosis and fatigue.[69] The researchers found that, in the short-term, ECM reduced the impact of fatigue and improved physical, social, and mental function.[69] The NCCN recommended a multimodal approach to managing fatigue that includes energy conservation strategies for patients with CRF.[52] Energy conservation is useful in reducing fatigue in patients undergoing cancer treatments as well as in those who have completed treatment.[68,70]

Strategies for conserving energy include identifying activities for which the patient wants to use energy. Providers should ask patients about their valued and enjoyable activities. Then, nonessential or less enjoyable activities can be eliminated or delegated. It becomes clear why fatigue management involves the patient's family or caregivers. Patients should be encouraged to incorporate rest periods throughout the day and use labor-saving devices such as walkers, commodes, and wheelchairs.[71] Saving energy now can allow participation in an enjoyable activity later. For example, the provider might recommend that someone use a wheelchair now to conserve energy to allow for family interaction once they arrive at the event.

Occupational therapists can be very helpful in educating patients about energy conservation. In addition, physical and occupational therapists can work with patients and families toward modifying their homes to maximize conservation of energy.

The loss of ability to be as active as one once was often is accompanied by the loss of significant factors of one's role, for example, as parent or partner, employee, or volunteer. That is, activity may be associated with self-worth. A loss of the ability to do some activity may diminish one's perception of self-worth. Similarly, the loss of self-sufficiency, the need for help in some or all ADLs can be very threatening to one's perceived self-worth or self-esteem. People are often reluctant to ask for help. This further impedes the ability to conserve energy. Providers must be willing to engage in discussions of self-esteem and perceived self-worth. Identification of core beliefs with a patient's willingness to ask for help, sort priorities, and reframe help-seeking as an adaptive strategy may be time-consuming but is crucial.[72] Involving family in these conversations may increase chances of success by establishing common goals based on an accurate understanding of fatigue.

Other Therapies

Chegeni, and colleagues assessed the effectiveness of progressive muscle relaxation (PMR) on fatigue and sleep quality in people with stage 3 and 4 COPD.[73] They found that while there was no improvement in overall sleep quality, patients did report improvement in fatigue, sleep duration, and habitual sleep efficiency.[73] Hassanzadeh and colleagues demonstrated that aromatherapy using 5% lavender essential oil decreased the level of fatigue in hemodialysis patients (before intervention: 6.49 ± 1.11; after intervention 3.64 ± 0.79; p. < 0.001).[74]

Behavioral and psychosocial Interventions

Several research teams have undertaken meta-analyses exploring the effectiveness of CBT as a tool in fatigue management. Researchers have uniformly concluded that CBT may be more effective than other psychological approaches in reducing fatigue symptoms.[59,66,75]

Researchers have also consistently found that mindfulness-based approaches for stress reduction also help relieve fatigue in cancer patients.[52,76] Recreation therapists or others with training in mindfulness, as well as online resources including various apps (e.g., Calm, Headspace, Breathe 2 Relax) are good options for patients. The advantage of a range of resources is that it gives people with fatigue some control and flexibility at a time when these might seem in short supply.

Other researchers have found weaker results. In a systematic review of 12 studies assessing the effect of psychosocial interventions versus usual care or other controls in patients with incurable cancer, Poort and colleagues found little evidence to suggest that these interventions reduce fatigue.[77] The authors also did not find support for the effectiveness of psychosocial interventions for improving social, role, emotional, or cognitive functioning. Furthermore, the authors found very low-quality evidence for the efficacy of psychosocial interventions in improving physical functioning.[77]

Pharmacologic Treatment of Fatigue

Pharmacological treatments can be beneficial to people living with fatigue. As with the nonpharmacologic options, much of the clinical decision-making is empirical due to the lack of data. Many clinical interventions are based on research with people living with cancer, and, of those, most are early in the disease trajectory.[78] Most of the medications that are used have been used for years.

In the most recent and largest narrative review, Klasson and colleagues evaluated 17 randomized controlled trials with 1,296 participants to explore the benefits of pharmacological interventions (including psychostimulants, corticosteroids, testosterone, and melatonin) on CRF in patients with advanced or metastatic cancer.[78] The authors concluded that the evidence remains weak for using pharmacological treatments on CRF in people with advanced disease, though they did find that methylphenidate and corticosteroids may improve CRF in this population. It is noteworthy that several studies included in this review found an improvement of fatigue in both the intervention and placebo arms.

In their randomized controlled trial comparing an open-label placebo to a control (treatment as usual) in 74 patients who had completed treatment for cancer and were living with at least moderate fatigue, Hoenemeyer and colleagues found participants in the placebo group reported a 29% improvement in fatigue severity (P = 0.008) and 39% improvement in fatigue-disruption on quality of life (P = 0.002) when compared to the usual care group.[79] Two recent systematic reviews with meta-analysis (29 and 30 studies, respectively) also found that placebo treatments had a significant effect on CRF and that predicting these effects may help design future studies for CRF.[80,81] Further exploration of these findings is important as treatment options that have any positive effect with virtually no adverse side effects are beneficial for the patient.

In the NCCN guidelines, methylphenidate and shorter courses of corticosteroids are recommended for management of CRF in people at end of life. Conversely, the European Society for Medical Oncology (ESMO) did not reach consensus on the benefits of methylphenidate, though they did recommend shorter courses of corticosteroids for patients in this population.[52,82]

Psychostimulants

Methylphenidate is a centrally acting stimulant with a short half-life (about 3 hours) and a rapid onset of action. In low doses, psychostimulants used in the palliative setting are often well tolerated and have no or only mild side effects.[78] The typical dose used for fatigue in most studies is methylphenidate 10 mg oral tablet given at 8 o'clock in the morning and 12 o'clock in the afternoon.[78,79,80,83,84] In clinical practice, the starting dose is usually 2.5–5 mg oral tablet given at the same times as above and titrated as necessary to 15–30 mg by mouth twice a day.[45] Few researchers who studies the effect of methylphenidate on fatigue found a significant effect on the primary outcome.[78,83–85] Most found a trend toward a positive effect or similar positive effects in both placebo and intervention groups, leading to lack of any consistent support for the use of methylphenidate in the treatment of fatigue in patients with advanced cancer.[84,86,87]

Some researchers have suggested that methylphenidate may reduce fatigue by reversing the sedating effects of opioids[88] and reducing depressive symptoms.[89] Conversely, in their pooled analysis of patients in two prospective controlled clinical trials who had received methylphenidate for CRF, Yennurajalingam and colleagues found a positive association between response to methylphenidate and higher intensity of baseline fatigue ($p < 0.001$). They did not, however, find increase in baseline depression or sedation.[90] This suggests that methylphenidate may be of particular benefit to patients with severe fatigue.

Modafinil is used less often. Although modafinil is a psychostimulant, studies conducted on its effect on CRF have shown conflicting or weak evidence to support its use for the treatment of CRF.[91–93]

Glucocorticoids

Glucocorticoids are widely used in patients with advanced cancers to treat symptoms such as inflammatory pain, nausea, edema, fatigue, and others.[94] Randomized controlled trials assessing the effects of glucocorticoids in alleviating CRF, however, have had mixed results. Of the four randomized controlled trials assessed in Klasson's review, three research teams showed positive effects of glucocorticoids on reducing fatigue in patients with advanced cancer ($p = 0.0306$, $p = 0.003$, $p = 0.008$, respectively).[78,95–97] Optimal dosing, length of treatment, and side effects of corticosteroids in this setting have not yet been established.[98] Reported regimens include prednisone 7.5–10 mg orally four times a day, dexamethasone 1–2 mg orally four times a day, and methylprednisolone 32 mg orally four times a day for 2–4 weeks.[45] It is important to consider the physiologic half-life of dexamethasone; avoiding around-the-clock dosing means the steroid would be less likely to interfere with the patient's sleep cycle.

Other Pharmacologic Treatments

Evidence for the effect of testosterone,[99] melatonin,[100] and vitamin D[101,102] on fatigue are not yet established. Their use in the treatment of fatigue at the end of life has not been integrated into any clinical guidelines.

Future Directions

Fatigue is complex, underrecognized, and often has insidious effects that affect not just the patient, but also the family. Patients with fatigue tire easily but also have generalized physical weakness and cognitive changes, including difficulty concentrating and even emotional lability. More research has been done in patients with cancer, but the symptom occurs across diseases and trajectories. Assiduous assessment is essential as a foundation for treatment. Perhaps even more importantly, *naming* fatigue, validating the myriad ways that it affects a person's life allows recognition of it as a part of disease and as a part of treatment. This is also a framework for recognizing the impact of fatigue on not just the patient, but also on the family. There is not one, ideal treatment for fatigue. An interdisciplinary team is essential for optimal management. Treatments must be better studied, especially in people with diseases other than cancer.

Fatigue affects the person's ability to engage with others, work, carry on usual roles (e.g., cook, breadwinner, Little League coach, pickle ball team member), and even care for oneself. The caregiver burden of fatigue is vastly underrecognized, as are the frustration, stress, and other responses of the affected individual *and* the family. Future study should encompass these dimensions. Perhaps of greater importance, providers must have the knowledge and take the time to name and explain the symptom of fatigue.

Key Points

- Fatigue is a complex symptom that is underrecognized and undertreated.
- Though most commonly studied in people with cancer, fatigue is also common in people with many chronic diseases, including chronic kidney disease, HIV/AIDS, heart disease, lung disease, and others.
- Fatigue has been assessed using unidimensional and multidimensional tools, though uniform screening is rare. Two more commonly used tools include the Brief Fatigue Inventory[11] and the Memorial Symptom Assessment Scale.[18,19]
- Nonpharmacologic measures (e.g., exercise, energy conservation) are first-line treatments in managing fatigue; however, pharmacologic measures (e.g., methylphenidate, corticosteroids) are also used. Treatment is often multimodal and may not be successful.
- Successful treatment is likely to involve an interdisciplinary team.

- Fatigue's encroachment on quality of life often necessitates changes not just for the patient, but also for the patient's family. If fatigue is not named, misunderstandings can affect the patient's and the family's responses.

References

1. Radbruch L, Strasser F, Elsner F, Goncalves JF, Loge J, Kassa S, et al. Fatigue in palliative care patients: An EAPC approach. *Palliat Med.* 2008;22(1):13–32. doi:10.1177/0269216307085183.

2. Yennurajalingam S, Frisbee-Hume S, Palmer JL, et al. Reduction of cancer-related fatigue with dexamethasone: A double-blind, randomized, placebo-controlled trial in patients with advanced cancer. *J Clin Oncol.* 2013;31(25):3076–3082. doi:10.1200/jco.2012.44.4661

3. Berger AM, Mooney K, Banerjee C, et al. *NCCN Clinical Practice Guidelines in Oncology (NCCN Guidelines): Cancer-Related Fatigue.* Fort Washington, PA: National Comprehensive CaSncer Network; 2017.

4. Mücke M, Mochamat, Cuhls H, et al. Pharmacological treatments for fatigue associated with palliative care: Executive summary of a Cochrane Collaboration systematic review. *J Cachexia Sarcopenia Muscle.* 2016;7(1):23–27. doi:10.1002/jcsm.12101

5. Picariello F, Moss-Morris R, Macdougall IC, Chilcot AJ. The role of psychological factors in fatigue among end-stage kidney disease patients: A critical review. *Clin Kidney J.* 2017;10(1):79–88. doi:10.1093/ckj/sfw113

6. Walthall H, Floegel T, Boulton M, Jenkinson C. Patients experience of fatigue in advanced heart failure. *Contemp Nurse.* 2019;55(1):71–82. doi:10.1080/10376178.2019.1604147

7. Artom M, Moss-Morris R, Caskey F, Chilcot J. Fatigue in advanced kidney disease. *Kidney Int.* 2014;86(3):497–505. doi:10.1038/ki.2014.86

8. Corbitt M, Eaton-Fitch N, Staines D, Cabanas H, Marshall-Gradisnik S. A systematic review of cytokines in chronic fatigue syndrome/myalgic encephalomyelitis/systemic exertion intolerance disease (CFS/ME/SEID). *BMC Neurol.* 2019;19(1):207. Published 2019 Aug 24. doi:10.1186/s12883-019-1433-0

9. Wang X. Cancer-related fatigue. *Palliat Care Support Onc Gynecol Oncol.* 2015 136:8446–452.

10. Hjollund NH, Andersen JH, Bech P. Assessment of fatigue in chronic disease: A bibliographic study of fatigue measurement scales. *Health Qual Life Outcomes.* 2007;5:12. Published 2007 Feb 27. doi:10.1186/1477-7525-5-12

11. Mendoza TR, Wang XS, Cleeland CS, et al. The rapid assessment of fatigue severity in cancer patients: Use of the Brief Fatigue Inventory. *Cancer.* 1999;85(5):1186–1196. doi:10.1002/(sici)1097-0142(19990301)85:5<1186::aid-cncr24>3.0.co;2-n

12. Hann DM, Denniston MM, Baker F. Measurement of fatigue in cancer patients: Further validation of the Fatigue Symptom Inventory. *Qual Life Res.* 2000;9(7):847–854. doi:10.1023/a:1008900413113

13. Minton O, Stone P. A systematic review of the scales used for the measurement of cancer-related fatigue (CRF). *Ann Oncol.* 2009;20(1):17–25. doi:10.1093/annonc/mdn537

14. Mock V, et al. Cancer-related fatigue. Clinical practice guidelines in oncology. *J Natl Comprehens Cancer Netw.* 2007;5:1054–1078.

15. Krupp LB, LaRocca NG, Muir-Nash J, Steinberg AD. The fatigue severity scale. Application to patients with multiple sclerosis and systemic lupus erythematosus. *Arch Neurol.* 1989;46(10):1121–1123. doi:10.1001/archneur.1989.00520460115022

16. Yellen SB, Cella DF, Webster K, Blendowski C, Kaplan E. Measuring fatigue and other anemia-related symptoms with the Functional Assessment of Cancer Therapy (FACT) measurement system. *J Pain Symptom Manage.* 1997;13(2):63–74. doi:10.1016/s0885-3924(96)00274-6

17. Smets EM, Garssen B, Bonke B, De Haes JC. The Multidimensional Fatigue Inventory (MFI) psychometric qualities of an instrument to assess fatigue. *J Psychosom Res.* 1995;39(3):315–325. doi:10.1016/0022-3999(94)00125-o

18. Portenoy RK, Thaler HT, Kornblith AB, et al. The Memorial Symptom Assessment Scale: An instrument for the evaluation of symptom prevalence, characteristics and distress. *Eur J Cancer.* 1994;30A(9):1326–1336. doi:10.1016/0959-8049(94)90182-1

19. Nekolaichuk CL, Bruera E, Spachynski K, MacEachern T, Hanson J, Maguire TO. A comparison of patient and proxy symptom assessments in advanced cancer patients. *Palliat Med.* 1999;13(4):311–323. doi:10.1191/026921699675854885

20. Pearson EJM, Morris ME, McKinstry CE. Cancer related fatigue: Implementing guidelines for optimal management. *BMC Health Serv Res.* 2017;17(1):496. doi:10.1186/s12913-017-2415-9

21. Berger AM, Mitchell SA, Jacobsen PB, Pirl WF. Screening, evaluation, and management of cancer-related fatigue: Ready for implementation to practice? *CA Cancer J Clin.* 2015;65(3):190–211. doi:10.3322/caac.21268

22. Abdalrahim MS, Herzallah M, Zeilani R, Alhalaiqa F. Jordanian nurses' knowledge and attitudes toward cancer-related fatigue as a barrier of fatigue management. *J Am Sci.* 2014;10:191–197.

23. Jones G, Rutkowski N, Trudel G, et al. Translating guidelines to practice: A training session about cancer-related fatigue. *Curr Oncol.* 2020;27(2):e163-e170. doi:10.3747/co.27.5681

24. Cella D, Davis K, Breitbart W, Curt G; Fatigue Coalition. Cancer-related fatigue: Prevalence of proposed diagnostic criteria in a United States sample of cancer survivors. *J Clin Oncol.* 2001;19(14):3385–3391. doi:10.1200/JCO.2001.19.14.3385

25. Radbruch L, Strasser F, Elsner F, et al. Fatigue in palliative care patients: An EAPC approach. *Palliat Med.* 2008;22(1):13–32. doi:10.1177/0269216307085183

26. Detmar SB, Muller MJ, Wever LD, Schornagel JH, Aaronson NK. The patient-physician relationship. Patient-physician communication during outpatient palliative treatment visits: An observational study. *JAMA.* 2001;285(10):1351–1357. doi:10.1001/jama.285.10.1351

27. Solano JP, Gomes B, Higginson IJ. A comparison of symptom prevalence in far advanced cancer, AIDS, heart disease, chronic obstructive pulmonary disease and renal disease. *J Pain Symptom Manage.* 2006;31(1):58–69. doi:10.1016/j.jpainsymman.2005.06.007

28. Ma Y, He B, Jiang M, et al. Prevalence and risk factors of cancer-related fatigue: A systematic review and meta-analysis. *Int J Nurs Stud.* 2020;111:103707. doi:10.1016/j.ijnurstu.2020.103707

29. Al Maqbali M, Al Sinani M, Al Naamani Z, Al Badi K, Tanash MI. Prevalence of fatigue in patients with cancer: A systematic review and meta-analysis. *J Pain Symptom Manage.* 2021;61(1):167–189.e14. doi:10.1016/j.jpainsymman.2020.07.037

30. Kutner JS, Kassner CT, Nowels DE. Symptom burden at the end of life: Hospice providers' perceptions. *J Pain Symptom Manage.* 2001;21(6):473–480. doi:10.1016/s0885-3924(01)00281-0

31. Hagelin CL, Wengström Y, Ahsberg E, Fürst CJ. Fatigue dimensions in patients with advanced cancer in relation to time of survival and quality of life. *Palliat Med.* 2009;23(2):171–178. doi:10.1177/0269216308098794

32. Ingham G, Urban K, Allingham SF, Blanchard M, Marston C, Currow DC. The level of distress from fatigue reported in the final two months of life by a palliative care population: An Australian national prospective, consecutive case series. *J Pain Symptom Manage.* 2021;61(6):1109–1117. doi:10.1016/j.jpainsymman.2020.10.031

33. Tranmer JE, Heyland D, Dudgeon D, Groll D, Squires-Graham M, Coulson K. Measuring the symptom experience of seriously ill cancer and noncancer hospitalized patients near the end of life with the memorial symptom assessment scale. *J Pain Symptom Manage.* 2003;25(5):420–429.

34. Grassi L, Indelli M, Marzola M, et al. Depressive symptoms and quality of life in home-care-assisted cancer patients. *J Pain Symptom Manage.* 1996;12(5):300–307. doi:10.1016/s0885-3924(96)00181-9

35. Della PN, Treisman G. HIV/AIDS. In: Levenson JL, ed., *Textbook of Psychosomatic medicine.* Arlington, VA: American Psychiatric Publishing, 2005:599–627.

36. National Collaborating Centre for Chronic Conditions. Chronic obstructive pulmonary disease. National clinical guideline on management of chronic obstructive pulmonary disease in adults in primary and secondary care. *Thorax.* 2004;59 Suppl 1(Suppl 1):1–232.

37. Cohen LM, Moss AH, Weisbord SD, Germain MJ. Renal palliative care. *J Palliat Med.* 2006;9(4):977–992. doi:10.1089/jpm.2006.9.977

38. Guck TP, Elsasser GN, Kavan MG, Barone EJ. Depression and congestive heart failure. *Congest Heart Fail.* 2003;9(3):163–169. doi:10.1111/j.1527-5299.2003.01356.x

39. Singh N, Gayowski T, Wagener MM, Marino IR. Depression in patients with cirrhosis. Impact on outcome. *Dig Dis Sci.* 1997;42(7):1421–1427. doi:10.1023/a:1018898106656

40. Hardcastle SL, Brenu EW, Johnston S, et al. Serum immune proteins in moderate and severe chronic fatigue syndrome/myalgic encephalomyelitis patients. *Int J Med Sci.* 2015;12(10):764–772. doi:10.7150/ijms.12399

41. Radbruch L, Strasser F, Elsner F, et al. Fatigue in palliative care patients: An EAPC approach. *Palliat Med.* 2008;22(1):13–32. doi:10.1177/0269216307085183

42. Wood LJ, Nail LM, Gilster A, Winters KA, Elsea CR. Cancer chemotherapy-related symptoms: Evidence to suggest a role for proinflammatory cytokines. *Oncol Nurs Forum.* 2006;33(3):535–542. doi:10.1188/06.ONF.535-542

43. Kurzrock R. The role of cytokines in cancer-related fatigue. *Cancer.* 2001;92(6 Suppl):1684–1688. doi:10.1002/1097-0142(20010915)92:6+<1684::aid-cncr1497>3.0.co;2-z

44. Golan D, Doniger GM, Wissemann K, et al. The impact of subjective cognitive fatigue and depression on cognitive function in patients with multiple sclerosis. *Mult Scler.* 2018;24(2):196–204. doi:10.1177/1352458517695470

45. Reisfield GM, Lowry MF, Wilson G. Palliative Care Network of Wisconsin, Fast Facts and Concepts #173 Cancer-Related Fatigue. 2007; https://www.mypcnow.org.fast-fact

46. Del Fabbro E, Dalal S, Bruera E. Symptom control in palliative care--Part II: Cachexia/anorexia and fatigue. *J Palliat Med.* 2006;9(2):409–421. doi:10.1089/jpm.2006.9.409

47. Yennurajalingam S, Bruera E. Review of clinical trials of pharmacologic interventions for cancer-related fatigue: Focus on psychostimulants and steroids. *Cancer J.* 2014;20(5):319–324. doi:10.1097/PPO.0000000000000069

48. Jacobsen PB, Donovan KA, Weitzner MA. Distinguishing fatigue and depression in patients with cancer. *Semin Clin Neuropsychiatry.* 2003;8(4):229–240.

49. Harvey SB, Wessely S, Kuh D, Hotopf M. The relationship between fatigue and psychiatric disorders: Evidence for the concept of neurasthenia. *J Psychosom Res.* 2009;66(5):445–454. doi:10.1016/j.jpsychores.2008.12.007

50. Curt GA, Breitbart W, Cella D, et al. Impact of cancer-related fatigue on the lives of patients: New findings from the Fatigue Coalition. *Oncologist.* 2000;5(5):353–360. doi:10.1634/theoncologist.5-5-353

51. Tchekmedyian NS, Kallich J, McDermott A, Fayers P, Erder MH. The relationship between psychologic distress and cancer-related fatigue. *Cancer.* 2003;98(1):198–203. doi:10.1002/cncr.11463

52. National Comprehensive Cancer Network. NCCN guidelines version 1.20201 cancer-related fatigue. 2020. https://www.nccn.org.guidelines

53. Lee SM, Choi HC, Hyun MK. An overview of systematic reviews: Complementary therapies for cancer patients. *Integr Cancer Ther.* 2019;18:1534735419890029. doi:10.1177/1534735419890029

54. Finnegan-John J, Molassiotis A, Richardson A, Ream E. A systematic review of complementary and alternative medicine interventions for the management of cancer-related fatigue. *Integr Cancer Ther.* 2013;12(4):276–290. doi:10.1177/1534735413485816

55. Koutoukidis DA, Land J, Hackshaw A, et al. Fatigue, quality of life and physical fitness following an exercise intervention in multiple myeloma survivors (MASCOT): An exploratory randomised Phase 2 trial utilising a modified Zelen design. *Br J Cancer.* 2020;123(2):187–195. doi:10.1038/s41416-020-0866-y

56. Langeskov-Christensen M, Bisson EJ, Finlayson ML, Dalgas U. Potential pathophysiological pathways that can explain the positive effects of exercise on fatigue in multiple sclerosis: A scoping review. *J Neurol Sci.* 2017;373:307–320. doi:10.1016/j.jns.2017.01.002

57. Mustian KM, Alfano CM, Heckler C, et al. Comparison of pharmaceutical, psychological, and exercise treatments for cancer-related fatigue: A meta-analysis. *JAMA Oncol.* 2017;3(7):961–968. doi:10.1001/jamaoncol.2016.6914

58. Gebruers N, Camberlin M, Theunissen F, et al. The effect of training interventions on physical performance, quality of life, and fatigue in patients receiving breast cancer treatment: A systematic review. *Support Care Cancer.* 2019;27(1):109–122. doi:10.1007/s00520-018-4490-9

59. Kangas M, Bovbjerg DH, Montgomery GH. Cancer-related fatigue: A systematic and meta-analytic review of nonpharmacological therapies for cancer patients [published correction appears in Psychol Bull. 2009 Jan;135(1):172]. *Psychol Bull*. 2008;134(5):700–741. doi:10.1037/a0012825

60. Schmitz KH, Holtzman J, Courneya KS, Mâsse LC, Duval S, Kane R. Controlled physical activity trials in cancer survivors: A systematic review and meta-analysis. *Cancer Epidemiol Biomarkers Prev*. 2005;14(7):1588–1595. doi:10.1158/1055-9965.EPI-04-0703

61. Mustian KM, Morrow GR, Carroll JK, Figueroa-Moseley CD, Jean-Pierre P, Williams GC. Integrative nonpharmacologic behavioral interventions for the management of cancer-related fatigue. *Oncologist*. 2007;12 Suppl 1:52–67. doi:10.1634/theoncologist.12-S1-52

62. Hilfiker R, Meichtry A, Eicher M, et al. Exercise and other nonpharmaceutical interventions for cancer-related fatigue in patients during or after cancer treatment: A systematic review incorporating an indirect-comparisons meta-analysis. *Br J Sports Med*. 2018;52(10):651–658. doi:10.1136/bjsports-2016-096422

63. Vadiraja SH, Rao MR, Nagendra RH, et al. Effects of yoga on symptom management in breast cancer patients: A randomized controlled trial. *Int J Yoga*. 2009;2(2):73–79. doi:10.4103/0973-6131.60048

64. Dong B, Xie C, Jing X, Lin L, Tian L. Yoga has a solid effect on cancer-related fatigue in patients with breast cancer: A meta-analysis. *Breast Cancer Res Treat*. 2019;177(1):5–16. doi:10.1007/s10549-019-05278-w

65. Wayne PM, Lee MS, Novakowski J, et al. Tai Chi and Qigong for cancer-related symptoms and quality of life: A systematic review and meta-analysis. *J Cancer Surviv*. 2018;12(2):256–267. doi:10.1007/s11764-017-0665-5

66. Wu C, Zheng Y, Duan Y, et al. Nonpharmacological interventions for cancer-related fatigue: A systematic review and Bayesian network meta-analysis. *Worldviews Evid Based Nurs*. 2019;16(2):102–110. doi:10.1111/wvn.12352

67. Oldervoll LM, Loge JH, Lydersen S, et al. Physical exercise for cancer patients with advanced disease: A randomized controlled trial. *Oncologist*. 2011;16(11):1649–1657. doi:10.1634/theoncologist.2011-0133

68. Barsevick AM, Dudley W, Beck S, Sweeney C, Whitmer K, Nail L. A randomized clinical trial of energy conservation for patients with cancer-related fatigue. *Cancer*. 2004;100(6):1302–1310. doi:10.1002/cncr.20111

69. Blikman LJ, Huisstede BM, Kooijmans H, Stam HJ, Bussmann JB, van Meeteren J. Effectiveness of energy conservation treatment in reducing fatigue in multiple sclerosis: A systematic review and meta-analysis. *Arch Phys Med Rehabil*. 2013;94(7):1360–1376.

70. Sadeghi E, Gozali N, Moghaddam Tabrizi F. Effects of energy conservation strategies on cancer related fatigue and health promotion lifestyle in breast cancer survivors: A randomized control trial. *Asian Pac J Cancer Prev*. 2016;17(10):4783–4790.

71. Lynch MT. Palliative care at the end of life. *Semin Oncol Nurs*. 2014;30(4):268–279. doi:10.1016/j.soncn.2014.08.009

72. Abbey, S. Psychiatric aspects of fatigue at the end of life. In: Chochinov M, Breitbart W, eds. *Handbook of Psychiatry in Palliative Medicine*. 2nd ed. New York: Oxford University Press. 2009:427–439.

73. Seyedi Chegeni P, Gholami M, Azargoon A, Hossein Pour AH, Birjandi M, Norollahi H. The effect of progressive muscle relaxation on the management of fatigue and quality of sleep in patients with chronic obstructive pulmonary disease: A randomized controlled clinical trial. *Complement Ther Clin Pract*. 2018;31:64–70. doi:10.1016/j.ctcp.2018.01.010

74. Hassanzadeh M, Kiani F, Bouya S, Zarei M. Comparing the effects of relaxation technique and inhalation aromatherapy on fatigue in patients undergoing hemodialysis. *Complement Ther Clin Pract*. 2018;31:210–214. doi:10.1016/j.ctcp.2018.02.019

75. Price JR, Mitchell E, Tidy E, Hunot V. Cognitive behaviour therapy for chronic fatigue syndrome in adults. *Cochrane Database Syst Rev*. 2008;2008(3):CD001027. doi:10.1002/14651858.CD001027.pub2

76. Hoffman CJ, Ersser SJ, Hopkinson JB, Nicholls PG, Harrington JE, Thomas PW. Effectiveness of mindfulness-based stress reduction in mood, breast- and endocrine-related quality of life, and well-being in stage 0 to III breast cancer: A randomized, controlled trial. *J Clin Oncol*. 2012;30(12):1335–1342.

77. Poort H, Peters M, Bleijenberg G, et al. Psychosocial interventions for fatigue during cancer treatment with palliative intent. *Cochrane Database Syst Rev*. 2017;7(7):CD012030. doi:10.1002/14651858.CD012030.pub2

78. Klasson C, Helde Frankling M, Lundh Hagelin C, Björkhem-Bergman L. Fatigue in cancer patients in palliative care: A review on pharmacological interventions. *Cancers (Basel)*. 2021;13(5):985. doi:10.3390/cancers13050985

79. Hoenemeyer TW, Kaptchuk TJ, Mehta TS, Fontaine KR. Open-label placebo treatment for cancer-related fatigue: A randomized-controlled clinical trial. *Sci Rep*. 2018;8(1):2784. doi:10.1038/s41598-018-20993-y

80. Junior PNA, Barreto CMN, de Iracema Gomes Cubero D, Del Giglio A. The efficacy of placebo for the treatment of cancer-related fatigue: A systematic review and meta-analysis. *Support Care Cancer*. 2020;28(4):1755–1764. doi:10.1007/s00520-019-04977-w

81. Roji R, Stone P, Ricciardi F, Candy B. Placebo response in trials of drug treatments for cancer-related fatigue: A systematic review, meta-analysis and meta-regression. *BMJ Support Palliat Care*. 2020;10(4):385–394. doi:10.1136/bmjspcare-2019-002163

82. Fabi A, Bhargava R, Fatigoni S, et al. Cancer-related fatigue: ESMO Clinical Practice Guidelines for diagnosis and treatment. *Ann Oncol*. 2020;31(6):713–723. doi:10.1016/j.annonc.2020.02.016

83. Pedersen L, Lund L, Petersen MA, Sjogren P, Groenvold M. Methylphenidate as needed for fatigue in patients with advanced cancer: A prospective, double-blind, and placebo-controlled study. *J Pain Symptom Manage*. 2020;60(5):992–1002. doi:10.1016/j.jpainsymman.2020.05.023

84. Richard PO, Fleshner NE, Bhatt JR, Hersey KM, Chahin R, Alibhai SM. Phase II, randomised, double-blind, placebo-controlled trial of methylphenidate for reduction of fatigue levels in patients with prostate cancer receiving LHRH-agonist therapy. *BJU Int*. 2015;116(5):744–752.

85. Roth AJ, Nelson C, Rosenfeld B, et al. Methylphenidate for fatigue in ambulatory men with prostate cancer. *Cancer*. 2010;116(21):5102–5110. doi:10.1002/cncr.25424

86. Mitchell GK, Hardy JR, Nikles CJ, et al. The effect of methylphenidate on fatigue in advanced cancer: An aggregated n-of-1 trial. *J Pain Symptom Manage*. 2015;50(3):289–296. doi:10.1016/j.jpainsymman.2015.03.009

87. Centeno C, Rojí R, Portela MA, De Santiago A, Cuervo MA, Ramos D, et al. Improved cancer-related fatigue in a randomised clinical trial: Methylphenidate no better than placebo. *BMJ Support Palliat Care*. 2022;12(2):226–234. doi:10.1136/bmjspcare-2020-002454

88. Bruera E, Miller MJ, Macmillan K, Kuehn N. Neuropsychological effects of methylphenidate in patients receiving a continuous infusion of narcotics for cancer pain. *Pain*. 1992;48(2):163–166. doi:10.1016/0304-3959(92)90053-E

89. Homsi J, Nelson KA, Sarhill N, et al. A phase II study of methylphenidate for depression in advanced cancer. *Am J Hosp Palliat Care*. 2001;18(6):403–407. doi:10.1177/104990910101800610

90. Yennurajalingam S, Palmer JL, Chacko R, Bruera E. Factors associated with response to methylphenidate in advanced cancer patients. *Oncology*. 2011;16:246–253.

91. Lee EQ, Muzikansky A, Drappatz J, et al. A randomized, placebo-controlled pilot trial of armodafinil for fatigue in patients with gliomas undergoing radiotherapy. *Neuro Oncol*. 2016;18(6):849–854. doi:10.1093/neuonc/now007

92. Spathis A, Fife K, Blackhall F, et al. Modafinil for the treatment of fatigue in lung cancer: Results of a placebo-controlled, double-blind, randomized trial. *J Clin Oncol*. 2014;32(18):1882–1888. doi:10.1200/JCO.2013.54.4346

93. Hovey E, de Souza P, Marx G, et al. Phase III, randomized, double-blind, placebo-controlled study of modafinil for fatigue in patients treated with docetaxel-based chemotherapy. *Support Care Cancer*. 2014;22(5):1233–1242. doi:10.1007/s00520-013-2076-0

94. Hardy J, Haywood A, Rickett K, Sallnow L, Good P. Practice review: Evidence-based quality use of corticosteroids in the palliative care of patients with advanced cancer. *Palliat Med*. 2021;35(3):461–472. doi:10.1177/0269216320986717

95. Tanioka, H., et al. Prophylactic effect of dexamethasone on regorafenib-related fatigue and/or malaise: A randomized, placebo-controlled, double-blind clinical study in patients with unresectable metastatic colorectal cancer. *Oncology*. 2018;94:289–296.

96. Paulsen O, Klepstad P, Rosland JH, et al. Efficacy of methylprednisolone on pain, fatigue, and appetite loss in patients with advanced cancer using opioids: A randomized, placebo-controlled, double-blind trial. *J Clin Oncol*. 2014;32(29):3221–3228. doi:10.1200/JCO.2013.54.3926

97. Yennurajalingam S, Frisbee-Hume S, Palmer JL, et al. Reduction of cancer-related fatigue with dexamethasone: A double-blind, randomized, placebo-controlled trial in patients with advanced cancer. *J Clin Oncol*. 2013;31(25):3076–3082. doi:10.1200/jco.2012.44.4661

98. Hatano Y, Matsuoka H, Lam L, Currow DC. Side effects of corticosteroids in patients with advanced cancer: A systematic review. *Support Care Cancer*. 2018;26(12):3979–3983. doi:10.1007/s00520-018-4339-2

99. Del Fabbro E, Garcia JM, Dev R, et al. Testosterone replacement for fatigue in hypogonadal ambulatory males with advanced cancer: A preliminary double-blind placebo-controlled trial. *Support Care Cancer*. 2013;21(9):2599–2607. doi:10.1007/s00520-013-1832-5

100. Lund Rasmussen C, Klee Olsen M, Thit Johnsen A, et al. Effects of melatonin on physical fatigue and other symptoms in patients with advanced cancer receiving palliative care: A double-blind placebo-controlled crossover trial. *Cancer*. 2015;121(20):3727–3736. doi:10.1002/cncr.29563

101. Björkhem-Bergman L, Bergman P. Vitamin D and patients with palliative cancer. *BMJ Support Palliat Care*. 2016;6(3):287–291. doi:10.1136/bmjspcare-2015-000921

102. Helde-Frankling M, Bergqvist J, Klasson C, et al. Vitamin D supplementation to palliative cancer patients: Protocol of a double-blind, randomised controlled trial "Palliative-D." *BMJ Support Palliat Care*. 2017;7(4):458–463. doi:10.1136/bmjspcare-2017-001429

Psychotherapeutic Interventions in Palliative Care

32

Psychodynamic Therapy in the Terminally Ill

Linda Emanuel and Stephanie Brody

Introduction

The central premise of palliative medicine is optimization of quality of life despite serious illness. Quality of dying is a unique process that affects the dying and the bereaved and ripples into the culture. Reckoning with death can result in enriching life's meaning by helping relationships overcome entanglements and by clarifying lasting values and intergenerational commitments.[1] The widespread experience that terminal processes can bring sustenance along with loss is widely acknowledged but little explained. In this chapter, we describe some of what psychodynamic approaches contribute to understanding and fostering these developments. We define "psychodynamic" as the combination of psychanalytic thought and contemporary derivatives from it that work predominantly with unconscious determinants of experience and behavior. That psychodynamic approaches bring relief to people facing existential challenge may be no surprise when we consider that key architects of the psychodynamic tradition placed great emphasis on mortality and loss.[2-5] One psychoanalytic scholar even posited that most of our unconscious lives are taken up with—creative or not creative—responses to death anxiety.[6] Though psychodynamic work can be long and intensive, shorter and less time-intensive dynamic work can still be profoundly useful for the palliative care patient, and more traditional dynamic work may be suitable for family members. To assist this work, we offer a theoretical explanation of well-accepted dynamic processes, here focused for this population. Then we set out, combining our experience, case-illustrated clinical approaches to working in this way.

Dynamic Therapy for Dealing with Mortality

Vacillation Between Opposing Experiences as Part of Psychological Processing

The fact of death brings a unique and confounding kind of distress. As observed in classical psychoanalytic literature, nonexistence seems impossible.[7] Yet fantasies of immortality fail the reality test. Furthermore, we have a profound sensation of fear about death. People respond to this two-sided experience in a process that involves oscillating back and forth between the opposing experiences. That process and what emerges from it are all important.

Psychodynamic literature recognizes how people oscillate between one state of mind and its opposite and accepts that such oscillation is part of an inherent process of forming and constantly reforming the mind. Consider the foundational concept of conflict in drive theory,[8] the notion of oscillating positions in early object relations theory,[3] the tension between separating and remaining merged or attached,[9,10] the deep-seated fear of falling apart assuaged by a nurturing figure,[11] the back-and-forth process of bringing raw feelings to a nurturing figure who helps make sense of the new experience,[12] or the sliding back and forth between more or less evolved states of mind,[13] etc. All major psychodynamic schools of thought presume or explicitly describe a process of going back and forth. This healthy back-and-forth process has the capacity to create in the mind of patients an integrated and effective way of managing feelings and thoughts such that they can respond optimally to the challenges of reality—especially the challenge of existence.

Palliative medicine also notes how patients vacillate back and forth in their prognostic awareness[14] (see also Chapter 21). Palliative clinicians have learned to allow this oscillation and harness it for its own product: adjustment. This shift from one awareness to another is central to the process as the person gains the emotional scaffolding and resources to bear reality even while struggling with denial, pain, and wishful thinking.

That process can also fail. A person can get stuck in fear or stuck in fantasy. Both entail suffering, and neither is as useful as an integrated state—including when facing death. Psychodynamic therapy uses its standard approaches to foster and if necessary restart a functioning oscillation. The process is described below, as applied to those facing mortality, and depicted in a more schematic construct in Figure 32.1.

How Oscillation Works to Process Difficult Reality

Oscillation, or vacillating between perceptions of reality or psychological positions, is necessary but not sufficient. It matters how the oscillation is being driven and whether the process is yielding understanding and integration. Repeated oscillation without change is more like repetition compulsion or obsessional processes. Indeed, it is more accurate to describe a healthy process as recursive oscillation since there is a forward-moving component.

What is happening for a person in the oscillation can be uniquely well-accessed by dynamic therapy. Dynamic therapy is exhaustively described in its own vast literature. In brief, it gains insight into what is entailed for a particular patient by paying attention, within the context of a therapeutic relationship in which the patient receives "evenly hovering attention" and "holding" from the therapist,[11] to evidence of how the deeper formations of

Visual depiction of model

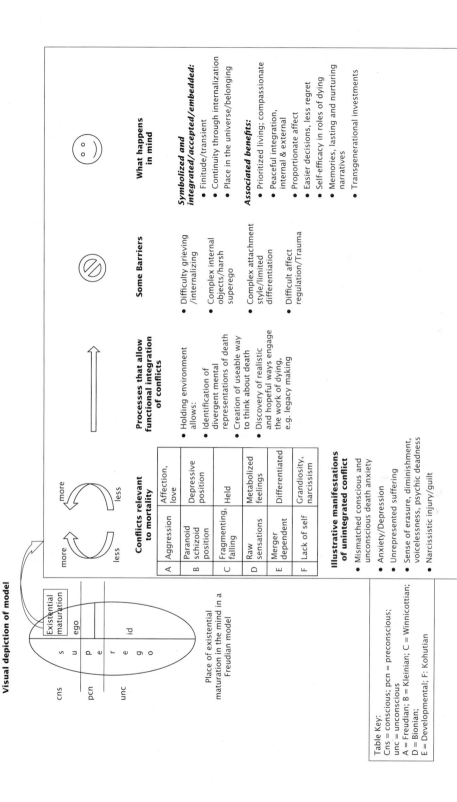

Place of existential maturation in the mind in a Freudian model

Table Key:
Cns = conscious; pcn = preconscious;
unc = unconscious
A = Freudian; B = Kleinian; C = Winnicottian;
D = Bionian;
E = Developmental; F: Kohutian

Conflicts relevant to mortality

		more	less
A	Aggression	Affection, love	
B	Paranoid schizoid position	Depressive position	
C	Fragmenting, falling	Held	
D	Raw sensations	Metabolized feelings	
E	Merger dependent	Differentiated	
F	Lack of self	Grandiosity, narcissism	

Illustrative manifestations of unintegrated conflict
- Mismatched conscious and unconscious death anxiety
- Anxiety/Depression
- Unrepresented suffering
- Sense of erasure, diminishment, voicelessness, psychic deadness
- Narcissistic injury/guilt

Processes that allow functional integration of conflicts
- Holding environment allows:
- Identification of divergent mental representations of death
- Creation of useable way to think about death
- Discovery of realistic and hopeful ways engage the work of dying, e.g. legacy making

Some Barriers
- Difficulty grieving /internalizing
- Complex internal objects/harsh superego
- Complex attachment style/limited differentiation
- Difficult affect regulation/Trauma

What happens in mind

Symbolized and integrated/accepted/embedded:
- Finitude/transient
- Continuity through internalization
- Place in the universe/belonging

Associated benefits:
- Prioritized living; compassionate
- Peaceful integration, internal & external
- Proportionate affect
- Easier decisions, less regret
- Self-efficacy in roles of dying
- Memories, lasting and nurturing narratives
- Transgenerational investments

FIGURE 32.1 Schematic depiction of existential maturation processes: Visual depiction of model.

that person's mind work. Sign posts to those deeper aspects come from many sources such as free association, dreams and reveries, parapraxes, transference and countertransference, affective states, somatic communications, manifest defenses, and how the patient navigates events. All these information sources provide for the therapist a dynamic formulation and very specific understandings of where the patient has gotten stuck or deviated into coping defenses that no longer serve. The utility (or not) of the insights becomes apparent from how, when shared or used in the therapeutic relationship, they resonate with the patient, deepen the treatment, and eventually yield for the patient a sense of liberating self-understanding, growth, and self-possession. In this process of learning, sharing, and reworking, new more usable understandings get created and laid down in the mind of the patient. All these processes can be applied for the benefit of patients facing dying and death. Opposing experiences related to death and dying must surface for this recreated understanding to emerge. Next we consider how they surface and what can happen in dynamic therapy.

Finding and Resolving Divergent Conceptions of Mortality

For palliative medicine patients and their family members, understanding how the person thinks and feels about their mortality, and the oscillations between opposing positions, is crucial. How people think and feel about mortality can be a surprise to themselves. The mind represents all relevant matters that it can in an effort to help us navigate the world of reality. Not least, it represents mortality. But representing mortality faces a unique dilemma in that nonexistence cannot be represented except by erasure or absence—something that depends for its perception on existence. Clinical experience suggests that people quite commonly, though not always, represent mortality rather differently in their conscious belief system and in their deeper systems. For instance, a person may consciously understand death as simply nothingness, but dreams and other pointers to a less conscious but operative conception may indicate that death is represented as home, or an embrace, a completion, a state of agony, being part of some other state of existence, etc. Dynamic therapy will "follow the trail," curious to understand where such representations come from, because understanding their origins seems to allow a re-visioning should that be needed.

Addressing Representations of Death That Come From Deadening Psychological Experiences

Psychologically, experiences of erasure, diminution, abandonment, emptiness, darkness, falling, and fragmentation or coming apart come close to representations of nonexistence or death. These are the most desperate and difficult, deadening, or terrifying sensations. They tend to be well covered by coping mechanisms (defenses). They are also the sensations that can occur from traumatizing experiences of any type and from failures in the early formation of the mind's existence.[15]

Apparently, people are prone to representing death in their minds in ways that reflect psychic deadening. This makes sense of common clinical experience that people approach mortality in ways that seem affected by early attachment, relational experiences, and trauma. It also makes sense of how difficult it can be to uncover these well-defended representations of terrible sensations.

Not everyone struggles with psychic deadening, but alertness to this area is usually indicated. More than a few dynamic therapy cases with palliative care patients that have pursued ordinary psychodynamic approaches also resulted in resolution of existential struggles. By that we mean that patients had developed not only an ability to terminate the treatment well, but, in the process, they had grieved the fantasy of immortality and resolved death anxieties enough to face mortality without becoming unmoored. They had done this through the ordinary evolution in dynamic therapy of developing understanding and creating more resilient ways of handling past injuries and difficult relationships. In the process, the patients faced their finitude, secured their connectedness, and bore their separateness from others.

Finding Reality-Based Ways to Balance Opposing Experiences of Death

An important counterpart component exists to the metabolizing or integrating process that hopefully occurs during oscillation. That is, people find sources of connectedness and continuity that make separateness and finitude less absolute. Typically, these are found in meaningful relationships and completing tasks of dying, such as legacy-making.

Importantly for dynamic therapy, these sources of connected continuity need to be realistic since failure of immortality fantasies to pass the reality test lies at the heart of death anxiety. Dynamic therapy uses its methods to provide patients with understanding about the place significant people have within them. Dynamic therapy focuses on those who may be deceased and have become internalized ("internal objects") and those who are still actively involved in the real world and are providing essential psychological functions ("external objects" providing "self-functions"). Through understanding these relationships and through experiencing a different kind of contribution to their psychological life in the therapeutic relationship, patients increasingly represent themselves in their own minds as part of a network of interconnecting, vital relationships. Patients start to see their significant relationships as "investments in their continuity" and as part of what defines their "place in the web of life."

Leaving some kind of legacy—whether by passing on cooking recipes, stories, material things, lessons, expressions of meaning, or something else—is a comforting part of the work of dying which provides realistic continuity in the face of death. (See also Chapter 35, "Dignity Therapy" and Chapter 36, "Meaning-Centered Psychotherapy.") Other jobs of dying, such as estate planning, making a living will, writing letters to be opened posthumously, settling difficult relationships, etc. all become part of optimizing the manner in which the dying person will live on as an internal presence in others. Since optimization of significant relationships is a major marker of change and signals readiness to end dynamic treatment, ordinary dynamic therapy is well aligned with having the ability to find reality-based ways to balance the absoluteness of death with the hope for finite life's generativity.

Symbolized and integrated/accepted/embedded:
- Finitude/transient
- Continuity through internalization
- Place in the universe/belonging

Associated benefits:
- Prioritized living; often of loving, respectful values
- Peaceful integration, internal and external
- Proportionate affect
- Easier decisions, less regret
- Self-efficacy in roles of dying
- Memories, lasting and nurturing narratives
- Transgenerational investments

Grief and Its Role in Adjusting to Mortality

Many barriers to digesting the warring feelings about death seem to have a common mechanism: they disrupt grieving. Grieving and internalization are not easy (see also Chapter 41). People who have had excessive loss without processing and replacement may find the experience of grief so painful that grieving itself, let alone the catharsis and healing it can bring, are beyond reach. To the extent that grief requires feeling, appreciating, and understanding painful feelings, it makes sense that people with difficult affect regulation, severe after-effects of posttraumatic stress disorder, and conflicted significant interpersonal relationships will have difficulty grieving. We find that people with these difficulties live, tragically, with the antithesis of existential maturity.

Dynamic therapy understands grief much as classical theory describes it.[4] We find it important to bring the oscillating and metabolizing processes of creating new structures (described above) together with those of grief.[16] Our experience with people engaged in grief is that, as they explore what the reality of loss means, they look for ways to retain or replace the internal role that belonged to the mourned person or capacity. If the grieving person can perform that role passably similarly, then the lost person or capacity has been internalized; the deceased person or lost capacity—perhaps through memory—has become a vitalized internal function. What cannot be sufficiently internalized must be replaced by another relationship of function. In the realization of need and the seeking of new ways to acquire the missing psychological nutrition, new relationships are formed. Something new is created by regenerating the inherent psychic growth and structure formation that happens between people in a meaningful relationship. Grief is more than letting go and moving on; successful grief entails psychic growth.

If the pain of remembering is insuperable or if reaching out to find new relationships fails or backfires, the grieving person may find that internalization fell short or seeking external sources generated more grief. That person may withdraw from the grieving process; mourning stops. A person in this painful, melancholic position has fewer ways to invest in continuing connections with the dead or the living and the harshness of mortality goes unassuaged; feeling peaceful about mortality is harder than ever except perhaps as a way out of suffering. Dynamic therapy for such a person will seek a careful and gentle return to bolstering internalization and seeking external sources, first through understanding what is underlying and the therapeutic relationship itself and then for other relationships.

Toward What Goals

Dynamic therapy aims to move mortality from a terrifying, impenetrable idea to an integrated and symbolized function in the mind that allows for acceptance and connection at the end of life. Broadly, these three understandings are central and transformative.

- Finitude and transience in capacity and time are accepted simply as reality for all.
- Continuity is possible through internalization.
- A sense of place or belonging in the universe is found that brings tranquility.

With these three understandings in place and active, people seem to experience acceptance, a sense of integration, and flourishing resilience even alongside pain, suffering, and loss.

Pediatrics

Pediatric palliative medicine clinicians observe that children face mortality with their own kind of equanimity, often greater than that of adults. This fits with our understanding that finding comfort in lasting, loving (internalized) relationships is crucial. Since children have as much or more active relatedness as adults and engage the processes of laying down psychic ways in the setting of those relationships from birth on, it is to be expected that continuity in the face of death is not more elusive to children than adults. Though stage-specific features may be dominant at a specific phase of life, essential capacities may also be acquired at any stage, especially through therapeutic interactions that integrate or focus on this central theme.

Illness-Related Suffering During Dying Processes

Death happens piecemeal for most people; indeed, some express the reality by noting that it is dying more than death that they fear. During an illness journey, early symptoms remind us of death's salience, then perhaps diagnosis removes hopes and dreams, then the illness and treatment usually cause physical suffering that challenges everything from thinking and feeling to relating and managing life, then perhaps lost capacities require letting sources of vitality go. Important relationships change; some people flee the difficulties and others come closer. All of these changes and more are pieces of dying that require mourning in both the person with illness and in those around. Beyond the moments of final systems shut down that we identify as death, losses continue piecemeal for the bereaved. For a while it feels like the person is just away. Rituals of mourning restore the person's place in the lives of others for a moment while marking their loss. The routines that they were a part of change, sometimes one by one; their smells fade. And so on.

Dynamic therapy, oriented as it is to making grief and mourning work toward the goal of laying down new, more adaptive psychological ways, is particularly well-suited to helping people through the processes of dying. A dynamic therapist will invite self-understanding about the meaning of each loss, hold the feelings of the very specific personal loss, and, through the presence of new or refocused shared understanding, invite exploration of new possibilities. Because the losses of dying need never be only losses but always grief and re-placement with new, realistic hope—even if the hope is for pain-free death—ordinary dynamic therapy applies hand-in-glove to the palliative care population.

Symptoms That Occur when the Realities of Mortality Are Unresolved

If a person cannot find a way to realistically bring together mortal hope and fear of death, it can pervasively affect many aspects of life and may manifest in varied symptoms. The following are a few of these symptoms, along with pointers about how a dynamic therapist might address them.

Anxiety and depression are nonspecific symptoms. We understand anxiety and depression as universal indicators of psychic duress.[17] Unmetabolized death fear and unrealistic vitality are both stressful conditions. Without the benefit of integration and adaptive defenses, anxiety and depression result. Anxiety may attach to other concerns, but death anxiety is the specific anxiety at play for many facing mortality. "Death anxiety" is a term that has been elaborated by scholars in terror management theory.[18] These scholars use it as Becker[6] intended: it is something all people have and, to some extent, require; death anxiety per se is not a symptom. Insufficiently mitigated death anxiety is a symptom of missing investment in realistic, continuing vitality. The psychic landscape can be one of lost reality, paralysis, or fragmentation. A person in this state finds relationships to others are overwhelmed by helplessness and fear, a sense of falling into a dark abyss, and panic signals disintegration which can border on psychosis. Aloneness is profound. These suffering states are often unrepresented in the mind and out of reach therefore of the reconciling possibilities from realistic conceptions of mortal life.

Depression related to facing mortality largely results from having withdrawn to melancholy from the mourning processes necessary to constantly adapt to the accelerating losses of dying. (See also the earlier section on "Grief and Its Role in Adjusting to Mortality.") The challenge to the dynamic therapist is finding what part of the grief process failed and rekindling it. Often the failed part has to do with patients finding that their main coping mechanism in life is not working and an alternate mode is not within reach. For instance, a person who approaches life's challenges largely successfully by being a fighter or a manager finds that cancer or Alzheimer's has won. If the dynamic therapist can help the person creatively find coping through, for instance, meaningful relationships despite serious capacity limitations, depression can lift.

Another manifestation of blocked processing is brittleness or rigidity that may belie a mismatch between a person's conscious and unconscious feelings. A person who engages death often, say in the line of duty, may have little fear of death on a conscious level, but unconscious fear is great. There may even be a form of defiance over death's authority, allowing a person to declare: "death has no power over me—I can do anything—I have no fear of death." Such compensatory mastery can point to unresolved unconscious matters.

Guilt enters early in psychic life and can play a role in many struggles around mortal life. Understandings put forward by early authors in object relations theory posit that guilt in response to aggressive appetite is one of the earliest elements in an infant's mind. Children suffering from parental psychic deadness can also fault themselves for being unable to vitalize that parent. When we foresee our death, we can feel guilty about leaving dependents. Or, when loved ones die, many feel that they killed them or failed to save them. Or, self-critical individuals may regard death as a final conviction—deserved condemnation for a transgression, failure, or limitation. Perhaps they even feel forgiveness is not possible, and death is a welcome alliance, an outcome based on an idea of punishment. Dynamic therapists generally view guilt as a response to aggressive drives that seemed overly impactful; as such, dynamic therapists are well positioned to address and resolve symptomatic guilt. Understanding both the aggressive drive and the assuaging, generative possibilities yields the integrated creativity that allows new psychic growth. Ideally, new or adjusted relationships form, compassion is possible, and the realistic continuity and part-taking that mortal life offers can be attained.

A long-standing experience of interpersonal annihilation interferes with the development of personal vitality. The process of existential maturation cannot be initiated if there has never been an experience of mutually reciprocated vitality, the experience of being valued, heard, or worthy of life. The dynamic therapist encountering a dying person or family member with such a history is likely to find them beset by raw, unrepresented suffering states. For such a person, the work is deep, difficult, and requires an intense presence in the therapeutic alliance that can touch the psychic deadness. As hard as this is, patients with such intense suffering can be highly motivated, and if the dynamic therapist can manage to be available, growth is possible. Accompanying a patient to their psychic deadness, feeling the rawness, may be the patient's first ever experience of vital relatedness in that part of their mind. It can feel to the therapist rather like being the proverbial boatman who crosses the psychic river Styx and can return with a psychically enlivened person. For some, it is then possible to invest in the relationships that offer mortal continuity beyond death.

Patients with personality disorders may have symptoms specific to their psychic organization. For instance, for a person with a narcissistic personality, mortality may be experienced as a narcissistic injury. That person may feel, in a form of grandiosity, "I am invulnerable to the forces of death." With a mortal diagnosis, then the question "How could this happen to me?" bedevils the sense of control and immortality. Their unwillingness to accept mortality can interfere with emotional intimacy and gratitude. The impact on loved ones, whose efforts to make amends may be thwarted, can interfere with grief and bereavement. Resolution of personality disorders is long and difficult work—though possible—in dynamic therapy. If the prognosis allows, intensive work is indicated. Sometimes the work moves remarkably fast, aided by the sword of Damocles that the patient powerfully feels. If not, the patient and their family may do better with behavior-oriented counseling to maximize the helpful work of dying and minimize the damage of unresolved conflict.

No matter the presenting symptom and the discovered matters to be resolved, our sense is that once a person has accepted finitude, found realistic forms of continuity, and has a way of thinking about their place in the grand scheme of things, they attain a kind of peaceful integration, both internally and in relationships with other.

How to Monitor and Recognize Progress in Treatment

The manner in which people resolve the dilemmas and suffering related to mortality is not linear, does not have set progressive stages or necessarily a state of arrival. But, in the same way dynamic therapists use markers of change to assess a patient's evolution, we also perceive markers relevant to maturation of an integrated relationship to mortality. These include

- Mutative moments such as re-experiencing psychic deadness, but now in the presence of the analyst's hovering and responsive attention.
- Reduction in the discrepancy between conscious and unconscious death anxiety
- More realistic conceptions of the future.
- Ability to contemplate death without becoming overwhelmed or detached from reality.
- Increased capacity to love, unimpeded or enhanced by mortality awareness.
- More flexible use of defenses against mortality awareness—dissociation, splitting, etc. are more moderate.
- More comfortable expressions about and ability to sit with feelings about death and dying.
- Realistic and creative directedness toward tasks of life's last stages—legacy making, etc.

Integrating Psychodynamic with Psychiatric Approaches

Psychodynamic approaches to facilitating a manageable relationship to death in the palliative medicine context are best used not as standalone but as part of integrated comprehensive care. For instance, understanding anxiety and depression as manifest symptoms, as we do, does not translate into opposing medical management. Biological disorders of the molecular physiology of anxiety and depression also exist. Furthermore, what may begin as manifest symptoms with a dynamic source can take on a life of their own. Whether in "split treatment" (when a psychiatrist prescribes self-administered medication and monitors NMDA or psychobilin categories of treatment or other electrophysiological treatments (Chapter 42) and a talk therapist engages dynamic therapy) or with a psychiatrist-analyst providing both, we acknowledge that, for many, optimal outcomes depend on medical intervention with talk therapy.

Case Examples

The case examples offered here are all fictitious but are based on real experiences with patients or modestly adapted from historical, documented cases.

Unconscious Representation and Anticipatory Grief as Part of Growth

In early work with a child analyst, a 10-year old boy whose mother had advanced cancer revealed through his drawings a distant relationship with his mother, anger directed at his father, and anxiety about social interactions. The next step for the therapist was now to trace the distance from his mother to its dynamic origins. Perhaps he is driven by fear of loss, anger, or displaced guilt and frustration that he and his father (with whom he identified) are unable to save his mother. Emerging anxiety led to the experience of anticipatory guilt over his (now understood) anger (expressed by acting out) at his mother for leaving him. While the child acquired these understandings, a meaningful relationship with the analyst was evolving. Within this stabilizing relationship, he accessed his capacity to grieve; he knew experientially that he has nurturing connection from someone other than his mother and father. The relationship to his parents was becoming embedded through internalization. Accepting his mother's mortality became easier because he could imagine life after her death. When his mother died, he was not beset by guilt at having been angry or distant, partly because both feelings reduced when he understood them and partly because he accepted the normalcy of the process. Those normalized feelings had ceased to be an impediment to being close with his mother before she died so actual intimacy with her allowed him to hold a lasting impression of expressed maternal love.

Narcissism

A middle-aged woman, shaped by her immigrant father's defensive narcissism and traumatic journey to this country, grappled with the origins of her own seductiveness and demand for merger relationships. She had disdain for anyone not willing to serve her needs, and this had left her isolated. A recent diagnosis of breast cancer brought her to dynamic therapy where she sought her usual merger relationship with her therapist. Setting a therapeutic limit, the therapist persisted in inviting her into the holding environment of dynamic work, demonstrating curiosity and optimism about her possibilities. As the patient explored the origins of her interpersonal style, she made a connection to her father's fight for psychic survival, and she realized that her mother's unmet needs in their marriage had left her deprived of psychic nutrition as well. Caring for herself through her cancer journey became an opportunity for individuation. Her understanding and re-experiencing of psychological life-and-death conflict was informed by and newly generated as she laid down new psychic structure. When her parents died and her own cancer treatment was successfully completed, her personal life began to flourish.

Trauma

A veteran with a history of trauma, now anticipating a decision about forgoing or accepting ventilator support for terminal emphysema, was offered the chance to utilize dynamic therapy to facilitate his ability to make this difficult decision. The smells of the hospital and the respirator revived his trauma-related panic episodes. He felt unable to assess whether his leaning to forgo mechanical respiration was overly influenced by his history. Anxiolytic and antidepressant treatment and additional medications prior to hospital trips reduced some of his trauma-related triggers and helped him to clarify that his leaning toward forgoing intervention had been about avoiding retraumatization and not based on death acceptance. As dynamic therapy progressed—fortunately, he remained well enough for long enough—he re-examined and restructured his important personal relationships. Ultimately, when he could no longer breathe without mechanical support he opted for intubation. But, with his few remaining friends and family around him, he soon felt ready to accept death and opted for extubation, something that was accomplished amid expressions of love and gratitude for the chance to be together.

Suicidality

A young man, born to a borderline psychotic and withholding mother and absent father, presented with borderline psychotic and schizoidal tendencies. He had been diagnosed with a curable cancer but refused chemotherapy. Furthermore, he sought to get his dynamic therapist to "join him in the darkness" by engaging in plausible suicide preparations. The therapist regarded this manifestation of suicidality as a symptom of psychic deadness, a consequence of parental psychic annihilation. When the therapist managed to find and name his pain, he felt understood, abandoned the suicide plans, and started anti-cancer treatment. But then the suicidality returned. The patient's psychic deadness could not be treated with one mutative turn-around. Mustering stamina and enough supportive consultation from colleagues, the therapist continued the slow process of fostering new psychological structures and organizing potential. Over time, the physical crisis receded and he was able to engage in a life, though inevitably finite, with less avoidance, less violence, and some real, affirming existence.

Resilience

A Catholic woman in her 80s reported a challenging reproductive and maternal history. She and her husband had eight pregnancies; two miscarried near term and six full-term babies died in infancy or early childhood of the same undiagnosed apparently genetic progressive condition. Some years before war broke out in her country the couple adopted an adolescent boy and, for a while, raised him. He was just beginning to manage the farm, despite his young age, when the war took her husband. Throughout this life of loss on loss, this woman was surrounded by a community of loving and supportive people, and her marriage was similarly so. Her relationship with the adopted son was deeply touching. Her dying was peaceful, with blessings expressed for each of her deceased children, her husband, her adopted son who inherited the farm, and what remained of the community. While she did not have psychotherapy she benefited from a many-layered holding environment. This is a form of extensive existential awakening and maturation that provided some resilient protection against repeated extremely harsh loss.

Future Directions

This chapter sets out a perspective on human struggles with mortality from a noncontroversial psychodynamic perspective; descriptions and clinical observations are shaped by extensive literature, research, and practice experience of psychodynamic clinicians.[19] However, something distinctive also emerges out of this application of settled psychodynamic understanding to this population: namely, a way to understand how people manage harsh mortality realities. This way of managing is an issue-specific process of growth, evolution, and perhaps maturation that elsewhere has been termed "existential maturity." Used elsewhere to describe phenomenologically what it is and how people find their way toward it,[20] this chapter describes the psychodynamic construct that offers more "psychophysiology." This above-described construct to describe how humans cope with mortality suggests some possible directions for future clinical inquiry.

Applications to Suicidality

Suicidality is far from a uniform condition, and its complex features are treated elsewhere, including in other chapters of this volume (Chapters 7 and 9). Its relevance to processes of existential maturation is the only aspect we consider now.

One of the barriers to existential maturation is profound suffering related to psychic deadness. Finding the source and understanding the nature of that psychic deadness is hard because deadness is such a powerful defense, masquerading as it does as "not there." Because the pain is powerful, an equally strong defensive "not-here anesthetic" is required. Probably the suffering is both unrepresented and as severe as it gets in existential matters.

Indescribable, by definition, people point to it with words of horror and represent it in dreams of incessant dying. Whether we think of this as psychic deadness, death anxiety or something else is less important than understanding that, for those individuals wracked by this kind of suffering, actual death is regarded as relief from it. This generates a type of suicidality that may be approachable through seeking to engage processes of existential maturation.

The safe holding environment focused on exploring mortality seems well suited to finding a person's psychic deadness. For many, psychic deadness is stumbled across. The analyst must be alert to such unexpected encounters, and indeed alert to the therapist's own difficulties that make for complicit deadness. If the analyst can find and then join the patient in that place of abandonment and suffering, witness it, name it, acknowledge its nature, and then respond with an attunement that shows what was originally missing, it can be mutative.

Applications to Trauma

Like suicidality, trauma is far from a uniform matter; it cannot be treated simply and is largely beyond the scope of this chapter. But with regards to existential maturation, trauma matters. In matters of mortality, trauma delivers an unmanageable dose of death experience. It may be unmanageable due to its nature, amount, duration, and inadequate follow-up processing response. Trauma describes the resulting psychological blockade that makes memories become uncontrollably intrusive rather than fade and relevant reactive affective states remain active in now quite different, inapplicable circumstances. The processing of the death experience is blocked, and the person becomes stuck, reliving the trauma. The process of existential maturation is blocked as well. Indeed, existential maturity is noted above to be a kind of obverse of trauma states. One implication is that it may be possible to use theories of existential maturation to develop approaches to treating trauma in matters related to mortality.

Existentially Mature Societies

Societies that invest in healthy attachment relationships, engage death-related cultural or religious rituals, and include understandings of mortality in education at all levels will likely be existentially mature societies, capable of resilience in the face of mortal challenge. The capacity to create memorials that address community loss and trauma are vital to the healing process. An absence of memorial can increase a sense of isolation and pervasive woundedness. Conversely, the balanced awareness of mortality and inclusion of expressions of it can integrate mental health benefits into institutional structure, health policy, and leadership.

Providers Need to Understand Their Own Existential Maturation to Provide It

Last but not least, we emphasize that providers need to know something about their own existential maturational journey. The burdens of providing dynamic therapy to people in palliative care settings activates mortal awareness that is bidirectional. Existential matura-tion is a process that will evolve for the patient and for the therapist, who will need enough capacity for mourning to help others gain their acceptance of loss. Patients imbibe the therapist's existential maturity through processes of idealization and internalization; these same processes (that also allow a therapy to end successfully) can also intensify grief and loss for the therapist. Dynamic therapists in palliative medicine working with mortality sa-lience all the time are always at risk of overdose.

Therapists are, of course, imperfect humans with unconscious matters that have re-mained unresolved. And work cannot wait until the therapist has attained perfect existen-tial maturity. That is not realistic. Indeed, psychoanalytic founders apparently had their own significant unresolved issues regarding mortality. For this reason, therapists working in this area should have their own therapist or consultant with whom to work on their own existential maturation. An absence of therapist self-exploration in this therapeutic context should sound a warning bell.

Key Points

- Psychodynamic understanding provides a model of how people grapple with and be-come more able to think about and manage mortality. By providing a facilitating en-vironment in which people can explore and oscillate between opposing thoughts and feelings about mortality, they can gain a way of understanding and accepting mortality that assuages fear and more realistically reconciles those positions.
- This process engages a great deal of active grief and mourning, and, for many, barriers to the process that come from attachment problems and/or trauma experiences must be addressed first—something dynamic therapy is well-suited for.
- A dynamic approach can be intense but can be modified to the time and energy available to seriously ill people and their family caregivers. Children can partake in the process in age-appropriate ways.
- Symptoms that reduce as a result of this process include anxiety and depression, guilt and feeling psychically dead, brittle, or relationally unresolved. A less turbulent way to think about mortality that this approach fosters results in a personal sense of cohesion and integration, more realistic conceptions of the future, an ability to contemplate death without becoming overwhelmed or detached from reality, and increased capacity to love unimpeded or enhanced by mortality awareness, more flexible use of defenses against mortality awareness, and more comfortable expressions about and ability to sit with feel-ings about death and dying.
- Psychodynamic care can be integrated with other psychiatric interventions.
- Future directions may include better approaches to suicidality and trauma treatment. Widespread existential maturation could lead to a welcome society-wide maturation. Providers need to understand where they are in their own existential maturation to be able to foster it in others.

References

1. Brody S. *Entering Night Country: Psychoanalytic Reflections on Loss and Resilience.* New York: Routledge; 2016.
2. Freud S. Beyond the pleasure principle. *Psychoanal Hist.*,2015;17(2):151–204.
3. Klein M. On the development of mental functioning. *Int J Psycho-Anal.* 1958;39:84–90.
4. Freud S. Mourning and melancholia. In: Strachey J, eds. *The Standard Edition of the Complete Psychological Works of Sigmund Freud Volume XIV (1914–1916).* London: The Hogarth Press; 1957.
5. Winnicott DW. Fear of breakdown. *Int Rev Psychoanalysis.* 1974; I:103–107.
6. Becker E. *The Denial of Death.* New York: Simon and Schuster; 1973.
7. Freud S. Thoughts for the times on War and Death. In: Strachey J, eds. *The Standard Edition of the Complete Psychological Works of Sigmund Freud (SE). Volume XIV (1914–1916).* London: The Hogarth Press; 1957.
8. Freud S. Frälein Elisabeth von R, Case Histories from Studies on Hysteria. In: Strachey J, eds. *The Standard Edition of the Complete Psychological Works of Sigmund Freud, Volume II (1893–1895).* London: The Hogarth Press; 1955.
9. Mahler MS. On human symbiosis and the vicissitudes of individuation. *J Am Psychoanal Assoc.*1967;15:740–763.
10. Bowlby J. The nature of the child's tie to his mother. *Int J Psycho-Anal.* 1958;39:350–373.
11. Winnicott DW. The maturational processes and the facilitating environment. *Int Psycho-Anal Lib.* 1965;64:1–276. London: The Hogarth Press and the Institute of Psycho-Analysis.
12. Bion WR. The psycho-analytic study of thinking. *Int J Psycho-Anal.* 1962;43:306–310.
13. Gedo JE, Goldberg A. *Models of the Mind: A Psychoanalytic Theory.* Chicago: University of Chicago Press; 1973.
14. Jackson VA, Jacobsen J, Greer JA, Pirl WF, Temel JS, Back AL. The cultivation of prognostic awareness through the provision of early palliative care in the ambulatory setting: A communication guide. *J Palliat Med* 2013;16:894–900.
15. Kohon G, ed. *The Dead Mother: The Work of Andre Green.* New York: Routledge; 1999.
16. Kris, A. Helping patients by analyzing self criticism. *J Am Psychoanal Assoc.* 1990;38:605–636.
17. McWilliams N, Grenyer BF, Shedler J. Personality in PDM-2: Controversial issues. *Psychoanal Psychol.* 2018;35(3):299–305.
18. Routledge C, Vess M, eds. *Handbook of Terror Management Theory.* Elsevier Academic Press; 2019.
19. Shedler J. The efficacy of psychodynamic psychotherapy. *J Am Psychol.* Feb–Mar 2010;65(2):98–109. doi:10.1037/a0018378. PMID: 20141265
20. Emanuel L, Reddy N, Hauser J, Sonnenfeld SB. "And yet it was a blessing": The case for existential maturity. *J Palliat Med.* 2017;20:318–327.

33

Narrative Medicine

Karen E. Steinhauser and Joseph G. Winger

Stories are a communal currency of humanity.
  —Tahir Shaw
There is no greater agony than bearing an untold story inside you.
  —Maya Angelou

Introduction

Stories serve as fundamental human currency, and, as such, they allow us to exchange contexts, causes, and consequences of illness and suffering as well as sources and paths of healing. They are as old as human history, incorporated in healing traditions across cultures and practices. In palliative care, stories hold data informing an understanding of whole-person pain. The capacity to elicit a patient's narrative—including illness understanding, history, hopes, and fears—is a central competency in the service of facilitating medical decision-making, informing a plan of care, and, in short, reducing suffering and increasing quality of life. In this chapter, we discuss the tradition of narrative medicine and its specific relationship to palliative care as both a clinical competency and an intervention for impacting patient, family caregiver, and provider well-being.

Definition and History

"Narrative medicine," as a term, has been in the literature for more than two decades and appears first in core clinical medicine journals in the early 2000s as one of its leaders, Rita Charon, defined narrative approaches to care as medicine that was practiced with the skills of "recognizing, absorbing, interpreting and being moved by stories of illness."[1]

The tradition of recording patient illness narratives is significantly longer, with case study and ethnography serving as standard tools for social scientists and clinicians, particularly nurses, drawing on qualitative methodologies. Arthur Kleinman's seminal work, *The Illness Narratives*, drew on his dual training as an anthropologist and physician to explore the power of patient story in relief of suffering and meaning-making in living with illness.[2]

Narrative medicine is rooted in the traditions of literature, history, anthropology, sociology, philosophy, theology, and the range of disciplines that value knowledge generated by local, particular, told experiences that in the telling reveal a more universal truth. This knowledge paradigm is complementary to the positivistic and "logicoscientific" knowledge, as Charon refers, that seeks objectively verifiable data that serve as foundations for testable propositions.[1] In the positivistic tradition, the particular experience gains value when translated into quantifiable, measurable traits that are one of many such observations within a sample representative and large enough to permit probabilistic estimates. In contrast, narrative knowledge seeks the outlier, the specific, and the local as valid indicators of experiences to be mined for thick descriptive content and explanations. The specific is the portal to the universal.[1]

Narrative knowledge requires a relationship between teller and listener or writer and reader to complete the transmission of knowledge.[1] In this manner, narrative knowledge is rooted in social phenomenology, which acknowledge and explores the ways meaning is *socially* constructed.[3] Meaning is constructed by social institutions and their norms, beliefs, and values and by individuals who interpret them. Individuals perpetually either meaning "make" or meaning "take," or most usually a combination of both. Meaning-taking comes from ingesting the traditions and explanations of a social institution such as a religion. Religions offer answers to questions of the meaning of life, the nature of illness, and the interpretation of death. Individuals interact with those institutions, ingesting part or all of those explanations. In addition, individuals confront events for which either the institutionally prescribed meaning does not exist or is deemed insufficient. In these instances, individuals in the context of family, culture, and other social interactions "make" meaning. Narrative medicine acknowledges these constructed stories and emphasizes their centrality in patient care and healing. For example, Cassell and Byock wrote extensively about the meaning of suffering and illness as created variously by individuals across their life course informed by social institutions such as religious and spiritual communities and familial and cultural affiliations.[4,5] A particular disease may have objective biomedical markers, but the meaning that illness holds for any given patient is constructed over a lifetime of socialization. "Why has this happened to me? Am I being punished? How will my family cope? Am I burden? What happens next?"

Eliciting and understanding that meaning is a necessary competency of skilled palliative care providers. The elicitation of that narrative may come within the clinical encounter. Increasingly, it may happen within programs that encourage patient story-telling and reflective writing. Whether tapped or untapped, the narrative holds power for the patient that is influencing decisions about care, approaches to recovery, and paths for living with illness.

Contexts for Narrative Medicine

When we look at the literature, within medicine, narrative knowledge unfolds in at least several common contexts: (1) between the provider and the patient or caregiver, (2) between the provider and themselves, and (3) between the provider and colleagues. Additionally, we see narrative knowledge shared between patient and caregiver and explored individually by patient or caregivers themselves. In short, all who engage in the clinical encounter bring a story and tell and re-tell that story either explicitly or implicitly. It may be shared with another or it may remain within. Competence with regard to navigating that story includes skills to (1) listen to the narrative to gain understanding, (2) listen to the narrative to "bear witness," and (3) listen to the narrative to build relationship.[6,7] These three are sometimes referenced as skills of attention, representation, and affiliation.[8] Charon argues that it is in these capacities that narrative medicine is a container for understanding, trust, and empathy.[1]

The clinician–patient/caregiver relationship is fiduciary, and the clinician is charged with gathering the patient's history, understanding their condition, and, ideally, exploring the meaning of that illness within a patient's personal context. Doing so builds understanding and rapport. However, given this expected professional dynamic, clinician's internal stories of caring for those with illness may fall prey to lack of exploration. Time constraints of busy clinics, pressures of attending, and responsibility for learners and patients in their care do not naturally give space for provider reflection. Recognizing its importance, institutions are incorporating efforts such as Swartz rounds, debriefings, narrative medicine clubs, and reflective writing as a means of applying the same narrative patient competencies to clinicians themselves. In doing so, there is the possibility of gaining understanding of clinician suffering, burnout, and well-being, bearing witness to one another within the profession and building new narratives around what it means to practice medicine.

The Evidence for Narrative Medicine

Within the framework of medicine more broadly, published work on narrative as intervention is most common with the focus on patient or caregiver as participant in that narrative approach. In 2016, a systematic review explored the latest evidence on use of narrative medicine as an intervention to enhance patient and caregiver experience.[6] Authors noted that such systematic reviews can be hampered by the lack of standard terminology within the field. First, finding such studies through literature searches is challenged by nomenclature of the intervention type. For example, some of the best research using narrative approaches, by Pennebaker, is referenced as "emotional self-disclosure."[9] Second, much of the literature is still theoretical or descriptive. Third, there are no standard outcomes used across studies that would permit comparison of settings, dosage, or populations. Of the more than 250 studies identified during the review period (1988–2015), only 10 met criteria for a systematic review.

Five studies used narrative medicine as an assessment or intervention tool. In one study, Cepeda conducted a randomized controlled trial (RCT) with patients with cancer to determine if writing about how cancer affected their lives, three times once a week, influenced pain levels as compared with an attention control (whose participants completed a pain questionnaire) and a true control receiving usual care.[10] While pain intensity did not differ among the three groups, patients with greater levels of emotional disclosure reported higher well-being. This confirms many other studies in emotional disclosure that show that an explanatory mechanism in this narrative technique is the frequency and level of emotion shared.[11] Additionally, statements of insight and causality versus venting without contextual meaning or more neutral statements that lack "meaning-making" elements are linked to changes in outcomes.[10,12]

Emotional Self-Disclosure

Several literature reviews and meta-syntheses of the self-disclosure literature summarize what is known about the efficacy of this narrative tool. A common technique within this method is to introduce reflective writing for participants who have experienced a health event or serious illness. Zhou et al. summarized the RCTs that employed expressive writing for women with breast cancer and found a statistically significant reduction in physical symptoms at up to 3 months following the intervention.[13] A meta-analysis of emotional self-disclosure in those with physical or psychiatric disorders also found improvements in physical health, with less impact on psychological health outcomes.[14] Another study by Houston et al. examined the use of narrative methods via storytelling to improve hypertension, finding improvements sustained for up to 9 months following the storytelling intervention among those with uncontrolled blood pressure (as reported by Fioretti).[6] Finally, a meta-analysis of 146 RCTs of emotional self-disclosure suggested the technique is effective, with an average effect size of .075.[15] Studies with higher doses (at least three sessions), increased spacing (at least weekly) between sessions, greater length (15 minutes), and with follow-up within the month had greater efficacy. Additionally, these studies conducted among populations experiencing current psychological or physical symptoms had strongest effect sizes.

While the emotional disclosure literature has been well-refined with regard to identifying best practices for study design, dosage, and potential mechanisms of effectiveness, the more broadly named narrative medicine literature is less well defined or mature with regard to standardized approaches. This may be in part because of the stance of an approach outside of the positivistic tradition of quantitative assessment. Second, narrative medicine is used more frequently as an approach to assessment or reflection and is less frequently subjected to randomized control design or more formal research designs.

Review of Palliative Care and Narrative Medicine

In palliative care, there have been several studies that employ techniques of emotional self-disclosure, primarily as an intervention tool to address emotional and existential well-being among seriously ill or end-of-life patient populations. Steinhauser et al. conducted an RCT, among patients eligible for hospice care, of the Outlook intervention as compared with an attention control condition.[12] The three sessions were spaced approximately 1 week apart and focused on issues of (1) life review, (2) forgiveness and peace, and (3) lessons learned and legacy. Because the patients were nearing end of life, the intervention was conducted verbally with a social worker rather than in writing, as Pennebaker had originally studied the modality. The attention control arm participants also met with the social worker for the same period of time (45 minutes to 1 hour) and listened to a guided relaxation meditation.

The Outlook intervention paired the techniques of emotional self-disclosure with content derived from previous empirical study of populations with advanced illness and the human development and life course literature demonstrating the benefit of life review.[15] This literature, founded in the work of Robert Butler, acknowledges the developmental tasks of each stage of life, including older adulthood. Older adults, when moving toward growth, cultivate generativity and legacy, often through a process of life review. The alternative to generativity, in the Eriksonian model of psychosocial growth, is stagnation. The Outlook intervention provided opportunities to review life and explore these opposing themes.

Study results demonstrated improvements among Outlook participants as compared with relaxation meditation in anxiety, depression, and preparation for end of life.[12] In a second trial of the intervention among those with earlier stage illness (not hospice eligible), we found no differences between Outlook and relaxation meditation, but both arms improved as compared with true control. The upstream palliative care population of this second study had low rates of baseline depression and anxiety.[16] Self-reports of benefit, generated qualitatively, were evident in both trials. This led the study team to conclude that this emotional self-disclosure intervention may be most useful in palliative care populations experiencing baseline distress. Furthermore, the outcomes being assessed should move beyond anxiety and depression to include aspects of reflection and growth.

Findings from qualitative recordings revealed two other sources of variation in the population that may have impacted the efficacy of the intervention for some. First, the intervention allowed participants to choose the level at which they wanted to discuss difficult times, and, for example, issues that may prompt a desire for forgiveness or experiences that spawned feelings of regret. The work of Pennebaker and the emotional disclosure literature suggests it is the expression of negative emotion that has the most impact on changing mood post intervention.[11] Refining questions to elicit challenges and the potentially difficult emotions that accompany them may improve changes in outcomes. The qualitative transcripts also showed broad variation in participant's capacity to make statements of insight and causality. Both of these are elements of self-expression most linked with changes in outcomes, as demonstrated in the self-disclosure literature. The study team concluded that some participants may benefit from a more active interventionist style that moves beyond reflective listening to include techniques of guiding cognitive reframing and other cognitive behavioral techniques. We present a new hybrid approach to narrative and cognitive behavioral therapy (CBT) in the "Future Directions" section.

In 2019, Laskow et al. conducted a scoping review of narrative intervention in palliative care as a means of providing a summary of this tool to the field and the depth and breadth of its designs, populations, and impact.[17] As with the state of the science in narrative medicine more broadly, the scholarship in this area applied to palliative care also would benefit from maturing study design, measurement, and outcomes selection.

In their review, they found 34 articles for inclusion. Of those, just under half (16 studies) used randomized control design. The majority of the 24 studies focused on patient or family reflection, 7 on trainee reflection, and 3 on provider communication with patient or family. In general, participants found the interventions acceptable. Many of those study focused primarily at the pilot stage of demonstrating feasibility of acceptability. Frequently, the main outcomes were self-report or single-item measures developed by the investigators. The exception includes work by Chochinov and another investigative team, Aldo et al.[17] Chochinov, in his enormous body of work via dignity therapy also employs tools of emotional self-disclosure by interviewing those with advanced illness about similar themes of generativity (see Chapter 36). Participants reflect on their lives and ultimately create a document—an ethical will to be shared, if desired, with family members. The study, also in the RCT format, compared dignity therapy with supportive counseling and found extensive self-report of benefit in the process, such as increased sense of dignity and how their family saw and appreciated them. There was improved spiritual well-being as compared with supportive counseling. The main outcome of distress did not change pre-post intervention. Both studies used the FACIT-sp as an outcomes measure. The Ando study reported significant effect sizes in the faith and meaning subscales.

The reviewers note some common challenges to narrative interventions in palliative care.[17] First, there is a lack of a gold standard or even common conceptual framework or lexicon. It is difficult to identify the range of studies that may use narrative-style techniques, albeit under a different name. Second, there is a dearth of understanding related to the best validated measures to assess comparable outcomes across studies. Thus, comparison is limited, and identifying evidence base gaps is impeded by the lack of standard assessment. Third, there is a crucial need to identify outcome measures that are most likely influenced by the intervention. For example, a number of studies assess influence on anxiety and depression. These are outcomes that health systems care about. However, many of the studies have been conducted in palliative populations with advanced illness but, on average, low rates of anxiety or depression. Additionally, many narrative medicine studies have weak to no influence on such outcomes, likely because the interventions have causal relationships with other factors such as capacity for reflection, goal setting, and sense of generativity. These are more positive psychology outcomes and linked to completing human developmental tasks, a crucial part of quality palliative care.

The review authors suggest, and we agree, that the focus of new work should be on identifying the particular methods that are best suited to palliative care and the means of objectively assessing those methods. We would add that more work is needed to understand (1) the mechanisms that link narrative methods with improved outcomes, (2) whether the methods' efficacy differs among subpopulations of illness types, and (3) whether the efficacy varies by stage of illness.

Additionally, the field would benefit from focused and rigorous study of the use of narrative medicine techniques as a tool for attention to, representation of, and affiliation among provider's experiences of care in the setting of life-limiting illness. Narrative medicine increasingly appears in medical school curricula, interest groups, or residency program special projects but has yet to be a standard approach in clinician training or longer term programming in career development. The literature includes examples of how such programs work, but only a handful of studies are subjected to empirical evaluation of the benefits of the program and potential mechanisms linking narrative and reflective techniques to changes in well-being. Two of the seven studies Laslow et al. describe in their scoping review covered provider reflection.[17] In one study by MacPherson, nurses were paired with one another to recount and listen to one another's narratives of grief and loss in the setting of pediatric oncology. The study showed the narrative technique influenced the capacity of sense-making but did not change outcomes of grief or loss. In a second study, the involved providers recorded a thought a day and debriefed those thoughts as a group. Participants reported valuing time for reflection and team building. Of note, narrative reflection as a tool for professional formation is a usual technique in chaplaincy training. Termed "verbatims," chaplains in training report interactions with patients and their own reflections on the interactions' impact on emotions, career, theological formation, and overall professional development as a care team provider. Reviewers posit that the mechanisms found to be operative among patient populations and community populations would be similar for clinicians, and the area represents a great opportunity for future investigation and program development.

Promising New Research

Some promising new work combines the tools of narrative medicine with the behavioral components of CBT. Winger et al. developed a psychosocial intervention called meaning-centered pain coping skills training (MCPC) to address the challenges of coping with pain from advanced cancer while preserving psychological, social, and spiritual well-being. MCPC is based on two efficacious intervention approaches: (1) pain coping skills training[18] for systematic instruction in cognitive behavioral pain management techniques and (2) meaning-centered psychotherapy[19] for enhancing a sense of meaning in life. The intervention's primary goal is to help patients reduce pain interference (i.e., the degree to which pain disrupts daily activities, social interactions, and family life) so that they can connect with life in ways that foster a sense of meaning and peace. This approach aims to enhance patients' confidence in their ability to manage pain through systematic training in cognitive behavioral skills such as activity pacing and guided imagery.[20]

The intervention was delivered by a clinical psychologist using videoconference technology over four, 45- to 60-minute weekly sessions. The trial results were quite promising. The intervention demonstrated exceptional feasibility and acceptability: 90% of participants completed all sessions and 100% rated the intervention's quality as "good" or "excellent." Participants also reported clinically meaningful reductions from baseline to postintervention in pain interference and significant improvement in anxiety symptoms, depressive symptoms, self-efficacy for pain management, and meaning in life and peace. Given the strength of these initial findings, the investigators are currently testing this approach in a larger study using an RCT design. If future studies support its efficacy, this approach could help alleviate suffering in patients facing pain from advanced cancer by using a hybrid intervention deeply rooted in the transmission of narrative knowledge.

Interdisciplinary Fluency and Narrative Medicine

An additional opportunity in narrative medicine within palliative care can be found in partnership with chaplain colleagues. Healthcare chaplains assess patient experiences and spiritual needs through narrative techniques. By eliciting the patient's story of illness, chaplains listen for various domains of need and subsequently formulate a plan of spiritual care. The story may also provide important information that can be shared with the interdisciplinary team to understand beliefs and values that may inform care. The narrative models include Pruyser's early work from a traditional Christian perspective exploring areas of Awareness of the Holy, Providence, Faith, Grace/Gratefulness, Repentance/Repenting, Communion/community, and Vocation. Broadening the focus to a more ecumenical perspective, Fitchett developed a 7 × 7 domain approach that focused on mapping the holistic context of a patient: medical context, psychological state, psychosocial, family system, ethnic and cultural, societal, and spiritual dimensions. Subsequently, the chaplain maps these onto corresponding spiritual needs in their respective order: beliefs and meaning, vocation and obligations, experience and motions, courage and growth, rituals and practice, community, authority, and guidance. Moving to a more spiritual versus religious approach, Susan Lyon's work emphasizes listening for seven domains of Celebration, Power, Rest, Dignity, Freedom, Love, and Meaning.[21] Chaplains listen to patient narratives and identify areas of need and resources in each dimension. While each model offers a differing language and sensitizing construct, the process of narrative assessment and narrative competencies, such as understanding, "bearing witness," and building relationship, are foundational and common across models.

Building on these models for use specific to palliative care, Kastenbaum et al. developed Spiritual Aim, a narrative assessment process that posits core spiritual needs, exhibited by all persons regardless of belief system, are either met or unmet.[16] Those needs include the need for meaning and direction, self-worth and belonging to community, and to love and be loved (termed "reconciliation"). The conceptual model underlying the intervention suggests that, in the time of serious illness, one of the core needs presents most predominantly and influences the individual's subjective experience as they confront the illness.[16] Only in listening to narrative does that chaplain discern patient's needs and resources.

A chaplain may write chart notes, referring to the elements of the narrative models listed above, that can appear as a foreign language to those team members not trained in theological studies and healthcare chaplaincy. However, within this disciplinary divide, there exists an opportunity. Chaplain colleagues may have the time, training, and inclination to bring narrative to the bedside. Partnering with chaplains to become aware of those skills (apart from the theological grounding), study their interventional power through rigorous design and evaluation, and share care responsibilities is an untapped resource for many palliative care teams. A recent article by Perry et al. cross-walks these three chaplain narrative assessment frameworks with existing psychometric and clinical quantitative measures of spirituality. Mapping narrative and quantitative assessments is one such example of interdisciplinary research and clinical opportunities.[21]

Future Directions

Narrative knowledge is a resource for palliative care clinicians. It is a source for generating understanding of experience, rapport, and trust with patients and families, and it is a tool for reflecting on one's own experience of what it means to provide care to those who are seriously ill and dying. The following Key Points come from a synthesis of the existing literature reviews and the chapter authors[6,17] and describe the most pressing needs of the field.

Key Points

- Identify a standard definition of what constitutes narrative methods.
- Identify a conceptual framework linking narrative methods with outcomes.
- Identify core validated outcomes that can be part of the conceptual framework and future studies.
- Conduct trials of patient- and caregiver-focused narrative medicine interventions in palliative care populations representing a variety of illness types and stages.
- Conduct large-scale, rigorously designed trials of narrative interventions in populations of clinicians to test their efficacy as a means of mitigating burnout and deepening professional meaning.
- Conduct large-scale training and evaluation of narrative competencies for palliative care clinicians.

References

1. Charon R. The patient-physician relationship. Narrative medicine: A model for empathy, reflection, profession, and trust. *JAMA*. 2001;286(15):1897–1902.
2. Kleinman A. *The Illness Narratives: Suffering, Healing and the Human Condition*. New York: Basic Books; 1988.
3. Berger P, Luckmann T. *The Social Construction of Reality*. New York: Doubleday; 1967.
4. Byock I. The nature of suffering and the nature of opportunity at the end of life. *Clin Ger Med*. 1996;12(2):237–252.
5. Cassell EJ. The nature of suffering: Physical, psychological, social, and spiritual aspects. *NLN Publ*. 1992(15-2461):1–10.
6. Fioretti C, Mazzocco K, Riva S, Oliveri S, Masiero M, Pravettoni G. Research studies on patients' illness experience using the Narrative Medicine approach: A systematic review. *BMJ Open*. 2016;6(7):e011220.
7. Arntfield SL, Slesar K, Dickson J, Charon R. Narrative medicine as a means of training medical students toward residency competencies. *Patient Educ Counsel*. 2013;91(3):280–286.
8. Vanstone M, Toledo F, Clarke F, Boyle A, Giacomini M, Swinton M, et al. Narrative medicine and death in the ICU: Word clouds as a visual legacy. *BMJ Support Palliat Care*. 2016; bmjspcare-2016-001179.

9. Pennebaker JW, Seagal JD. Forming a story: The health benefits of narrative. *J Clin Psychol.* 1999;55(10):1243–1254.

10. Cepeda MS, Chapman CR, Miranda N, Sanchez R, Rodriguez CH, Restrepo AE, et al. Emotional disclosure through patient narrative may improve pain and well-being: Results of a randomized controlled trial in patients with cancer pain. *J Pain Symptom Manage.* 2008;35(6):623–631.

11. Pennebaker JW, Seagal JD. Forming a story: The health benefits of narrative. *J Clin Psychol.* 1999;55(10):1243–1254.

12. Steinhauser KE, Alexander SC, Byock IR, George LK, Olsen MK, Tulsky JA. Do preparation and life completion discussions improve functioning and quality of life in seriously ill patients? A pilot randomized control trial. *J Palliat Med.* 2008;11(9):1234–1240.

13. Zhou C, Wu Y, An S, Li X. Effect of expressive writing intervention on health outcomes in breast cancer patients: A systematic review and meta-analysis of randomized controlled trials. *PLoS One.* 2015;10(7):e0131802.

14. Frisina PG, Borod JC, Lepore SJ. A meta-analysis of the effects of written emotional disclosure on the health outcomes of clinical populations. *J Nerv Mental Dis.* 2004;192(9):629–634.

15. Fratorolli J. Experimental disclosure and its moderators: A meta-analysis. *Pyschol Bull.* 2006;132(6):823–865.

16. Kestenbaum A, Shields M, James J, Hocker W, Morgan S, Karve S, et al. What impact do chaplains have? A pilot study of spiritual AIM for advanced cancer patients in outpatient palliative care. *J Pain Symptom Manage.* 2017;54(5):707–714.

17. Laskow T, Small L, Wu DS. Narrative interventions in the palliative care setting: A scoping review. *J Pain Symptom Manage.* 2019;58(4):696–706.

18. Kelleher SA, Winger JG, Dorfman CS, Ingle KK, Moskovich AA, Abernethy AP, et al. A behavioral cancer pain intervention: A randomized noninferiority trial comparing in-person to videoconference delivery. *Psychooncology.* 2019;28:1671–1678.

19. Breitbart WS. *Meaning-Centered Psychotherapy in the Cancer Setting: Finding Meaning and Hope in the Face of Suffering* New York: Oxford University Press; 2017.

20. Winger JG, Ramos K, Kelleher SA, Somers TJ, Steinhauser KE, Porter LS, et al. Meaning-centered pain coping skills training: A pilot feasibility trial of a psychosocial pain management intervention for patients with advanced cancer. *J Palliat Med.* 2022;25(1):60–69.

21. Perry KR, King HA, Parker R, Steinhauser KE. Coordinating assessment of spiritual needs: A crosswalk of narrative and psychometric assessment tools used in palliative care. *J Health Care Chaplain.* 2021:1–14.

34

Cognitive Behavioral Therapy in Palliative Care

Meghan McDarby, Kelly Trevino, and Elissa Kozlov

Introduction

The cognitive behavioral therapy (CBT) framework facilitates patient insight into the relationships among cognitions, emotions, and behaviors, as well as how these relationships function to exacerbate or attenuate symptoms of psychopathology. CBT has a robust evidence base for treating many psychological disorders, including depression, generalized anxiety, health anxiety, social anxiety, panic disorder, and obsessive-compulsive disorder.[1] These psychological disorders—and other psychological challenges, including prognostic uncertainty and existential distress—are highly prevalent in patients with serious, life-limiting illness and can be the precipitating reason behind a palliative care referral.[2] Thus, there has been great interest in understanding the potential application of CBT to palliative care.

Until the past decade, questions remained about the feasibility, acceptability, and efficacy of CBT for individuals with life-limiting illnesses, stemming largely from concerns that illness-related physical and functional limitations would create insurmountable obstacles to receiving multisession, structured psychological treatments as they are typically imagined. However, CBT has been successfully incorporated into care for a range of patients with palliative needs, and meta-analytic evidence indicates that CBT is both feasible and acceptable to these patients.[3] Furthermore, data indicate that CBT can effectively treat psychological suffering associated with life-limiting illness for patients[4] and their care partners.[5] Due to this strong evidence, the National Institute of Health and Care Excellence guidelines for best treatment practices recommend CBT for use in palliative and cancer populations.[6]

The goal of this chapter is to offer a comprehensive summary of CBT as it is applied to patients with palliative care needs and to provide a series of structured but adaptable recommendations for implementing a CBT approach in palliative settings. To achieve this goal, we provide background on the theoretical underpinnings of CBT, offer recommendations for providing CBT to patients across the palliative trajectory, and enumerate special considerations for practicing CBT with patients receiving palliative care using illustrative case examples. We also acknowledge the limitations of CBT in palliative care settings and offer recommendations for simple modifications to maximize the utility of CBT with this patient population.

Cognitive Behavioral Therapy: An Overview

The foundational principles of CBT posit that thoughts, feelings, and actions build on one another: beliefs and thoughts affect how a person feels and may shape the behaviors in which they choose to engage. Similarly, actions and behaviors influence how one feels and thinks. Broadly, the target mechanisms of CBT are (a) the ability to challenge maladaptive, biased, or unhelpful thoughts and (b) behavior modification. According to the CBT framework, it is through these primary mechanisms—and the enduring skill sets which develop as a result— that symptom reduction and psychological adjustment occur. The interconnectedness between these primary targets of treatment is depicted in Figure 34.1. The length of traditional CBT treatment varies across patients and disorders, but CBT is flexible in that greater or lesser time can be devoted to covering certain topics as deemed necessary by the patient– provider team, and the CBT approach can be integrated across settings and modalities.

CBT is intended to be a short-term psychotherapy that prioritizes skill development and patient independence. The ultimate goal of CBT treatment is for patients to become equipped with tools and strategies to break the thoughts-feelings-behaviors cycle that leads to psychological distress.

One type of CBT skill helps the patient challenge and reframe negative, maladaptive automatic thoughts, which are often distorted or exaggerated in some way (e.g., "Nobody will want to take care of me once I'm incontinent") and that typically derive from corresponding

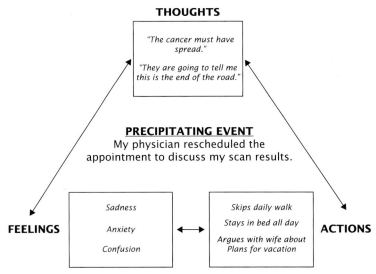

FIGURE 34.1 Example cognitive behavioral therapy (CBT) thought triangle depicting relations among thoughts, feelings, and actions in serious illness.

core beliefs the patient holds about the self as a whole (e.g., "I am undeserving and worth-less"). This process is often referred to as *cognitive restructuring*: it encourages the patient to determine the veracity of a thought after they have considered all evidence that supports or opposes that thought[7] and to establish a less biased thought which accommodates *all* of the information pertaining to the original, distorted thought (see Table 34.1). CBT providers work with patients to identify the range of negative automatic thoughts that they experience in order to understand the underlying core beliefs that have contributed to the development of their distorted, negative thinking. After these thoughts and beliefs are identified, the provider teaches patients to challenge automatic thoughts by re-examining core beliefs, including evidence that supports and refutes those core beliefs. Patients are also encouraged to identify common cognitive distortions like black-and-white thinking, catastrophizing, and mind reading—which reinforce maladaptive patterns of thinking—and to understand how those distortions contribute to thoughts that are unbalanced and biased. Table 34.2 describes some common cognitive distortions and sample distorted beliefs endorsed by patients.

TABLE 34.1 Example cognitive behavioral therapy (CBT) exercise to be used by patients to examine the antecedents of maladaptive thoughts and behavioral and emotional responses to those thoughts.

Situation	Emotions	Automatic Thoughts	Examining Your Thinking	Outcome
Where were you and what was happening at the time?	What emotions did you feel? Rate the intensity of each (0-100%)	What thoughts and/or image went through your mind? Rate your beliefs in each thought (0-100%)	Describe evidence for and against each thought. Identify thinking traps/cognitive distortions and alternative explanations for each thought.	Write your new, reframed thought. Then, re-rate your beliefs in your automatic thoughts (0-100%) and the intensity of your emotions (0-100%)
Walked to the bathroom and couldn't breathe by the time I got there	Scared 100%	My oxygen isn't working 75%	**Evidence:** *For:* No oxygen = death *Against:* I often feel like this after I walk a similar distance	Sometimes it feels like I can't breathe after I walk a short distance, but that's because I have COPD.
	Upset 70%	I'm going to die 90%		People with COPD often get short of breath, but it doesn't mean I will die.
	Fear of dying 90%	I've never been this short of breath– something serious is definitely wrong 90%	I've never died after walking to the bathroom before **Thinking traps/ distortions:** Jumping to conclusions **Alternative Explanations?** Short of breath because I was sitting for the past 2 hours	It makes me anxious to feel short of breath, but I can tolerate my anxiety until my breathing returns to normal– I know it will eventually.

Used http://med.standford.edu/fastlab/research/imapp/wkst.html to develop this figure

TABLE 34.2 Common cognitive distortions, definitions, and examples

Cognitive distortion	Definition	Sample distorted thought
Mind reading	Guessing or jumping to conclusions about what another person is thinking or feeling	My sister wishes that she didn't have to take care of me and that I could just take care of myself.
Black-and-white thinking	"All or nothing" mentality; situations are viewed as extremes, and there is no middle or "gray" area	If I start dialysis, I'll never be able to work again. If I don't start dialysis, I'll be able to maintain my usual schedule.
Catastrophizing	Belief that the worst possible outcome is certain to happen, even if the likelihood of that outcome is low	Getting an ostomy bag will ruin my life: people will be able to see it, and I'll never be able to go out in public.
Fortune-telling	Belief that one knows what will happen in a particular situation	I'll never make it to see my granddaughter if I don't start treatment this week.
Overgeneralization	Attributing an extreme description or interpretation based on a single circumstance or single piece of evidence	I was exhausted today after chemotherapy. I'm always going to be exhausted after chemotherapy.
Should statements	Thoughts and beliefs (private or vocalized) that underscore dismay at not having done something in an ideal way	I should have quit smoking years ago. Then I wouldn't have to use this oxygen machine all the time.

Other CBT skills target behavior. These approaches include *behavioral activation*, a method by which patients strategically incorporate activities that promote feelings of pleasure or a sense of mastery into their daily routine. Behavioral activation involves a preliminary functional behavioral analysis to help the provider gather information about antecedents and consequences of maladaptive behaviors in the patient's life. Providers may request that patients track their daily activities over the course of a week to understand how the patient uses their time on an average day. The provider then uses this information to support the patient in identifying activities that may perpetuate negative symptomatology (e.g., sleeping all day) and that may promote a positive mood (e.g., playing with grandchildren). Patients are asked to brainstorm their own list of activities that have cultivated a positive mood in the past, including pleasurable activities (e.g., taking a bath) and activities that promote a sense of accomplishment or achievement (e.g., sewing). Patients then work with their provider to incorporate a select number of these activities into their daily routine, with modifications as needed to accommodate the patient's physical functioning (e.g., a simple sewing project). The patient schedules specific times to complete each activity and tracks their relative mood before, during, and after completing the activity. Through this process, patients gather evidence about what activities make them feel better or worse, ultimately learning that activities intended to evoke mastery and pleasure generally help to improve mood and break the depressive cycle.

CBT also offers therapeutic strategies that target physiological symptoms. For example, progressive muscle relaxation (PMR)[8] is used to provide the patient with a way to quickly "relax" when symptoms of anxiety become overwhelming. The PMR protocol trains the patient to sequentially tense, then relax, 16 separate muscle groups. Over time, patients reduce the number of muscle groups from 16 to 12, 8, and then 4 to simplify the technique. At the end of the protocol, the patient is theoretically prepared to *relax* in one single step by tensing, then relaxing, the entire body, all at once. This technique is usually offered in combination with other cognitive and behavioral treatment strategies.[9]

Several meta-analyses provide strong evidence for CBT's efficacy in treating mood[10] and anxiety[11] disorders. The evidence that has accumulated in support of CBT is so strong that it is recommended by multiple national organizations as a preferred approach to the treatment of depressive and anxiety disorders.[6,12] CBT includes a combination of cognitive, behavioral, and physiological strategies to manage psychological symptoms, making it a robust, comprehensive treatment approach for individuals with mood, anxiety, sleep, and even psychotic disorders.

CBT and Palliative Care

CBT can be a valuable resource for patients in palliative settings as cognitive distortions and negative self-talk that arise in the context of life-limiting illness directly shape patterns of behaviors and emotions. More importantly, cognitions exacerbate behavioral and emotional challenges that are principally resultant from the underlying disease. In fact, the cognitive model of adjustment to cancer[13] suggests that the ways in which a patient appraises, interprets, and evaluates their disease trajectory shapes their psychological adjustment to the disease course and to their "new normal" of life. A number of factors, including beliefs that a patient holds about their disease trajectory, the patient's general outlook about their disease trajectory, and attitudes toward remaining time left to live, as well as their overall appraisal of what their illness represents, converge to shed light on how a patient is likely to cope with and adjust to the course of their illness. For example, a patient with cancer who has a very positive outlook about their prognosis, believes in treatment effectiveness, and feels confident that they can continue with life as usual in spite of their diagnosis (e.g., working, raising children, living independently) is likely to cope more effectively compared to a demographically similar patient with a negative outlook about the disease trajectory, uncertainty about treatment effectiveness, and loss of hope with regard to maintaining function in everyday life. Patients who persist with a realistic, but hopeful attitude are likely to adjust more successfully.

The CBT framework—with thoughts, feelings, and behaviors shaping one another in a multidirectional fashion—maps directly onto patient experiences across the trajectory of palliative care. Because CBT approaches are firmly rooted in an empirical evidence base but increasingly adaptable across a number of presenting problems and disease trajectories,[14] they are invaluable in palliative care settings. CBT can be incorporated early in the illness trajectory to promote and facilitate coping with worries, fears, and maladaptive thoughts. For example, at the point of diagnosis, a patient with ALS might describe anxiety resulting from prognostic uncertainty. Cognitive approaches might be used in these situations to help patients develop balanced beliefs, as opposed to catastrophizing thoughts, about treatment options, functional decline, and quality of life. Behavioral techniques might also be applied to circumvent anhedonia or amotivation resultant from a poor prognosis, as well as to offer relaxation from physiological symptoms of anxiety. As one example, daily scheduling could be used to ensure that a patient maintains engagement with valued activities as well as with activities central to general well-being, including nutrition, exercise, and personal care.

For patients diagnosed with a terminal disease, CBT interventions can be applied to address fears about treatment efficacy and disease recurrence as well as to support the patient in coping with disease symptoms and treatment side effects. Cognitive work with patients with cancer might also center on prognostic uncertainty and could include practice with identifying and restructuring core beliefs about treatment options and treatment efficacy. In major organ failure (e.g., chronic obstructive pulmonary disease, heart failure), CBT might emphasize skill-building during periods when the patient is faring well in order to support the patient during potential future periods of distress and disruption to daily life, including during hospitalizations. For example, practice with progressive muscle relaxation and breathing exercises can prepare patients to handle periods of high physiological arousal (e.g., episodes of severe respiratory distress). Cognitive exercises, including identifying cognitive distortions ("I'm going to have a panic attack and die if I can't catch my breath") and reframing them ("I might feel anxious when I have trouble breathing, but I'll catch my breath eventually once I sit down"), may also support patients in balancing the truth about their functional status with the reality of their decline. Last, diseases characterized by progressive frailty (e.g., dementia) may also benefit from CBT interventions. Behavioral approaches are useful, especially earlier in the illness trajectory, to maintain a patient's engagement in valued, meaningful activities, thereby reducing the risk of depressive symptoms. In the context of known limited life expectancy, beliefs about the imminence of death may be accurate and therefore not appropriate for cognitive restructuring. Validating these thoughts and emotions, as well as being present with the patient in these moments, is a vital component of any psychotherapy. In addition, CBT techniques can be used to challenge cognitive distortions that are further exacerbating this distress ("I didn't make a difference during my life") and increase engagement in meaningful activities such as important conversations with loved ones. Notably, CBT interventions may also be applicable to caregivers supporting individuals with terminal illnesses and caregivers who are outsourcing care for their loved one. Cognitive approaches especially may help caregivers grapple with feelings of guilt, blame, and responsibility, while behavioral approaches such as increasing engagement in self-care activities and enlisting help from others can support management of caregiver burden and strain.[15]

Specific Issues to Treat with CBT in Palliative Care

Physical Symptoms

CBT is useful in the treatment and management of disease-related symptoms, including shortness of breath and fatigue.[16] The prevalence of these symptoms is high among patients with palliative needs, especially for patients with diseases affecting the cardiopulmonary system. Both behavioral and cognitive strategies, such as aligning activities to patients' energy level and challenging catastrophic thoughts about the impact of physical symptoms on functional status, are useful in managing burdensome symptoms and may be incorporated separately or in combination, on a case-by-case basis.

CBT could also be applied to address complaints about insomnia and difficultly sleeping. In fact, CBT for insomnia (CBT-I) is an evidence-based treatment approach that is specifically designed for patients with insomnia. As part of the CBT-I protocol, providers offer psychoeducation about sleep hygiene to patients and their care partners in order to support best sleep practices. Providers working in palliative settings might also help patients brainstorm ways to be more physically and cognitively engaged throughout the day to prevent napping. Activity scheduling, as well as setting strict wake and sleep times, are core CBT-I strategies used to treat insomnia. CBT-I has robust support for the treatment of insomnia in patients with cancer[17] and other patients with palliative care needs[18] and is considered the gold standard treatment for insomnia.

Pain

CBT can also be applied to support patients in managing illness-related pain.[19] For patients reporting mood dysregulation or anxiety as a result of pain, cognitive restructuring can support those with distorted beliefs about how their pain will shape their daily life ("I'll never be able to attend my daughter's concert with this pain") or about how they should manage their pain more broadly ("I shouldn't take medicine for this pain because I might get addicted to it"). Additionally, behavior-oriented interventions, like a daily schedule, can support patients whose routines would otherwise be disrupted because of concerns about pain. Both types of interventions can stave off depressed mood and offer opportunities for patients to challenge anxious thoughts about the impact of their pain.

Psychological Adjustment to the Disease

Psychological concerns that are inherently rooted in adjustment to serious illness—including overall adjustment to a life-limiting diagnosis, existential distress, prognostic uncertainty, beliefs about the treatment and illness trajectory, coping with treatment, and anticipatory grief—respond to CBT strategies. In fact, these issues may be best addressed using a cognitive behavioral lens that supports the patient's approach to such concerns by reframing beliefs and optimizing behaviors to enact the most meaningful outcomes. For example, management of anxiety surrounding an uncertain prognosis might be approached with relaxation strategies (e.g., PMR), while distorted beliefs about side effects of treatment ("I'm going to feel nauseated all the time after my first round of chemotherapy") could be targeted by developing balanced beliefs and coping statements ("I might feel nauseated *sometimes* after my first chemotherapy treatment, but I have tools that I can use and activities that I can do that will help to take my mind off of the nausea"). In the context of a life-limiting illness, distressing thoughts such as "I'm not going to see my granddaughter get married" may be accurate. Validating these difficult thoughts and the emotions they generate, in addition to being present with the patient during these difficult times, is important in the psychotherapeutic approach. Furthermore, CBT strategies can be applicable even if some distressing thoughts are rational. For example, patients may endorse distress-inducing, maladaptive thoughts such as "after I die, my family will forget about me." Identifying and reframing these thoughts may reduce the distress associated with a poor prognosis. In addition, behavioral strategies can be used to help the patient define how they would like to spend their remaining time and generate a plan for engaging in these meaningful activities.

Preexisting Psychopathology

CBT might be beneficial for a patient with symptoms of psychopathology that preceded disease onset. Lifetime diagnoses of depressive disorders, anxiety or trauma disorders, and sleep disorders may be approached using a CBT lens that addresses preexisting psychopathology and illness context. In fact, these patients with palliative care needs may have a history of treatment with CBT and thus may only require a "refresher course" which they could then apply independently moving forward and across the disease trajectory. Regardless of the extent to which these patients have previously been treated using principles of CBT, strategies including behavioral activation, behavioral modification, and cognitive restructuring can benefit those with preexisting mood and anxiety disorders. In sum, CBT offers approaches and patient-focused skills to support navigating symptoms, psychological challenges, and psychopathology throughout the illness trajectory and across diseases.

Indications for Specific Approaches with Patients in Palliative Settings

CBT is effective in palliative care settings when cognitive-only, behavioral-only, or a combination of cognitive and behavioral approaches are incorporated as part of treatment. Behavioral interventions may be indicated in certain patient populations, for example, among individuals with mild cognitive impairment or cognitive deficits who may have difficulty with the more abstract cognitive restructuring techniques. Behavioral strategies may also be a more straightforward approach to treatment for individuals presenting primarily with anhedonia and amotivation, as the evidence for behavioral approaches alone in treating these symptoms is robust.[20] Such approaches include activity scheduling and basic behavioral experiments (e.g., "How did I feel *before* I listened to music from my wedding compared to *after* I listened to music from my wedding?"). Behavior-focused interventions may also be more attainable when time or number of sessions available is limited. For example, helping the patient create a list of valued activities that can be pursued anytime they are feeling anxious or depressed (e.g., snuggling with a pet, preparing a cup of tea) is an intervention that would be sustainable even without routine therapy appointments.

In other circumstances, cognitive-only approaches may be more strongly indicated. For patients with core beliefs that permeate multiple aspects of their lives, skills targeting maladaptive thinking may be more beneficial. For example, a patient with ALS who feels depressed because they are "a worthless person who is a burden to their children and family" is likely to benefit from cognitive work to identify and restructure distorted cognitions. Such an approach would include dedicated time pinpointing which cognitive distortions are at play (see Table 34.2) and how those distortions shape behaviors and emotions. In the case of the patient with ALS, *mind reading*, or predicting what another person is thinking or feeling, might be identified as the most influential distortion contributing to the patient's depressed mood around their family and their reluctance to participate in family activities. Patients should be encouraged to examine evidence for and against distorted thoughts ("My family has never actually said that I'm a burden," and "My daughter told me she's so happy that I'm around to play with my grandbaby") and to consider alternate beliefs and hypotheses ("Maybe my family is grateful that I'm still around at all since my son mentioned that the other day at dinner").

Finally, many professionals will find that an approach that combines both cognitive and behavioral interventions is the most comprehensive and adaptable, especially for patients in palliative settings whose needs and abilities may vary across the disease trajectory. Importantly, drawing on techniques that are both cognitive and behavioral may provide patients with a wider range of potential skills that can be applied in various circumstances.

Challenges and Special Considerations

Providers will need to account for a number of special considerations when planning to use a cognitive behavioral therapeutic approach in palliative settings. Broadly, reflection upon the ways in which CBT has been successfully modified for patients with palliative needs—including reduced number of total sessions, reduced length of individual sessions, and inclusion of care partners in therapy sessions—may be useful at the onset of treatment. More specifically, providers should integrate their full working knowledge of patient and logistical factors that might shape the treatment approach.

At the patient level, illness-related factors including disease severity, physical limitations, functional limitations, and cognitive limitations should be taken into account before treatment commences. Providers should conduct a thorough intake interview to understand how the patient's condition may shape their ability to engage in treatment and CBT exercises. Other treatment factors, including psychiatric and other medications that may interfere with CBT approaches, should be considered when determining whether CBT is appropriate. To this end, interprofessional communication and teamwork with the patient's other treating providers is essential for care coordination. Finally, the intersection of factors unique to patients at the individual level, including gender, sexuality, religion, culture, social support system, and attitudes toward psychological symptoms, may also inform a provider's approach to CBT in palliative care. For example, patients for whom faith is prominent might benefit from cognitive and behavioral treatment approaches that integrate religion. Cognitive restructuring of distorted beliefs could include information that corresponds to a patient's use of faith to cope with symptoms ("Even though I'm anxious about my scan results, I can't predict for sure what they will say. I can pray for peace—like I have in the past—to help me stay calm when I start to worry too much."). Similarly, behavioral activation strategies for patients with strong religious beliefs could include modified versions of important practices (e.g., watch a service on television every morning).

Similarly, providers should consider attributes of care partners and caregivers that may inform approaches to treatment. For example, understanding the patient's preference for the role of the care partner during therapy (e.g., whether they will be in the room with the patient, whether any of the patient's presenting concerns involve relationships with these individuals) and outside of therapy (e.g., whether they will be involved in supporting the patient with therapy-related assignments) is important, especially for patients with cognitive deficits who could benefit from assistance with CBT-related tasks between therapy sessions. Discussions about the role of care partners are likely to provide more insight about dynamics within the patient's closest relationships, which will also ultimately inform treatment approaches.

Treatment setting can also inform approaches to CBT in palliative care. Tailored approaches may be especially important for inpatients when a number of factors outside of the patient's control could affect the structure of treatment. Such factors include whether there is a private area within which to conduct treatment, whether the patient has regular access to resources that might be used to supplement treatment (e.g., a device that offers access to mHealth apps and other internet-based resources), and how much time will be available to conduct therapy during each session. When working with inpatients, providers should be prepared to deliver abbreviated sessions and offer self-help resources that can be used by the patient independently outside of the therapy session. Although therapy in the outpatient setting may be more structured, with clear goals for treatment followed across a regular schedule and course, providers should still consider how the patient's other symptoms and medical treatment regimen may create barriers to consistent treatment. Because gaps in treatment are possible due to extenuating patient factors (e.g., multiple appointments, etc.), providers may cover topics in such a way that accounts for lapses in treatment and offers opportunities for patients to engage in self-help outside of therapy.

Teletherapy is another way to overcome logistical barriers such as symptom burden, multiple outpatient appointments, and transportation issues. If patients are willing, providers can conduct CBT therapy sessions via telephone or video. There are also several mHealth applications available to help with CBT skills, including mood and activity tracker apps, relaxation apps that include progressive muscle relaxation and meditation, and psychoeducation apps for CBT. Telemedicine offers great potential to extend the role of the provider outside of psychotherapy sessions, when appropriate.

Case Example

Mr. Cross is a 59-year-old Latino man with end-stage renal disease (ESRD). He was diagnosed with type 2 diabetes mellitus at age 45. Mr. Cross reports that his irregular work schedule made it difficult to consistently manage his insulin levels. Shortly after his ESRD diagnosis, Mr. Cross started dialysis thrice weekly. This decision was established as his preferred course of treatment after multiple conversations with his primary care physician and his nephrologist. Mr. Cross understands that his life-expectancy is likely 1 year or less.

After 1 month of dialysis, Mr. Cross expressed concern to his nephrologist that the treatment approach had taken a toll on his quality of life. Mr. Cross missed his younger son's championship lacrosse game, and he was unsure whether he would make it to his granddaughter's baptism because he had "no energy" most days. Following this conversation, Mr. Cross's nephrologist consulted the palliative care team.

During his initial visit with palliative care, Mr. Cross expressed concern about his decision to pursue dialysis. He described fears of becoming a burden to his family throughout his decline and feared that he already was a burden. He shared concern about his wife whose activities and opportunities for work were becoming increasingly limited due to his dialysis schedule. His score on the Beck Depression Inventory was 30, indicating severe depression characterized by difficulty sleeping, decreased appetite, bouts of tearfulness, and passive suicidal ideation. At several points during the conversation with the team, Mr. Cross stated that he felt like he was "waiting to die" and that he lived in fear of being a burden to his family and "wasting their time when they could be doing more important things without me." In addition, Mr. Cross endorsed sadness regarding his limited life expectancy and reported worries that his family would forget about him after he died.

Mr. Cross began work with the palliative care team psychologist immediately; they met once weekly during dialysis. Given the psychologist's understanding of Mr. Cross's high functional status, she opted to incorporate both cognitive and behavioral strategies in their work together. However, because Mr. Cross's negative beliefs about his condition were evidently the primary factor precluding him from engaging in valued activities, the psychologist worked to help him challenge these distorted thoughts first. She focused on his core beliefs about (a) his disease state, (b) being a burden on his family, and (c) deciding to pursue dialysis. She took time to understand Mr. Cross's core beliefs about himself and his disease ("I am a burden to my family," "My family would be able to do more things if I weren't here; Dialysis is ruining my wife's life and her future") and asked Mr. Cross to carefully consider the truthfulness of and evidence for these beliefs over several sessions. Mr. Cross identified which distortions characterized his cognitions (fortune telling, catastrophizing, mind reading) and worked to restructure those beliefs after fully weighing all of the evidence ("Sometimes I worry that I'm a burden to my family, but they've never told me that, and they always act like they're happy to have me around to do things with them," "I can't read my wife's mind, so I don't know that my condition is ruining her career, and nothing she's ever said to me suggests that I'm ruining her life"). When Mr. Cross endorsed sadness regarding his limited life expectancy, the psychologist validated these feelings and provided time for Mr. Cross to express and experience his sadness and grief. In addition, Mr. Cross was able to challenge his thought that his family would forget him. While he still felt sad about his prognosis, restructuring this belief ("I will always be a part of my family's experiences") reduced his concern about being forgotten.

After Mr. Cross had become skilled at recognizing distorted thoughts and coming up with evidence that supported or refuted them, the psychologist slowly introduced behavioral strategies to increase Mr. Cross's engagement in activities. First, she conducted a functional behavior analysis to develop a clearer picture of (a) how Mr. Cross's overall behavior had changed since the start of dialysis, (b) what activities Mr. Cross engaged in on an average day, and (c) how engagement with different activities seemed to affect Mr. Cross's overall well-being. This behavior analysis focused on activities Mr. Cross found particularly meaningful and important to engage in over his remaining time. The psychologist learned that Mr. Cross had discontinued nearly all activities that he had previously enjoyed (e.g., short walks with his wife, babysitting his granddaughter, attending his son's lacrosse games) and that, on an average day, he spent most of the day sleeping or watching TV. In response, the psychologist provided psychoeducation about the reinforcement value of pleasurable activities. She asked Mr. Cross to track his daily activities and reflect on his mood state before and after completing each activity. The psychologist and Mr. Cross worked together to establish a "short list" of activities that Mr. Cross could incorporate into his schedule. He started with abbreviated activities like FaceTiming with his granddaughter for 15 minutes, sitting outside in his backyard, and going for a drive around the neighborhood. After realizing that he felt good after these activities, Mr. Cross was open to trying more "advanced" activities including going over to his son's home to spend time with his grandchild and even attending the semi-final lacrosse game. Over time, Mr. Cross worked to incorporate a manageable number of pleasurable activities back into his schedule, which significantly increased his time spent awake and resulted in his leaving the house significantly more often. Mr. Cross continued to work with the team psychologist on his beliefs about dialysis and his prognosis moving forward, as well as what those things would mean for his family. However, foundational CBT skills created a space within which Mr. Cross could challenge his thoughts independently and modify maladaptive behaviors in real time outside of therapy.

Future Directions

Although the relevance of CBT to patients receiving palliative care is now widely understood, researchers and clinicians continue to investigate the feasibility, acceptability, and efficacy of CBT in palliative care. As the range of illness types treated in palliative settings continues to grow, the need for additional trials to establish the utility of CBT approaches across disease types remains increasingly important. Additionally, as the scope of palliative care as a service grows (e.g., an increase in the provision of outpatient palliative care, palliative care delivered via teletherapy), continued work is needed to demonstrate the validity of CBT for patients with palliative care needs across treatment settings and modalities.

Perhaps most importantly, there is a strong need to train physicians and other palliative care providers in the basic principles of CBT. The majority of inpatient palliative care teams in the United States do not employ a psychologist, and palliative care social workers—who may have training in evidence-based psychological treatments—often fill other roles on palliative care teams and do not have protected time for providing psychological services to patients. Initiatives that promote basic training in CBT for all palliative care providers could be delivered in the form of weekend workshops or professional development seminars and would not only instruct providers on the primary principles of CBT, but would also offer opportunities for providers to practice basic CBT skills in a setting with experienced providers who can provide scaffolding and constructive feedback.

Key Points

- Cognitive behavioral therapy (CBT) is an evidence-based therapy with robust empirical support that is often appropriate for patients receiving palliative care.
- CBT supports patients in developing skills to address symptoms using cognitive, behavioral, and physiological approaches.
- Patients across the palliative care trajectory—from the point of serious illness diagnosis to the very end of life—can benefit from CBT and the skills emphasized in CBT treatment.
- Providers should consider patient-, illness-, and context-specific factors that could shape the way in which CBT is conducted with individual patients.
- CBT is flexible in that it can be modified to accommodate patients with different abilities and resources, and it can be modified across settings.

References

1. Hofmann SG, Asnaani A, Vonk IJ, Sawyer AT, Fang A. The efficacy of cognitive behavioral therapy: A review of meta-analyses. *Cognit Ther Res.* 2012;36(5):427–440.
2. Kozlov E, Phongtankuel V, Prigerson H, Adelman R, Shalev A, Czaja S, et al. Prevalence, severity, and correlates of symptoms of anxiety and depression at the very end of life. *J Pain Symptom Manage.* 2019;58(1):80–85.
3. Greer JA, Traeger L, Bemis H, Solis J, Hendriksen ES, Park ER, et al. A pilot randomized controlled trial of brief cognitive-behavioral therapy for anxiety in patients with terminal cancer. *Oncologist.* 2012;17(10):1337–1345.
4. Fulton JJ, Newins AR, Porter LS, Ramos K. Psychotherapy targeting depression and anxiety for use in palliative care: A meta-analysis. *J Palliat Med.* 2018;21(7):1024–1037.
5. Chi N, Demiris G, Lewis FM, Walker AJ, Langer SL. Behavioral and educational interventions to support family caregivers in end-of-life care: A systematic review. *Am J Hosp Palliat Care,* 2016;33(9):894–908.
6. National Institute for Health and Care Excellence. End of life care for adults. NICE guideline (QS13). 2016. https://www.nice.org.uk/guidance/qs13.
7. Beck JS, Beck AT. *Cognitive Behavior Therapy: Basics and Beyond.* New York: Guilford; 2011.
8. Jacobson E. Progressive muscle relaxation. *J Abnorm Psychol.* 1938;75(1):18–19.
9. Pelekasis P, Matsouka I, Koumarianou A. Progressive muscle relaxation as a supportive intervention for cancer patients undergoing chemotherapy: A systematic review. *Palliat Support Care,* 2017;15(4):465–473.
10. Cuijpers P, Berking M, Andersson G, Quigley L, Kleiboer A, Dobson KS. A meta-analysis of cognitive-behavioural therapy for adult depression, alone and in comparison with other treatments. *Can J Psychiatry.* 2013;58(7):376–385.
11. Hofmann SG, Smits JA. Cognitive-behavioral therapy for adult anxiety disorders: A meta-analysis of randomized placebo-controlled trials. *J Clin Psychiatry.* 2008;69(4):621–632.
12. APA Presidential Task Force on Evidence-Based Practice. Evidence-based practice in psychology. *Am Psychol.* 2006;61(4):271–285.

13. Moorey S, Greer S. A cognitive model of adjustment to cancer. 2nd ed. In: Moorey S, Greer S, eds. *Oxford Guide to CBT for People with Cancer*. Oxford: Oxford University Press; 2011:11–27.

14. Beatty L, Koczwara B, Wade T. Evaluating the efficacy of a self-guided Web-based CBT intervention for reducing cancer-distress: A randomised controlled trial. *Support Care Cancer*. 2016;24(3):1043–1051.

15. Wilz G, Reder M, Meichsner F, Soellner R. The Tele.TAnDem intervention: Telephone-based CBT for family caregivers of people with dementia. *Gerontologist*. 2018;58(2):e118-e129.

16. Hundt NE, Renn BN, Sansgiry S, Petersen NJ, Stanley MA, Kauth MR, et al. Predictors of response to brief CBT in patients with cardiopulmonary conditions. *Health Psychol*, 2018;37(9):866–873.

17. Garland SN, Johnson JA, Savard J, Gehrman P, Perlis M, Carlson L, Campbell T. Sleeping well with cancer: A systematic review of cognitive behavioral therapy for insomnia in cancer patients. *Neuropsychiatr Dis and Treat*. 2014;10:1113–1124.

18. Lebrun C, Gély-Nargeot MC, Rossignol A, Geny C, Bayard S. Efficacy of cognitive behavioral therapy for insomnia comorbid to Parkinson's disease: A focus on psychological and daytime functioning with a single-case design with multiple baselines. *J Clin Psychol*. 2020;76(3):356–376.

19. Knoerl R, Lavoie Smith EM, Weisberg J. Chronic pain and cognitive behavioral therapy: An integrative review. *West J Nurs Res*. 2016;38(5):596–628.

20. Cuijpers P, Van Straten A, Warmerdam L. Behavioral activation treatments of depression: A meta-analysis. *Clin Psychol Rev*. 2007;27(3):318–326.

35

Meaning-Centered Psychotherapy

Allison J. Applebaum, Wendy G. Lichtenthal, Hayley Pessin, and William Breitbart

Introduction

For patients, their loved ones, and caregivers, a diagnosis of an advanced, life-limiting cancer often brings with it a sense of fear and despair. The impact of cancer and its treatment often leads to significant physical limitations and changes in patients' capacity to carry out important roles and activities, which subsequently contributes to a sense of hopelessness and even a desire for hastened death. Such patients may not be suffering from a clinical depression[1] but rather may be confronting an existential crisis of loss of meaning, value, and purpose due their advanced disease. Meaning-centered psychotherapy (MCP) arose from a need to address this specific challenging clinical problem—a problem for which no effective intervention was yet available. Inspired primarily by the works of Viktor Frankl[2] and further informed by the contributions of Irvin Yalom,[3] our research group utilized Frankl's "logotherapy" as the foundation of our approach. We created a brief, manualized intervention centered on the importance of meaning in human existence to help patients with advanced cancer cultivate a sense of meaning and purpose in their lives, even in the face of death. MCP is based heavily on Frankl's concepts of meaning, and incorporates other fundamental existential principles related to the search for, connection with, and creation of meaning. Through a series of didactics and experiential exercises, therapists and patients work together to help patients understand the importance and relevance of sustaining, re-connecting with, and creating meaning in their lives.[4-7] Importantly, they explore how various sources of meaning in patients' lives can serve as *resources* to help patients cope with and diminish feelings of despair that emerge at particularly challenging times.

The Importance of Meaning and Spiritual Well-Being

The provision of psychiatric, psychosocial, existential, and spiritual care is critical to the provision of high-quality, comprehensive end-of-life care.[8] In this context, our conceptualization of spirituality is aligned with the definition offered by the Consensus Conference on Improving Spiritual Care as a Dimension of Palliative Care, which described it as "the aspect of humanity that refers to the way individuals seek and express meaning and purpose and the way they experience their connectedness to the moment, to self, to others, to nature, and to the significant or sacred."[8] There is growing evidence that spirituality plays an important role for patients coping with cancer, particularly at the end of life. Our research group has demonstrated a central role for spiritual well-being, one that includes a sustained sense of meaning, as a buffering agent that protects against depression, hopelessness, and desire for hastened death among terminally ill cancer patients.[1] For example, patients who are able to maintain a sense of meaning report higher satisfaction with their quality of life and tolerate severe physical symptoms better than those reporting lower levels of meaning.[9]

Given the significant impact of spiritual well-being on psychosocial outcomes in advanced cancer, it is unsurprising that cancer patients report needs related to meaning, spirituality, and hope as among the most important aspects of end-of-life care. In a study of the psychosocial needs of 248 patients with cancer, 51% reported that they needed help overcoming fears, 41% needed help finding hope, 40% needed help finding meaning in life, 43% needed help finding peace of mind, and 39% needed help finding spiritual resources.[10] As such, addressing such spiritual and existential concerns is critical to quality end-of-life care.

Theoretical Framework

Frankl highlighted the spiritual component of the human experience and underscored the central importance of meaning. He conceptualized the will to find meaning as a driving force or instinct in human psychology. The understanding that humans are driven to find and cultivate meaning in life is at the core of the theoretical framework of MCP.[4–7] Some of the specific meaning-related concepts that are highlighted in MCP include

1. *Meaning of life*: Life has meaning and never ceases to have meaning, from the very first moment of life, up to our very last breath. While meaning may change in its context, it never ceases to exist. When we feel our lives lack meaning, it is because we have become disconnected from meaning in our lives, not because it no longer exists. This concept is interpreted and expressed in MCP in the following way: *The possibility of creating or experiencing meaning exists throughout life, even up to the last moments of life.*

2. *Will to find meaning*: The desire to find meaning in human existence is a primary motivating force in human behavior. Human beings are creatures who innately search for and create meaning in their lives and are thereby conceptualized as meaning-making creatures.

3. *Freedom of will*: We have the freedom to find meaning in existence and choose our attitude toward suffering. We have the capacity to choose how we respond to limitations, obstacles, losses, and uncertainty. Moreover, we have the responsibility to create

an existence of meaning, direction, and identity. We must respond to the fact of our existence and create the "essence" of what makes us human.

4. *Sources of meaning*: Meaning in life has specific and available sources (Box 35.1). The four main sources of meaning in life that are explored in MCP are derived from legacy (meaning exists in a historical context, thus legacy—past, present, and future—is a critical element in sustaining or enhancing meaning), attitude (the attitude one takes toward suffering and existential problems), creativity (work, deeds, dedication to causes), and experiences (connection through love, beauty, humor).

Drawing from these principles, MCP seeks to enhance patients' sense of personal meaning by helping them to reflect on, understand, and use various sources of meaning in their lives as resources for coping with challenging times.[4–7] The resulting enhancement in meaning plays a role in improving other psychosocial outcomes, such as quality of life, psychological distress, and despair.[11] As such, meaning is conceptualized as an intermediary outcome and a mediator of change for these other important psychosocial outcomes.

In MCP, we discuss with patients how having a sense that one's life has meaning involves the conviction that one is fulfilling a unique role and purpose in a life that is a gift.[2] It comes with a responsibility to live to one's full potential as a human being; in so doing, one is able to achieve a sense of peace, contentment, or even transcendence through connectedness with something greater than one's self.[2] Faith is differentiated from meaning as it reflects a belief in a higher transcendent power, not necessarily identified as God, and not necessarily through participation in the rituals or beliefs of a specific organized religion.

Although the emphasis of MCP is on meaning and sources of meaning, the psychotherapeutic work is enriched when therapists are well versed in basic conceptual framework

---

BOX 35.1 Sources of Meaning in Meaning-Centered Psychotherapy

Historical: *Legacy given (past), lived (present), and to give (future)*. Examples include our story, our family history, traditions, the history of our name, our accomplishments, and whatever we hope to pass on to others.

Attitudinal: *Encountering life's limitations* by turning personal tragedy into triumph, things we have achieved despite adversity, rising above or transcending difficult circumstances. Examples include achieving an education despite personal/financial challenges, persevering through cancer treatment, grief and loss, etc.

Creative: *Engaging in life* through work, deeds, causes, artistic endeavors, hobbies, etc. Examples include our careers/job, volunteer work, involvement with faith or religious communities, engagement in political and social activism, etc.

Experiential: *Connecting with life* through love, beauty, and humor. Examples include our family, children, loved ones, watching the sunset, gardening, beaches, museums, playing with pets, etc.

and theories of existential philosophy and psychotherapy.[2,3] Existential concepts such as freedom, responsibility, choice, creativity, identity, authenticity, engagement, existential guilt, care, transcendence, transformation, direction, being unto death, being and temporality, and existential isolation are incorporated in the theoretical framework of MCP and are utilized throughout treatment.

Park and Folkman's "meaning-focused coping"[12] is also relevant to the theoretical framework of MCP and can involve re-evaluating an event as positive, enumerating ways in which life changed because of an event, answering the question of *why* an event occurred (or "Why me?"), and stating the extent to which one has "made sense of" or "found meaning" in an event. Frankl[2] also viewed suffering as a catalyst for both the need for meaning and an opportunity for finding it. Therefore, the diagnosis of an incurable illness may be viewed as a crisis in the fullest sense—an experience of distress or even despair that may offer an opportunity for growth and meaning. In the face of a crisis, one may experience a loss of meaning and purpose in life, or one may sustain or even heighten a sense of meaning, purpose, and peace, which can allow one to more positively appraise events and to more profoundly value life. Frankl[2] viewed meaning as a state and believed that individuals can move from feeling demoralized and as if their lives hold no value, to recognizing their personal sense of meaning and purpose. This conceptualization of meaning as a state subject to change helps patients to recognize their agency in constructing meaning and suggests that personal meaning may be a target that is particularly responsive to intervention.

Formats and Existential Themes

MCP is a brief (7 weeks for Individual Meaning-Centered Psychotherapy [IMCP], 8 weeks for Meaning-Centered Group Psychotherapy [MCGP]) intervention that integrates didactics, discussions, and experiential exercises focused on finding and sustaining a sense of meaning in the context of advanced cancer. (See Table 35.1 for an outline of session content, and see Breitbart[4] for additional details.) Through MCP, patients are taught to identify sources of meaning in their lives and to use those most meaningful aspects of their lives as resources for coping. Discussions reinforce the importance of connecting and reconnecting to sources of meaning when patients feel disconnected because of their illness-related concerns. Existential concepts such as freedom, responsibility, authenticity, existential guilt, transcendence, and choice are also highlighted and attended to as they emerge. Throughout each MCP session, while the focus is primarily on how one makes meaning of that suffering and utilizes sources of meaning to cope, therapists support the expression of emotion and validate patients' suffering as it arises.

Humans are creators who construct values, roles, responsibilities, and, ultimately, their lives. Therefore, therapists should incorporate additional existential concepts such as responsibility, transformation, authenticity, and existential guilt, as these often emerge as patients engage in the experiential exercises. Therapists may strive to *detoxify death* by speaking openly about death as the ultimate limitation that causes suffering and for which meaning can be derived through the attitude that one takes toward suffering (e.g.,

TABLE 35.1 Meaning-centered psychotherapy session content

Session	Session title	Content
1	Concepts and Sources of Meaning	Introductions; review of concepts and sources of meaning; *Meaningful Moments* experiential exercise; homework is to read *Man's Search for Meaning* and to reflect on Session 2 experiential exercise
2	Cancer and Meaning	Discussion of sense of identity before and after cancer diagnosis; *Who am I?* experiential exercise; homework is to reflect on Session 3 experiential exercise
3	Historical Sources of Meaning (Past Legacy)	Discussion of life as a legacy that has been given (past); *Historical Sources of Meaning-Past* experiential exercise; homework is to reflect on Session 4 experiential exercise
4	Historical Sources of Meaning (Present and Future Legacy)	Discussion of life as a legacy that one lives (present) and gives (future); *Historical Sources of Meaning-Present and Future* experiential exercise; homework is to share one's story with someone and to reflect on Session 5 experiential exercise
5	Attitudinal Sources of Meaning: Encountering Life's Limitations	Discussion of confronting limitations imposed by cancer, prognosis, and death; *Encountering Life's Limitations* experiential exercise; introduction to Legacy Project; homework is to reflect on Session 6 experiential exercise
6	Creative Sources of Meaning: Engaging in Life Fully	Discussion of creativity, courage, and responsibility; *Creative Sources of Meaning* experiential exercise; homework is to reflect on Session 7 experiential exercise
7	Experiential Sources of Meaning: Connecting with Life	Discussion of experiences as sources of meaning, such as love, nature, art, and humor; *Love, Beauty, & Humor* experiential exercise; homework is to complete Legacy Project for presentation in Session 8
8	Transitions: Reflections, and Hopes for the Future	Review of sources of meaning, as resources, reflections on lessons learned; *Hopes for the Future* experiential exercise; goodbyes

* In individual Meaning-Centered Psychotherapy, which consists of seven sessions, Sessions 3 and 4 are combined into a single session on Historical Sources of Meaning.

transcendence, choice). Therapists may also employ an *existential nudge* to gently challenge the resistance of patients to explore difficult existential realities, such as the ultimate limitation of death or existential guilt.

Administration of Meaning-Centered Group Psychotherapy

In MCGP, each patient shares their responses to the experiential exercises with the group, and the process of experiential learning is reinforced through the comments of the facilitator(s) and patients. Commonalities among patients' responses are highlighted. Therapists should be aware of the "co-creation of meaning" between therapists and patients, as well as between group members. Therapists and participants serve as "witnesses" or repositories of meaning for one another and, as such, become part of a meaningful legacy created by each MCGP participant. MCGP groups have the advantage of patients offering multiple and varied examples of the sources of meaning, enabling members to learn from each other. In addition, therapists are able to reflect on the common existential concerns that are frequently shared by patients with cancer, which can provide patients with a sense of validation.

Attention to the basic tenets of group processes, dynamics, and etiquette remains important in facilitating MCGP groups, and therapists should promote group cohesion and a safe and open atmosphere. While MCGP is not intended to be primarily a supportive group intervention, therapists inevitably provide support as patients share and express emotion.

Administration of Individual Meaning-Centered Psychotherapy

One of the primary challenges in delivering MCGP to patients with advanced cancer is that participants cannot always commit to and regularly attend weekly sessions at a specified day and time. As a one-on-one intervention, IMCP addresses this issue by affording more flexibility in the delivery of the meaning-centered work. The individual format also allows therapists to delve more deeply into the patient's past and personal goals. However, since there is more time and space in the session, it is easier to get "off track," and so therapists should be mindful of accomplishing each session's goals. It is recommended that patients still attend sessions weekly or bi-weekly if feasible.

Psychoeducation Through Didactics and Experiential Exercises

In many ways, MCP is a psychoeducational intervention. Therapists teach patients about concepts of meaning and their applications as one faces a terminal illness, and each session includes didactic portions focused on specific meaning-centered topics followed by an experiential exercise that is designed to facilitate learning of these abstract concepts through patients' own emotional experiences. Through exploration, these sources of meaning (see Box 35.1) ultimately become resources for patients as they cope with advanced cancer. Throughout, therapists emphasize flexibility in drawing on sources of meaning, as certain sources of meaning may become unavailable due to disease progression and other sources may become more pertinent to the patient over time. Importantly, therapists support *moving from ways of doing* to *ways of being* to assist patients with recognizing that meaning can be derived in more passive ways. Therapists also call attention to *meaning shifts* when patients begin to incorporate the vocabulary and conceptual framework of meaning into the material they share.

While there is a logical progression to the presentation of content as sessions unfold, therapists are encouraged to deliver MCP flexibly. It is ideal for patients to attend all sessions in their specified order to theoretically obtain the optimal response. However, if all the material designated for a specific session is not completed, discussion and exercises can be carried over to the subsequent session.

Empirical Support for Meaning-Centered Psychotherapy

Research on interventions focusing on existential or spiritual issues, particularly in patients with advanced cancer, was limited before the development of MCP. Thus, we conducted several large-scale trials of MCP, focusing on advanced cancer patients with stage III or IV solid tumor cancers. We also focused on patients with elevated distress as indicated by a score of 4 or higher on the Distress Thermometer from the National Comprehensive Cancer Network (NCCN) Clinical Practice Guidelines in Oncology[13]—particularly if issues involved emotional problems and spiritual/religious concerns. In these trials, we excluded patients with significant physical, psychiatric, or cognitive limitations sufficient to preclude participation in outpatient psychotherapy as they are not ideal candidates for this intervention.

An initial trial compared eight sessions of either MCGP or a standardized supportive group psychotherapy (SGP).[6] A total of 90 patients with advanced cancer were randomized, and 55 patients completed one of the eight-session interventions.[6] Thirty-eight patients completed a follow-up assessment 2 months later, with attrition due largely to patient death or physical deterioration. Results demonstrated significantly greater benefits of MCGP as compared to SGP, particularly in enhancing a sense of meaning and spiritual well-being. Notably, improvements in patients who received MCGP appeared even stronger at the 2-month follow-up assessment, while patients who received SGP failed to demonstrate any such improvements, either post-treatment or at follow-up. In a larger randomized controlled trial of MCGP versus SGP in 253 patients with advanced cancer, results similarly demonstrated significantly greater benefits from MCGP as compared to SGP in improvement in depression, hopelessness, desire for hastened death, spiritual well-being, and quality of life.[7]

A separate pilot randomized controlled trial evaluated individually delivered MCP, comparing seven sessions of IMCP to therapeutic massage (TM). Patients with advanced cancer who received IMCP demonstrated significantly greater improvements in spiritual well-being, symptom burden, and symptom-related distress among participants than those who received TM.[5] Importantly, attrition from this study was lower than that reported in the pilot randomized controlled trial of MCGP (43%): of the 120 patients with advanced cancer randomly assigned to receive either IMCP or TM, 65% completed the 2-month follow-up assessment.[5] In a second, large-scale randomized controlled trial of IMCP, 321 patients with advanced cancer were randomly assigned to IMCP, supportive psychotherapy, or enhanced usual care. Assessments were conducted before the intervention, mid-treatment (4 weeks), 8 weeks after treatment, and 16 weeks after treatment.[14] When compared to enhanced usual care, patients who received IMCP demonstrated significant improvements in quality of life, sense of meaning, and spiritual well-being and significant reductions in anxiety and desire for hastened death. Furthermore, the effect of IMCP was significantly greater than the effect of supportive psychotherapy for quality of life and sense of meaning. As in our previous studies, the strongest treatment effects for IMCP were observed for measures of sense of meaning, spiritual well-being, and overall quality of life.[14]

Research has consistently demonstrated stronger effects for MCP compared to supportive psychotherapy. To examine the extent to which the effectiveness of MCP is due to its theoretical mechanism of change—improvement in a sense of meaning—a recent analysis of a combined sample from the two randomized controlled trials of MCGP[6,7] explored the extent to which improvement in sense of meaning and peace accounted for improvement in psychosocial outcomes.[11] This study provided strong support for the theoretical foundation underlying MCP as an improved sense of meaning and peace mediated improvement in distress and, specifically, improved quality of life and decreased depression.[11]

Meaning-Centered Psychotherapy Adaptations

While MCP was designed originally for patients with advanced cancer, the approach has broad applicability across a range of patient, caregiver, and family populations. Multiple adaptations of MCP are in development, and several have already demonstrated efficacy in improving the quality of life in various patient populations.

Cancer Survivors

MCP has been adapted for the treatment of cancer survivors,[15-17] who often face significant challenges to their sense of meaning in life as they strive to move forward in life after active cancer treatment concludes. Survivors frequently report feeling "stuck" as they experience a heightened desire to live meaningfully and intentionally but struggle in coping with negative treatment sideeffects and physical changes, fear of cancer recurrence, and losses in physical, social, and occupational domains.[17] van der Spek and colleagues[15,16] adapted MCP and developed MCGP-Cancer Survivors (MCGP-CS). MCGP-CS has demonstrated efficacy in improving personal meaning, psychological well-being, and psychological adjustment to cancer while reducing distress and depressive symptoms among cancer survivors.[15] In collaboration with the American Cancer Society, Lichtenthal et al.[16,17] developed a version of MCGP specifically for breast cancer survivors (MCGP-BCS) and found that distressed breast cancer survivors randomized to receive eight sessions of MCGP-BCS evidenced a greater sense of meaning than those who received eight sessions of a standardized support group.

Cancer Caregivers

Given the universal will to find and sustain meaning in life, the utility of MCP extends beyond the treatment of medically ill populations. One such population for which MCP has been adapted is cancer caregivers, the family members and friends who provide care to patients with cancer and are increasingly playing a critical role on treatment teams, often with minimal training and support.[18] Caregivers face numerous physical, psychological, and existential challenges as a result of their enormous responsibilities. These challenges may be compounded by existential distress, including guilt and powerlessness, which is likely a driving force behind the burden that is so well documented in the caregiving literature.[19] For example, the competing demands of cancer caregiving, other caregiving responsibilities (i.e., childcare), paid employment, and personal life goals have the potential to lead to psychological, spiritual and existential distress. Such distress may lead caregivers to become disconnected from important aspects of their identity, prioritized activities, and relationships and result in an overall sense of meaning and purpose.[18] Such loss of meaning ultimately increases suffering and burden and negatively impacts the quality of care provided to patients. This suffering, however, may exist concurrently with positive emotions, connectedness, and growth and therefore cancer caregiving may be looked on as an opportunity for meaning-making and growth.[20] Through an exploration of the unique experience of providing care for a patient with cancer, including caregivers' previous experiences of illness, loss, and care; the manner in which caregivers respond to limitations of the caregiving role; how providing care for another may serve as a catalyst for improved self-care; and relationship with oneself and the care recipient, caregivers may find great meaning in the caregiving role, which will ultimately improve their quality of life.

MCP-Cancer Caregivers (MCP-C) was therefore developed to help caregivers connect to a sense of meaning and purpose in the caregiving role, mitigate caregiver burden, and improve their overall quality of life. Modeled after MCP for delivery among patients with advanced cancer, in its original format, MCP-C includes seven individually delivered sessions. While the topics and themes are similar to MCP, MCP-C specifically addresses the unique existential challenges of caregiving. For example, in discussions of *legacy* in Session 3, a key focus is on caregivers' previous experiences with or familial examples of caregiving and loss. While most caregivers feel that they did not have a choice in becoming a caregiver, the discussion of *attitude* in Session 4 assists caregivers in recognizing how they are choosing to face current limitations and ways in which such choice can engender a sense of pride in one's caregiving role. In lieu of exploring what a good death would be for caregivers specifically, this session allows for a discussion of advance care planning through exploration of what a good or meaningful death would mean for their loved one and steps caregivers may take to ensure such outcomes. In Session 5, responsibility to the self and self-care is emphasized, and, in addition to the *Legacy Project* introduced in Session 4, caregivers are specifically asked in Session 5 to complete a *Self-Care Project* to facilitate a commitment to self-care. Exploration of the *experiential* source of meaning in Session 6 specifically addresses how connecting to life through the five senses and through experiences of love, beauty, and humor may be used in service of self-care. Together, these sources of meaning are presented as resources to which caregivers may connect throughout—and after—their caregiving journey.

Like patients with cancer, cancer caregivers report barriers to psychosocial service use, including limited time to travel to and from treatment centers, financial constraints, and guilt. As such, supportive services are generally underutilized by caregivers, and telehealth is increasingly relied upon for the delivery of support.[21] Therefore, in addition to delivery of MCP-C in person, we adapted MCP-C for web-based delivery. In lieu of seven individually delivered sessions, this adaptation consists of a series of five self-administered webcasts, each of which includes didactic components, video clips of therapeutic interaction of MCP-C therapists and (trained actors portraying) caregivers demonstrating the MCP-C principles, and a message board where participants post responses to the experiential exercise questions that form the backbone of MCP-C.[22] Results from a randomized controlled trial evaluating the efficacy of web-based MCP-C indicated that, at 3 months follow-up, participants randomized to MCP-C demonstrated significant improvement in meaning and benefit-finding as compared to caregivers randomized to enhanced usual care.[22]

The benefits of MCP-C have also been explored in unique groups of caregivers, such as those of patients with malignant brain tumors like glioblastoma multiforme (GBM). Such caregivers are at risk for existential distress and burden due to the devastating neurologic and oncologic sequelae of these diseases. Personality changes, mood disturbances, and cognitive limitations are ubiquitous in the course of illness and make caregiving particularly challenging. The care needs of patients are complex due to cognitive and language deficits, diminished decision-making abilities, and progressive personality changes. This places tremendous responsibility on caregivers to attend increasingly to activities of daily living and engage in treatment decision-making and advance care planning. Our group is currently evaluating the efficacy of MCP-C delivered to caregivers of patients with GBM, and our preliminary results are promising: caregivers who engage in MCP-C experience clinically meaningful improvements in a sense of meaning and purpose, spiritual well-being, ranxiety, depression, and benefit finding.[23]

Meaning-Centered Grief Therapy

Given the challenges to caregivers' sense of meaning and purpose that can occur following the patient's death, an adaptation of MCP for grieving individuals has also been developed. Efforts to develop meaning-centered grief therapy (MCGT) were initially focused on parents who lost a child to cancer because of the unique struggles they often experience in finding meaning in their child's illness and untimely death and in their lives following their loss.[24,25] It was developed with the input of bereaved parents to enhance its relevance and sensitivity. MCGT is a one-on-one intervention that incorporates the principles of MCP as well as meaning reconstruction and cognitive behavioral approaches to help grievers adaptively find meaning in their loss and enhance their sense of meaning to help them coexist with their grief.[24,25] Over 16 sessions, MCGT systematically explores aspects of meaning commonly challenged by loss, highlighting the choices parents have in how they face their pain, how they tell their and their child's story, and how they connect to sources of meaning in their lives, including their child's legacy.[24] Sources of meaning are used as "lighthouses" to help the grieving parents find their way, offering them a "why" to continue to engage in life despite the profound pain they face. MCGT has demonstrated promise in improving bereaved parents' sense of meaning, connection with their child, and symptoms of prolonged grief, depression, and hopelessness.[24] Efforts to adapt MCGT for other grieving populations are currently under way.

Future Directions

Overall, there is strong support for the efficacy of MCP as a treatment for psychological and existential/spiritual distress among patients with advanced cancer. Both the group and individual formats of MCP are novel and effective interventions for the enhancement of quality of life for patients with advanced cancer at the end of life. Given the importance of spiritual well-being and sense of meaning among patients confronting a terminal illness, the availability of a manualized, empirically supported intervention, such as MCP, has tremendous potential for improving patient quality of life at the end of life.

Given the efficacy of MCP demonstrated in randomized controlled trials, replication studies of MCP are being conducted national and internationally, and several other adaptations of MCP have been developed.[4] MCP has also been adapted in a brief three-session version designed for inpatient palliative care and hospice patients.[4,26] Other applications are being developed for oncology care providers, as well as various for cultural groups, with intervention manual transcreation in several languages.[4] Efforts are now focused on disseminating MCP through workshops and a federally funded multidisciplinary training program that recruits psychosocial care providers worldwide who are interested in learning and implementing MCP in their clinical settings. The goal of the training is to expand the availability of MCP across a broad range of cancer and palliative care settings so that its accessibility to cancer patients is optimized.[27] As the network of MCP providers continues to grow, the goal is to develop a sustainable MCP community of clinicians who can support and learn from each other and continue to build on these effort to enhance meaning and reduce suffering in the lives of those impacted by cancer.

Key Points

- Existential distress and suffering are common among patients with advanced cancer.
- Meaning-centered psychotherapy (MCP) is an existential therapeutic approach that was developed originally to help patients with advanced cancer sustain or enhance a sense of meaning, peace, and purpose in their lives in the face of the challenges and limitations they commonly face.
- MCP focuses on four sources of meaning the historical, attitudinal, creative, and experiential that can become resources for patients as they face the challenges and limitations of their illness.
- The efficacy of MCP has been well-established in trials evaluating the approach delivered in seven individual and eight group sessions.
- MCP has been adapted for delivery among other groups, including cancer survivors, cancer caregivers, and those who have lost a child to cancer.

References

1. Breitbart W, Rosenfeld B, Pessin H, Kaim M, Funesti-Esch J, Galietta M, et al. Depression, hopelessness, and desire for hastened death in terminally ill patients with cancer. *JAMA*. 2000;284:2907–2911.
2. Frankl VE. *Man's Search for Meaning*. Revised ed. New York: Washington Square Press; 1959/1984.
3. Yalom ID. *Existential Psychotherapy*. New York: Basic Books; 1980.
4. Breitbart W. *Meaning-Centered Psychotherapy in the Cancer Setting: Finding Meaning and Hope in the Face of Suffering*. New York: Oxford University Press; 2017.

5. Breitbart W, Poppito S, Rosenfeld B, et al. Pilot randomized controlled trial of individual meaning-centered psychotherapy for patients with advanced cancer. *J Clin Oncol.* 2012;30:1304–1309.

6. Breitbart W, Rosenfeld B, Gibson C, et al. Meaning-centered group psychotherapy for patients with advanced cancer: A pilot randomized controlled trial. *Psychooncology.* 2010;19:21–28.

7. Breitbart W, Rosenfeld B, Pessin H, et al. Meaning-centered group psychotherapy: An effective intervention for improving psychological well-being in patients with advanced cancer. *J Clin Oncol.* 2015;33:749–754.

8. Puchalski C, Ferrell B, Virani R, et al. Improving the quality of spiritual care as a dimension of palliative care: The report of the Consensus Conference. *J Palliat Med.* 2009;12:885–904.

9. Nelson CJ, Rosenfeld B, Breitbart W, et al. Spirituality, religion, and depression in the terminally ill. *Psychosomatics.* 2002;43:213–220.

10. Moadel A, Morgan C, Fatone A, et al. Seeking meaning and hope: Self-reported spiritual and existential needs among an ethnically-diverse cancer patient population. *Psychooncology.* 1999;8:378–385.

11. Rosenfeld B, Cham H, Pessin H, et al. Why is meaning-centered group psychotherapy (MCGP) effective? Enhanced sense of meaning as the mechanism of change for advanced cancer patients. *Psychooncology.* 2018;27:654–660.

12. Park CL, Folkman S. Meaning in the context of stress and coping. *Rev Gen Psychol.* 1997;1:115–144.

13. NCCN. Distress management. Clinical practice guidelines. *J Natl Compr Canc Netw.* 2003;1:344–374.

14. Breitbart W, Pessin H, Rosenfeld B, et al. Individual meaning-centered psychotherapy for the treatment of psychological and existential distress: A randomized controlled trial in patients with advanced cancer. *Cancer.* 2018;124(15):3231–3239.

15. van der Spek N, Vos J, van Uden-Kraan CF, et al. Efficacy of meaning-centered group psychotherapy for cancer survivors: A randomized controlled trial. *Psychol Med.* 2017;47:1990–2001.

16. van der Spek N, Lichtenthal WG, Holtmaat K, et al. Meaning-centered group psychotherapy for cancer survivors. In: Breitbart W, Butow P, et al., eds. *Psychooncology.* New York: Oxford University Press; 2021: 521–527.

17. Lichtenthal WG, Roberts KE, Jankauskaite G, et al. Meaning-centered group psychotherapy for breast cancer survivors. In: Breitbart WS, ed. *Meaning-Centered Psychotherapy in the Cancer Setting.* New York: Oxford University Press; 2017:54–66.

18. Applebaum AJ, Kulikowski JR, Breitbart W. Meaning-centered psychotherapy for cancer caregivers (MCP-C): Rationale and overview. *Palliat Support Care.* 2015;13:1631–1641.

19. Jadalla A, Ginex P, Coleman M, et al. Family caregiver strain and burden: A systematic review of evidence-based interventions when caring for patients with cancer. *Clin J Oncol Nurs.* 2020;24:31–50.

20. Folkman S, Chesney MA, Christopher-Richards A. Stress and coping in caregiving partners of men with AIDS. *Psychiatr Clin North Am.* 1994;17:35–53.

21. Dionne-Odom JN, Lyons KD, Akyar I, et al. Coaching family caregivers to become better problem solvers when caring for persons with advanced cancer. *J Soc Work End Life Palliat Care.* 2016;12:63–81.

22. Applebaum AJ, Buda KL, Schofield E, et al. Exploring the cancer caregiver's journey through web-based Meaning-Centered Psychotherapy. *Psychooncology.* 2018;27:847–856.

23. Applebaum AJ, Haque N, Baser R, et al. *Improving Palliative Care of Caregivers of Patients with Glioblastoma Multiforme.* Paper presented at Kathleen Foley Palliative Care Retreat and Research Symposium, Jackson Hole, WY; 2019.

24. Lichtenthal WG, Catarozoli C, Masterson M, et al. An open trial of meaning-centered grief therapy: Rationale and preliminary evaluation. *Palliat Support Care.* 2019;17(1):2–12.

25. Lichtenthal WG, Breitbart W. The central role of meaning in adjustment to the loss of a child to cancer: Implications for the development of meaning-centered grief therapy. *Curr Opin Support Palliat Care.* 2015;9:46–51.

26. Rosenfeld B, Saracino R, Tobias K, et al. Adapting meaning-centered psychotherapy for the palliative care setting: Results of a pilot study. *Palliat Med.* 2017;31:140–146.

27. Polacek LC, Reisch S, Saracino RM, et al. Implementation of a meaning-centered psychotherapy training (MCPT) program for oncology clinicians: A qualitative analysis of facilitators and barriers. *Transl Behav Med.* 2021;11:270–275.

36

Dignity Therapy

Tasha Mari Schoppee and Harvey Max Chochinov

Introduction

Amazing strides have been made in the past century in the development of diagnostics, medical interventions, and curative modalities. Despite these advances, patients have not necessarily felt a greater sense of being cared for and valued. "Dignity" has been defined as "the quality or state of being worthy, honored, or esteemed."[1] Research suggests that many patients facing advancing age, debilitation, terminal illness, or end of life do not experience dignity conserving care. Nearly 30 years ago, this author (HMC) and colleagues began exploring the subjective healthcare experiences of patients nearing death. While this research initially focused on more traditional psychiatric topics such as depression, hopelessness, and desire for death, it eventually shifted to studies examining dignity and personhood. The resulting research led to the development of and extensive research on a brief individualized psychotherapy coined "dignity therapy" (DT). In this chapter we lay out the evidentiary pathway that led to the development of DT, report the state of the science of the intervention, and present the treatment process.

The Case for Dignity Therapy

The last decade of the 20th century was in a time when death with dignity had found a place in the literature.[2-5] Often, the notion of dying with dignity has been conflated with ideas about the rights of patients to hasten death by suicide or euthanasia.[6,7] Appreciating dignity toward the end of life requires a perspective that goes beyond considerations of how to control the timing and circumstances of one's hastened death. Studies examining this broader perspective were predated by research examining psychiatric dimensions of palliative care.

Early research by Chochinov and colleagues revealed an association between desire for death and clinical depression.[8] When explored more deeply, among those terminally ill patients who had wishes for death to come soon, only 19% indicated a pervasive desire to die.[9] This same study noted that the pervasive desire to die was transient even within a 2-week period. This underscores the imperative to consider the person holistically to understand the various causes of distress, their impact on desire for death, and how they could be addressed. We also discovered that will to live fluctuated in response to various diverse influences, depending on where patients were along the trajectory toward death. Further research illuminated that hopelessness was more highly correlated with suicidal ideation than was the level of depression in patients with advanced terminal cancer.[10] The study authors recommended the need for additional research regarding the nature of hope and its impact on persons facing the end of life.

These findings led to questions about what might provide stabilizing effects on hopefulness and will to live for patients approaching the end of life. The progression of this research was not simply theoretical, but was also informed and defined by the insights and experiences of patients facing death.[11] This growing body of evidence indicated that psychological and existential distress had a profound impact on how patients approached and perceived their end-of-life journey and suggested important insights for how to mitigate that distress.

In response to this gap and given its prominence in requests for hastened death, Chochinov and colleagues began exploring how dying patients understood dignity. The experiences and perceptions patients shared led to identifying primary categories pertinent to dignity, which included illness-related concerns, dignity-conserving repertoire, and the social dignity inventory.[12] These categories, along with themes and sub-themes that were captured in the Model of Dignity in the Terminally Ill (Figure 36.1), provided a foundation to understand and promote dignity in caring for patients nearing death. The category of illness-related concerns recognized the impact of dependency and symptom distress had on dignity. Dignity-conserving repertoire was the category that described the perspectives and practices that assisted patients to protect and reinforce their sense of dignity. The social dignity inventory was the third emergent dignity category, one that delineated social and relational elements that either enhanced or detracted from sense of dignity.[12]

This evidence-based model of dignity provided a broad framework within which to understand the whole person. Understanding a patient's notion of dignity can guide and shape their care, providers' interactions, and the plan of care while keeping the person at the center. This is in contrast to a medical model in which providers seek to fit the patient into an intervention structure. Dignity looks at the individual's sense of meaning and values, within *all* areas of life, physical, psychological, spiritual, and relational. The themes and subthemes subsumed within the model of dignity provide raw material to explore how *dignity-conserving* **care** might look. Dignity-conserving care is meant to help clinicians attend to patients by guiding them to affirm patient choice, validate personhood, and introduce practices to reinforce sense of dignity.[13] The Dignity Model recognized that every patient has their own story thread, the narrative they use to make sense of life.[14] Very often the patient's thread may be unrecognizable or apt to get lost within the environment of a

MAJOR DIGNITY CATEGORIES, THEMES, AND SUB-THEMES

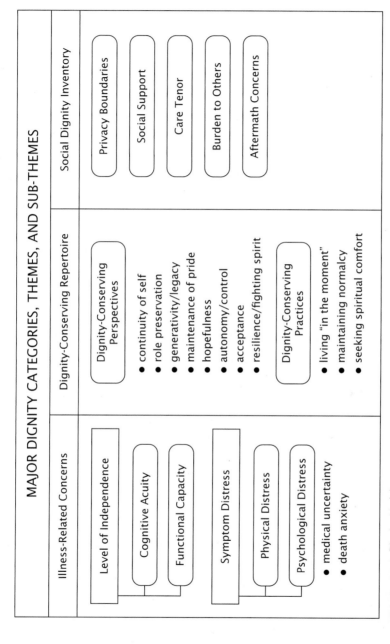

FIGURE 36.1 Dignity Model.

complex medical system. It often requires intentionality to extricate the person from the patient.[14] And this very disentanglement may be necessary to assist the patient to recover their authentic sense of self.

Dignity Therapy as a Psychotherapeutic Intervention

From the empirical Model of Dignity in the Terminally Ill was born DT, which includes a question framework (Box 36.1) intended to guide the patient through an interview that affirms personhood and draws out the individual's own story thread.[13,14] DT allows the patient to express dignity in their own words and reminiscences, with an eye toward the goal of creating a legacy document. The purpose of the questions was not to itemize a rote interview, but to provide a framework that would create the space in which patients could express the thread of their own stories. Within this therapeutic encounter, the therapist supports the patient in pursuit of sharing words of love and hope, offering words of advice or wisdom, and preparing a legacy document to communicate memories and values.[15]

BOX 36.1 Dignity therapy protocol questions

- Tell me a little about your life history, particularly the parts that you either remember most or think are the most important? When did you feel most alive?
- Are there specific things that you would want your family to know about you, and are there particular things you would want them to remember?
- What are the most important roles you have had in life (e.g., family roles, vocational roles, community-service roles)? Why were they so important to you and what do you think you accomplished in those roles?
- What are your most important accomplishments, and what do you feel most proud of?
- Are there particular things that you feel still need to be said to your loved ones or things that you would want to take the time to say once again?
- What are your hopes and dreams for your loved ones?
- What have you learned about life that you would want to pass along to others? What advice or words of guidance would you wish to pass along to your son, daughter, husband, wife, parents, or other(s)?
- Are there words or perhaps even instructions that you would like to offer your family to help prepare them for the future?
- In creating this permanent record, are there other things that you would like included?

State of the Science of Dignity Therapy

DT has been implemented and studied for two decades in 11 countries (Table 36.1). A rich wealth of literature has documented the progression and impact of both the practice and the intervention. The initial populations within which DT was implemented were persons in North America and Australia with cancer and terminal illness.[5,12,16–19] Interest steadily grew, and the application of DT broadened to include other serious, chronic, and progressive diagnoses.

Patients with motor neuron disease and their family caregivers reported high satisfaction with DT.[20,21] The intervention was well-received by people with chronic obstructive pulmonary disease (COPD), and the recipients described improved sense of well-being.[22]

This overarching view of distress is integral to the holistic construct of dignity. DT pays attention to the needs and goals of the whole person, including the physical, psychological, emotional, spiritual, and relational aspects of their lives. DT supports providers in attending to the existential domains of the person that are often forgotten or neglected within the medical arena.[12,13,23] Addressing these existential issues are vital to alleviating suffering as this is the realm wherein sense of meaning and purpose are nurtured or forgotten.[13,18] Patients receiving DT have reported increased sense of meaning and purpose,[15] and an association between higher levels of baseline spiritual[24] stress and greater experience of meaning-making has been reported.[25] Sense of dignity and well-being have been noted to have significant improvement with DT, although there has not been the same improvement noted in areas of depression and anxiety,[26] except where higher base rates of the latter have been reported.[24] Results regarding changes in quality of life have been inconsistent, indicating a need for further research.[26,27] A large study currently under way is looking into this more deeply.[28]

Issues related to family, culture, and living environment are central to a sense of dignity. Evidence has demonstrated that DT is helpful to families in studies from Canada, Australia, the United States, Japan, and Poland.[15,17,29,30] DT and the Chochinov construct of dignity have also been studied in Denmark,[31] Singapore,[32] Mexico,[27] Italy,[33–36] Portugal,[37–40] and Kenya.[41] One Italian study even explored the implementation of DT within a prison: the resulting themes included common human rights the right to work, experience health, pursue education, and to love.[36] Each of these studies has enriched the cultural understanding regarding the construct of dignity.

DT has also been implemented with both young and old persons with positive results. Older people have reported alleviation of psychospiritual distress and beneficial meaning-making.[25] Adolescents reported they believed telling their stories would help their parents to positively impact care.[37] The open nature of DT, inviting the individual to express their own concept of what brings them a sense of worth and value, makes it flexible to apply to people of varying demographic backgrounds.

Whether for the purpose of preparing to introduce DT to a new population or seeking to ensure intervention fidelity, the operationalization of the treatment is of significant importance. One study of older patients with cancer has evaluated early attrition and found that the reasons include death, withdrawal from the study, and loss to follow-up; these

TABLE 36.1 Dignity and dignity therapy literature review

Year Region[a]	Title	Findings (F), Recommendations (R), and Contributions (C[b])
2002	Dignity-conserving care – a new model for palliative care: helping the patient feel valued.[59]	R – The concept of dignity at the end of life should be incorporated into the lexicon of palliative care. Dignity-conserving care should be validated in diverse populations. C – Presentation of a model to help providers incorporate dignity-supporting conversation into care and the first presentation of the Dignity Question Protocol.
2002	Dignity in the Terminally Ill: A Developing Empirical Model.[12]	F – Three major categories emerged in how patients define dignity: illness-related concerns; dignity conserving repertoire; and, social dignity inventory. R – The concept of dignity provides a framework to guide providers, patients and families in considering options and making care plans. C – Dignity Model presented.
2002	Dignity in the terminally ill: A cross-sectional, cohort study.[5]	F – Loss of dignity associated with higher likelihood for psychological and symptom distress R – Preservation of dignity should be goal in care for those approaching death
2004	Dignity and psychotherapeutic considerations in end-of-life care.[57]	R – Good palliative care must move beyond adequate pain and symptom management and must address the needs of the whole person; the construct of dignity should be utilized to guide care. C – Dignity Therapy (DT) term first presented in the literature; rationale and basic premise of DT provided.
2004	Dignity and the Eye of the Beholder[13]	R – Dignity Model can assist care provider to be present and actively listening to the patient in order to understand what comprises dignity for the individual. C – Illumination of question regarding how physically focused care alone can address suffering that is primarily in the existential realm.
2004 Canada	Defining dignity in terminally ill cancer patients: A factor-analytic approach.[16]	F – 213 patients with <6 months to live: 46% reported some/occasional loss of dignity; 7.5% reported loss of dignity as a significant problem. 6 primary factors identified: (1) Pain, (2) Intimate Dependency, (3) Hopelessness/Depression, (4) Informal Support Network, (5) Formal Support Network, and (6) Quality of Life. R – End-of-life care should include treatment of depression, foster hope, and facilitate functional independence. C – Empirical support for Dignity Model.
2005 Canada Australia	Dignity therapy: A novel psychotherapeutic intervention for patients near the end of life.[52]	F – 100 patients. Reported: satisfied w/DT (91%), heightened sense of dignity (76%), increased sense of purpose (68%), heightened sense of meaning (67%), increased will to live (47%), and helpful to family (81%). Measures of suffering showed significant improvement (P = .023) and reduced depressive symptoms (P = .05). R – DT is feasible and effective for end-of-life care; Providers should use every contact to support patients' dignity. C – Full DT treatment first published.

TABLE 36.1 Continued

Year Region[a]	Title	Findings (F), Recommendations (R), and Contributions (C[b])
2005	Interventions to enhance the spiritual aspects of dying.[60]	R – Research to examine constructs of spiritual well-being, transcendence, hope, meaning, and dignity; correlation of these with quality of life, pain control, coping with loss, and acceptance. Also, research regarding personhood, and longitudinal studies. C – Summary of evidence related to spirituality, dying patients, care providers, and caregivers.
2007 Canada	Dignity therapy: family member perspectives.[61]	F – 60 family members of diseased persons who received DT reported: DT was helpful (95%), heightened sense of dignity (78%), heightened sense of purpose (72%), helped patient prepare for death (65%), as important as any other aspect of the patient's care (65%), reduced patient's suffering (43%). Regarding family, members reported that generativity document helped them during time of grief (78%), document would continue to be a source of comfort (77%), and they would recommend DT to others (95%). C – Family members endorse use of DT.
2007	Dignity and the essence of medicine: the A, B, C, and D of dignity-conserving care.[45]	C – ABCD mnemonic of dignity care; framework to remind clinicians and operationalize dignity in patient care.
2008 Canada Australia	The patient dignity inventory: A novel way of measuring dignity-related distress in palliative care.[47]	F – 253 patients. Results: Cronbach's coefficient α for PDI 0.93; test-retest reliability r = 0.85. Four-factor analysis resulted in a five-factor solution: Symptom Distress, Existential Distress, Dependency, Peace of Mind, and Social Support; this accounted for 58% of the overall variance. R – Use of PDI for clinicians to identify areas of distress that may otherwise go unrecognized. C – 25-item Patient Dignity Inventory (PDI) is a valid and reliable measure.
2008	Dignity-based approaches in the care of terminally ill patients.[62]	R – DT is robust model to help direct improvement of care at end-of-life. C – Review of dignity-based approaches.
2009 Canada Australia	The landscape of distress in the terminally ill.[18]	F – 253 patients. Reported the prevalence of dignity-related distress in patients receiving palliative care: An average of 5.74 problems (SD 5.49; range, 0–24). Dimensions: physical, psychological, existential, and spiritual challenges. The existential dimension (sense of meaning and purpose) was associated with lessening distress. R – Further research to focus on aspects of religiosity, including beliefs and practices.
2009	A Phase II randomized controlled trial assessing the feasibility, acceptability and potential effectiveness of dignity therapy for older people in care homes: study protocol.[63]	R – Research is needed to rigorously evaluate treatment to address psychological and spiritual distress for older patients in care home. C – Study protocol for DT in nursing homes.

(continued)

TABLE 36.1   Continued

Year Region[a]	Title	Findings (F), Recommendations (R), and Contributions (C[b])
2009	Assessing the feasibility, acceptability and potential effectiveness of Dignity Therapy for people with advanced cancer referred to a hospital-based palliative care team: Study protocol.[19]	R – Research is needed to rigorously evaluate treatment to address psychological and spiritual distress for patients with advanced cancer. C – Study protocol for DT with people with advanced cancer.
2010	Humility and the practice of medicine: tasting humble pie.[23]	C – Essay addressing the importance of humility in clinical practice.
2010 Canada Australia	Learning from dying patients during their final days: life reflections gleaned from dignity therapy [54]	F – 50 randomly selected DT transcripts. Most common themes were Family, Pleasure, Caring, Sense of Accomplishment, True Friendship, and Rich Experience.
2010 Denmark	Testing the feasibility of the Dignity Therapy interview: Adaptation for the Danish culture.[31]	F – DT perceived by Danish professionals and patients as comprehensive and relevant. R – DT is acceptable and relevant for Danish patients. The authors recommend minor adjustments prior to larger study with this population.
2011 Canada Australia USA	Effect of dignity therapy on distress and end-of-life experience in terminally ill patients: A randomized controlled trial.[29]	F – DT ($n = 108$) and client-centered care ($n = 107$), and standard palliative care ($n = 111$). As compared to client-centered care and standard palliative care, DT reported to be more likely to be helpful ($\chi2 = 35.501$, 2 df; p<0.001), improve quality of life ($\chi2 = 14.520$, 2 df; p<0.001), improve sense of dignity ($\chi2 = 12.655$, 2 df; p = 0.002), be helpful to family ($\chi2 = 33.864$, 2 df; p < 0.001), and change how family sees patient ($\chi2 = 33.811$, 2 df; p < 0.001). R – Future research to explore DT as mitigating factor for depression, desire for death, and suicidality.
2012 Japan	Dignity therapy: preliminary cross-cultural findings regarding implementation among Japanese advanced cancer patients.[17]	F – Preliminary findings: DT useful to improve dignity (67%), beneficial (56%), improved sense of meaning (56%), improved sense of purpose (44%), useful for decreasing suffering (44%), helpful for family (78%), improved sense of well-being (56%), burden (0%), and recommendation for other patients (33%). Higher than usual rate of refusal to participate indicated possible cultural preference not to be aware of impending death; also noted importance to recognize some cultures are use less direct language around death. C – Early report of study to explore feasibility of DT in Japanese population.
2012 Australia	Is dignity therapy feasible to enhance the end of life experience for people with motor neuron disease and their family carers?[20]	F – Study protocol: Study to explore feasibility, acceptability, and potential effectiveness for persons with motor neuron disease and their caregivers. Hopefulness, dignity, and spiritual well-being. R – Report indicates need for research to identify interventions for people with motor neuron disease that will support hopefulness, sense of meaning, and dignity. This article provides a study protocol. C – Study protocol to implement DT with persons with motor neuron disease and their families.

TABLE 36.1 Continued

Year Region[a]	Title	Findings (F), Recommendations (R), and Contributions (C[b])
2012 Canada	Dignity therapy: A feasibility study of elders in long-term care.[64]	F – Providers reported improved perceptions of patients, more knowledge of the patients, and inclination to recommend DT for other patients. R – Results were consistent between non-impaired patients and proxies who spoke on behalf of patients, indicating this area merits future research.
2013 USA	Hospice staff perspectives on Dignity Therapy.[65]	F – 92% of staff believe DT will help patients' families in future; 100% of staff desire to recommend DT R – future studies: contentment; gratitude; connectedness to family; DT ability to enhance staff job satisfaction.
2013 Canada	Health care provider communication: An empirical model of therapeutic effectiveness.[46]	F – 78 psychosocial clinicians across 24 healthcare centers in Canada; 3 primary therapeutic domains emerged: (1) personal growth and self-care, (2) therapeutic approaches, and (3) creation of a safe space. An empirical model comprised of these three domains provides insight regarding communication and psychosocial care of patients. R – Future research is merited regarding how model might inform pedagogy of communication and psychosocial care of patients.
2014 Denmark	A prospective evaluation of Dignity Therapy in advanced cancer patients admitted to palliative care.[66]	F – 80 patients. Test/retest. DT helpful, satisfactory and of help to relatives (73–89%); heightened sense of purpose, dignity, and will to live 47–56%. Substantial subset of advanced cancer patients reported DT relevant and beneficial.
2015 Australia	Dignity therapy for people with motor neuron disease and their family caregivers: A feasibility study.[21]	F – 27 patient and 18 family caregivers. High satisfaction and endorsement was reported by patients with motor neuron disease; generativity was found to be important for this population. Family caregivers reported DT is helpful to them and will continue to provide comfort. R – Research for patients with other neurodegenerative diseases may be of merit.
2015	Care of the human spirit and the role of dignity therapy: A systematic review of dignity therapy research.[15]	F – 17 articles (12 quantitative) reviewed. Patients report high satisfaction with DT, increased sense of meaning and purpose; effects on physical and emotional symptoms were inconsistent. R – Future research: consider spiritual nature of intervention; implantation of DT in real world settings; impact of illness on family. C – Systematic review.
2015 Canada	Eliciting Personhood Within Clinical Practice: Effects on Patients, Families, and Health Care Providers.[15]	F – 126 patients: 99% indicated information was accurate; 93% felt it was important for providers to know. 137 providers: 90% indicated they learned something new; 64% were emotionally impacted by it; 44% their care was impacted. R – Patient Dignity Question (PDQ) is a good tool to begin patient conversations and is an effective way for providers to get a brief insight into the personhood of the patient. C – Evaluation of impact of PDQ.

(continued)

TABLE 36.1 Continued

Year Region[a]	Title	Findings (F), Recommendations (R), and Contributions (C[b])
2016 Canada	Dignity and Distress towards the End of Life across Four Non-Cancer Populations.[48]	F – 404 patients: ALS ($n = 101$), COPD ($n = 100$), ESRD ($n = 101$), and frail aging ($n = 102$). Patient Dignity Inventory (PDI) results indicated no significant different across the four populations, the number of PDI items varied, indicating unique challenges are faced across populations R – PDI can assist providers to assess particular sources of patient distress.
2016	Effects of dignity therapy on terminally ill patients: A systematic review.[67]	F – Review of 10 articles. Studies have reported increased sense of dignity, sense of purpose, and will to live. Results indicate not a close association between DT and depression, anxiety, spirituality, and physical symptoms. R – Further studies needed to increase knowledge of DT. C – Systematic review.
2017	A narrative review of Dignity Therapy Research.[68]	F – 39 articles reviewed. DT is often effective, but may not always be the most appropriate treatment. Careful assessment should be made to determine if DT is the best intervention for a given population/patient. R – Future research needed to evaluate DT for various cultural populations and to compare DT with other EOL psychotherapeutic interventions. C – Narrative review.
2017 Asia	A novel Family Dignity Intervention (FDI) for enhancing and informing holistic palliative care in Asia: study protocol for a randomized controlled trial.[32]	C – Study protocol for application of DT to care of family. With attention to Asian cultural considerations, and building on foundation of DT, this article reports regarding an intervention developed for an interview and legacy document including conversation with both the patient and the caregiver.
2017	Dignity Therapy, a promising intervention in palliative care: A comprehensive systematic literature review.[58]	F – 28 articles reviewed. DT is beneficial, with respect to effectiveness, satisfaction, feasibility, and adaptability to various cultures. However, results were not always consistent between studies, indicating some recommendations for future studies. R – Recommendations for future research to define characteristics of the patients for whom DT is most appropriate. Also, for consideration: exploration of whether patients with high distress can have the most benefit from DT and exploration of the mechanisms of impact for DT. C – Systematic review.
2018 Canada	Development and evaluation of the Dignity Talk question framework for palliative patients and their families: A mixed-methods study.[51]	F – The Dignity Talk questions were tested with 20 patients, 20 family members, and 34 healthcare providers. >70% of patients and family members endorsed the framework. This framework may provide supportive guidance for facilitating end-of-life conversations. R – Additional research is needed. C – Based on concepts of dignity, the Dignity Talk model is explored with regard to its impact.

TABLE 36.1　Continued

Year Region[a]	Title	Findings (F), Recommendations (R), and Contributions (C[b])
2018 Poland	Application of dignity therapy in an advanced cancer patient; wider therapeutic implications.[30]	F – Case review. DT was found effective to support patient's sense of dignity and to facilitate communication within family. R – Merits research to explore impact of DT to support family relationships. C – Exploration of adaptation of DT within Polish hospital.
2018 Canada Australia USA	Dignity Impact as a Primary Outcome Measure for Dignity Therapy.[49]	F – 326 patients. Patients received standard palliative care ($n = 111$), client-centered care ($n = 107$), or DT ($n = 108$). DIS score for patients who received DT (21.4 + 5.0) was higher than for those who received standard palliative care (17.7 + 5.5; t ¼ 5.2, df ¼ 216, $P < .001$) or client-centered care e (17.9 + 4.9; t ¼ 5.2, df ¼ 213, $P < .001$). R – Recommendation DIS be used as primary outcome measure in DT research. C – Presentation of a new outcome measure, the Dignity Impact Scale (DIS).
2018	Effects of Dignity Therapy on Family Members: A Systematic Review.[56]	F – 18 articles. Aim to identify strengths and gaps in DT research related to impact on family. Gaps identified with regard to: feasibility, acceptability, and effects of DT for family members; how family members benefit from receiving legacy document. R – Further research needed to explore impact of DT on family members. C – Systematic review looking at impact on family members.
2019 Poland	Dignity Therapy as an aid to coping for patients with chronic obstructive pulmonary disease (COPD) at their end-of-life stage.[22]	F – 10 patients received DT. Satisfaction 3.9 (on a 5-point Likert scale. Report of improved sense of well-being and is well-received by patients with COPD. R – Further research needed to identify impact of DT to larger COPD population.
2019 USA	Dignity Therapy Led by Nurses or Chaplains for Elderly Cancer Palliative Care Outpatients: Protocol for a Randomized Controlled Trial.[28]	C – Study protocol for rigorous RCT DT study.
2019	Psychotherapy at the End of Life.[43]	R – Optimization of training and dissemination of psychotherapeutic studies merits future study. C – A review of DT and meaning-centered therapy.
2019 Italy	Dignity as wisdom at the end of life: sacrifice as value emerging from a qualitative analysis of generativity documents.[34]	F – 5 DT legacy documents were evaluated. Significant finding of identification of sacrifice as a value. R – The identification of sacrifice as a value could have implications for both end-of-life care and other fields. This merits further exploration.
2019	Effects of dignity therapy on dignity, psychological well-being, and quality of life among palliative care cancer patients: A systematic review and meta-analysis.[26]	F – Review of English and Chinese DT studies. Significant improvement in domains of existential distress and social support, but not in areas of depression and anxiety. Positive impact was reported with regard to dignity, psychological well-being, and quality of life. R – Further studies recommended with regard to psychological well-being and DT within a cultural context. C – Systematic review of English and Chinese DT studies.

(continued)

TABLE 36.1 Continued

Year Region[a]	Title	Findings (F), Recommendations (R), and Contributions (C[b])
2020 Italy	Dignity Therapy Helps Terminally Ill Patients Maintain a Sense of Peace: Early Results of a Randomized Controlled Trial.[69]	F – Decrease in peace over time post intervention for terminally ill people following standard palliative care, but no decrease in peace over time for DT group.
2020 Portugal	Adapting the Portuguese dignity question framework for adolescents: Ages 10-18.[37]	F – 20 adolescents (10–18 years old). Adolescents indicated belief that their participation could provide information to parents and friends and would positively impact their care. R – Recommend this tool be considered in pediatric palliative care. C – Adaptation of Portuguese DT for adolescents.
2020 Portugal	Operationalizing dignity therapy for adolescents.[40]	C – Letter to the Editor (in a palliative journal) to inform providers of the adaptation of DT to a framework applicable for adolescents in Portugal.
2020	Psychotherapeutic Considerations for Patients With Terminal Illness.[70]	R – Research to compare efficacy and feasibility of DT, meaning-centered psychotherapy, acceptance and commitment therapy, and cognitive behavioral therapy is merited. C – Review of psychological, spiritual, existential, and physical factors impacting patients at EOL.
2020 Italy	The Sense of Dignity at the End of Life: Reflections on Lifetime Values through the Family Photo Album.[33]	F – Three main themes: relationship between self and family values, characterization of personal dignity, hope and generativity. R – Study indicates continued use of photograph album metaphor.
2020 Italy	The Value of Dignity in Prison: A Qualitative Study with Life Convicts.[36]	F – Participants highlighted values related to right to work, health, education, and love. Of note was the limitation that audio recordings were not allowable in the setting. R – This topic merits additional research in different prison settings.
2020 Kenya	Randomized control trial of advanced cancer patients at a private hospital in Kenya and the impact of dignity therapy on quality of life.[41]	F – 144 patients (72 received DT; 72 received usual care). The largest effects were improvement of appetite, decreased anxiety, and improved well-being. R – Future studies should include sociodemographic factors.
2021 Italy	Dignity Therapy and the past that matters: Dialogues with older people on values and photos.[35]	F – Feasibility for this approach was confirmed. C – Feasibility exploration with regard to use of photo album metaphor to help older persons process loss of sense of dignity and past trauma.
2021	Quality of Life for Older Cancer Patients: Relation of Psychospiritual Distress to Meaning-Making During Dignity Therapy.[25]	F – Narrative analysis. Greater baseline psychospiritual distress, dignity-related distress ($r = .46$), greater spiritual distress ($r = .44$), and lower quality of life ($r = -.56$), was associated with greater meaning-making for older cancer patients who received DT.
2021 Italy	Meanings Emerging From Dignity Therapy Among Cancer Patients.[53]	F – Three themes emerged: meanings regarding life, illness, and suffering; Thoughts and actions toward self; Thoughts and actions toward others. R – Generativity conversations could support clinicians' communication with patients about existential and meaning issues across continuum of illness.

TABLE 36.1 Continued

Year Region[a]	Title	Findings (F), Recommendations (R), and Contributions (C[b])
2021 Mexico	Dignity therapy in Mexican lung cancer patients with emotional distress: Impact on psychological symptoms and quality of life.[27]	F – 24 patients. Report that DT was helpful, increased meaning and purpose, improved sense of dignity and will to live, and decreased suffering. No changes were noted in quality of life. R – Further research to confirm results. C – First DT study in a Latin American population; suggests effectiveness with Latin American population.
2021	Interim Analysis of Attrition Rates in Palliative Care Study on Dignity Therapy.[42]	F – For the 76 individuals (24% of enrollees), the most common reasons for attrition were death (47%), withdrawal from study (21%), and lost to follow-up (21%). These results will be compared to analysis at the end of the study.
2021	Conserving dignity and facilitating adaptation to dependency with intimate hygiene for people with advanced disease: A qualitative study.[71]	F – Adjustment to dependence is individually mediated; four patterns of adaptation identified related to relationships with caregivers: (1) there is a way of doing and a way of asking, (2) helping each other be at ease, (3) "it's just how it is," (4) achieving and maintaining control. R – Caregivers are central to the care of patients at the end of life and conserving person's dignity.
2021 USA	Description of a Training Protocol to Improve Research Reproducibility for Dignity Therapy, an Interview-Based Intervention.[44]	F – Eight areas of needed support/reinforcement in training for DT therapist trainees were identified. C – Training protocol for DT therapists

[a] The region/country has been noted for any study in which this information was clearly noted.
[b] The authors recognize the valuable contributions of all Findings (F) and Recommendations (R), but the additional Contribution (C) designation is intended to acknowledge those contributions that may not fall into the other categories.

highlight the importance of screening individuals to be sure they are appropriate candidates for participation.[42] The importance of training has also been emphasized in a recent study protocol.[28] A review of DT and meaning-centered therapy made the recommendation for optimization of training and dissemination of psychotherapeutic studies.[43] A recent study has documented a systematized training protocol to support DT reproducibility.[44]

In addition to the many evidentiary contributions and guidelines regarding DT, the program of research regarding dignity and DT has provided a foundation for several concepts and models that are supportive of therapeutic communication. The first of these is the *ABCDs of Dignity Conserving Care*, which delineates the concepts integral to the construct of dignity: Attitude; Behavior; Compassions; and, Dialogue.[45] These components may be described as: "(A) is *attitude* that is subject to self-awareness and self-reflection and their influence on patients' perceptions of care; (B) is *behavior* that is kind, respectful, and attentive; (C) is expressed *compassion* for the suffering and experience of the individual, including strategies to mitigate suffering; and, (D) is *dialogue* that connects with the person beyond the illness or frailty."[44] Also, in support of psychotherapeutic communication was a study in which 78 experienced psychosocial clinicians were queried regarding factors they deemed impactful in alleviating distress; they identified three areas personal growth and self-care, therapeutic approaches, and creation of a safe place—that were vital to understand in the communication with patients experiencing distress.[46]

The Patient Dignity Inventory (PDI) measure is a validated tool that helps clinicians to identify areas of distress that may otherwise go unrecognized.[47] The PDI concepts of dignity were explored with regard to four non-cancer populations, and it was discovered that although the level of distress was not significantly different, the particular causes of dignity-related distress varied, including physical, psychological, and emotional factors.[48] Another measure, the Dignity Impact Score (DIS), is a measure based on selected items from the PDI; it has been recommended as the primary outcome measure for patient dignity in DT research.[49]

To facilitate the weaving of dignity support into communication, the Patient Dignity Question (PDQ) and Dignity Talk were developed. In using the PDQ, the clinician poses the question, "What do I need to know about you as a person to give you the best care possible?"[50] Dignity Talk is a question framework that provides patients and their families a means of enhancing communication between them to affirm personhood and dignity and improve the dignity-supporting nature of all communications.[51]

Additional insights include the recognition that dignity competence and generativity work can open dialogue between providers and patients that goes far beyond the mere medical details that often are the locus of healthcare communication.[12,13,52,53] Knowing and understanding the essence of personhood for each individual enables providers to guide decision-making in a way that meets the highest goals of the patient and family. Staff perspectives have offered insight into the impact that DT and dignity competence have in their patient encounters, stating that they had not only more understanding, but improved perceptions including empathy, connectedness, and respect.[47-49]

Some of the richest and most profound results have been the insights and revelations shared by the patients themselves. Most common themes in life reflections of persons receiving DT have included family, pleasure, caring, sense of accomplishment, friendship, life experiences, and the value of sacrifice.[34,54] Other themes have included relationships with self and others, personal dignity, and generativity.[33]

How Do You Do Dignity Therapy?

Dignity Therapy Intervention

Central to the DT implementation is focus on the dual goals of the intervention: creating an interactive communication within which the individual's dignity is validated and honored and capturing the patient's story thread so that it may be woven into a legacy document, which the individual may choose to give to a significant other. The intervention process flow, which is delineated below (and in Table 36.2), as well as further details of this process, may be found in the book, *Dignity Therapy: Final Words for Final Days*.[55] Details regarding therapist training and operationalization are also available in cited references.[44]

TABLE 36.2 Overview of steps and responsible team member

Step	Team member
Identification of participant	Clinician
Introduction of dignity therapy (DT) to the participant	Dignity therapist
Framing conversation	Dignity therapist
Interview (audio-recorded)	Dignity therapist
Transcription of audio recording	Transcriptionist
Creation of legacy document	Dignity therapist (or editor)
Editing (review of legacy document draft with the individual)	Dignity therapist
Revisions to legacy document	Dignity therapist
Delivery of legacy document to individual (or designee)	Dignity therapist

1. *Identify the participant.* When considering the appropriateness of DT, the clinician should be aware of the individual's level of reflective and prognostic awareness. It is not the role of the dignity therapist to reveal to the individual details of prognosis. As noted previously, DT need not be limited only to those who are facing the end of life, although approaching death does often increase the individual's quality and depth of reflection and existential readiness. Also of note is that it is not necessary that the individual discuss details of approaching death. The focus is always on the patient's story thread, the life experiences that have been most meaningful, and the messages they want to share with significant others.

It is imperative to verify that the individual understands the goal of DT and has an interest in creating a legacy document. Expressed motivation to engage in the creation of a legacy document is a strong indicator toward identifying individuals who are suitable for this brief, individualized psychotherapeutic treatment.

When identifying appropriate participants, there are several factors the clinician must consider to avoid barriers to completion of the intervention. It is vital that the individual, the therapist, and the transcriptionist all speak the same language. Individuals who feel too ill to engage in the interview and those who are not expected to live long enough to complete the full process should not be enrolled in DT; generally, the timeframe is at least 2 weeks, depending on the expediency of the transcription and editing process. Also, individuals who lack the cognitive ability to participate in a reflective and meaningful conversation should be excluded.

2. *Introduction of DT to the participant.* The clinician may communicate to the individual the opportunity to participate in a conversation that will allow them to share some important parts of their story, which can then be gathered into a legacy document that they may share with a significant other. If this individual is interested, the clinician will make a referral to the dignity therapist. The dignity therapist (or a trained designated administrative assistant) will provide greater detail regarding the steps of the process and answer any questions. During this conversation, the therapist will provide a copy of the questions to the individual so they may think about them prior to the interview. Alternatively, if this contact

is by phone, the therapist will obtain an email/mailing address and notify the individual that they will send the Dignity Questions to them.

3. *Framing conversation.* A day or two before the scheduled interview, the therapist should call the individual for a "framing conversation" to review the process and the purpose of DT, as well as to verify that they have a copy of the Dignity Questions. During this conversation, the therapist should seek information to prepare a "frame" for what the interview will look like. This includes identifying the specific goals the participant has for the legacy document. The therapist should ask participants if there are particular messages they want to include in the document for the people in their life. This isn't the time to gather the text of the specific messages, but it is the time for the therapist to be sure they know the participant's reasons for participating. It is recommended that the therapist make some notes during this conversation for reference during the interview. It is important to ask the individual to share the names and relationships of significant others. Some therapists have found it helpful to make a rough family tree to help keep track of the significant people who need to be mentioned and remembered as the document is developed. In other words, the framing interview establishes what the patient hopes to accomplish and who the legacy document is being created for. The therapist should also confirm that the participant has the date and time of the interview, as well as the location and directions (or the link if the interview will be conducted via a secure online platform). If this will be a virtual interview, all technology (virtual link, recording, etc.) should be tested by the therapist prior to the interview.

4. *Interview (audio-recorded).* The interview should last approximately 60 minutes. Roughly the first half of this time will be gathering biographical elements of the story. This is important for two reasons: it gives an overall detailed flow of the person's life, and it also helps the person step back and look at the overall flow so that they are best prepared for the second portion of the interview. The second half will focus on getting to the depth of the story thread via the Dignity Question protocol. These questions are more emotionally evocative, asking about hopes, wishes, or dreams for loved ones and sharing words of wisdom or advice and final messages they wish to impart. During the interview the therapist will guide the participant through the conversation using the Dignity Questions (Box 36.1). The therapist should have a list of the Dignity Questions and any notes made during the framing call. The questions are designed in the spirit of inquiry rather than to mandate an inflexible script for the therapist. The therapist has the responsibility to use the question framework but also be malleable in following the patient's cues, guiding the patient to communicate their own story thread. The question protocol is a tool, a guide to provide structure. Patients are invited to engage regarding the questions with which they identify. If sensitive material is presented, the therapist should explore whether the patient wishes the details to be included in the document. Clarifying questions and techniques to draw out the participant's elaboration are vital to ensure that the intended message is being heard and to mine out the gems within the story, giving it depth and richness.

An example of one especially effective technique that therapists use is that of the "photo album metaphor," which is helpful in assisting patients to become present with their own story thread. This tool is particularly useful in eliciting biographical detail and things they would want remembered. The therapist asks the participant to, "imagine you are showing me a photo album of your life." The individual is asked to look toward the beginning of the album and identify a "picture" that stands out as something they would want to share. When the therapist needs to facilitate moving the story forward, the therapist can ask, "If we think back to the photo album, what would be the next picture you would want to share?" This technique helps the participant to recall meaningful memories and weave them into the thread of the story.

The role of the therapist is to maintain a dignity-affirming stance, always remaining an active listener. Through compassionate engagement the therapist affirms the worth and value of the individual, thus validating the person's dignity. Through attention to the Dignity Question Framework, the therapist ensures that the goal of creating a legacy document remains the focus. This interview is audio-recorded so that it may next be transcribed verbatim. It is important to note that the more focused the therapist is during the interview—keeping the interview on track with the information from the framing conversation, following the question protocol, clarifying information, verifying whether sensitive details should be included—the more streamlined and time-efficient the creation of the legacy document and the editing process will be.

5. *Transcription of audio-recording.* The recording should then be transcribed into a verbatim transcript. This will provide a working copy for the next step—the process in which the legacy document will be developed.

6. *Creation of the legacy document.* Either the therapist or an editor will next work with the verbatim transcript to streamline the words of the interviewer and weave the participant's words into a story. The therapist's voice should only be heard when it provides clarity to the document. Although the order of the statements made by the individual may be shifted to develop a coherent flow, the authentic "voice" of the participant must remain intact. It is imperative that when the participant, and later their significant others, read the document, it "sounds" like the individual. Some editors pull out a fitting phrase or theme from the interview and suggest it as a title for the document.

7. *Editing (review of legacy document draft with the individual).* The therapist will next meet with the patient to review the draft of the legacy document. The document should be read to the patient unless the patient decides to read it themselves. This will give the person a chance to hear and read the story and make any additions or remove any details they do not wish to share. This is also the time for the therapist to discuss what the person would like as the title for their document, such as the suggestion provided by the editor or a quote that is meaningful to the person.

8. *Revisions to legacy document.* The therapist will make any needed revisions to the document. The document will then be printed on nice parchment-type paper with a cover page and placed in a folder or report cover. If the person has elected to receive an electronic copy, the document should be formatted with the cover page.

9. *Delivery of legacy document to individual (or designee).* The document will be delivered to the individual via the previously selected method—hard copy, electronic copy, or both. If the patient is no longer available to receive the document, it should be delivered to whomever they designated (during the initial interview) as an alternate recipient for the document.

Personhood and the Dignity Question

As noted earlier in this chapter, there is enormous risk for people facing serious illness to lose their sense of self and become overwhelmed with the identity of simply being a patient. It is this loss of self that erodes dignity. The demise of hope and engagement in life are often next in line. They become caught in the trap of "patienthood," which sees their sense of self overwhelmed by diagnoses, debility, hospitals, and treatments. They become the proverbial "amputee" or the "renal failure in room 213" or the "COPDer"—personhood becomes overshadowed by patienthood.[23] Helping people reconnect to personhood validates their worth and value. Acknowledging their experiences and accomplishments—recognizing that they are people with interests, passions, areas of expertise and wisdom, that they are spouses, parents, and friends—is a vital pathway leading back toward dignity.

Beyond the specialized DT intervention, the concepts of dignity and personhood may be woven into the usual daily practice of clinicians by use of the simple Dignity Question: "What do I need to know about you as a person to give you the best care possible?"[50] The response can provide the lens to see who the patient really is—not only illness and disability—and this clearer, more complete perspective enables clinicians to work more effectively. The time in life when persons are facing serious illness or end of life is fraught with many challenges, and they need to have access to their greatest strengths—their hopes, their experiences, their wisdom, and their memories. These riches—the wealth of their dignity—will support them as they navigate their way toward the end of life.

Future Directions

In considering the future of DT research, it is imperative that we look to those who are often not seen or heard. People who are incarcerated are often marginalized from dignity-affirming interventions, and DT may have applications for this group.[36] Special attention is needed to evaluate the impact of DT with the pediatric population.[37] It has been recommended that sociodemographic factors be considered in research studies to identify underserved subgroups of many populations (e.g., the poor, racialized, marginalized, disenfranchised).[41] Often the family caregivers are lost in the burdens of care and grief, and it will be important to explore the impact of DT on their functioning and the processing of their grief.[56] To broaden the cultural appropriateness, future research should explore application of DT within diverse cultural context.[26,27] Additionally, it has been recommended that future research compare the efficacy of DT with other psychotherapeutic models[57] and explore mechanisms for the effectiveness of DT.[58]

Key Points

- Dignity has been explored and defined over the past quarter-century.
- Chochinov and colleagues turned to patients to inform their construct of dignity and the concepts comprising dignity.

- The Dignity Model was developed around the empirical concepts of illness-related concerns, dignity-conserving repertoire, and social dignity inventory.
- The Dignity Model was used to inform the DT psychotherapeutic treatment, an interview developed with the dual goals of: creating an interactive communication within which the individual's dignity is validated and honored and capturing their story thread so that it can be woven into a legacy document.
- DT has been implemented and researched in 11 countries, in a variety of inpatient and outpatient environments, over the past two decades.
- Evidence has demonstrated DT to have application across various cultures, ages, and diagnoses; high satisfaction with patients and families; and impact to increase sense of meaning, purpose, and will to live.

References

1. Merriam-Webster. Definition of dignity; 2018. https://www.merriam-webster.com/dictionary/dignity.
2. Abiven M. Dying with dignity. *World Health Forum.* 1991;12:375–381.
3. Pullman D. Dying with dignity and the death of dignity. *Health L J.* 1996;4:197–219.
4. Madan TN. Dying with dignity. *Soc Sci Med.* 1992;35:425–432.
5. Chochinov HM, Hack T, Hassard T, Kristjanson LJ, McClement S, Harlos M. Dignity in the terminally ill: A cross-sectional, cohort study. *Lancet.* 2002;360(9350):2026–2030.
6. Back AL, Wallace JI, Starks HE, Pearlman RA. Physician-assisted suicide and euthanasia in Washington State; Patient requests and physician responses. *JAMA.* 1996;275(12):919–925.
7. Emanuel EJ, Fairclough EL, Daniels ER, Clarridge BR. Euthanasia and physician-assisted suicide: Attitudes and experiences of oncology patients, oncologists, and the public. *Lancet.* 1996;347(9018):1805–1810.
8. Chochinov HM, Wilson KG. The euthanasia debate. *Can J Psychiatry.* 1995;40(10):593–602.
9. Chochinov HM, Wilson KG, Enns M, Mowchun N, Lander S, Levitt M, et al. Desire for death in the terminally ill. *Am J Psychiatry.* 1995;152(9):1185–1191.
10. Chochinov HM, Wilson KG, Enns M, Lander S. Depression, hopelessness, and suicidal ideation in the terminally ill. *Psychosomatics.* 1998;39(4):366–370.
11. Chochinov HM, Tataryn D, Clinch JJ, Dudgeon D. Will to live in the terminally ill. *Lancet.* 1999;354(9181):816–819.
12. Chochinov H, Hack T, McClement S, Kristjanson LJ, Harlos M. Dignity in the terminally ill: Developing empirical model. *Soc Sci Med.* 2002(54):433–443.
13. Chochinov HM. Dignity and the eye of the beholder. *J Clin Oncol.* 2004;22(7):1336–1340.
14. Chochinov HM. The art of medicine: Health-care provider as witness. *Lancet.* 2016;388:1272–1273.
15. Fitchett G, Emanuel L, Handzo G, Boyken L, Wilkie DJ. Care of the human spirit and the role of dignity therapy: A systematic review of dignity therapy research. *BMC Palliative Care.* 2015;14:8.
16. Hack TF, Hassard T, Kristjanson LJ, McClement S, Harlos M. Defining dignity in terminally ill cancer patients: A factor-analytic approach. *Psychooncology.* 2004;13(10):700–708.
17. Akechi T, Akazawa T, Komori Y, Morita T, Otani H, Shinjo T, et al. Dignity therapy: Preliminary cross-cultural findings regarding implementation among Japanese advanced cancer patients. *Palliat Med.* 2012;26(5):768–769.
18. Chochinov HM, Hassard T, McClement S, Hack T, Kristjanson LJ, Harlos M, et al. The landscape of distress in the terminally ill. *J Pain Sympt Manage.* 2009;38(5):641–649.
19. Hall S, Edmonds P, harding R, Chochinov H, Higginson IJ. Assessing the feasibility, acceptability and potential effectiveness of Dignity Therapy for people with advanced cancer referred to a hospital-based palliative care team: Study protocol. *BMC Palliat Care.* 2009;5(5):1–8.

20. Bentley B, Aoun SM, O'Conner MO, Breen LJ, Chochinov H. Is dignity therapy feasible to enhance the end of life experience for people with motor neuron disease and their family carers? *BMC Palliat Care.* 2012;11(18):1–7.

21. Aoun SM, Chochinov HM, Kristjanson LJ. Dignity therapy for people with motor neuron disease and their family caregivers: A feasibility study. *J Palliat Med.* 2015;18(1):31–37.

22. Brozek B, Fopka-Kowalczyk M, Łabuś-Centek M, Damps-Konstańska I, Ratajska A, Jassem E, et al. Dignity therapy as an aid to coping for COPD patients at their end-of-life stage. *Adv Respir Med.* 2019;87(3):135–145.

23. Chochinov HM. Humility and the practice of medicine: Tasting humble pie. *Can Med Assoc J.* 2010:1217–1218.

24. Juliao M, Oliveira F, Nunes B, Vaz Carneiro A, Barbosa A. Efficacy of dignity therapy on depression and anxiety in Portuguese terminally ill patients: A phase II randomized controlled trial. *J Palliat Med.* 2014;17(6):688–695.

25. Bluck S, Mroz EL, Wilkie DJ, Emanuel L, Handzo G, Fitchett G, et al. Quality of life for older cancer patients: Relation of psychospiritual distress to meaning-making during dignity therapy. *Am J Hospice Palliat Care.* 2022;39(1):54–61.

26. Xiao J, Chow KM, Liu Y, Chan CWH. Effects of dignity therapy on dignity, psychological well-being, and quality of life among palliative care cancer patients: A systematic review and meta-analysis. *Psychooncology.* 2019;28(9):1791–1802.

27. Gonzalez-Ling A, Vazquez OG, Rascon-Gasca ML, Robles R, Chochinov HM. Dignity therapy in Mexican lung cancer patients with emotional distress: Impact on psychological symptoms and quality of life. *Palliat Support Care.* 2021:1–7.

28. Kittelson S, Scarton L, Barker P, Hauser J, O'Mahony S, Rabow M, et al. Dignity therapy led by nurses or chaplains for elderly cancer palliative care outpatients: Protocol for a randomized controlled trial. *J Med Internet Res.* 2019;8(4):e12213.

29. Chochinov HM, Kristjanson LJ, Breitbart W, McClement S, Hack TF, Hassard T, et al. Effect of dignity therapy on distress and end-of-life experience in terminally ill patients: A randomised controlled trial. *Lancet Oncol.* 2011;12(8):753–762.

30. Labus-Centek M, Adamczyk A, Jagielska A, Brożek B, Graczyk M, Larkin P, et al. Application of dignity therapy in an advanced cancer patient: Wider therapeutic implications. *Palliat Med Pract.* 2018;12(4):218–223.

31. Houmann LJ, Rydahl-hanson S, Chochinov HM, Kristjanson LJ, Groenvold M. Testing the feasibility of the dignity therapy interview: Adaptation for the Danish culture. *BMC Palliat Care.* 2010;9(21):1–11.

32. Ho AHY, Car J, Ho MH, Tan-Ho G, Choo PY, Patinadan PV, et al. A novel Family Dignity Intervention (FDI) for enhancing and informing holistic palliative care in Asia: Study protocol for a randomized controlled trial. *Trials.* 2017;18(1):587.

33. Testoni I, Baroni V, Iacona E, Zamperini A, Keisari S, Ronconi L, et al. The sense of dignity at the end of life: Reflections on lifetime values through the family photo album. *MDPI Behav Sci.* 2020;10:1–14.

34. Testoni I, Bingaman KA, D'Iapico G, Marinoni GL, Zamperini A, Grassi L, et al. Dignity as wisdom at the end of life: Sacrifice as value emerging from a qualitative analysis of generativity documents. *Pastoral Psychol.* 2019(68):479–489.

35. Testoni I, D'Ippolito M, Iacona E, Zamperini A, Mencacci E, Chochinov HM, et al. Dignity Therapy and the past that matters: Dialogues with older people on values and photos. *J Loss Trauma.* 2021:1–8.

36. Testoni I, Marrella F, Biancalani G, Cottone P, Alemanno F, Mamo D, et al. The value of dignity in prison: A qualitative study with life convicts. *MDPI Behav Sci.* 2020;10(6):1–11.

37. Juliao M, Antunes B, Santos A, Sobral MA, Albuquerque S, Fareleira F, et al. Adapting the Portuguese dignity question framework for adolescents: Ages 10–18. *Palliat Support Care.* 2020;18(2):199–205.

38. Juliao M, Barbosa A, Oliveira F, Nunes B, Vaz Carneiro A. Efficacy of dignity therapy for depression and anxiety in terminally ill patients: Early results of a randomized controlled trial. *Palliat Support Care.* 2013;11(6):481–489.

39. Juliao M, Nunes B, Barbosa A. Dignity therapy and its effects on the survival of terminally ill Portuguese patients. *Psychother Psychosomatics.* 2015;84(1):57–58.

40. Juliao M, Santos A, Albuquerque S, Antunes B, Crujo M, Sobral MA, et al. Operationalizing dignity therapy for adolescents. *Palliat Support Care.* 2020;18(5):626–631.

41. Weru J, Gatehi M, Musibi A. Randomized control trial of advanced cancer patients at a private hospital in Kenya and the impact of dignity therapy on quality of life. *BMC Palliat Care.* 2020;19(114):1–12.

42. Samuels V, Schoppee TM, Greenlee A, Gordon D, Jean S, Smith V, et al. Interim analysis of attrition rates in palliative care study on dignity therapy. *Am J Hospice Palliat Care.* 2021;38(12):1503–1508.

43. Saracino RM, Rosenfeld B, Brietbart W, Chochinov HM. Psychotherapy at the end of life. *Am J Bioethics.* 2019;19(12):19–28.

44. Schoppee TM, Scarton L, Bluck S, Yao Y, Keenan G, Handzo G, et al. Description of a training protocol to improve research reproducibility for dignity therapy, an interview-based intervention. *Palliat Support Care.* 2022;20(2):178–188.

45. Chochinov H. Dignity and the essence of medicine: The A, B, C and D of dignity conserving care. *BMJ.* 2007;335:184–187.

46. Chochinov HM, McClement SE, Hack TF, McKeen NA, Rach AM, Gagnon P, et al. Health care provider communication: An empirical model of therapeutic effectiveness. *Cancer.* 2013;119(9):1706–1713.

47. Chochinov HM, Hassard T, McClement S, Hack T, Kristjanson LJ, Harlos M, et al. The patient dignity inventory: A novel way of measuring dignity-related distress in palliative care. *J Pain Sympt Manage.* 2008;36(6):559–571.

48. Chochinov HM, Johnston W, McClement SE, Hack TF, Dufault B, Enns M, et al. Dignity and distress towards the end of life across four non-cancer populations. *PLoS One.* 2016;11(1):e0147607.

49. Scarton L, Oh S, Sylvera A, Lamonge R, Yao Y, Chochinov H, et al. Dignity impact as a primary outcome measure for dignity therapy. *Am J Hosp Palliat Care.* 2018:1049909118777987.

50. Chochinov HM, McClement S, Hack T, Thompson G, Dufault B, Harlos M. Eliciting personhood within clinical practice: Effects on patients, families, and health care providers. *J Pain Sympt Manage.* 2015;49(6):974–980.

51. Guo Q, Chochinov HM, McClement S, Thompson G, Hack T. Development and evaluation of the Dignity Talk question framework for palliative patients and their families: A mixed-methods study. *Palliat Med.* 2018;32(1):195–205.

52. Chochinov HM, Hack T, Hassard T, Kristjanson LJ, McClement S, Harlos M. Dignity therapy: A novel psychotherapeutic intervention for patients near the end of life. *J Clin Oncology.* 2005;23(24):5520–5525.

53. Buonaccorso L, Tanzi S, De Panfilis L, Ghirotto L, Autelitano C, Chochinov HM, et al. Meanings emerging from Dignity Therapy among cancer patients. *J Pain Sympt Manage.* 2021;21.

54. Hack TF, McClement SE, Chochinov HM, Cann BJ, Hassard TH, Kristjanson LJ, et al. Learning from dying patients during their final days: Life reflections gleaned from dignity therapy. *Palliat Med.* 2010;24(7):715–723.

55. Chochinov H. *Dignity Therapy: Final Words for Final Days.* New York: Oxford University Press; 2012.

56. Scarton LJ, Boyken L, Lucero R, Fitchett G, Handzo G, Emanuel L, et al. Effects of dignity therapy on family members: A systematic review. *J Hospice Palliat Nurs.* 2018;20(6):542–547.

57. Chochinov HM, Hack T, Hassard T, Kristjanson LJ, McClement S, Harlos M. Dignity and psychotherapeutic considerations in end-of-life care. *J Palliat Care.* 2004;20(3):134–142.

58. Martinez M, Arantzamendi M, Belar A, Carrasco JM, Carvajal A, Rullán M, et al. "Dignity therapy," a promising intervention in palliative care: A comprehensive systematic literature review. *PalliatMed.* 2017;31(6):492–509.

59. Chochinov HM. Dignity-conserving care: A new model for palliative care. *JAMA.* 2002;287(17):2253–2261.

60. Chochinov HM, Cann BJ. Interventions to enhance the spiritual aspects of dying. *J Palliat Med.* 2005;8 Suppl 1:S103–115.

61. McClement S, Chochinov HM, Hack T, Hassard T, Kristjanson LJ, Harlos M. Dignity therapy: Family member perspectives. *J Palliat Med.* 2007;10(5):1076–1082.

62. Thompson G, Chochinov H. Dignity-based approaches in the care of terminally ill patients. *Support Palliat Care.* 2008;2(1):49–53.

63. Hall S, Chochinov H, Harding R, Murray S, Richardson A, Higginson IJ. A Phase II randomised controlled trial assessing the feasibility, acceptability and potential effectiveness of dignity therapy for older people in care homes: Study protocol. *BMC Geriatr.* 2009;9:9.

64. Chochinov HM, Cann B, Cullihall K, Kristjanson L, Harlos M, McClement SE, et al. Dignity therapy: A feasibility study of elders in long-term care. *Palliat Support Care.* 2012;10(1):3–15.

65. Montross LP, Meier EA, De Cervantes-Monteith K, Vashistha V, Irwin SA. Hospice staff perspectives on dignity therapy. *J Palliat Med.* 2013;16(9):1118–1120.

66. Houmann LJ, Chochinov HM, Kristjanson LJ, Petersen MA, Groenvold M. A prospective evaluation of Dignity Therapy in advanced cancer patients admitted to palliative care. *Palliat Med.* 2014;28(5):448–458.

67. Donato SC, Matuoka JY, Yamashita CC, Salvetti MG. Effects of dignity therapy on terminally ill patients: A systematic review. *Revista da Escola de Enfermagem da U S P.* 2016;50(6):1014–1024.

68. Bentley B, O'Connor M, Shaw J, Breen L. A narrative review of Dignity Therapy research. *Australian Psychologist.* 2017;52(5):354–362.

69. Ianai L, De Vincenzo F, Maruelli A, Chochinov HM, Ragghianti M, Durante S, et al. Dignity therapy helps terminally ill patients maintain a sense of peace: Early results of a randomized controlled trial. *Front Psychol.* 2020;11:1–9.

70. Kredenster MS, Chochinov HM. Psychotherapeutic considerations for patients with terminal illness. *Am J Psychother.* 2020;4:137–143.

71. Morgan DD, Marston C, Barnard E, Farrow C. Conserving dignity and facilitating adaptation to dependency with intimate hygiene for people with advanced disease: A qualitative study. *Palliat Med.* 2021:1–12.

37

Managing Cancer and Living Meaningfully (CALM) Therapy

Carmine Malfitano, Sarah Hales, and Gary Rodin

Introduction

Individuals living with advanced cancer experience multiple challenges, including the progressive burden of disease, complex treatment decisions, an increasing requirement to depend on others, the loss of meaning in life, and fears about dying and death. These challenges contribute to the occurrence of clinically significant symptoms of depression and demoralization, which we found in one-quarter of these individuals at any point in the disease trajectory.[1] Furthermore, we demonstrated that, without psychological treatment, depression becomes three times more common in such individuals toward the end of life compared to its prevalence earlier in the course of the disease.[2] Distress about dying and death may be an even more common manifestation of distress in this population, reported by more than 40% of patients living with advanced cancer.[3] We have proposed that depression and death anxiety can be understood as a final common pathway of distress in this context, one related to the interaction of the burden of disease, individual, and psychosocial factors, and the threat of impending mortality.[1]

The psychological distress reported by the family partners of individuals facing a life-threatening cancer is often equal to or even greater than that reported by patients and tends to persist or increase over time.[4] These informal caregivers frequently assume key roles in complex and often burdensome tasks, such as the coordination of care, management of symptoms, administration of various treatments, and provision of direct personal care. Such tasks must often be performed along with other ongoing responsibilities, such as those related to finance, employment, or caring for other dependents. With the progression of disease, informal caregivers often increasingly become the primary source of practical, social, and emotional support for patients, with a consequent narrowing of their social interactions and heightening of their sense of isolation. However, despite growing aware-ness of the physical and psychological burden of caregiving in such individuals, caregivers' distress is often missed and untreated in cancer care settings and access to interventions to relieve their distress or their caregiving burden is limited in most community or institu-tional settings.

Although advancing disease may trigger profound distress in individuals and their family members, it may also provide an opportunity for psychological growth and devel-opment, or what has been termed as *posttraumatic growth*. The perceived shortness of time may trigger a "now moment" that is associated with a search for authenticity, the desire to re-evaluate life priorities, and the longing to make meaningful changes in life goals and in important relationships. Drawing on terror management theory,[5] we have shown that the psychological pillars that protect individuals from depression and death anxiety in the con-text of advanced disease are attachment security (i.e., confidence about the availability and benefit of emotional support from significant others); self-esteem, or the sense of being a person of value in the world; and the capacity to find a sense of meaning in life.[5] Managing Cancer and Living Meaningfully (CALM) is guided by and intended to strengthen this tri-partite psychological system that serves to manage the terror of death anxiety.

CALM is a brief, individual- and couple-based, supportive-expressive, psychothera-peutic intervention that emerged from a longitudinal program of research informed by the theoretical foundations of relational theory,[6] attachment theory,[7] and existential theory.[8] It addresses both the practical and profound issues faced by individuals with advanced cancer and their informal caregivers, and it was designed and manualized[9] to relieve distress and promote psychological growth in individuals with advanced cancer. The perceived short-ness of time in this context often heightens the motivation of those affected to seek help, reflect, and engage authentically in the therapeutic process. The relatively brief format of CALM, the evidence for its effectiveness, and the possibility for it to be delivered by a wide range of healthcare providers make it feasible and beneficial to become a standard of care in oncology and palliative care settings.

The focus on existential, spiritual, and meaning-centered issues in CALM is shared with other interventions that have been developed for patients with advanced disease.[10] These include supportive-expressive,[11] cognitive-existential,[12] and meaning-centered[13] psychotherapies. In contrast to some of the group interventions that have been developed for this population, the individual and couple-based format of CALM allows for greater privacy in the discussion of sensitive personal issues that may arise and greater flexibility regarding the content and timing of the sessions. The last is important for these patients who typically struggle with fluctuating health status, complicated treatment schedules, fre-quent investigations, and hospitalizations and who may be unable to participate in group interventions that occur on a fixed day and time. Furthermore, many individuals with met-astatic cancer have difficulty absorbing the emotional distress of other patients that emerges in group interventions.

CALM shares with dignity therapy[14] a focus on identity, self-concept, and life closure for patients near the end of life. However, CALM is intended for patients earlier in the course of the illness, usually with at least 6 months of expected survival, when they are as engaged with living as they are with facing the end of life. CALM aims to support both life engagement and the contemplation and planning for the progression of disease and the end of life, a capacity that has been referred to as "double awareness."[15] A measure to assess this construct, the Double Awareness Scale, has been developed and is currently undergoing validity testing.[16]

Structure of Calm

CALM typically consists of three to six individual or couple-based sessions, each lasting 45–60 minutes, delivered over a 3- to 6-month period, although the number of sessions may vary depending on the patient's clinical circumstances. The CALM sessions address four broad domains: (1) symptom management and communication with healthcare providers, (2) changes in self and relations with close others, (3) spiritual well-being and the sense of meaning and purpose, and (4) preparing for the future, sustaining hope, and facing mortality (see Figure 37.1). These domains should be considered with all patients at some point during the intervention, although the sequence in which they are addressed and the degree of attention to each will vary based on their relative importance in each case. The CALM domains are not mutually exclusive but provide an overarching framework for therapists regarding issues that are likely to be important for this population. Each participant's primary caregiver (e.g., spouse, adult son or daughter, friend) is invited to participate in one or more sessions to facilitate the exploration of relational dynamics and support the dyad in anticipating and preparing for the future. When mutually agreed upon, caregivers may attend all sessions.

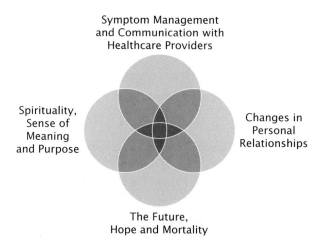

FIGURE 37.1 Managing cancer and living meaningfully (CALM) therapy. From: Hales S, Lo C, Rodin G. Managing cancer and living meaningfully (CALM) therapy. In: Holland JC, Breitbart WS, Butow PN, Jacobsen, Loscalzo MJ, McCorkle R, eds., *Psycho-Oncology*, 3rd ed. New York: Oxford University Press; 2015:487, figure 32.1. © Oxford University Press 2015. Reproduced with permission of the Licensor through PlSclear.

The CALM Patient

CALM is intended for patients with advanced and life-threatening cancer who have some interest in and capacity for reflection and who are physically and cognitively well enough to engage in psychotherapeutic sessions over a 3- to 6-month period. With the recent introduction of immunotherapy and other targeted therapies and more prolonged survival of many patients with advanced disease, CALM may continue over a longer period of time. Depending on the patient's interest or capacity for reflection, the therapy may focus more in some cases on practical issues in the management of their disease and its impact on themselves and their families, whereas in others it may be characterized by more reflection on profound existential issues. However, CALM may not be suitable or appropriate for individuals who insist on thinking only in positive terms about their condition, although this coping style becomes increasingly untenable with disease progression.

The CALM Process

The aim of the CALM therapist is to address the four content domains of CALM while also promoting affect regulation, reflection, decision-making, and renegotiation of attachment relationships in the context of increased dependency needs. The therapeutic posture is intended to support patients' capacity to engage in life while also helping them to face the challenges of cancer and its treatment and planning for the end of life. CALM is intended to create reflective space for patients to consider the implications and meaning of their condition and to help them consider multiple potential perspectives on their situation. CALM differs from some other psychotherapeutic modalities in which the therapeutic process focuses more on prescriptive goals, positivity, reassurance, or the correction of cognitive distortions. The following elements of the therapeutic process can be regarded as active ingredients of CALM therapy that support exploration of the relevant domains and that contribute to its therapeutic effect.

The Supportive Relationship: A central component of the CALM process is the establishment of a therapeutic relationship that provides attachment security and supports the capacity of the patient to reflect on their experience and to consider their circumstance from multiple perspectives. The openness of the therapist to the experience of the patient and the therapist's engagement with the patient at this time of tragedy and crisis often allows depth in the relationship to develop in a relatively short period of time. CALM therapists consistently work to engage empathically with patients and communicate their understanding of the patients' felt experience. In this way, therapists become witness to the patient's experience, helping them to address their fears of isolation and dependency, manage feelings of grief and loss, and identify strengths and potential adaptive coping strategies.

Authenticity: The therapeutic stance is one of genuineness and honesty in relation to the patient. Authenticity in this context refers neither to self-disclosure nor to the communication of prognostic information, but to being emotionally present and open to the patient, accepting their fears without false reassurance or with dismissal. Therapists may help patients to distinguish facts from feelings and consider multiple perspectives, a capacity that has been referred to as mentalization.[17] This may allow patients to understand that assumptions that they may make, such as that their life is not worth living or that they are an unwanted burden on others, are ways of thinking rather than immutable truths or beliefs shared by close others or by the therapist.

Shifting Frame and Flexibility: Fluctuations in the patients' clinical state, symptom control, or the receipt of test results or other prognostic information may drastically alter patients' capacity or motivation for self-reflection. Such changes may necessitate shifts in the therapy between supportive and exploratory approaches and adjustments in the content and timing of sessions. Brief or intermittent sessions after the formal conclusion of the CALM intervention may be of great value in some cases because of the trust in the therapist that has developed during the treatment. However, clinical deterioration or death can occur unexpectedly or suddenly, preventing the opportunity for a planned end to treatment and for processing feelings of the patient about the ending.

Modulation of Affect: Fluctuations in the emotional state of the patient are common during the course of advanced disease and may be evident even within sessions depending on content of the sessions and recent events that have occurred. The goal of the CALM therapist is to help patients modulate the intensity of their emotions so that patients' emotional arousal remains within a tolerable range. With patients who are overwhelmed by affect, the therapist aims at reducing its intensity with structuring interventions and a focus on practical tasks. With patients whose affect is constricted, the aim is to facilitate the emergence of the emotional experience. Facilitating the communication of emotions within an atmosphere of support and understanding allows patients to be less afraid that they will be flooded by distressing emotions. This process fosters a greater capacity and confidence in the ability to manage, understand, and differentiate the complex emotions that may arise in the context of a life-threatening illness.

Renegotiation of Attachment Security: Individuals vary in their capacity to seek, expect, accept, or rely on emotional support. This capacity is captured in the construct of attachment security and can be assessed on the dimensions of *attachment avoidance* and *attachment anxiety*.[18] The former reflects the tendency toward compulsive self-sufficiency with the minimization of distress, while the latter refers to the tendency to fear that support will not be available and that distress cannot be managed. The threat to life in the context of advanced disease heightens attachment needs and makes attachment security more salient. Those who are less securely attached may have greater difficulty adjusting in response to these changes, leaving these individuals fearful of isolation or threatened by dependency. Individuals with a tendency to be self-sufficient and/or more comfortable with giving rather than receiving care, characteristics of the avoidantly attached, may feel threatened by the growing dependency imposed by the progressive disease. Individuals who tend to worry about the availability of others, a feature of the anxiously attached, may become increasingly worried about the availability of support as their needs increase.

CALM therapy helps patients with advanced disease to manage the disruption caused by these attachment crises and re-establish equilibrium in their attachment relationships. This is accomplished by helping patients and their family members understand the changes in their needs that have occurred because of the illness. The CALM therapist may help to legitimize increased dependency needs of patients in the context of the disease and facilitate the communication of these needs to partners or other family members. This is particularly important in those patients who have tended to be caregivers, with insufficient attention to their own needs. Therapists may help family members to understand the need for predictability and reliability of support in patients who are anxiously attached. Finally, the therapist may come to be an attachment figure for both patients and caregivers, which may help to resolve the disease-related attachment crisis.

The Joint Creation of Meaning: Whereas traditional psychodynamic approaches assign to the therapist the task of interpreting to the patient the meaning of their symptoms and behavior, relational theory emphasizes that meaning is co-created in the collaboration of the therapist and the patient.[6] The meanings that patients attach to their life history, their accomplishments and failures, and the disease are explored in CALM therapy. This may result in a reframing of the patients' life narrative and, more importantly, in the creation of new meanings and new priorities in the context of the patients' present life circumstances. New understandings may follow from this dialogue and exchange between therapists and patients and are offered tentatively and in the spirit of collaboration.

Mentalization and Double Awareness: *Mentalization* refers to the capacity to reflect on feeling states, distinguish them from literal facts, and accept the possibility of multiple perspectives.[19] This capacity may be challenged in the context of advanced disease because of the dominating impact of the illness and of impending mortality. This may obscure that what is experienced as a "fact" about the situation is actually a mental construction, or one of multiple ways in which it can be viewed. Supporting the mentalization of such feelings states allows individuals to sustain what we have termed a "double awareness"[15] of possibilities for both living and for facing and planning for the end of life. The CALM therapist supports this duality by understanding and validating the experience of patients while also helping them to entertain the possibility of multiple psychological responses to a physical circumstance that cannot be eliminated. Paradoxically, understanding and validating the unique personal meaning of patients' experience opens the possibility for other ways of thinking and feeling to be considered.

The Content of CALM

Domain One: Disease Management and Relationships with Healthcare Providers

"I don't understand what is wrong with me. Lately my breathing is worse and twice I've had to go to the emergency room. They did investigations, said my oxygen levels were fine, and sent me home saying it was just a panic attack." This experience was described by Amara, a 41-year-old woman with breast cancer and recent metastases to her lungs and bones. She had been relatively asymptomatic from her cancer for many years, but her current intermittent shortness of breath led to a cascade of anxiety and sometimes full panic attacks. It became clear she was deeply worried about suffering and asphyxiation, and a referral to palliative care provided helpful education about potential medical management of dyspnea and pain. CALM therapy provided an opportunity for validation of her distress and need for medical attention and for the modulation of her anxiety. After just a few CALM sessions, the panic attacks ceased.

The disease, symptoms, process of cancer treatment, and decision-making that is required are central concerns of patients with advanced cancer and their families. The opportunity for patients to reflect on these issues outside of the cancer clinic has been an important and beneficial dimension of CALM. Such issues that may be related to the first domain of CALM include the following.

Understanding the Disease and Managing Symptoms: Treatment decisions and management of the disease and the complications of treatment are challenging for patients, particularly as medical treatments and diagnostic processes have become more complex. CALM therapy provides an opportunity for patients to discuss information that they have received from their healthcare providers and others and alternative treatments that they are considering but may not feel comfortable discussing with their oncology providers. CALM therapists aim to support patients in communicating and negotiating effectively with the patients' healthcare providers. They may also help to correct misunderstandings about treatment and direct patients to appropriate sources of information, including to other healthcare providers.

Supporting Medical Decision-Making: Decisions about cancer treatment and clinical trials are difficult for many patients with advanced disease, particularly when the recommendations from their oncologist are ambiguous or when there is diminishing likelihood of benefit and greater potential for toxicity. A collaborative decision-making process between patients and their medical team has many benefits, but some patients feel overwhelmed by the perceived obligation to participate in complex treatment decisions. Some patients have difficulty understanding the information that they have received or balancing the adverse effects of toxicity and the potential benefit of certain treatments. Others may perceive pressures from their family or their healthcare providers to make a particular decision. Declining further treatment or clinical trials that are offered is difficult for many individuals with advanced disease and can seem to them like "giving up," even when the likelihood of benefit from such interventions is vanishingly small.

CALM therapists can help patients to explore the range of feelings that they may have in relation to treatment decisions and distinguish their views from those of their healthcare providers, family, or friends. The unique role of CALM therapists as "insiders" in the cancer system, ones who are separate from the cancer treatment team and from the family, often makes them uniquely valuable in the decision-making process.[20] However, therapists must monitor their own feelings and vicarious preferences as they engage with patients in their questions and decisions about treatments in which the stakes are high.

Supporting Collaborative Relationships with Healthcare Providers: The relationship with the cancer treatment team is profoundly important to most patients with cancer, and the sense of partnership with their treatment team often has a positive impact on their emotional well-being and adaptation to the disease and treatment. Helping patients to find an appropriate and tolerable balance between self-management and seeking help, support, and advice from their healthcare team is an important goal of CALM. The former may require patients to become more able to tolerate the inherent uncertainties in their treatment, a challenging task for many patients with advanced disease. Even in well-organized treatment settings, the fallibility of healthcare providers, lapses in continuity of care, and inevitable limitations in healthcare resources may be frustrating and distressing to patients and their families. The CALM therapist can listen empathically to such experiences of disappointment and find ways to support or repair the alliance of patients with the treatment team.

Domain Two: Changes in Self-Concept and Relationships with Close Others

"I think we understand what we're facing but I can't imagine dumping this on our kids. They're too young. Why destroy their lives by telling them about my cancer?" These reflected the concern about what to communicate to his children of Nico, who was a 50-year-old man with metastatic pancreatic cancer. He also had great difficulty accepting support for himself, being more comfortable taking care of others. After some encouragement from his wife, he attended CALM therapy sessions and soon found it beneficial to speak more openly about his fears for the future. CALM therapy provided an opportunity for Nico to accept support from his wife and from the therapist, and it helped them to consider together the needs and perspective of their son. Through this process, they eventually developed practical strategies for conversations with him about Nico's condition.

Caregiving and Care-receiving: The experience of advanced disease often leads to dramatic changes within primary relationships, including in the household division of labor, financial responsibilities, parenting roles, and/or emotional and physical intimacy. Many patients with advanced disease are able to seek and obtain emotional and practical support, as needed, from loved ones. However, fears of abandonment or of dependency on others may contribute to anxious clinging or dismissive avoidance of needs. These relational tendencies may interfere with the ability to seek or obtain support from caregivers or take their needs into account, resulting in tension and disequilibrium in these relationships. Identifying and acknowledging the relational tendencies of patients and their caregivers can facilitate mutual understanding of the adjustments that are required to restore attachment security and facilitate more satisfying and supportive relationship experiences.

Supporting Children and Other Family: When there are younger children in the family, a question that commonly arises is what to tell them about the disease, when to tell them, and how to support them throughout the illness process. CALM therapy provides an opportunity for patients to consider what and how to communicate information about their illness to their family. This includes a consideration of the developmental capacity and needs of children in the family and attention to the timing and readiness of children to receive this information. Patients may also benefit from the reminder that discussions of illness and dying comprise a process that occurs over time rather than a single event. CALM therapy sessions do not typically include younger children or extended family, but joint sessions can be held when needed.

Domain Three: Spirituality, Sense of Meaning and Purpose

"It's surreal. I know this cancer will end my life some day but I feel well now, and sometimes like a fraud. I'm probably able to work but I don't think I want to focus on my career any longer." This was the distressing and confusing experience reported by Felix, a 45-year-old man with metastatic melanoma. The initial diagnosis of this disease was devastating for him and his wife, but he felt better and became calmer as immunotherapy began to be effective. Felix acknowledged that he had a tendency to focus more on the needs of others than his own and had continued to work in a high-pressure environment throughout the period of his initial diagnosis and treatment. He did not want to let down his employer and colleagues, and he was reluctant to discuss the future openly with his wife for fear of upsetting her. CALM therapy provided an opportunity for Felix to reflect on his own wishes and take them into account and then for Felix and his wife to consider together how they wanted to spend the time while he was still relatively well.

The Personal Meaning of the Disease: The meaning of the disease and the fears associated with it are determined by a variety of factors, including its nature and course, the symptoms and visible sequelae associated with it, the support and communication of medical caregivers, and the psychological organizing principles of the patient. For some, the cancer may represent the frailty and transience of human life, an unfair or unjust burden, a punishment from God, or either predetermination or randomness of human destiny. Some attribute their disease to stress that they or others imposed on them, to their lifestyle, to the environment, or to medical caregivers whom they perceive to have failed them. Such meaning-making, a human response to trauma and uncertainty, which may be more or less adaptive, can be reframed in the therapeutic process.

Questions related to meaning, purpose, and faith become more salient for many in the context of impending mortality. For some, the crisis of illness and the thought of dying may strengthen long-held religious or philosophical views. For others, it may challenge these beliefs and questions such as "Why me?", "What comes next?", "Why must my family suffer?" may emerge. By exploring how individual patients make sense of their situation, therapists can facilitate and support meaning-making as an adaptive way to cope with a situation that is beyond one's control.

The Life Narrative: Helping individuals with advanced disease to create a life narrative may be an important task that helps them to find meaning in their past and present life, process feelings of disappointment or regret, and face the end of their life. Helping patients to weave together the narrative of their life and their illness may help them to experience a sense of coherence about their past and present life. This may also allow patients to perceive a sense of accomplishment and achievement about their lives and about their legacy and also to process feelings of regret or disappointment about aspects of their life.

Evaluate Priorities and Goals in the Face of Advanced Disease: The experience of advanced disease and end of life often leads patients to re-evaluate their priorities and life goals. Activities or attributes that previously supported the sense of identity and the sense of meaning in life may have been dramatically undermined, and the perceived shortness of time impels many patients with advanced disease to reconsider how to spend the time that remains.[7] By encouraging reflection on priorities and goals, therapists can help patients to remain engaged in life while also planning for and facing the end of life.

Domain 4: Thinking of the Future, Hope, and Mortality

Acknowledgment of Anticipatory Fears: Fears about dying and death are common in many with advanced disease,[3] although there are few interventions that have been designed specifically to focus on this problem. In fact, the emphasis on hope and positive thinking that is common in the community, media, cancer charities, and even in healthcare may cause some patients to feel that their fears have been silenced. Distress about death and dying may be shaped by past experiences with illness and death of close others, the extent to which support is perceived to be present, and the nature of the disease. It may also be heightened by specific physical symptoms, such as dyspnea, pain, or dysphagia. The CALM therapist provides opportunities for patients to speak openly about dying and death and consider advance care planning and for therapists to normalize and validate the anxiety of patients about the future. Such approaches may alleviate death anxiety in patients with advanced cancer, and the authors of a recent systematic review concluded that CALM is the only psychotherapeutic intervention that has thus far been shown to have this effect.[21]

Balance of Living and Dying

CALM is intended not only to diminish death-related distress and facilitate death acceptance, but also to support "double awareness."[15] Patients who are unable to consider mortality-related issues may neglect important decision-making and practical planning, such as making a will or arranging personal financial matters. However, those who are overly preoccupied with death may not be able to enjoy or attend to life in the present. The CALM therapist does not insist on exploration of dying and death but provides opportunities for the patient and caregivers to explore their feelings and concerns about the future, helping them to sustain the balance of living and dying.

Advance Care Planning, Life Closure, and Death Preparation: Research exploring the concept of the good death with patients and families has consistently identified advance care planning, life closure, and death preparation activities as important components of a positive dying experience.[22] Making treatment wishes explicit, making funeral and financial plans, taking the opportunity to say goodbye to closed loved ones, or "legacy projects" such as letters, videos, or gifts for loved ones, are examples of life closure or death preparation activities that may be helpful. By supporting exploration about hopes and fears for the future, the CALM therapist encourages an active approach to end of life, supporting what the patient can control while also helping the patient to prepare for the end of life.

CALM Therapist Selection, Training, and Supervision

The CALM therapist should be an individual who has experience with cancer and its treatment and thus be a knowledgeable "insider" in cancer care. Clinicians from different disciplines and backgrounds, including psychiatrists, psychologists, palliative care physicians, nurses, social workers, and spiritual care providers, have been successfully trained to deliver CALM. Each of these disciplines may bring unique and valuable skills and insights to the care of patients with advanced disease.

CALM training includes both didactic teaching and case treatment under supervision. To achieve competence in CALM delivery, participants must complete an interactive, case-based workshop, and treat at least two cases satisfactorily under supervision of a qualified CALM supervisor. Regular ongoing peer supervision is considered an integral part of the CALM therapy model and the maintenance of competence. This provides an opportunity for therapist support, validation, and monitoring to ensure the ongoing quality and integrity of treatment and advanced skill development. Ongoing peer supervision may also allow CALM therapists to experience the benefits of sharing the ongoing experience of being exposed to the universal and inescapable dilemma of mortality and protected from emotional depletion or burnout.

Evidence for CALM Therapy

A rigorous body of research on CALM has emerged over the past 15 years through the work of clinicians and scholars from North and South America, Europe, and Asia. This research has demonstrated that CALM is effective in reducing distress and improving psychological well-being and is applicable and feasible across diverse cultures.[20,23–30] We initially demonstrated the feasibility and preliminary efficacy of CALM in a phase 2 pilot study, in which we found significant improvements in depressive symptoms, death anxiety, and spiritual well-being over the 6-month follow-up period.[31] In qualitative interviews, therapy participants indicated that CALM provided them with (1) a safe place to process the experience of advanced cancer, (2) the permission to talk about death and dying, (3) assistance in managing the illness and navigating the healthcare system, (4) the resolution of relational strain, and (5) the opportunity to "be seen as a whole person" within the healthcare system.[20]

We subsequently conducted a large randomized controlled trial of CALM plus usual care versus usual care alone, in which we recruited 305 patients with an expected survival of 12–18.[25] We demonstrated that participants in the CALM group reported significant improvements in depressive symptoms and end-of-life preparation compared to those in the usual care group. We also found that individuals in the CALM group who were not depressed at baseline were less likely to become depressed at the 3- and 6-month follow-ups, indicating a preventive effect of the intervention. Patients in the CALM group with moderate levels of distress about dying and death at baseline reported greater reduction of death-related distress at both endpoints.

Future Directions

Despite recognition of the psychological suffering among patients and families facing advanced disease, evidence-based psychological care for this population has lagged behind physical symptom care. Psychological interventions are not yet well-integrated or standard within oncology or palliative care, and access to psychosocial resources in cancer treatment settings remains highly variable. To address this lack, a global network of clinicians and researchers has been established to support adaptation and implementation of CALM within diverse cultural and clinical settings. Evidence of benefit from CALM has been found in research trials in Germany[32] and Italy,[23] and pilot studies are now under way in other sites within North America, the Netherlands, Portugal, China, Japan, and Australia. This growing network is creating momentum to heighten awareness and implement standards for the psychological dimensions of palliative care. To further increase access to the CALM approach, we have developed with colleagues in Ulm, Germany, a digital version of CALM referred to as iCALM. A clinical trial evaluating the feasibility and acceptability of iCALM is now under way.

There is growing evidence that psychotherapeutic interventions developed for the advanced disease population can address the unique challenges that contribute to depression, death anxiety, and other forms of distress. However, the treatment of patients with cancer and other medical conditions in all parts of the world is much more focused on biomedicine than it is on the "soul of medicine."[33] Advocacy is needed to heighten awareness among clinicians and policymakers about the need for the prevention and treatment of psychological distress in patients with advanced disease and for interventions such as CALM to be adopted as the standard of care for such conditions. Global collaborative efforts aimed at teaching, training, and adaptation of interventions such as CALM may provide a path to more universal patient and family-centered care that addresses all dimensions of suffering and well-being until the end of life.

Key Points

- Individuals living with advanced cancer experience great physical and psychological distress, and those who care for them are often equally or even more distressed.
- Depression and death anxiety are common in this population and can be understood as a final common pathway of distress
- CALM is a brief, individual- and couple-based, supportive-expressive psychotherapeutic intervention that addresses the practical and profound issues faced by individuals with advanced cancer and their informal caregivers. It was designed and manualized to relieve distress and promote psychological growth in these individuals.

- CALM therapy addresses four content domains while also supporting reflection, affect regulation, mentalization, and the renegotiation of attachment security. CALM enhances the capacity of patients to sustain a "double awareness" of the possibilities for engagement in life while also preparing for its ending.
- A rigorous program of research on CALM conducted in diverse cultural contexts demonstrates that CALM is effective in reducing and preventing distress and in facilitating the adjustment and well-being of patients with advanced cancer.

References

1. Rodin G, Lo C, Mikulincer M, Donner A, Gagliese L, Zimmermann C. Pathways to distress: The multiple determinants of depression, hopelessness, and the desire for hastened death in metastatic cancer patients. *Soc Sci Med*. 2009;68(3):562–569.
2. Lo C, Zimmermann C, Rydall A, Walsh A, Jones JM, Moore MJ, et al. Longitudinal study of depressive symptoms in patients with metastatic gastrointestinal and lung cancer. *J Clin Oncol*. 2010;28(18):3084–3089.
3. Eggen AC, Richard NM, Bosma I, Jalving M, Natasha B, Liu G, et al. Factors associated with cognitive impairment and cognitive concerns in patients with metastatic non-small cell lung cancer. *Neuro-Oncol Pract*. 2021;9(1):50–58.
4. Braun M, Mikulincer M, Rydall A, Walsh A, Rodin G. Hidden morbidity in cancer: Spouse caregivers. J Clin Oncol. 2007;25(30):4829–4834.
5. Willis E, Mah K, Shapiro GK, Hales S, Li M, An E, Zimmermann C, Schultebraucks K, Rodin G. Testing terror management theory in advanced cancer. *Death Studies*. 2021;1–10. doi:10.1080/07481187.2021.2019145
6. Mitchell SA. *Relational Concepts in Psychoanalysis: An Integration*. Cambridge, MA: Harvard University Press; 1988.
7. Bowlby J. *Attachment*. 2nd ed. New York: Basic Books; 1982.
8. Yalom I. *Existential Psychotherapy*. New York: Basic Books. 1980.
9. Rodin G, Hales S. *Managing Cancer and Living Meaningfully: An Evidence-Based Intervention for Cancer Patients and Their Caregivers*. Oxford: Oxford University Press; 2021.
10. Rodin G, An E, Shnall J, Malfitano C. Psychological interventions for patients with advanced disease: Implications for oncology and palliative care. *J Clin Oncol*. 2020;38(9):885–904.
11. Spiegel D, Bloom JR, Yalom I. Group support for patients with metastatic cancer: A randomized prospective outcome study. *Arch Gen Psychiatry*. 1981;38(5):527–533.
12. Kissane DW, Bloch S, Smith GC, Miach P, Clarke DM, Ikin J, et al. Cognitive-existential group psychotherapy for women with primary breast cancer: A randomised controlled trial. *Psycho-Oncology J Psychol Soc Behav Dimens Cancer*. 2003;12(6):532–546.
13. Breitbart W, Rosenfeld B, Pessin H, Applebaum A, Kulikowski J, Lichtenthal WG. Meaning-centered group psychotherapy: An effective intervention for improving psychological well-being in patients with advanced cancer. *J Clin Oncol*. 2015;33(7):749.
14. Chochinov HM, Hack T, Hassard T, Kristjanson LJ, McClement S, Harlos M. Dignity therapy: A novel psychotherapeutic intervention for patients near the end of life. *J Clin Oncol*. 2005;23(24):5520–5525.
15. Rodin G, Zimmermann C. Psychoanalytic reflections on mortality: A reconsideration. *J Am Acad Psychoanal Dyn Psychiatry*. 2008;36(1):181–196.
16. Miljanovski M, McConnell M, Mak E, Zimmermann C, Hannon B, Rodin G. Double awareness in advanced cancer: Preliminary psychometric evaluation of a novel self-report measure. Poster presentation presented at 17th World Congress, European Association for Palliative Care; Oct 6, 2021.
17. Shaw C, Chrysikou V, Lanceley A, Lo C, Hales S, Rodin G. Mentalization in CALM psychotherapy sessions: Helping patients engage with alternative perspectives at the end of life. *Patient Educ Couns*. 2019;102(2):188–197.

18. Rodin G, Hales S. Attachment security. In: Rodin G, Hales S, eds., *Managing Cancer and Living Meaningfully: An Evidence-Based Intervention for Cancer Patients and Their Caregivers*. Oxford: Oxford University Press; 2021:45–50.

19. Rodin G, Hales S. Mentalization and mortality. In: Rodin G, Hales S, eds., *Managing Cancer and Living Meaningfully: An Evidence-Based Intervention for Cancer Patients and Their Caregivers*. Oxford: Oxford University Press; 2021:53–65.

20. Nissim R, Freeman E, Lo C, Zimmermann C, Gagliese L, Rydall A, et al. Managing Cancer and Living Meaningfully (CALM): A qualitative study of a brief individual psychotherapy for individuals with advanced cancer. *Palliat Med*. 2012;26(5):713–721.

21. Grossman CH, Brooker J, Michael N, Kissane D. Death anxiety interventions in patients with advanced cancer: A systematic review. *Palliat Med*. 2018;32(1):172–184.

22. Hales S, Zimmermann C, Rodin G. The quality of dying and death. *Arch Intern Med*. 2008;168(9):912–918.

23. Caruso R, Sabato S, Nanni MG, Hales S, Rodin G, Malfitano C, et al. Application of Managing Cancer and Living Meaningfully (CALM) in advanced cancer patients: An Italian pilot study. *Psychother Psychosom*. 2020;89(6):402–404.

24. Lo C, Hales S, Chiu A, Panday T, Malfitano C, Jung J, et al. Managing Cancer and Living Meaningfully (CALM): Randomised feasibility trial in patients with advanced cancer. *BMJ Support Palliat Care*. 2019;9(2):209–218.

25. Rodin G, Lo C, Rydall A, Shnall J, Malfitano C, Chiu A, et al. Managing cancer and living meaningfully (CALM): A randomized controlled trial of a psychological intervention for patients with advanced cancer. *J Clin Oncol*. 2018;36(23):2422.

26. Mehnert A, Koranyi S, Philipp R, Scheffold K, Kriston L, Lehmann-Laue A, et al. Efficacy of the Managing Cancer and Living Meaningfully (CALM) individual psychotherapy for patients with advanced cancer: A single-blind randomized controlled trial. *Psycho-Oncology*. 2020;29(11):1895–1904.

27. Ding K, Zhang X, Zhao J, Zuo H, Bi Z, Cheng H. Managing Cancer and Living Meaningfully (CALM) intervention on chemotherapy-related cognitive impairment in breast cancer survivors. *Integr Cancer Ther*. 2020;19:1534735420938450.

28. Fernández-González L, Namías MR, Bravo P. Facilitators and barriers perceived by health professionals in the implementation of Managing Cancer and Living Meaningfully (CALM) psychotherapy in Santiago. *ecancermedicalscience*. 2021;15.

29. Rodin G. From evidence to implementation: The global challenge for psychosocial oncology. *Psycho-Oncology*. 2018;27(10):2310–2316.

30. Troncoso P, Rydall A, Hales S, Rodin G. A review of psychosocial interventions in patients with advanced cancer in Latin America and the value of CALM therapy in this setting. *Am J Psychiatry Neurosci*. 2019;7(4):108.

31. Lo C, Hales S, Jung J, Chiu A, Panday T, Rydall A, et al. Managing Cancer and Living Meaningfully (CALM): Phase 2 trial of a brief individual psychotherapy for patients with advanced cancer. *Palliat Med*. 2014;28(3):234–242.

32. Scheffold K, Wollbrück D, Schulz-Kindermann F, et al. Pilot results of the German Managing Cancer and Living Meaningfully (CALM) RCT: A brief individual psychotherapy for advanced cancer patients. *BMC Cancer*. 2015;15:592.

33. Rodin G, Ntizimira C, Sullivan R. Biomedicine and the soul of medicine: Optimising the balance. *Lancet Oncol*. 2021;22(7):907–909.

38

Mindfulness-Based Interventions

Linda E. Carlson, Chelsea Moran, and Mohamad Baydoun

Introduction

In this chapter, we address the potential and actual uses of mindfulness-based interventions (MBIs) for people with chronic progressive illness and those nearing end of life. We begin by introducing the concept of *mindfulness*, and we provide a high-level overview of the areas of medicine that have already seen an influx of research in and application of MBIs. Following that, we briefly summarize the major psychosocial issues facing people nearing end of life and their caregivers, focusing on those most likely to be responsive to MBIs. After this theoretical overview of the needs most likely amenable to a mindfulness-based therapeutic approach, we summarize the research in this area in more detail, followed by a critique of the current literature. The chapter wraps up by summarizing gaps and opportunities, with suggestions for adaptation of traditional MBIs for palliative populations and promising areas for future application.

What Is Mindfulness?

Mindfulness itself is often defined as nonjudgmentally paying attention, on purpose, in the present moment. It can be thought of in two ways: as a way of being in the world and as a skill or practice one learns over time. As a way of being, one can be more or less mindful at any given time, no matter what activity one may be engaged in. It doesn't take extra time to live life in a mindful way, and indeed people report feeling happier when they are more fully engaged in the present moment. The problem is that most people are not socialized, and our minds are not trained, to be mindful of the present moment. Rather, most people spend a good deal of mental energy and focus either reliving the past, worrying about the future, or judging and analyzing events. Dwelling in the past leads to feelings of regret, anger, resentment, and depression. Constantly worrying about the future and all the potential dangers ahead leads to anxiety and stress. Mindfulness teachers often say that so much time is spent in the past or the future that we often miss the only time we actually have to live our lives—the present.

Hence, in order to train the capacity to become more mindful in everyday life, we turn to the second type of mindfulness, a skill that we build through the practice of mindfulness training, usually in the form of various meditation practices and exercises. One model that encompasses this is called the IAA model of mindfulness.[1] The "I" stands for "Intention," which is the "Why" of the practice. To be mindful we first have to do it on purpose, or intentionally. Intention is considered the guiding star for one's mindfulness practice and may vary over time. A beginning intention may be simply to learn to be more present for oneself and in one's relationships; others may desire to learn to be more mindful because they've heard it might help them manage stress, sleep better, cope with pain, gain a sense of meaning and purpose in life, etc. Whatever the intention, lightly held, it serves as motivation and direction for sustaining the practice.

The fist "A" stands for "Attention," the "What" of the practice. The core of the training is building the capacity to direct attention when and where one chooses, for sustained periods of time. Meditation focusing on the breath or the body is often used to train this capacity. Cultivating attention requires repeated sustained practice, most often 20–45 minutes daily, as recommended in most standardized mindfulness training programs. Constantly returning to the focal point when the mind wanders retrains the brain and enhances the capacity of the mind to stay focused in the present; this training not only improves the capacity to pay attention, but also has repercussions in the neuronal wiring of the brain.[2]

The second "A" is for "Attitude," the "How" of the practice. It is essential to apply attitudes of kindness, curiosity, openness, patience, and acceptance to the learning process because it can be difficult and frustrating, and this can lead to discontinuation of mindfulness training if one does not apply these attitudes. People need to recognize that retraining the mind in the capacity to pay kind attention is not easy, despite its simplicity, and be kind to themselves when their minds inevitably wander and they struggle to sustain attention. Without these attitudes, people are much more likely to give up on mindfulness meditation programs. Applying acceptance, non-striving, and letting go of the need to control life events that are outside of one's control are also keys to adjusting to serious illness.

What Are Mindfulness-Based Interventions?

"MBIs" is the collective term for standardized mindfulness training programs based on the Mindfulness-Based Stress Reduction (MBSR) model developed by Jon Kabat-Zinn at the University of Massachusetts Medical Center in 1979.[3] At that time, Kabat-Zinn and colleagues integrated intensive training in mindfulness meditation modeled on Eastern

Buddhist approaches with current popular cognitive behavioral methods of stress reduction to create a standardized 8-week group training program. This program included daily practice of 45-minute home mindfulness meditation and gentle Hatha yoga (a popular form of yoga practiced in North America consisting of breathing exercises [*pranayama*] and gentle physical postures [*asanas*]), along with weekly group discussion, inquiry around embodied practice, and didactic learning. The group was first offered to people with a variety of intractable medical conditions and symptoms including chronic pain, anxiety, cardiovascular disease, and fibromyalgia. Kabat-Zinn documents the benefits and transformations associated with this program in his book *Full Catastrophe Living*.[3]

Since that time, MBSR has steadily grown in popularity, and many clinicians and researchers have been trained in the MBSR model, going on to create their own adaptations specific to many psychological and medical conditions. The most well-known of these is mindfulness-based cognitive therapy (MBCT), which was intentionally and theoretically developed to address the maladaptive cognitions that serve as risk factors for depression relapse.[4] Other adaptations include mindfulness-based relapse prevention for addictions,[5] our program mindfulness-based cancer recovery for people living with cancer,[6] mindfulness-based eating awareness training for eating disorders,[7] and many others[1] (see Table 38.1). Research investigating the efficacy of these programs across a wide range of conditions has grown exponentially since the first few studies appeared in the late 1990s.

Acceptance and commitment therapy (ACT)[8] and existential behavior therapy (EBT)[9] are two individually delivered psychological interventions that incorporate mindfulness skills but include more emphasis on cognitive processes and behavior change strategies. They are sometimes included in reviews of MBIs, although typically only adaptations of the MBSR group model are included under this umbrella term. ACT is designed to bring language and cognition to heel, with psychological flexibility as the ultimate goal of treatment.[10] Psychological flexibility refers to the ability to change one's behavior in ways that

TABLE 38.1 A summary list of adapted mindfulness-based interventions (MBIs) and the conditions for which they have been tailored

Mindfulness-based intervention	Condition adapted for	Other applications
Mindfulness-Based Cognitive Therapy[4]	Preventing depression relapse	Treating depression and anxiety symptoms in other psychological conditions
Mindfulness-Based Relapse Prevention[1]	Addictions (alcohol/drug dependence)	Smoking cessation
Mindfulness-Based Cancer Recovery[6]	Cancer survivors	Patients during treatment, family members
Mindfulness-Based Eating Awareness Training/ Mindful Eating-Conscious Living[7]	Binge eating disorder	Obesity
Mindfulness-Based Art Therapy[1]	Medical conditions	Wide application
Mindful Self-Compassion[1]	People with low self-compassion	Wide application
Mindfulness-Based Awareness Training (M-BAT)[1]	First responders/military	Business

serve one's goals and values, in a context of mindfully attending to the internal and external experiences occurring at the present moment.[10] Similarly, EBT involves a mindfulness approach to help explore human reality from the perspective of the patient to achieve therapeutic goals.[11] The literature on the value of ACT and EBT across a wide range of conditions shows promising results across various psychological and medical outcomes.[12,13]

How Have Mindfulness-Based Interventions Been Integrated into Medical Care?

The work of Kabat-Zinn in developing MBSR and creating a training pathway for MBSR teachers at the UMass Center for Mindfulness spearheaded the widespread adoption of MBIs into Western medicine, beginning in the 1990s and quickly escalating in the 21st century. Along with widespread clinical adoption and adaptation of MBIs, research efforts also increased exponentially (see Figure 38.1), to the point where hundreds and even thousands of scientific papers are published each year pertaining to some form of mindfulness or MBIs.

A recent meta-synthesis of meta-analyses included 28 separate meta-analyses of randomized controlled trials assessing the effects of meditation on health outcomes, which collectively included more than 31,000 participants.[14] A medium-sized effect of meditation on health was obtained after aggregating across meta-analyses (d = 0.50) on aggregate measures of both mental health (e.g., anxiety, depression, stress) and physical health (e.g., blood pressure, blood sugar, hemoglobin, pain, diagnosed health conditions, insomnia) across an extremely wide range of clinical populations.

All told, the literature on the value of MBIs across a wide range of physical and mental health conditions shows myriad potential benefits for addressing common features of

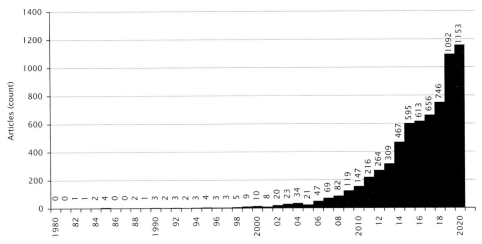

FIGURE 38.1 Articles in scientific journals with mindfulness in the title, published by year: 1980–2020. Source: goAMRA.org.

illness—uncertainty, feelings of loss of control, fear of disease recurrence or progression, symptom management, and diminished overall quality of life.

The question remains as to how much of this body of research is relevant or applicable in the context of palliative care. We conceptualize the palliative care team as consisting of the patient, informal caregiver(s), and healthcare providers (HCPs)/healthcare system and have organized the following sections accordingly. In the next section, we summarize the major psychosocial issues in palliative care and address how a mindfulness approach may be beneficial in addressing psychosocial issues specific to those facing chronic progressive disease and end-of-life.

What Are the Major Psychosocial Issues in Palliative Care?

Patients

Psychosocial health issues are common among palliative populations. While estimates of distress vary depending on the underlying condition, the rates are generally high. In one study of end-of-life patients, 46.4% had moderate to severe anxiety, and 43% had moderate to severe symptoms of depression.[15] A systematic review of the literature on chronic pain also reports psychiatric morbidity rates between 20% and 30% and depression rates between 6% and 30% using operationalized diagnostic criteria, such as the *Diagnostic and Statistical Manual of Mental Disorders* (DSM-IV) or International Classification of Diseases (ICD-10).[16] Higher prevalence rates are observed in terminally ill patients: 10–15% require professional psychiatric treatment or psychological counseling.[16] Additionally, palliative patients can experience functional impairment, and many need to depend on others for their basic needs (e.g., toileting), potentially undermining their sense of dignity. Healthcare costs in many countries impose a substantial financial burden on high-need patients such as those receiving palliative care, creating additional distress.

Palliative care recipients experience a broad range of medical symptoms. For instance, the prevalence of pain in this population has been estimated at 55–100%.[16] Other symptoms commonly associated with a terminal, advanced, or metastatic disease include fatigue, weakness, poor appetite, constipation, breathing difficulties, and nausea and vomiting. Poor pain and symptom management is associated with increased depression and insomnia, more suicidal thoughts, and worsening in quality of life.[16]

In people confronting end-of-life, distress can result from anticipatory grief and fear of death and the unknown in terms of what to expect in the afterlife. Patients can experience negative emotions such as stress, anxiety, and sadness due to impending separation from loved ones. Adolescents and young adults with a terminal prognosis may encounter major existential conflicts which can precipitate a period of urgency to complete milestones of early adulthood. In children, understanding the concept and finality of death and coping with their own life-threatening disease can be very challenging.

Informal Caregivers

Informal palliative caregivers provide physical, emotional, and practical support to a person with advanced, incurable, or progressive illness. They typically have a preexisting relationship with the patient by kinship or social ties (e.g., spouse, partner, family relative or friend) and are not financially compensated for their caregiving duties. Caring for palliative patients can be emotionally draining. It is estimated that 40–60% of informal caregivers experience heightened levels of psychological distress, which can result in greater distancing and poorer communication with patients.[17] Informal caregivers not only need to cope with the severe illness or possible death of a loved one, but also adapt to role changes within the family and new caregiving responsibilities. They are often expected to perform and engage in nursing-related activities as well as to play an active role in patient care and treatment decisions. Anxiety about the patient's comfort, disruption of their own work and social lives, financial concerns related to healthcare costs, and anticipatory grief are all additional factors that can contribute to informal caregiver distress.

Healthcare Providers

HCPs bear responsibility for attending to the comfort of patients. Those working in palliative care may experience high levels of distress and burnout while trying to meet the emotional, physical, and spiritual needs of people whose illness cannot be cured and who may be nearing the end of life. HCPs witness the pain and suffering of patients, sometimes in an intimate way. They often encounter situations of moral distress while trying to address ethical problems around decision-making (e.g., whether to discontinue mechanical life support for the terminally ill), which may involve uncertainties about patient wishes and quality of life. Families may hold unreasonable expectations about the patient's prognosis or be waiting for a "miracle," making them perceive palliative care as inadequate and thus place unreasonable demands upon HCPs. In these conditions, HCPs may understandably learn to use avoidant coping to manage these overwhelming negative emotions, thus diminishing the quality of patient care.

How Can Mindfulness Approaches Be Useful for Palliative Care Populations?

Patients

The primary goal of palliative care is to relieve pain and suffering. By paying attention to experiences occurring in the present moment with a nonjudgmental attitude, MBIs can enhance trait mindfulness (i.e., one's predisposition to be mindful in daily life) which leads to higher momentary awareness of thoughts and feelings and develops the capacity to better identify and regulate emotional responses to pain and other physical symptoms. Since palliative patients may not always have control over their physical symptoms, MBIs may also help them develop a more accepting and self-compassionate attitude toward suffering and enhance coping. For example, MBIs make clear the distinction between pain and suffering, noting that overall suffering is a product of pain itself, amplified by resistance to pain, both mental and physical. An individual may not be able to change the physiological causes of pain sensations, but by releasing physical (e.g., muscle clenching) and mental (e.g., aversion) resistance, suffering can be lessened through softening and acceptance, even in the face of continued pain.

In addition to enhancing higher quality moment-to-moment experiences and better pain management, mindfulness may give the person a greater sense of control by directing cognitive processes in more skillful and effective ways. For example, rather than focusing on things one cannot control or worrying about the unknown future, directing efforts toward more immediate, quality interactions with loved ones, creating legacy projects, for example, which usually decreases feelings of regret, depression, and worry caused by excessive past or future focus.

Symptoms in palliative patients may be related to spiritual and existential needs in addition to physical and psychological ones. To this end, mindfulness has long been associated with enhanced spiritual growth, defined as feeling a profound sense of connection to something larger than oneself (however defined), along with a clear sense of meaning and purpose in life. Through cultivating a nonreactive and stable awareness and seeing the self as part of a much larger whole, MBIs have been shown to enhance a sense of inner peace and thereby improve spiritual well-being and quality of life. Mindfulness practice can also help address existential concerns of palliative patients through acceptance and attention to life's most meaningful elements. Cultivating a level of comfort and peace with "not knowing" what the future will bring or what to expect after death can also decrease death anxiety in those near the end of life who struggle with these questions.

While spirituality and religion are related to one another, they are distinct concepts, with spirituality focusing more on one's sense of meaning and purpose in life and connection to a larger whole. Mindfulness is typically practiced within a secular context, which makes it suitable for enhancing spirituality in patients with different religious beliefs as well as those who are agnostic or not affiliated with any religion or set of organized beliefs. MBIs can also be adapted to palliative patients who find comfort and inner peace in their faith, by adding religious content as appropriate to strengthen spirituality, reduce distress, and improve end-of-life experiences.

Furthermore, MBIs place few demands on patients in terms of formal practice frequency as well as physical strength and mobility. As many palliative patients experience physical deconditioning and moderate to severe fatigue and pain, the availability of a gentle yet potentially effective supportive care intervention is crucial.

Informal Caregivers

Without adequate supportive interventions, informal caregivers of patients undergoing palliative care may be at high risk of psychological morbidity and poor health outcomes, especially if they have preexisting health conditions that compromise their ability to cope effectively with stress. MBIs can be easily integrated into daily routines of caregivers to mitigate psychological distress and foster more positive coping strategies. In end-of-life care, MBIs can help caregivers process and accept the approaching death of a loved one and deal with associated feelings such as loss and anger. As noted above, MBIs have the potential to direct mental processes in useful ways, promoting the emergence of positive immediate responses to stressors to improve general well-being. When the well-being of informal caregivers is enhanced, patient outcomes also improve.

Healthcare System

In-house evidence-based MBI programs may be beneficial in managing emotional and psychological distress in palliative patients and their families, as well as in reducing burnout and posttraumatic stress in HCPs working in palliative care settings, to equip them to provide optimal patient care. Adaptations in mindfulness style and intensity are possible for various populations (patients, informal caregivers, HCPs) with regard to preference, demographics, and physical condition. In addition, virtual (live and pre-recorded) and smartphone app–based MBIs are available and may promote uptake and maintenance of mindfulness practice by eliminating barriers of time and distance that often preclude in-person MBI programs.

Mindfulness practice can also be self-delivered at any time and from any place, which makes it accessible by patients in acute and hospice care settings as well as those being cared for at home. In the following section, we summarize and evaluate evidence available on the effects of MBIs on outcomes in palliative care for patients, informal caregivers, and HCPs.

Literature Review: Mindfulness-Based Interventions in Palliative Care

The psychosocial and existential issues faced by patients, informal caregivers, and HCPs working in palliative care are amenable targets for MBIs. The majority of the research to date has focused on adapting multicomponent MBIs that have been evaluated in other health populations, such as cancer patients, to the unique needs and requirements of end-of-life care.

Patients

A systematic review by Latorraca et al.[18] summarized the results of four randomized controlled trials ($N = 234$) examining the efficacy of mindfulness meditation for improving psychosocial outcomes of adults in palliative care. Three studies included palliative cancer patients while one study included patients with moderate to severe chronic obstructive pulmonary disease (COPD). The four studies evaluated four different MBIs: two studies examined the effects of a single session of mindfulness teaching and/or practice (e.g., 5-minute MBSR exercises and 90 minutes of guided body scan training), and two studies examined the effects of weekly sessions (e.g., six weekly 45-minute sessions of mindfulness-based training and eight weekly 2.5-hour sessions of MBSR with relaxation training). All studies but the 5-minute single session also encouraged participants to engage in daily practice. Furthermore, various HCPs (e.g., nurses, physicians) or mindfulness facilitators were involved in intervention delivery at home or the hospital.

Interestingly, the only study from this review that reported a statistically significant outcome in favor of the intervention group was the 5-minute single session of MBSR teaching.[19] In that study, 60 patients with cancer were randomized, and those who received the brief MBSR delivered by a physician experienced a significant reduction in perceived stress 10 minutes after the intervention when compared to the active control group receiving 5 minutes of active listening. This finding is likely an artifact of the immediate follow-up, and the persistence of this effect is unknown since longer-term follow-up data are not available.

The studies reported in the Latorraca et al.[18] review were criticized for being generally of low quality, at high risk of bias, and underpowered. The authors also caution that none of the studies analyzed adverse events or the safety of MBIs in palliative care settings. Furthermore, the search criteria for the Latorraca et al.[18] systematic review only included randomized controlled studies and thereby did not retrieve reports of alternate study designs like uncontrolled prospective studies (e.g., with pre-post assessment) or mixed-method designs. Such early phase research is also important to summarize as it provides information about the feasibility and patient acceptability of MBIs in palliative care.

For instance, a mixed-method study by Poletti et al.[20] examined the feasibility, acceptability, and preliminary effectiveness of an 8-week MBSR intervention for individuals with metastatic cancer attending an early palliative care program. The MBSR program followed the standard format, and consisted of 8 weekly meetings of 2.5 hours each, a 4.5-hour session between week 6 and 7, and 30 minutes of daily home practice. Adherence to home practice among the 16 participants that completed the program was 75%, and two participants could only attend six sessions due to illness progression.

Additionally, we have identified three further randomized controlled studies published since the 2017 Latorraca et al.[12] review, evaluating the effects of MBIs in palliative care. Building on the finding that a brief intervention may be sufficient to have a clinically significant short-term impact on psychosocial outcomes, all three studies investigated the effects of brief, 20-minute single session MBI's based on mindful breathing principles and MBSR, designed to be adjuncts to palliative care.

Beng et al.[21] recruited palliative patients with a suffering score of 4 or above on the Suffering Pictogram. Forty participants were randomly assigned to receive a 20-minute single session of mindful breathing with a trained physician or 20-minutes of active listening. Perceived level of suffering and pain was assessed at baseline, minute 5, 15 and 20 of the intervention. Both groups experienced a significant reduction in suffering between baseline and post-intervention, while the mindful breathing group experienced a significant reduction in pain compared to the active control group.

Next, Look et al.[22] randomized 40 patients, and the experimental condition participated in a 20-minute session of mindful breathing during which they were guided by the investigator to identify the in and out-breath, follow the length of the breath, bring attention back to the body, and engage in relaxation, compared to the control group receiving usual care. Participants randomized to the mindful breathing session experienced a significant reduction in the total Edmonton Symptoms Assessment Scale (ESAS) score, which assessed a range of symptoms including pain, tiredness, drowsiness, lack of appetite, shortness of breath, depression and anxiety, compared to control.

Finally, Warth et al.[23] conducted a crossover trial evaluating the effects of a pre-recorded excerpt of MBSR delivered at bedside compared to a resting state control comparison. The aim of the MBI was to shift attention away from symptom burden to the patient's breath and the present moment. This trial collected psychophysiological data in the form of heart rate variability (HRV), a measure of the variation in the time interval between heartbeats that can be used to infer the extent of sympathetic and parasympathetic nervous system activation, in addition to self-report information on stress and well-being. Forty-two participants were randomized and they found a significant reduction in self-rated stress, which persisted 20 to 40 minutes after the intervention compared to the control condition. HRV also increased immediately after the mindfulness intervention, indicating increase parasympathetic nervous system activation. There were no significant differences between groups on self-rated well-being.

Overall, participants experienced a mean reduction in pain and improvement in mood between baseline and post-intervention, similar to results in other MBSR program participants often reported in the literature. Specifically, participants reported a statistically significant reduction in fatigue and depression, as measured by the Profile of Mood States (POMS), and a trend towards reduction in cancer-related pain at post-intervention and 4-month follow-up. Results from qualitative interviews explicated that the MBSR program helped participants develop a more accepting attitude toward their illness, increased their attunement to emotions and face anxiety and cancer-related pain, and developed an openness to spiritual beliefs and values at end-of-life.

Overall, the available evidence to date suggests that MBIs may be beneficial for mitigating pain and distress in palliative patients. However, significant biases were possible in some of the studies identified due to design shortcomings. Though lack of evidence does not necessarily indicate a lack of effect, the mostly null results reported by this systematic review can likely be explained by the low quality of individual studies and reliance on small convenience samples. These limitations of the literature are worth noting. However they are not surprising given the early stage of research in this area.

Research reviewed seems to suggest that brief MBI programs that are shorter than the standard 8-week MBSR curriculum may be preferred by palliative populations, possibly due to limitations on energy and mobility and symptoms associated with disease progression. As a first step toward testing the effectiveness of MBIs, some of the reviewed studies also showed that MBI programs in palliative patients were feasible, providing the foundation needed for further investigations.

Informal Caregivers

Like the patient literature, investigating MBIs for informal caregivers is a relatively new field of inquiry. Jaffray et al.[24] performed a systematic review of MBIs for informal palliative caregivers and identified 13 articles reporting on 10 studies ($N = 432$). In contrast to the review by Latorraca et al.[18] of the patient literature, Jaffray et al.[24] did not limit their search by study design and thus retrieved four randomized controlled trials, four pre-post uncontrolled studies, and two wait-list controlled trials. Most studies (7 out of 10) investigated recruited caregivers of people with dementia, and the majority of caregivers in identified studies were female, White, and caring for spouses or partners. A wide range of MBI interventions were delivered, including MBSR ($n = 6$), MBCT ($n = 2$), ACT ($n = 1$), and EBT ($n = 1$), with protocols varying from 4 to 10 weekly sessions ranging from 1 to 2.5 hours and 10–45 minutes of assigned formal home practice. Five of seven studies found a significant reduction in depression, two of three found a significant increase in quality of life, and four out of five studies demonstrated a significant reduction in caregiver burden. Qualitative findings from an uncontrolled study of a "lower dose" (i.e., four weekly sessions) of MBSR with eight dementia caregivers identified that valued intervention effects included increased acceptance of the care recipient's illness, increased acceptance and decreased judgment toward self and family, increased sense of presence, peace and reduced stress, and decreased reactivity to challenging care recipient behavior. Furthermore, social support and self-regulation were identified as the most helpful elements of the EBT intervention by 16 caregivers of patients with advanced cancer or neurological conditions who were interviewed about their experience participating in the intervention.

Taken together, MBIs for informal palliative caregivers appear to decrease depression, increase quality of life and reduce caregiver burden. Jaffray et al.[24] point out, however, that the effects reported in these studies are less robust than those reported in the overall MBI literature, where effects on a variety of psychological and physical health outcomes are well-established. Furthermore, the use of small convenience samples likely compromises the generalizability of these findings to other palliative populations, and effects were generally inconsistent across studies making concrete conclusions difficult.

Healthcare Providers

Developing, evaluating, and implementing MBIs for HCPs in palliative care settings is an emerging field of research, complementary to ongoing research using a variety of therapeutic orientations and interventions to improve resilience in HCPs. Much of the research on MBIs to manage distress in palliative HCPs has focused on mindful communication practices. *Mindful communication* combines the core principles of mindfulness (present-centered and nonjudgmental awareness) with skills training to teach HCPs how to actively and attentively interact with patients. The purpose is to promote reflective, genuine, and adaptive communication, which may help HCPs develop flexibility and confidence in their ability to effectively communicate with patients while also feeling more in control over their emotional responses while engaging with their patient's suffering.

The effect of mindfulness-based communication training for palliative care professionals was evaluated in the pilot study of the Aware Compassionate Communication: An Experiential Provider Training Series (ACCEPTS) for Palliative Care Providers.[25] ACCEPTS was an 8-week (10 session) group-based training intervention that tailored mindfulness and acceptance-based strategies to the needs of HCPs working with chronically ill and palliative patients. The goal of the intervention was to reduce depression, burnout, and symptoms of posttraumatic stress by enhancing mindful communication and psychological flexibility. Psychological flexibility was selected as a key treatment target for HCPs because experiential avoidance and inflexibility in subjective beliefs are theoretically associated with increased distress, poor communication, and detachment from professional and personal values of compassion and beneficence. Beyond promoting communication and flexibility, ACCEPTS aimed to help HCPs learn to normalize and reduce judgmental reactions to uncomfortable experiences within professional settings in palliative care.[25]

ACCEPTS is a multicomponent program delivered in a group format by a psychologist, a palliative care physician, and meditation instructors. Each session is 1.5–2 hours in duration and composed of didactic content, mindfulness practice and skill acquisition, and discussion. Topics include mindfulness of the present moment, contemplating impermanence, thinking of own death/funeral, values and tension between patient and provider values, committed action, cultural competence, working with silence, listening skills, mindful communication, and mindfulness of difficult emotions.[25]

In total, 21 palliative care providers participated in the ACCEPTS intervention. The intervention significantly reduced depressive symptoms ($d = -.64$), posttraumatic stress disorder (PTSD) re-experiencing ($d = -.34$) and work-related depersonalization ($d = -.83$) post-treatment. There was also a significant decrease in cognitive fusion ($d = -.54$), which is the tendency to experience distressing thoughts as true. There were no significant post-treatment reductions in experiential avoidance ($d = -.29$), PTSD avoidance ($d = .04$) and hyperarousal ($d = -.29$), or work-related emotional exhaustion ($d = -.70$).[25]

Similarly, in a single group pilot study, Heeter et al.[26] evaluated a 6-week MBI program, consisting of five 10- to 12-minute meditations delivered via a smartphone app to palliative and hospice professionals ($n = 36$). Meditation exercises integrated focused attention, synchronized breath, and gentle movements. Participating HCPs used the meditations an average of 17 times during the intervention period. Results showed significant improvements in compassion fatigue, burnout, and interoceptive awareness. Participation also significantly increased active body listening, awareness of physical sensations, and perceived ability to direct attention to bodily sensations.

Overall, MBI programs appear to be acceptable and beneficial for palliative HCPs, reducing depressive and posttraumatic stress symptoms, and improving cognitive processes related to mindfulness practice such as cognitive fusion and interoceptive awareness. Despite the encouraging findings from these investigations, studies were generally nonrandomized, with small sample sizes. In contrast to the patient literature, much of the MBI studies in HCPs used similar intervention duration to the 8-week MBSR curriculum, and thus examination of effects of shorter intervention packages may be beneficial to account for time constraints typically faced by HCPs.

Future Directions

Over the past 10 years, an increasing number of studies have suggested that MBIs can reduce distress and improve quality of life in palliative and end-of-life patients and may help address psychosocial issues faced by their informal caregivers and HCPs. However, this body of research is nascent and has several limitations. First, despite encouraging findings from the reviewed investigations, many studies are of low quality with small sample sizes. Heterogeneity is also noticed in MBI program intensity, frequency, length, and training of facilitators, limiting the replicability of findings. Programs do not seem to have been adapted based on theory or to address specific symptoms common to the target population. Future research should employ more robust designs that use standardized MBI protocols tailored to the needs of palliative populations. For convenience and immediacy, they should be individualized (not group based) and available at the bedside, perhaps with a combination of professional in-person or videoconference delivery along with supportive app-based practice/teaching material. Short, single sessions may relieve symptoms in the short term, but likely ongoing access to guided meditations or professionally led sessions would be required to sustain relief over time.

A further limitation of this literature is the lack of patient-oriented research. It is crucial to engage patient partners in the development of MBI studies, involving them in the selection of outcomes, including those that are most important to patients at end of life, and intervention formats that would be appealing and acceptable to them. Such knowledge can ensure evaluating outcomes that are relevant to palliative populations and interventions that are feasible. Research is also needed to understand the mechanisms of mindfulness-related improvement in outcomes in palliative care. For instance, the field would benefit from studies to explore the most important skills or elements to teach within MBI programs offered to patients, informal caregivers, and clinicians to improve benefits and effectiveness. Qualitative and mixed-method research could provide a deep understanding of participants' perceptions of MBIs in great detail, including mechanisms of action as well as barriers to implementation of mindfulness in palliative care.

Additionally, participant samples in the reviewed studies appear to include primarily White women, which is a commonly cited limitation of mindfulness research more generally. Future studies may need to examine the efficacy of MBIs in more diverse samples to improve the generalizability of the results. Empirical investigation into long-term benefits and trajectories of effects of MBI programs in palliative care is another good prospect for future study to understand whether additional mindfulness sessions/intervention boosters are required to maintain benefits, bolster treatment effects, and prevent practice decay. Much of the research in this area also seems to involve in-person MBI programs. More research is needed to evaluate online MBIs that offer advantages over those in-person in terms of time and convenience. Online MBIs can be more accessible to palliative patients and their informal caregivers in rural areas. More importantly, online MBIs could be useful for palliative patients who are not able to receive in-person supportive care interventions due to deteriorating health or the current COVID-19 pandemic.

Last, as most MBI studies in palliative patients have used brief interventions, researchers may wish to examine the role of palliative HCPs in delivering mindfulness sessions versus more experienced professional mindfulness instructors to help address implementation barriers, including assessment of what types of HCPs have the required expertise, skill, and time to deliver MBIs. Given the importance of moving from efficacy to effectiveness for successful implementation of MBIs into palliative care settings, this is a crucial question to address.

Key Points

- Mindfulness meditation is one supportive approach that involves nonjudgmentally paying attention to the internal and external experiences occurring in the present moment. It has been suggested that mindfulness techniques can mitigate stress-related symptomatology and help patients cope with chronic pain through cultivating a nonjudgmental awareness to everyday stressful situations.

- In addition to heightened levels of distress, palliative patients can experience a broad range of unpleasant symptoms, most notably pain. Attention to emotional distress and physical symptoms can often allow for improvement in functioning and quality of life even at the very end of life.

- Informal caregivers bear responsibility to provide support to their loved ones, often accompanied by distress. HCPs working in palliative care settings are repeatedly exposed to the trauma and distress of their patients and their caregivers, and they may spend less time with patients and their families as a way to reduce contact with events that trigger emotional sequelae.

- Within the context of palliative and end-of-life care, preliminary evidence has accumulated in support of the psychosocial benefits of MBIs for patients, informal caregivers, and HCPs. Brief MBIs can be implemented easily in hospitals and healthcare clinics and seem to be appealing to patients. More research is needed that addresses the limitations of existing research, especially with regard to enhanced methodological quality (e.g., adequately powered trials, active controls) and more representative samples.

- The techniques of mindfulness meditation may represent an effective adjunct intervention for transforming the ways in which palliative populations are cared for, and they are easily adaptable to the needs of various populations including patients, informal caregivers, and HCPs. More research is needed to identify and address barriers to sustainability and scalability.

References

1. Shapiro SL, Carlson LE. *The Art and Science of Mindfulness: Integrating Mindfulness Into Psychology and the Helping Professions, Second Edition*. Washington, DC: American Psychological Association; 2017.

2. Hölzel BK, Hoge EA, Greve DN, Gard T, Creswell JD, Brown KW et al. Neural mechanisms of symptom improvements in generalized anxiety disorder following mindfulness training. *NeuroImage Clin.* 2013;2:448–458. doi:10.1016/j.nicl.2013.03.011

3. Kabat-Zinn J. *Full Catastrophe Living: Using the Wisdom of Your Body and Mind to Face Stress, Pain, and Illness (Revised Edition)*. New York: Delacourt; 2013.

4. Segal Z V., Williams M, Teasdale J, Kabat-Zinn J. *Mindfulness-Based Cognitive Therapy for Depression, Second Edition*. New York: Guilford; 2002.

5. Bowen S, Chawla N, Marlatt G. *Mindfulness-Based Relapse Prevention for Addictive Behaviors: A Clinician's Guide*. New York: Guilford; 2010.

6. Carlson LE, Speca M. *Mindfulness-Based Cancer Recovery: A Step-by-Step MBSR Approach to Help You Cope with Treatment and Reclaim Your Life*. New York: Harbinger; 2011.

7. Kristeller JL, Wolever RQ. Mindfulness-based eating awareness training for treating binge eating disorder: The conceptual foundation. *Eat Disord.* 2011;19(1):49–61. doi:10.1080/10640266.2011.533605

8. Hayes SC, Strosahl K, Wilson KG. *Acceptance and Commitment Therapy. An Experiential Approach to Behavior Change.* New York: Guilford; 1999.

9. Spinelli E. *Tales of Un-Knowing: Therapeutic Encounters from an Existential Perspective.* London: Duckworth; 1997.

10. McCracken LM, Vowles KE. Acceptance and commitment therapy and mindfulness for chronic pain: Model, process, and progress. *Am Psychol.* 2014;69(2):178–187. doi:10.1037/a0035623

11. Corbett L, Milton M. Existential therapy: A useful approach to trauma? *Counselling Psychology Review.* 2011;26(1):62–74.

12. Vos J, Cooper M, Correia EA, Craig M. Existential therapies: A review of their scientific foundations and efficacy. *Existential Analysis.* 2015;26(1)49–69.

13. Veehof MM, Trompetter HR, Bohlmeijer ET, Schreurs KMG. Acceptance- and mindfulness-based interventions for the treatment of chronic pain: A meta-analytic review. *Cogn Behav Ther.* 2016;45(1):5–31. doi:10.1080/16506073.2015.1098724

14. Rose S, Zell E, Strickhouser J. The effect of meditation on health: A metasynthesis of randomized controlled trials. *Mindfulness (N Y).* 2020;11. doi:10.1007/s12671-019-01277-6

15. Kozlov E, Phongtankuel V, Prigerson H, Adelman R, Shalev A, Czaja S, et al. Prevalence, severity, and correlates of symptoms of anxiety and depression at the very end of life. *J Pain Symptom Manage.* 2019;58(1):80–85. doi:10.1016/j.jpainsymman.2019.04.012

16. Thekkumpurath P, Venkateswaran C, Kumar M, Bennett MI. Screening for psychological distress in palliative care: A systematic review. *J Pain Symptom Manage.* 2008;36(5):520–528. doi:10.1016/j.jpainsymman.2007.11.010

17. Dumont S, Turgeon J, Allard P, Gagnon P, Charbonneau C, Vézina L. Caring for a loved one with advanced cancer: Determinants of psychological distress in family caregivers. *J Palliat Med.* 2006;9(4):912–921. doi:10.1089/jpm.2006.9.912

18. Latorraca C de OC, Martimbianco ALC, Pachito DV, Pacheco RL, Riera R. Mindfulness for palliative care patients: Systematic review. *Int J Clin Pract.* 2017;71(12):e13034. doi:10.1111/ijcp.13034

19. Ng CG, Lai KT, Tan SB, Sulaiman AH, Zainal NZ. The effect of 5 minutes of mindful breathing to the perception of distress and physiological responses in palliative care cancer patients: A randomized controlled study. *J Palliat Med.* 2016;19(9):917–924. doi:10.1089/jpm.2016.0046

20. Poletti S, Razzini G, Ferrari R, Ricchieri MP, Spedicato GA, Pasqualini A, et al. Mindfulness-based stress reduction in early palliative care for people with metastatic cancer: A mixed-method study. *Complement Ther Med.* 2019;47:102218. doi:10.1016/j.ctim.2019.102218

21. Beng TS, Jie HW, Yan LH, Ni CX, Capelle DP, Yee A, et al. The effect of 20-minute mindful breathing on the perception of suffering and changes in bispectral index score in palliative care patients: A randomized controlled study. *Am J Hosp Palliat Care.* 2019;36(6):478–484. doi:10.1177/1049909118812860

22. Look ML, Tan SB, Hong LL, Ng CG, Yee HA, Lim LY, et al. Symptom reduction in palliative care from single session mindful breathing: A randomised controlled trial. *BMJ Support Palliat Care.* 2021;11(4):433-439. doi:10.1136/bmjspcare-2020-002382

23. Warth M, Koehler F, Aguilar-Raab C, Bardenheuer HJ, Ditzen B, Kessler J. Stress-reducing effects of a brief mindfulness intervention in palliative care: Results from a randomised, crossover study. *Eur J Cancer Care (Engl).* 2020;29(4):e13249. doi:10.1111/ecc.13249

24. Jaffray L, Bridgman H, Stephens M, Skinner T. Evaluating the effects of mindfulness-based interventions for informal palliative caregivers: A systematic literature review. *Palliat Med.* 2016;30(2):117–131. doi:10.1177/0269216315600331

25. Gerhart J, Omahony S, Abrams I, Grosse J, Greene M, Levy M. A pilot test of a mindfulness-based communication training to enhance resilience in palliative care professionals. *J Context Behav Sci.* 2016;5. doi:10.1016/j.jcbs.2016.04.003

26. Heeter C, Lehto R. Meditation app benefits hospice and palliative care clinicians. *Oncology Nursing News.* Published online July 31, 2018. https://www.oncnursingnews.com/view/meditation-app-benefits-hospice-and-palliative-care-clinicians

39

Acceptance and Commitment Therapy

Nicholas J. Hulbert-Williams and Lee Hulbert-Williams

There has been a substantial growth in both awareness and use of acceptance and commitment therapy (ACT) within palliative care. In this chapter, we outline the conceptual background of ACT, particularly focusing on how this fits with and differs from other types of psychotherapeutic intervention. Following this, we describe why ACT seems suitable for those affected by life-limiting illness, reflecting on our knowledge as researchers and Dr. Nick Hulbert-Williams's experience as an applied coaching psychologist with experience of working directly with this client group. We close the chapter with a review of the evidence base. In some regards this evidence base is scant and so one might think that ACT remains relatively unused within palliative care settings. But that is not the case: as is happening in other therapeutic approaches, a recent increase in training opportunities has meant a growth in use by practitioners working in palliative care. While we do not discourage this, we will use this chapter to advocate for more research to ensure that ACT is being applied in the most appropriate and efficacious way for this specific population.

A Conceptual Introduction to ACT

In our experience, the best way to familiarize oneself with the ACT model may be to contrast it against an earlier and now dominant approach to psychotherapy—cognitive behavioral therapy (CBT). Aaron Beck's seminal work in the 1960s was intended to provide an alternative to the psychodynamic way of understanding the neuroses—and especially depression. Borrowing heavily from the Stoic philosophers, one of Beck's chief insights was that his client's thinking patterns were largely responsible for the way they felt: "People are not disturbed by things, but by the view they take of them" (Epictetus).

By changing a client's thoughts about events, themselves, or the wider world, the therapist might bring about lasting change in how the client *felt* about various things. This approach is now widely known as *cognitive restructuring*, and a large number of clinical techniques have been developed to help in the process. (For an excellent overview, see Beck.)[1] CBT has substantial empirical support, including within palliative care (see Chapter 34 of this textbook). Nonetheless, there are reasons to believe that this focus on cognitive restructuring can sometimes be unhelpful.

In early work that would later inform ACT, Hayes[2] drew on clinical experience to suggest that clients' thinking patterns often take on the function of reason-giving for behaviors done and left undone. Much though we are all taught as children to give socially acceptable reasons for our behaviours, this does not mean that we always have an accurate awareness of what is actually *causing* our behaviours. For instance, a client might report that they want to engage in a frank conversation with their loved ones about the end of life. They might report deep ambivalence—feeling torn to the point of anguish. They might also report their reason for not doing so—perhaps that their loved ones could not cope. The CBT approach, and indeed the common approach in our society, might be to appeal to the person's logic, analyze the situation, and attempt to help them act in accordance with their own values. Engaging in cognitive restructuring like this might be futile if, in fact, the client has other reasons—of which they may be hardly aware—for holding back from such conversations. To be brief: reasons are not always causes.

A second factor which might lead us to be skeptical of cognitive refutation is that, under certain circumstances, such attempts can backfire. There is now a broad evidence base, mostly from experimental cognitive psychology, showing that deliberate efforts *not* to think a certain thought can often result in that thought becoming more frequent and believable.[3] This is not to say that cognitive restructuring cannot work, only that it brings with it the risk of such "paradoxical" effects.

If the therapist is not to use logic, visual imagery, and a dozen other techniques to change how the client thinks about things, then how does ACT suggest one ought to proceed?

The ACT approach rests on an insight regarding the centrality of experiential avoidance to a wide range of psychological problems and differing forms of distress. The co-developers of ACT have argued that "many forms of psychopathology can be conceptualized as unhealthy efforts to escape and avoid emotions, thoughts, memories."[4] (p. 1152) This is where the "acceptance" in ACT comes from. It is not an invitation to accept events as they are or to take a fatalistic attitude to life. Rather, the client is invited to recognize that unpleasant feelings and thoughts are an inevitable part of life.

Everything that we value in life brings inherently the risk for unwelcome emotions, thoughts, and physical sensations. Hard work risks fatigue, ambition risks failure, and love risks grief, opening oneself up to another person risks rejection, and so on. The contrary belief, that unpleasant feelings and thoughts are avoidable, even pathological, can initiate a devastating narrowing of one's behavioral repertoire. ACT's various processes aim at teaching "psychological flexibility"—the ability and willingness to experience the inevitable suffering that comes along with choosing to pursue what we value.

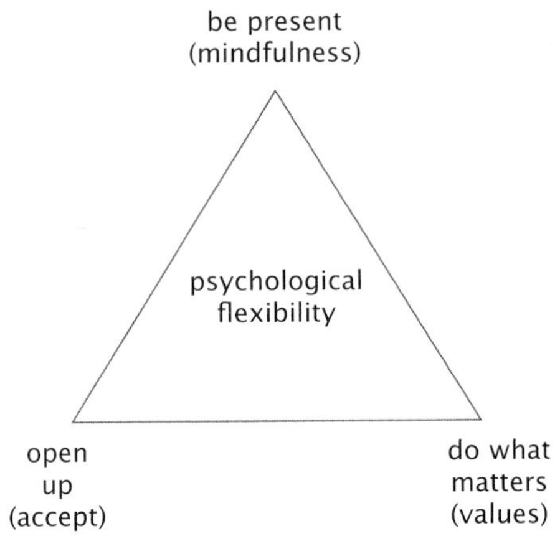

FIGURE 39.1 The "triflex" model of acceptance and commitment therapy (ACT).

ACT therapists make liberal use of conceptual diagrams which act as *aides memoires* and which can also function as basic case conceptualization tools. The most accessible such model is the"'triflex" (see Figure 39.1).

One important component of this model is mindfulness, which of course has its own stand-alone evidence base within palliative care (see Chapter 38). ACT is fundamentally a mindfulness-based intervention approach, though the degree to which different practitioners teach mindfulness practice as a formal part of ACT varies considerably. Even for those ACT practitioners who do not engage in long meditation sessions with clients, the basic philosophy of mindfulness is present. ACT is intertwined with a substantial body of basic research in human cognition, and this research supports the common-sense view that human beings often get carried away with their own thoughts about an event or situation, even to the point of losing psychological contact with that event or situation. We have a great many expressions in common parlance for experiences of this sort: "I felt like I was on another planet. I felt like nothing was real. I was just in my head the whole time." Such experiences might represent the extreme point of such phenomena, where the person themself becomes aware that they are paying more attention to their thoughts about a situation than to the situation itself. The research on this kind of metacognition is in its infancy, but clinical experience suggests that this kind of overanalysis, of living in one's head, is unhelpful. This claim seems to be backed up by related work showing that rumination is linked to psychopathology[5] and that attempting to experience events without overanalysis is generally salutary.[6]

The above "triflex" is often broken down into six components in order to better reflect the types of exercises ACT practitioners actually use with clients (see Figure 39.2).[7] Here you'll see that *doing what matters* has been broken down into *values* and *committed action*. *Opening up* and *being present* in the triflex map directly onto *acceptance* and *contact with the present moment* respectively on the "hexaflex."

The resulting hexaflex also includes, for instance, the process of *defusion*, which describes a group of exercises and techniques designed to undermine the literality of

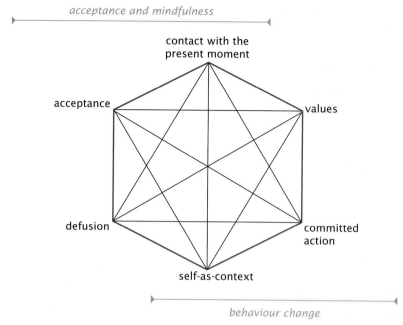

acceptance and mindfulness

contact with the
present moment

acceptance

values

defusion

committed
action

self-as-context

behaviour change

FIGURE 39.2 The "hexaflex" model of acceptance and commitment therapy (ACT).

language-based thinking. Whereas a traditional CBT approach might involve attempting to change the *content* of unpleasant thoughts, an ACT approach would more likely focus on changing the *relationship* of the client to that thought. The most common defusion exercises involve either meditation techniques or physical metaphors where the person is encouraged to see that the thought is not inherently part of them and to experience the thought as something that happens to them.[8]

Defusion techniques can be somewhat difficult to teach, and some clients find they have relatively little patience for learning them initially. Nonetheless, ACT-consistent work can be done by focusing on whichever processes seem most achievable at the time. There is no strict order for applying the processes, and some of the ACT processes have an evidence base in their own right. Taken together, intervening on the various components of the ACT model increases the individual's level of *psychological flexibility*.

While *defusion* (and, indeed *self-as-context*) are established and important ACT processes which both relate closely to mindfulness, it's not altogether clear from the empirical literature how they fit within the distinct constructs on the triflex model. Described abstractly, it can also be difficult to see how ACT can be applied when working with individual clients, but the next section will hopefully clarify that. Before moving on we recommend reading the metaphor presented in Box 39.1: developed for clients with noncurative illness, this metaphor represents what psychological flexibility is, and isn't, and is often a good "conversation starter" when beginning ACT-based work with clients.

BOX 39.1 The BEACHeS Metaphor

ACT makes considerable use of metaphor as therapeutic strategy. In developing our BEACHeS (Brief Engagement and Acceptance Coaching for Hospice and Community Settings) intervention,[9] we adapted a metaphor shared with us by a psychologist who worked in palliative care. The script below is a simplified version of that metaphor and will give you a sense of how psychological flexibility is conceptualized within ACT interventions.

Imagine you go to the beach one day. When you arrive, the tide is way out and you have a very wide space of beach to enjoy. Maybe you set up your camp, perhaps walking on the flat wet sand, making a little cricket or football pitch, sitting and reading, sun bathing etc. [Help the client to then generate the kinds of things they would like to do at the beach].

After a while, you notice that the tide has turned and is beginning to come up the beach toward you. What might your reactions be to the tide turning? [Generate thoughts and feelings about the tide turning].

You have choices about how you deal with knowing that the tide has turned. You could pack up and leave the beach, you could turn your back on the tide and pretend like it's not coming in, you could stand shouting at the tide, fighting it to go back, or just move your things up the beach and carry on doing what you were doing, with less space. [At this point see if you can get the patient to generate as many different options of what they actually could do in that scenario].

Maybe you need to change what you are doing several times as the tide comes in, perhaps it happens that there isn't enough room left for football, but you can still do something else, maybe at the last you are sitting on a tiny strip of beach, by a campfire, watching the sun go down.

What if our work could be about learning how to let go of strategies that aren't working, like turning your back on the sea, packing up and going home early, and instead clarifying how you want to be, what you most want to be doing and finding ways to do that, even as the tide slowly reduces the amount of space you have to play? [Give the client time to absorb it, space to reflect].

Thanks to David Gillanders and Nick Hulbert-Williams for giving permission for this to be shared from the BEACHeS Intervention Manual.

Special Considerations for Using ACT in Palliative Care

When delivering psychosocial care to those with chronic or potentially curative illness, our goals are often focused on helping clients to manage short-term distress and training skills to help them to self-manage psychological complications that may arise from their illness at some future point. However, the nature of palliative illness means that some of these therapeutic goals have to change simply because the context is different for this client group.

For example, rather than working with clients on managing their distressing emotional reactions to the thought that their cancer may return in an untreatable way at some unknown point in the future, we are instead working with a group for whom the end of life is inevitable and may be not far away. Grounding those clients in the present moment can be beneficial (e.g., to reduce worry about future symptoms) but is also a considerable challenge where that requires confronting—rather than avoiding—that inevitable outcome. For this reason, other ACT processes go hand in hand to helping clients to be in the present moment while having the necessary skills to manage the psychological suffering that that concurrently might bring up for them.

One of the particular difficulties in teaching ACT-based skills to a client with palliative illness is that so much of our work is about committing to making values-driven choices about what to do with their life. We are often confronted with responses like "But my life is now too short to do those things that I really wanted to do? What's the point if I'm going to die anyway?" In any ACT intervention we work with clients to help them to understand the difference between goals and values, and that is especially important for those approaching end of life. While it is true that their lives may now be too curtailed to achieve some of those big life goals, in understanding *why* those were important goals to begin with, we can work with a client to enact those same underlying values in a different way. There are psychological benefits to engaging with life more purposefully, even if we can only do that for brief spells of 10 or 20 minutes each day. Making these values-driven choices brings a sense of control to a client's life, and this is sometimes important for those who feel that decisions in other domains of life are now outside of their control.

It is in the very essence of being a social species that a vast majority of clients identify "family" as a core value. This can be particularly challenging for younger people at the end of life. Prof. Nick Hulbert-Williams worked with a client in her late 30s—Sophie (a pseudonym)—some years ago who was being treated for stage IV breast cancer.

One skill that is easily overlooked in general ACT training, but that is often crucial when working with clients at the end of life, is in not only identifying and committing to values, but communicating those wishes to others. While relevant to anyone undergoing ACT, and particularly for those re-engaging with values that necessitate considerable changes to usual activities, for those with advanced and progressing illness, the time span to make those changes is often short. The end of life is often (though not always) a time where clients increase time spent with family and close friends, and so any change in chosen activities may have a potentially bigger impact beyond just the client whom we are working with. It is, therefore, important to discuss how our clients may broach the outcomes of those values-based exercises with other people who might also be affected. This is often challenging for clients who may feel torn between (a) doing what's going to bring most value and personal meaning and (b) doing what's going to best prepare loved ones for their future grief. Supporting the client to communicate with their family about their therapeutic work can therefore be profoundly important.

Legacy Building

Sophie had been seeking psychological support for many years since receiving her palliative diagnosis. She wasn't depressed or anxious, but told me that she couldn't shift the thought that her life will have been meaningless because she hadn't left a legacy behind. None of the therapists she had worked with had been able to help her with that, and so she came to me for coaching support instead.

We did some initial work to explore what "legacy" meant to Sophie, exploring whether this could be achieved through some kind of work-related achievement or goals related to her hobbies. But for Sophie, legacy came from having children, something that her illness and treatment had rendered her unable to do. Over a few brief sessions, we explored what values underpinned this now unachievable goal of being a mother.

This was not easy work for Sophie, but when we explored this deeply we developed a shared understanding that this was about "passing on her life lessons" and of "not being forgotten."

Once we knew that these were the underpinning values we brainstormed potential ideas for how Sophie might feel that her life was more aligned to achieving these outcomes. She tried a number of things, such as volunteering in a nursery, but many of these didn't work for her. She later told me that she had a 10-year-old god-daughter who she had distanced from when she was diagnosed with cancer because she "didn't want her to see her looking poorly and without hair." Sophie decided to reconnect with her friend (the mother) to explore how to also reconnect with her god-daughter.

When Sophie returned for a follow-up some weeks later, she explained that she had seen her god-daughter a number of times. She smiled when explaining how much she enjoyed "spoiling her" with gifts and trips out and that she now looked after her, on her own, for a few hours each week when she felt well enough.

This was my last session with Sophie. She said shortly before the end of that session, "It really hurts that I can't have children of my own, but at least I now know that my god-daughter and her family will remember me after I die." She declined any further sessions at the cancer center because she "had never needed therapy"; she just needed "someone to help [her] find a way to do something to give her life some meaning despite her illness."

This is often complicated by the fast-moving and rapidly changing nature of palliative illness. Often, we'll encourage clients to "try on" different ways of committing to their values to establish what will bring most purpose to that individual. But interventions that last several weeks can be burdensome for this client group, particularly when these need coordinating around other care appointments and treatments. Furthermore, the accelerating nature of palliative illness might mean that some clients may not be well enough to complete an 8- (or more) week intervention program. As a result, we have to think creatively about brief and innovative delivery methods in palliative care.

Prof. Nick Hulbert-Williams has delivered a single-day, group-based, ACT coaching workshop for people with cancer. He recalls working with Brenda (a pseudonym), a client with end-stage lung cancer who attended one of these workshops some years ago.

We share this case study for two reasons. First, to counter concerns that we've frequently heard from colleagues that the therapeutic goals of ACT are just too challenging and difficult for those approaching the end of life. This is certainly not our experience—whether a client has days or years left to live, enacting a values-driven choice about how to spend the next couple of hours even is possible and can be empowering. ACT gives people the skills, and permission, to be able to make choices for themselves where they are still able to.

Second, when we have trained practitioners in using ACT, one of the frequent concerns raised is how values work might lead clients to make selfish choices that benefit only themselves, when the goals of palliative care should instead be about supporting whole family for the end of life. This case study demonstrates how effectively delivered ACT can be beneficial beyond just the client who we are working with; enacting her values meant that Brenda could finally have difficult—and previously avoided—conversations with her family. They were secondary beneficiaries of Brenda's experience with ACT.

What Is the Evidence for ACT?

Since its inception in the 1980s, ACT has been subject to an exponential increase in clinical trials. The professional body most closely connected with ACT (the Association for Contextual Behavioural Science) now lists more than 800 published randomized controlled trials.[9] Though the results are encouraging, no large set of clinical trials is without ambiguity, and so it is equally important that these findings have now been grouped and summarized in more than 200 reviews and meta-analyses.[9]

Gloster and colleagues[10] produced a meta-review which is useful as a jumping-off point for practitioners wanting to navigate this evidence base. They identified 20 meta-analyses which provided a meta-analytic effect size estimate specifically comparing ACT to another treatment or non-treatment control. They concluded that ACT is better than or equivalent to other active treatments across a range of conditions and outcomes including anxiety, depression, and chronic pain.

Some notable critics of ACT have also reviewed the evidence. For instance, a review and meta-analysis published in 2014 reported that there was, at the time, little evidence of ACT's superiority over traditional CBT.[11] Furthermore, as with many other types of psychotherapy, the methodological quality of many ACT trials is less than ideal.[11]

A number of professional bodies now list ACT as an evidence-based intervention for a range of disorders and client issues. Division 12 of the American Psychological Association (the clinical psychology division) rate the evidence base as "modest" for mixed anxiety disorders, as "modest" for depression, and as "strong" for chronic or persistent pain (see https://div12.org/psychological-treatments/). The UK National Institute for Health and Care Excellence also recommends ACT for chronic pain (see https://www.nice.org.uk/

Finding Values

I was trepidatious about how a workshop initially designed for cancer survivors would work for her, but I spoke to Brenda to explain that some parts may be emotionally difficult and that the day could feel long, so she should take breaks or leave early if she needed to. She remained quiet throughout the day, engaging with exercises but not group discussions. (She later explained that because most other group members were cancer survivors, she didn't want to tell her story and remove their hope.) I checked in with Brenda during scheduled breaks, and she told me that she was getting a lot out of the day and wanted to stay.

Brenda stayed behind after everyone had left at the end. I remember her thanking me for "opening her eyes" to the opportunities still available to her at the end of life. She told me that while other members of her care team had spoken compassionately and empathically, she had interpreted those discussions as psychologically preparing her to accept that her life was coming to end. By contrast, Brenda explained that the ACT approach made her realize that there was still life left to life, and she still had control over what that looked like.

I saw Brenda at the cancer center around 3 weeks later. She was visibly more symptomatic and doing poorly. She told me that she had spent more time outside and even though she couldn't walk far it was better than being "cooped-up" inside the house. Brenda had also had important conversations with family members about her hopes for their lives after she had died. She described how difficult these were, but that they were more meaningful than "just discussing shared memories of her life." She explained how she hoped remembering those conversations would help her family with their grief and described feeling more "at peace" with her approaching death.

Brenda died a short while later. I was told that her family (who had never previously visited the center) came in to express their thanks for the support that was provided to the whole family.

guidance/ng193), while the Australian Psychological Society has concluded that ACT enjoys "Level II" support (involving "an independent, blinded comparison with a valid reference standard, among consecutive persons with a defined clinical presentation") across a broad range of conditions and outcomes (see https://psychology.org.au/getmedia/23c6a11b-2600-4e19-9a1d-6ff9c2f26fae/evidence-based-psych-interventions.pdf).

ACT Interventions for People with Life-Limiting Illness

Despite the growth of interest in using ACT within palliative care, we remain surprised at the lack of evidence currently available and the focus, almost exclusively, on people with advanced cancer and not other types of palliative illness.

Two cross-sectional surveys explore potential therapeutic mechanisms of ACT-based processes within palliative samples. Low and colleagues[12] recruited participants from palliative day therapy units and report significant correlations between psychological flexibility and both psychological morbidity and physical function (2-minute walking test and 1-minute sit-to-stand test) outcomes. In one of our own forthcoming papers we have surveyed 178 people with cancer, including a subsample of 51 with palliative diagnoses. Across our full sample, preliminary analysis suggests that psychological flexibility moderates the relationships between fighting spirit and desire for hastened death, and between fear of cancer progression and depression.

Modeling work aside, the intervention evidence for using ACT in palliative care is in its infancy. A number of programs of work, primarily from North America and the United Kingdom, have reported results from early-phase acceptability, pilot, or feasibility studies for those with advanced cancer; we have selected a few which best demonstrate the breadth of work in development.

O'Hayer and colleagues[13] report a case study of using ACT for a client with end-stage metastatic pancreatic cancer, reporting acceptability and improvements in anxiety, depression, and treatment side effect coping ability. In our own BEACHeS study,[14] which used a mixed-methods single-case design, we demonstrated the acceptability of a brief intervention protocol and initial effectiveness data, including qualitative reports of a number of perceived benefits. Psychological well-being remained stable for most participants, thus demonstrating a potential buffering effect against the increased distress often associated with physical health deterioration at the end of life. Arch and colleagues[15] report feasibility findings from a mixed-modality (combined in-person and online delivery) ACT intervention for clients with metastatic cancer: high acceptability and satisfaction were reported, with those completing the intervention showing notable reductions in anxiety and depression but not pain interference. Importantly, this study explored some palliative-specific outcomes, noting positive impacts on fear of death, sense of life meaning, and increased engagement with advanced care planning.

Although the sample size is still relatively small, Rost et al.[16] provide more convincing evidence by comparing ACT against traditional CBT in women with advanced-stage ovarian cancer. They demonstrated that both treatment approaches were efficacious at improving distress and quality of life, and, though significant between-group differences were not found, those improvements were greater and had more rapid onset in the ACT group.

We know of only one study which explores the benefits of ACT in a generic palliative care population. The Life Programme[17] is a group-based intervention including both traditional CBT and ACT elements. Though the study design is single-arm, the authors report clinically meaningful change over time in symptom severity for depression, anxiety, and stress outcomes.

Other studies, for example Mosher et al.'s[18] feasibility study of telephone-based ACT for those with advanced lung cancer (and their caregivers) and Serfaty et al.'s CanACT feasibility trial[19] of an eight-session in-person ACT program, demonstrate feasibility and acceptability but are less conclusive in demonstrating improvements in patient-reported outcomes. This may be a methodological artifact: these kinds of early-phase trial are not designed to fully power analysis of efficacy, but rather to establish the feasibility of methodological design for later clinical trials. Further work is needed, though with the ongoing challenge of obtaining funding for psychosocial palliative care research, outcomes from fully powered trials may be some way off.

Other Applications of ACT in Palliative Settings

Though this chapter has primarily focused on using ACT for the person with palliative illness, it would be remiss not to give some space to the benefits of ACT for other people affected by advanced and end-of-life illness (e.g., Davis and colleagues'[20] feasibility randomized controlled trial of self-help ACT to support caregivers' grief and psychological distress). Preliminary efficacy data failed to demonstrate significant between-group differences and only small effects on acceptance, valued living, and grief outcomes. While differences in distress were also non-significant, within-group analysis demonstrated a significant reduction from baseline to 6-month post-grief follow-up, which was not observed in the control group. Though a fully powered trial is needed, this points to potential efficacy of ACT for supporting caregivers through their transition to life following the loss of a loved one to palliative illness.

Recognizing the high cost of providing psychosocial palliative care, we have an ongoing program of research exploring how non-psychologist members of the care team can be trained in ACT. Our ACT-enhanced communication skills training program has been delivered to more than 350 cancer and palliative care professionals in the United States, Canada, and Australia. We aim to up-skill the broader clinical care team to improve day-to-day clinical conversations with patients and their families by providing knowledge of the ACT model and basic, brief intervention techniques. We recently evaluated three iterations of our training program,[21] finding a high level of satisfaction. At 3-month follow-up, 46% of our trainees reported feeling better placed to provide an improved clinical service to their patients. We believe this work offers an important insight into how ACT might be effectively used by *all* members of the palliative care team, not just highly trained psychologists.

Future Directions

In the short term at least, the lack of a strong evidence base for ACT in palliative settings will likely be a barrier to widespread implementation, with financially stretched palliative care services unlikely to invest in training staff without more convincing efficacy data. Many individual practitioners have, however, already shifted toward more ACT-consistent approaches, and while we await conclusive trial evidence, we encourage those practitioners to disseminate their work to generate further dialogue and documentation of just how widely ACT is being used.

The palliative care setting presents specific challenges around resourcing and time. The unpredictable nature of life-limiting illness might mean, for example, that long manualized interventions are too burdensome or that end of life comes before the intervention is "complete." It is encouraging to see feasibility studies are exploring briefer[9] and more cost-effective delivery methods, such as group[17] or telephone-based[19] interventions, and we recommend this as a research priority moving forward.

We are surprised that most of the available evidence focuses on clients with non-curative cancer. While this group remains one of the largest within palliative care, other client groups might equally benefit from ACT, for example those with palliative coronary, respiratory, and neurological conditions. The nature of other palliative illnesses may necessitate tailoring of content or delivery mode, and so it is important that research explores this important issue, too.

What often marks a palliative care client from others that we have personally worked with is that their concerns are often much greater than simply living better in the present moment. The existential suffering of approaching end of life and the grief and demoralization that often accompany this can be equally, if not more, challenging. ACT seems well-placed to help clients to navigate this, coping better with distress and with more quality of life, no matter how short that life might be. However, more research which explores impacts on other palliative care–specific outcomes—existential or spiritual distress and grief, for example—is needed.

One final perspective we wish to close this chapter on is a reflection on what better psychological coping might enable regarding other aspects of supportive and palliative care. A core goal of palliative care is to enable a person-centered approach to discussing end-of-life care, but heightened distress often acts as a barrier to advance care planning. Having worked with a number of clients approaching end of life, we strongly believe that ACT-based approaches can facilitate this, enabling those conversations to occur earlier and in a more open forum. If this can be achieved, it is likely that symptom management will be more suited to individual needs and perhaps even more cost- and resource-effective. It is encouraging that engagement with anticipatory care planning was explored in Arch et al.'s feasibility study,[15] and we strongly encourage researchers to consider embedding these kinds of outcomes into future trials given the weight that such evidence might have for later implementation into clinical care.

Key Points

- ACT is becoming more commonly used in palliative care and may be more conceptually suited to the nature of distress in clients approaching end of life than other intervention approaches.
- Values-based work is especially helpful for maximize opportunities for more meaningful living and increased sense of purpose.
- While ACT enjoys a robust evidence base overall, there remain few fully powered trials of ACT in palliative care populations.
- Future research needs to consider the challenging nature of palliative care and specific tailoring requirements that might be needed to better reflect the full range and variety of client presentations in palliative care.

References

1. Beck JS. *Cognitive Behavior Therapy: Basics and Beyond*. 2nd ed. New York: Guilford; 2011.

2. Hayes SC. A contextual approach to therapeutic change. In: NS Jacobson, ed., *Psychotherapists in Clinical Practice: Cognitive and Behavioral Perspectives*. New York: Guilford; 1987:327–387.

3. Abramowitz JS, Tolin DF, Street GP. Paradoxical effects of thought suppression: A meta-analysis of controlled studies. *Clin Psychol Rev*. 2011;21(5):683–703. https://doi.org/10.1016/S0272-7358(00)00057-X

4. Hayes SC, Wilson KG, Gifford EV, Follette VM, Strosahl K. Experiential avoidance and behavioral disorders: A functional dimensional approach to diagnosis and treatment. *J Consult Clin Psychol*. 1996;64(6):1152. https://doi.org/10.1037/0022-006X.64.6.1152

5. Nolen-Hoeksema S. The role of rumination in depressive disorders and mixed anxiety/depressive symptoms. *J Abnorm Psychol*. 2000;109(3):504. https://doi.org/10.1037/0021-843X.109.3.504

6. Goldberg SB, Tucker RP, Greene PA, Davidson RJ, Wampold BE, Kearney DJ, Simpson TL. Mindfulness-based interventions for psychiatric disorders: A systematic review and meta-analysis. *Clin Psychol Rev*. 2018;59:52–60. https://doi.org/10.1016/j.cpr.2017.10.011

7. Hayes SC, Luoma JB, Bond FW, Masuda A, Lillis J. Acceptance and commitment therapy: Model, processes and outcomes. *Behav Res Ther*. 2006;44(1):1–25. https://doi.org/10.1016/j.brat.2005.06.006

8. Assaz DA, Roche B, Kanter JW, Oshiro CKB. Cognitive defusion in acceptance and commitment therapy: What are the basic processes of change. *Psychol Record*. 2018. https://doi.org/10.1007/s40732-017-0254-z

9. Hayes SC. State of the ACT evidence | association for contextual behavioral science. 2021. http://contextualscience.org/state_of_the_act_evidence

10. Gloster AT, Walder N, Levin ME, Twohig MP, Karekla M. The empirical status of acceptance and commitment therapy: A review of meta-analyses. *J Contextual Behav Sci*. 2020;18:181–192. https://doi.org/10.1016/j.jcbs.2020.09.009

11. Öst LG. The efficacy of acceptance and commitment therapy: An updated systematic review and meta-analysis. *Behav Res Ther*. 2014;61:105–121. https://doi.org/10.1016/j.brat.2014.07.018

12. Low J, Davis S, Drake R, King M, Tookman A, Turner K, et al. The role of acceptance in rehabilitation in life-threatening illness. *J Pain Symptom Manage*. 2012;43(1):20–28. https://doi.org/10.1016/j.jpainsymman.2011.03.020

13. O'Hayer CVF, O'Hayer KM, Sama A. Acceptance and commitment therapy with pancreatic cancer: An integrative model of palliative care—A case report. *J Pancreat Cancer*. 2018;4(1):1–3. https://www.liebertpub.com/doi/10.1089/pancan.2017.0021

14. Hulbert-Williams NJ, Norwood S, Gillanders D, Finucane A, Spiller J, Strachan J, et al. Brief Engagement and Acceptance Coaching for Hospice Settings (the BEACHeS study): Results from a Phase I study of acceptability and initial effectiveness in people with non-curative cancer. *BMC Palliat Care*. 2021;20(1):96. https://doi.org/10.1186/s12904-021-00801-7

15. Arch JJ, Fishbein JN, Ferris MC, Mitchell JL, Levin ME, Slivjak ET, et al. Acceptability, feasibility, and efficacy potential of a multimodal acceptance and commitment therapy intervention to address psychosocial and advance care planning needs among anxious and depressed adults with metastatic cancer. *J Palliat Med*. 2020;23(10):1380–1385. http://doi.org/10.1089/jpm.2019.0398

16. Rost AD, Wilson K, Buchanan E, Hildebrandt MJ, Mutch D. Improving psychological adjustment among late-stage ovarian cancer patients: Examining the role of avoidance in treatment. *Cogn Behav Pract*. 2012;19(4):508–517. https://doi.org/10.1016/j.cbpra.2012.01.003

17. Ramos KS. Hastings N, Bosworth HB, Fulton JJ. Life program: Pilot testing a palliative psychology group intervention. *J Palliat Med*. 2018;21(11):1641–1645. https://doi.org/10.1089/jpm.2017.0454

18. Mosher CE, Secinti E, Hirsh AT, Hanna N, Einhorn LH, Jalal SI, et al. Acceptance and commitment therapy for symptom interference in advanced lung cancer and caregiver distress: A pilot randomized trial. *J Pain Symptom Manage*. 2019;58(4):632–644. https://doi.org/10.1016/j.jpainsymman.2019.06.021

19. Serfaty M, Armstrong M, Vickerstaff V, Davis S, Gola A, McNamee P, et al. Acceptance and commitment therapy for adults with advanced cancer (CanACT): A feasibility randomised controlled trial. *PsychoOncology*. 2018;28:488–496. https://doi.org/10.1002/pon.4960

20. Davis EL, Deane FP, Lyons GC, Barclay GD, Bourne J, Connolly V. Feasibility randomised controlled trial of a self-help acceptance and commitment therapy intervention for grief and psychological distress in carers of palliative care patients. *J Health Psychol*. 2020;25(3):322–339.https://doi.org/10.1177/13591 05317715091

21. Hulbert-Williams N, Hulbert-Williams L, Patterson P, Suleman S, Howells L. Acceptance and Commitment Therapy (ACT) enhanced communication skills: Development and evaluation of a novel training programme. *BMJ Support Palliat Care*. 2021. https://doi.org/10.1136/bmjspcare-2020-002786.

40

Supportive-Expressive Group Therapy and the Terminally Ill

David Spiegel and Manuela Kogon

Introduction

Supportive-expressive group therapy (SEGT) was designed to provide emotional, social, cognitive, and symptomatic support for people coping with advancing and terminal cancer. It has been offered most frequently to women with advanced breast cancer, but it has been helpful to those with early-stage disease and with other cancer types as well. SEGT has been used widely worldwide, successfully adapted to other cultures and languages, and has been found to decrease anxiety, depression, and pain and increase quality of life, functioning and satisfaction with treatment.[1-7] The need for such support comes from the fact that life does not adequately prepare us to deal with a life-threatening illness and the rigors of treatment, including surgery, radiotherapy, chemotherapy, hormonal treatments, and other biomedical interventions. Effective support for the emotional, existential, physical, social, and financial burdens that accompany progressive cancer is crucial, regardless of continuing advances being made in treatment efficacy. Group psychotherapy can help in educating patients about their illness and its effects on their lives, processing emotions inextricably intertwined with the disease, and enhancing social support, which is often adversely affected by the presence of the disease. Group intervention has the benefit of positioning those with cancer in the roles of both recipients and providers of emotional and informational support to one another, allowing them to both witness and experience strategies designed to enhance coping and emotional support in the course of group therapy.

The social-cognitive processing model of adjustment to trauma points out that it is not merely the act of thinking about trauma-related information that facilitates processing, but it is disclosure and active contemplation of meanings, feelings, and thoughts with supportive others that is pivotal.[8] A social environment that inhibits such disclosure may cause patients to avoid thinking and talking about the stressful experience and interfere with cognitive processing, resulting in prolonged distress and a failure to come to terms with the cognitive and emotional implications of advancing cancer. These social constraints cause cancer patients to feel unsupported, misunderstood, or otherwise alienated from their social networks and have been associated with greater cancer-related intrusive ideation and avoidance. A similar construct, *aversive emotional response*,[9] has been found to amplify the impact of past stressful life events on current traumatic stress symptoms in cancer patients. Treatment-related changes in patients' perception of social constraints would therefore result in enhanced processing of the cancer experience.

Living with the traumatic stressor of cancer creates an unending series of existential challenges.[10] The threat to life is continuous, and reminders are constant through symptoms such as pain, treatments and their side effects, loss of social roles, and the response of others to the condition. Thus, the successful treatment of symptoms and the enhancement of quality of life for cancer patients requires interventions that focus on social, emotional, and cognitive processing of the cancer experience and address the themes and issues that are specific to living with and dying of cancer. Successful treatment of cancer-related symptoms and improvements in quality of life[11,12] are mediated by engaging cancer-related fears and other aversive emotions, increasing patient emotional self-efficacy for coping with the challenges of living with the illness,[13] processing of existential cancer-related concerns and stressful cancer-related events,[14] reducing social constraints that inhibit processing, reorganizing life priorities and living more fully in the present, and utilizing techniques such as self-hypnosis for pain and anxiety control.[15,16] Many of the psychotherapies that have shown promise in improving emotional adjustment and even influencing survival time encourage open expression of emotion and assertiveness in assuming control over the course of treatment, life decisions, and relationships.

Supportive-Expressive Group Therapy Treatment Content

There are seven themes that constitute the core of the therapeutic work in SEGT.[1] While originally developed and evaluated among women with metastatic breast cancer, the themes are salient to all types of cancer. SEGT has been utilized with people with a variety of cancers, usually in groups consisting homogeneous types of disease. It was developed to be an ongoing weekly treatment, 90 minutes in length, over the course of a year or more, with rolling recruitment of members as some die or leave. It has also been evaluated as a shorter program of 12–20 sessions, usually for more recently diagnosed patients. It has been successfully run with one or two co-therapists. The treatment is semi-structured: the therapist(s) encourage open interaction rather than a series of recitations of problems, but direct the discussion toward the following themes:

1. *Social support.* Psychotherapy, especially in groups, can provide a new social network with the common bond of facing similar problems. Just at a time when the illness makes

a person feel removed from the flow of life and many withdraw out of awkwardness or fear, psychotherapeutic support provides a new and important social connection. The very thing that alienates others is the ticket of admission to such groups, providing a surprising intensity of caring among members from the very beginning. Furthermore, members find that the process of giving help to others enhances their own sense of mastery of the role of cancer patient and their self-esteem, giving meaning to an otherwise meaningless tragedy. This has been called the "helper-therapy principle."

2. *Emotional expression.* The expression of emotion is important in reducing social isolation and improving coping. Yet it is often an aspect of cancer patient adjustment which is overlooked or suppressed. Emotional suppression and avoidance are associated with poorer coping. At the same time, there is much that can be done in both group and individual psychotherapies to facilitate the expression of emotion appropriate to the disease. Doing so seems to reduce the repressive coping strategy, which reduces expression of positive as well as negative emotion. Emotional suppression, often referred to in common parlance as "being strong," also reduces intimacy in families, limiting opportunities for direct expression of affection and concern. There is evidence that those who are able to ventilate strong feelings directly cope better with cancer.[13]

   The use of the psychotherapeutic setting to deal with painful affect also provides an organizing context for handling it. When unbidden thoughts involving fears of dying and death intrude, they can be better managed by patients who know that there is a finite time and place during which such feelings will be expressed, acknowledged, and dealt with. Furthermore, disease-related dysphoria is more intense when amplified by isolation, leaving the patient to feel understandably alone with the sense of anxiety, loss, and fear. Death, a fundamentally unknowable experience, is often conceptualized as isolation, so being in a group where many others express similar distress normalizes their reactions, making them less alien and overwhelming.

3. *Detoxifying dying: Processing existential concerns.* Exploring and processing existential concerns is a primary focus of supportive-expressive therapy. Yalom has described the ultimate existential concerns as death, freedom, isolation, and meaning.[14] Rather than avoiding painful or anxiety-provoking topics in attempts to "stay positive," this form of group therapy addresses these concerns head-on with the intent of helping group members to make better use of the time they have left. This component of the therapy involves looking the threat of death in the eye rather than avoiding it. The goal is to help those facing the threat of death to see it from a different point of view. When processed, life-threatening problems can come to seem real but not overwhelming. Conversely, denial and avoidance have their costs, including an increase in anxiety and isolation. Directly facing life-threatening fears can help patients shift from emotion-focused to problem-focused coping. The process of dying, with its associated fear of suffering and uncertainty, is often more threatening than death itself. Open communication can help overcome the patients' reluctance to discuss death-related concerns to "protect: their loved ones or themselves from distress. Discussion of these concerns can lead to means of addressing if not completely resolving each of these issues. Talking openly about death anxiety can help to divide the fear of death into a series of problems: loss of control

over treatment decisions, fear of separation from loved ones, anxiety about pain. Thus, even facing death can result in positive life changes. One woman with metastatic breast cancer described her experience in this way:

> What I found is that talking about death in the group is like looking down into the Grand Canyon (I don't like heights). You know that if you fell down, it would be a disaster, but you feel better about yourself because you're able to look. That is how I feel about death in the group: I can't say I feel serene, but I can look at it.[1]

Even the process of grieving can be reassuring at the same time that it is threatening. The experience of grieving others who have died of the same condition constitutes a deeply personal experience of the depth of loss that will be experienced by others after one's own death. With a smile, one group member reported having called a local cemetery to inquire about the cost of being buried there. "I was shocked by the price, so I said, 'actually, I represent a group of women looking for a place to be buried.' I was told: "Skylawn Park does not offer group discounts." The story elicited a good laugh from the group.

4. *Reorganizing life priorities and living in the present.* Acceptance of the possibility of illness shortening life carries with it an opportunity for re-evaluating life priorities. When cure is not possible, a realistic evaluation of the future can help those with life-threatening illness make the best use of their remaining time. One of the costs of unrealistic optimism is the failure to accomplish important life projects, communicate openly with family and friends, and set affairs in order. Facing the threat of death can aid in making the most of life. This can help patients take control of those aspects of their lives they can influence while grieving and relinquishing those they cannot. Having a domain of control can be reassuring. Previous studies of the sequelae of past traumatic events indicate that long-term psychological distress is associated with a temporal orientation that is focused on the past rather than the present or future. For cancer patients who are experiencing the traumatic stressor of their past diagnosis and treatment while anticipating their imminent death and its impact on their loved ones, oddly enough, adjustment can be enhanced with a focus on the present and the future. Acknowledging that their lives have been shortened can actually enrich the present and help them to make the most of their foreshortened future. Progress in life goal reappraisal, reorganization of life priorities, and attention to the preciousness of the life and relationships they have may also mediate improvement in symptoms and enhance quality of life.

5. *Enhancing family support.* Psychotherapeutic interventions can also be quite helpful in improving communication, identifying needs, increasing role flexibility, and adjusting to new medical social, vocational, and financial realities. An atmosphere of open and shared problem-solving in families results in reduced anxiety and depression among cancer patients. Thus, facilitating the development of such open discussion of common problems is a useful therapeutic tool. The group format is especially helpful for such a task in that problems expressing needs and wishes can be examined among group members as a model for clarifying communication in their families.

Mary was clearly becoming more frail, but always arrived perfectly coiffed and dressed. One day she said: "My husband is a banker but not a teller—he doesn't talk. I think he is getting to the point where I am just a burden, so I am thinking of trying to end my life." Rather than discussing her relationship with her husband, the group leader commented: "I think Mary is posing a question to us: Would we prefer to be without her?" The group members immediately told her how much they admired her not yielding an inch more than necessary to the progression of her illness, how much they appreciated her presence and wanted her to be with them as long as possible. Mary died naturally several months later and had a provision in her will that a limousine would pick up the group members and bring them to her memorial service.

In addition to enhancing communication, group participants are encouraged to develop role flexibility, a capacity to exchange roles or develop new ones as the illness progresses. One woman, for example, who became unable to carry out her usual household chores, wrote an "owner's manual" to the care of the house so that her husband could better help her and carry on after her death. Others wrote letters to friends asking them to cook an extra bit of dinner on one evening a month to share with them and their families.

6. *Improving communication with physicians.* Supportive-expressive groups facilitate better communication with physicians and other healthcare professionals. Groups provide mutual encouragement to get questions answered, participate actively in treatment decisions, and consider alternatives carefully. The three crucial elements are communication, control, and caring: improving communication, enhancing patients' sense of control over treatment decisions, and finding caring physicians and other healthcare professionals who are interested in the patient as a person. Engagement in planning the final stages of life rather than withdrawal is a powerful communication of the value of the patient as a person rather than as a "treatment failure."

7. *Symptom control.* Many treatment approaches involve teaching cognitive techniques to manage distress. These include learning to identify emotions as they develop, analyze sources of emotional response, and move from emotion-focused to problem-focused coping. These approaches help the patient take a more active stance toward their illness. Rather than feeling overwhelmed by an insoluble problem, they learn to divide problems into smaller and more manageable ones, such as: "If I don't have much time left, how do I want to spend it? What effect will further chemotherapy have on my quality of life?"

Many group and individual psychotherapy programs teach specific coping skills designed to help patients reduce cancer-related symptoms such as anxiety, insomnia, and pain. In SEGT, hypnosis is utilized at the end of each session. Hypnosis is used for pain and anxiety control in cancer to attenuate the experience of pain and suffering and to allow painful emotional material to be examined. Group sessions involving instruction in self-hypnosis provide an effective means of reducing pain and anxiety and consolidating the major themes of discussion in the group.

Hypnosis is an altered state of consciousness, composed of heightened absorption in focal attention, dissociation of peripheral awareness, and enhanced responsiveness to social cues.[17,18] It has a long tradition of effectiveness in controlling somatic symptoms such as pain and anxiety. Patients with the requisite hypnotic capacity can be taught to utilize self-hypnosis to reduce or eliminate pain and the tension that accompanies it. Hypnotic techniques have been shown to effectively reduce cancer pain in the context of SEGT[15,19] and to facilitate medical procedures.[20]

In a recent study of 16 weekly sessions of SEGT, participants reported that the most helpful aspects were the expression and normalization of feelings, thoughts, and reactions; the improvement of social support; and the learning opportunities obtained through sharing of experiences among participants.[5]

Implementation

Discussion of these seven themes in the group is implemented utilizing four primary strategies designed to stimulate and direct emotion-focused interaction (Table 40.1).

1. *Personalization.* Leaders are taught to bring group discussions "into the room" by keeping the focus on interactions occurring among group members, rather than directing discussion toward people and events outside the group. While some discussion of family, friends, and outside events in inevitable, the processing of issues raised on the "outside" is best done on the "inside." Thus, as noted above, when one patient mentioned how she feels that she is a burden to her husband, the discussion is better directed toward the question, "Do you feel like a burden here in the group?" "Do other group members feel that you are a burden?"

2. *Affective expression.* Leaders should "follow the affect" in the room rather than the content. If a silent group member shows signs of emotion, the leader should respectfully direct attention toward her: "You seem upset now—what are you feeling?" Expression of emotion involves revealing vulnerability, and it is important to make sure that those who express feelings are heard and acknowledged. Group members find that open expression of emotion of all kinds is liberating and helpful, facilitating sharing of positive reactions even to negative feelings and thereby enhancing cohesion.[5,21]

TABLE 40.1 Group process goals for leaders

Personalization	Facilitating an examination of personal and specific cancer-related issues.
Affective expression	Facilitating the expression of here-and-now feelings
Supporting group interaction:	Facilitating supportive interactions among group members Sharing group time and access to group attention Avoiding scapegoating Maintaining boundaries
Active coping	Facilitating the use of active coping strategies

3. *Supportive group interactions.* The leader is responsible for starting and ending the group on time and seeing that there are few interruptions of the group's time. Each member should be made to feel that her problems are as important as anyone else's. It is necessary to inquire about missing members and make sure that very silent members have a chance to talk. Also, dealing with scapegoating—the group's attempts to "fix" one member as a displacement of dealing with their own problems—is critical. Leaders must remember that their "patient" is the group, not just a series of individuals.

4. *Active coping.* As problems are discussed, it is helpful for the leader to direct the group toward means of responding to them, rather than merely accumulating a series of unresolved difficulties or avoiding discussing them. Finding a strategy for addressing specific problems reduces the helplessness engendered by them.

Outcome

Randomized clinical trials have demonstrated the benefit of group therapy for breast cancer patients facing dying and death,[14,22–25] notably reducing pain[15,19] and emotional distress;[3,12] increasing personal growth and mastery;[24] and providing significant help in quality of life, depression, hopelessness, sense of dignity, and spiritual well-being.[25,26] A systematic review of the literature that included two meta-analyses and nine well-designed randomized controlled trials indicated that psychoeducational interventions not only enhance patient knowledge about their cancer and its treatments, but also reduce depression, anxiety, nausea, and pain.[27] A Cochrane database review concluded that group psychotherapy for cancer patients, including SEGT, significantly reduces depression even in the setting of advanced disease.[28] It is especially important to be able to offer effective psychotherapeutic support since antidepressants tend to be less effective among those with metastatic illness.[29]

Implications for Cancer Progression and Mortality

While it is well established that psychosocial interventions improve quality of life and satisfaction with treatment and decrease depression and anxiety, there have been mixed results with SEGT effects on survival time. Our initial RCT demonstrated a significant 18 month survival advantage for women randomized to SEGT versus routine care,[30] and the differences in disease course between the control and treatment groups appeared to be independent of any differences in medical treatment received.[31] Our follow-up trial showed no overall survival advantage but a significant interaction with disease receptor status, such that ER-positive patients showed equal survival while ER-negative ones lived longer in the treatment group.[32] Our recent meta-analysis of 12 trials involving 2,439 cancer patients found an overall cancer survival effect favoring group treatment (HR = 0.71; 95% confidence interval [CI] 0.58–0.88; P = 0.002). In particular, an effect size favoring the treatment group was observed in studies sampling lower versus higher percentage of married patients' (NNT = 4.3 vs. NNT = 15.4), when cognitive behavioral therapy was applied for early versus late cancer stage (NNT = 2.3 vs. NNT = −28.6), and among patients older versus younger than 50 (NNT = 4.2 vs. NNT = −20.5).[33] Similarly, reduction in depression over the course of a year predicts significantly longer survival among women with metastatic breast cancer.[34] Psychosocial effects on survival time seem most pronounced when medical treatments have become less effective.[35] Furthermore, no study has found that psychotherapy, even involving direct confrontation with dying and death, shortens survival. In addition, there are data showing the impact of SEGT on physiology. In a comparison study of SEGT and mindfulness-based group therapy, both resulted in more normative diurnal cortisol profiles than in the control condition, and both treatment types maintained telomere length over the 3-month intervention period whereas women in the control condition demonstrated a trend toward decreases in relative telomere length that are associated with more rapid physiological aging.[36]

Other interventions that contain psychosocial treatment elements have shown survival benefits. A randomized trial of a palliative care intervention involving an average of four visits that focused on choices about resuscitation preference, pain control, and quality of life among 151 patients with non-small-cell lung cancer demonstrated a significant reduction of depression and pain and also a significant 2.7-month improvement in survival time (median survival, 11.85 vs. 8.9 months; $p = 0.02$).[37]

The potential benefit of psychotherapeutic support on cancer progression receives further support from evidence that being married is associated with a 12–33% improvement in overall survival, which constitutes an average of 4 months.[38] The authors noted that this was comparable to the overall effect of chemotherapy. This study involved analysis of Surveillance, Epidemiology, and End Results (SEER) data in the United States from 2004 to 2008 involving 734,889 cancer patients with lung, colorectal, breast, pancreatic, prostate, liver/intrahepatic bile duct, non-Hodgkin lymphoma, head/neck, ovarian, or esophageal cancer. Being married was associated with better outcome with each of these cancer types, independent of demographics, stage, and treatment. Thus, social support would seem to have a tangible effect on disease progression and survival time.

Future Directions

SEGT mobilizes powerful emotional, social, and coping skills to help those with cancer face medical, social, and existential problems in a way that is effective and interactive. The close bonds that develop in the course of treatment provide a sense of belonging and meaning, even as these groups face and grieve the loss of members. SEGT provides an opportunity for those with advancing cancer to feel like experts in living and facing the disease, to give as well as receive help. As virtual group interactions have proliferated in response to the COVID-19 pandemic, there is reason to believe that the reach of SEGT and other effective group psychotherapies for cancer patients can be substantially expanded, especially given early evidence of its effectiveness online.[39] SEGT is one of a number of psychotherapeutic treatments that have proved benefit in helping those with cancer live better, and perhaps even longer, in the face of life-shortening disease.

Key Points

- SEGT mobilizes powerful emotional, social, and coping skills to help those with cancer face medical, social, and existential problems in a way that is effective and interactive
- SEGT can serve as a core component of supportive oncology and psycho-oncology.
- SEGT is an effective treatment to alleviate pain, depression, and anxiety in cancer patients and increase quality of life and satisfaction with treatment
- A group setting facilitates mutual support, emotional expression, and behavior modeling; enhances problem-solving; eases existential concerns; and creates social networks.
- SEGT is applicable to diverse settings independent of culture, language, gender, or age and can be widely disseminated via electronic technology.

References

1. Spiegel D, Classen C. *Group Therapy for Cancer Patients: A Research Based Handbook of Psychosocial Care.* New York: Basic Books; 2000.
2. Akechi T, Okuyama T, Onishi J, Morita T, Furukawa TA. Psychotherapy for depression among incurable cancer patients. *Cochrane Database Syst Rev.* 2008;(2):CD005537.
3. Classen C, Butler LD, Koopman C, Miller E, DiMiceli S, Giese-Davis J, et al. Supportive-expressive group therapy reduces distress in metastatic breast cancer patients: A randomized clinical intervention trial. *Arch Gen Psychiatry.* 2001;58:494–501.
4. Butler LD, Koopman C, Neri E, Giese-Davis J, Palesh O, Thorne-Yocam KA, et al. Effects of supportive-expressive group therapy on pain in women with metastatic breast cancer. *Health Psychol.* 2009;28(5):579–587.
5. Brandao T, Tavares R, Schulz MS, Matos PM. Experiences of breast cancer patients and helpful aspects of supportive-expressive group therapy: A qualitative study. *Eur J Cancer Care (Engl).* 2019;28(5):e13078.
6. Goodwin PJ, Leszcz M, Koopmans J, Arnold A, Doll R, Chochinov H, et al. Randomized trial of group psychosocial support in metastatic breast cancer: The BEST study: Breast-Expressive Supportive Therapy study. *Cancer Treatm Rev.* 1996;22 Suppl A:91–96.
7. Ye ZJ, Qiu HZ, Liang MZ, Liu ML, Li PF, Chen P, et al. Effect of a mentor-based, supportive-expressive program, Be Resilient to Breast Cancer, on survival in metastatic breast cancer: A randomised, controlled intervention trial. *Br J Cancer.* 2017;117(10):1486–1494.
8. Lepore SJ, Helgeson VS. Social constraints, intrusive thoughts, and mental health after prostate cancer. *J Soc Clin Psychol.* 1998;17:89–106.
9. Butler LD, Koopman C, Classen C, Spiegel D. Traumatic stress, life events, and emotional support in women with metastatic breast cancer: Cancer-related traumatic stress symptoms associated with past and current stressors. *Health Psychol.* 1999;18(6):555–560.
10. Spiegel D. A 43-year-old woman coping with cancer [clinical conference] [see comments]. *JAMA.* 1999;282(4):371–378.
11. Classen C, Butler LD, Koopman C, Miller E, DiMiceli S, Giese-Davis J, Fobair P, Carlson RW, Kraemer HC, Spiegel D, et al. Supportive-expressive group therapy and distress in patients with metastatic breast cancer: A randomized clinical intervention trial. *Arch Gen Psychiatry.* 2001;58:494–501.
12. Spiegel D, Bloom JR, Yalom I. Group support for patients with metastatic cancer: A randomized outcome study. *Arch Gen Psychiatry.* 1981;38(5):527–533.
13. Giese-Davis J, Koopman C, Butler LD, Classen C, Cordova M, Fobair P, et al. Change in emotion-regulation strategy for women with metastatic breast cancer following supportive-expressive group therapy. *J Consult Clin Psychol.* 2002;70(4):916–925.
14. Yalom ID. *Existential Psychotherapy.* New York: Basic Books; 1980.

15. Spiegel D, Bloom JR. Group therapy and hypnosis reduce metastatic breast carcinoma pain. *Psychosomatic Med.* 1983;45(4):333–339.

16. Butler LD, Symons BK, Henderson SL, Shortliffe LD, Spiegel D. Hypnosis reduces distress and duration of an invasive medical procedure for children. *Pediatrics.* 2005;115(1):e77–85.

17. Elkins GR, Barabasz AF, Council JR, Spiegel D. Advancing research and practice: The revised APA Division 30 definition of hypnosis. *Int J Clin Exp Hypnosis.* 2015;63(1):1–9.

18. Spiegel H, Spiegel D. *Trance and Treatment: Clinical Uses of Hypnosis.* Washington, DC: American Psychiatric Publishing; 2004.

19. Butler LD, Koopman C, Neri E, Giese-Davis J, Palesh O, Thorne-Yocam KA, et al. Effects of supportive-expressive group therapy on pain in women with metastatic breast cancer. *Health Psychol.* 2009;28(5):579–587.

20. Lang EV, Benotsch EG, Fick LJ, Lutgendorf S, Berbaum ML, Berbaum KS, et al. Adjunctive non-pharmacological analgesia for invasive medical procedures: A randomised trial. *Lancet.* 2000;355:1486–1490.

21. Giese-Davis J, Koopman C, Butler LD, Classen C, Cordova M, Fobair P, et al. Change in emotion-regulation strategy for women with metastatic breast cancer following supportive-expressive group therapy. *J Consult Clin Psychol.* 2002;70(4):916–925.

22. Carlson LE, Doll R, Stephen J, Faris P, Tamagawa R, Drysdale E, et al. Randomized controlled trial of mindfulness-based cancer recovery versus supportive expressive group therapy for distressed survivors of breast cancer. *J Clin Oncol.* 2013;31(25):3119–3126.

23. Cunningham AJ, Edmonds CV, Jenkins GP, Pollack H, Lockwood GA, Warr D. A randomized controlled trial of the effects of group psychological therapy on survival in women with metastatic breast cancer. *Psycho-Oncology.* 1998;7(6):508–517.

24. van der Spek N, Vos J, van Uden-Kraan CF, Breitbart W, Cuijpers P, Holtmaat K, et al. Efficacy of meaning-centered group psychotherapy for cancer survivors: A randomized controlled trial. *Psychol Med.* 2017;47(11):1990–2001.

25. Breitbart W, Rosenfeld B, Pessin H, Applebaum A, Kulikowski J, Lichtenthal WG. Meaning-centered group psychotherapy: An effective intervention for improving psychological well-being in patients with advanced cancer. *J Clin Oncol.* 2015;33(7):749–754.

26. Chochinov HM, Kristjanson LJ, Breitbart W, McClement S, Hack TF, Hassard T, et al. Effect of dignity therapy on distress and end-of-life experience in terminally ill patients: A randomised controlled trial. *Lancet Oncol.* 2011;12(8):753–762.

27. Devine EC, Westlake SK. The effects of psychoeducational care provided to adults with cancer: Meta-analysis of 116 studies. *Oncol Nurs Forum.* 1995;22(9):1369–1381.

28. Akechi T, Okuyama T, Onishi J, Morita T, Furukawa TA. Psychotherapy for depression among incurable cancer patients. *Cochrane Database Syst Rev.* 2008;(2):CD005537.

29. Lloyd-Williams M, Payne S, Reeve J, Kolamunnage Dona R. Antidepressant medication in patients with advanced cancer--An observational study. *QJM.* 2013;106(11):995–1001.

30. Spiegel D, Bloom JR, Kraemer HC, Gottheil E. Effect of psychosocial treatment on survival of patients with metastatic breast cancer. *Lancet.* 1989;2(8668):888–891.

31. Kogon MM, Biswas A, Pearl D, Carlson RW, Spiegel D. Effects of medical and psychotherapeutic treatment on the survival of women with metastatic breast carcinoma. *Cancer.* 1997;80(2):225–230.

32. Spiegel D, Butler LD, Giese-Davis J, Koopman C, Miller E, DiMiceli S, et al. Effects of supportive-expressive group therapy on survival of patients with metastatic breast cancer: A randomized prospective trial. *Cancer.* 2007;110(5):1130–1138.

33. Mirosevic S, Jo B, Kraemer HC, Ershadi M, Neri E, Spiegel D. "Not just another meta-analysis": Sources of heterogeneity in psychosocial treatment effect on cancer survival. *Cancer Med.* 2019;8(1):363–373.

34. Giese-Davis J, Collie K, Rancourt KM, Neri E, Kraemer HC, Spiegel D. Decrease in depression symptoms is associated with longer survival in patients with metastatic breast cancer: A secondary analysis. *J Clin Oncol.* 2011;29(4):413–420.

35. Spiegel D. Mind matters in cancer survival. *JAMA.* 2011;305(5):502–503.

36. Carlson LE, Beattie TL, Giese-Davis J, Faris P, Tamagawa R, Fick LJ, et al. Mindfulness-based cancer recovery and supportive-expressive therapy maintain telomere length relative to controls in distressed breast cancer survivors. *Cancer.* 2015;121(3):476–484.
37. Temel JS, Greer JA, Muzikansky A, Gallagher ER, Admane S, Jackson VA, et al. Early palliative care for patients with metastatic non-small-cell lung cancer. *N Engl J Med.* 2010;363(8):733–742.
38. Aizer AA, Chen MH, McCarthy EP, Mendu ML, Koo S, Wilhite TJ, et al. Marital status and survival in patients with cancer. *J Clin Oncol.* 2013;31(31):3869–3876.
39. Lieberman MA, Golant M, Giese-Davis J, Winzlenberg A, Benjamin H, Humphreys K, et al. Electronic support groups for breast carcinoma: A clinical trial of effectiveness. *Cancer.* 2003;97(4):920–925.

41

Grief Interventions in Palliative Care

Wendy G. Lichtenthal, Kailey E. Roberts,
Madeline Rogers, Carol Fadalla, William E. Rosa,
and Robert A. Neimeyer

National guidelines highlight that continuity of care from end of life through bereavement is an integral component of palliative care.[1] Grief support is a common psychosocial need for palliative care patients' chosen family (which may include relatives, partners, and close friends), and familiarity with various intervention approaches can help clinicians offer evidence-based family-centered care. In this chapter, we provide a broad overview of interventions designed to support family members experiencing grief before and after the death of a patient with a life-limiting illness. We describe both psychotherapeutic and psychopharmacological interventions and, where relevant, research findings suggesting their efficacy. This chapter concludes by highlighting the ongoing need to develop and evaluate grief interventions for special populations in palliative care, including bereaved parents and palliative care clinicians.

Though grief support approaches and targets may vary, key tenets of care are important to keep in mind when delivering interventions to grieving families.[2,3] They should first and foremost aim to support family members in their natural grief process.[2] This means adopting a nonpathologizing stance; offering an empathic, validating presence; and providing psychoeducation about grief. Clinicians working with grieving family members in palliative care often serve a critical role as they bear witness to the griever's pain and hold space for stories about the deceased. It is important to develop comfort with silence "in the room" and to understand that there is no way to "fix" or resolve grief.[4] For many family members, this type of empathic support is sufficient scaffolding as they naturally adapt to their loss,[2,5] while others may need more targeted therapeutic techniques to address impairing psychological symptoms, such as anxiety, depression, or prolonged grief disorder (PGD).[6]

As described in Chapter 17, grief in family members can begin long before a patient receiving palliative care dies and often continues many years after the patient's death. Thus, grief support, including formal interventions when appropriate, should be made available during the patient's illness, around the time of death, and throughout bereavement. Clinicians may offer individual and family therapy, psychiatric medication, and group interventions pre- and post-loss.[7,8]

Importantly, while family members should be provided with access to evidence-based grief interventions if needed, most bereaved individuals will adapt without intervention, learning to coexist with their grief with time and general support.[5] Thus, although this chapter describes several intervention approaches, before attempting intervention with grieving individuals, assessment of the appropriateness and necessity of targeted treatment is critical. Chapter 17 provides additional information on the phenomenology of grief to assist palliative care clinicians in differentiating between normative and pathological grief presentations, both pre- and post-loss.

Pre-Loss Grief Interventions

As noted in Chapter 17, family members may experience grief around current losses, such as the patient's physical abilities and valued roles, as well as the anticipated death of the patient. Supportive counseling may offer families a place to process their natural grief responses to these losses. However, family members characterized by such risk factors as lower education, poor grief support, proneness to anxiety, spiritual struggle, and especially high dependency on the dying patient and inability to make sense of the loss have been found to experience more anguishing pre-loss grief and accordingly merit closer evaluation for enhanced professional support.[9] Likewise, for family members who have experienced traumatic circumstances or are struggling with end-of-life decisions, more targeted pre-loss grief interventions may be warranted to reduce current distress and prevent bereavement-related mental health challenges following the patient's death.

The importance of preparing family members for the patient's death by communicating about the patient's end-of-life care plan and the dying process has been highlighted in proposed standards of bereavement support in palliative care.[10] However, research on palliative care interventions for family members has focused on addressing practical needs (e.g., problem-solving, communication skills) and coping with other aspects of caregiving rather than grief.[11] This said, to the extent that existing pre-loss interventions aim to improve the end-of-life experience and increase the family's preparedness for the loss,[11] they can reduce the likelihood of poor bereavement outcomes and therefore are, in essence, bereavement interventions.

Below, we describe the limited literature on pre-loss interventions that specifically address pre-death grief.[11,12] Of note, maximizing flexibility of intervention delivery is important as families are often burdened with many caregiving responsibilities.[12] Families appear to appreciate the option of delivery of pre-loss interventions through telehealth, which has not been found to adversely affect outcomes.[12]

Empower

Enhancing and Mobilizing the POtential for Wellness and Emotional Resilience (EMPOWER) is a modular intervention for surrogate decision-makers of patients at the end of life who are in intensive care units (ICUs).[13] Its modular design allows for flexible delivery in person or via telehealth to accommodate the interruptions common to the ICU environment. EMPOWER utilizes components of cognitive behavioral therapy (CBT; see Chapter 34), acceptance and commitment therapy (ACT; see Chapter 39), psychoeducation, and mind-body tools to support surrogates who are often grieving amid decision-making and potentially traumatic conditions in the ICU. EMPOWER aims to reduce *experiential avoidance* (i.e., the tendency to avoid distressing, uncomfortable thoughts and feelings) which can impede value-concordant decision-making and can maintain grief and trauma-related symptoms in the longer term. In addition to introducing coping tools to decrease physiological reactivity and increase distress tolerance, EMPOWER also brings in the voice of the patient, using an approach from Gestalt and grief therapy to aid in medical decision-making and encourage adaptive coping. Facilitating connection to the patient's voice can further serve to mitigate current or future regret and guilt and help the surrogate recognize that the voice of the patient is always available to them as they continue to navigate the hospitalization and bereavement. Meaning-centered grief therapy (MCGT) principles are incorporated to highlight the surrogate's ability to choose their response to match their circumstances, increasing their sense of agency and sense of empowerment in an out-of-control situation.[14] While EMPOWER's content largely focuses on coping with pre-loss grief, it can easily be adapted to provide post-loss care. Preliminary findings from the EMPOWER open trial and pilot randomized controlled trial (RCT) demonstrate its superior efficacy as compared to enhanced usual care. Reductions in anxiety, peritraumatic distress, and experiential avoidance have been observed immediately post-invention, with improvements in experiential avoidance and prolonged grief, depression, and anxiety symptoms at a 3-month follow-up assessment.[13]

Family-Focused Grief Therapy

Family-focused grief therapy (FFGT) is a time-limited intervention that begins pre-loss, guiding families of patients receiving palliative care in processing anticipatory grief and exploration of family dynamics, values, beliefs, individual roles, and conflicts.[15] It may consist of 4–10 sessions lasting 90 minutes each and continues through bereavement, promoting continuity of care beyond the patient's death. FFGT targets at-risk families exhibiting dysfunction in the domains of communication, conflict, or cohesion and thus demonstrates the value of screening families who may be in need of support. Promoting adaptive communication and the sharing of grief among family members, the goal of FFGT is to help families create a sense of cohesion, reduce distress in family members pre-loss, and prevent later challenges in bereavement.[15] For families with a mild to intermediate level of dysfunction, FFGT has shown significant effect in reducing depression and distress.[15]

Pre-Loss Grief Interventions in Pediatrics

The families of children receiving palliative care have unique grief support needs, both before and after their child's death. These needs are described in depth in Chapter 44, but here we briefly note ways to support parents in their pre-death grief. End-of-life decision-making in pediatrics can be particularly complex and, if parents are not provided with adequate support, can contribute to negative bereavement outcomes such as impairing regret, ruminations, and guilt.[16] Providing parents with support in making difficult decisions about their child's care can provide them with a sense of control, a way to reduce their child's suffering, increase their trust in providers and satisfaction with the care their child received, and thus reduce their risk for negative bereavement outcomes such as regret, anger, guilt, and posttraumatic stress reactions.[16] The care team can support parents as they engage in end-of-life decision-making, including speaking to their child about what is important to them and providing the appropriate psychoeducation to both parents and their child as it pertains to the child's age and development level. In addition, clinicians may consider use of interventions like EMPOWER and FFGT, which have been used in pediatrics settings.

Acute Post-Loss Support

When a patient dies, there is often abrupt discontinuation of contact with the treatment team and inconsistent and impersonal bereavement follow-up.[10] Psychiatrists working in palliative care can help address this by reaching out to the family soon after the patient's death, beginning with offering condolences and support through a phone call or card that highlights how the patient touched them and that they mattered. Chapter 17 offers detailed guidelines for condolence calls. Persistent outreach is often appreciated.

During supportive encounters with acutely grieving individuals, it is important for providers to be aware that family members may be experiencing profound pain, anxiety, tearfulness, numbness, and cognitive challenges. Such clinical presentation is in many cases considered normative in the weeks and months after a significant loss, and the intensity of symptoms often dissipates with time. Clinicians should be mindful of any impulses to "fix" the pain[3] and can instead offer empathic validation and normalization, psychoeducation about the grief process and the importance of giving oneself compassionate permission to grieve, and bereavement support resources that the family member may use at a later time (e.g., support groups, memorial services).

Clinicians must take care not to pathologize and overtreat (e.g., prescribe medications without a thorough assessment) during the first several months of bereavement. With that said, it is also important to assess for support needs as well as evidence of suicidality risk.[3] Bereavement risk screening can help clinicians determine when treatment may be appropriate.[10,17] It can also be useful for triaging limited bereavement support resources to family members at greatest risk of poor outcomes, as not everyone needs formal grief interventions.[5,10,17] See Chapter 17 for risk factors to consider in bereavement.

Bereavement Interventions

For those family members who develop bereavement-related mental health challenges such as PGD,[6] targeted grief intervention may be appropriate. However, research has shown that there is no "one size fits all" approach for bereavement care.[5] When possible, grief interventions should be tailored to kinship type, cause of death, geographical location, cultural background, and careful consideration about the family member's needs. Bereavement interventions can include groups, individual counseling or psychotherapy, or psychiatric intervention.[7,8,18] They may be delivered via telehealth to increase accessibility, particularly for family members facing emotional or logistical barriers to returning to the institution where the patient received care.

Systematic reviews have demonstrated there are few extensively studied grief interventions,[8,18] and meta-analyses suggest that, comparable to other psychotherapeutic interventions, they have small to moderate effects. One-on-one treatments targeting high-risk or symptomatic individuals, particularly those who are at least 6 months post-loss, seem to yield stronger effects.[7,8] Interventions that have been subject to rigorous study include prolonged grief disorder therapy (PGDT),[19] CBT, and FFGT. Meaning-based approaches such as MCGT[14] and creative therapies can also be invaluable.[4] Though the theoretical foundations of these grief interventions and their foci vary, some common elements include enhancing social support, psychoeducation, stress reduction skills, cognitive reframing, expressive writing, exposure, continuing bonds, and meaning-making.[8,18] There are several resources available describing specific grief therapies,[2,4] but here we describe those with the strongest evidence base to date.

Meaning Reconstruction

A prominent theoretical grief intervention approach involves facilitating the process of meaning reconstruction through development of a narrative about the lost relationship and the loss event.[20] Meaning reconstruction can be useful when loss disrupts the griever's assumptive worldviews, such as beliefs in justice, control, or predictability in life, which may be especially applicable when deaths are untimely (e.g., the death of a child) or traumatic. Clinicians can apply techniques such as narrative retelling and directed journaling to process the event story of the death. Imaginal conversations using empty chair exercises and letter writing may be helpful in assisting the griever with incorporating the back story of their relationship with the patient.[20] This may be particularly useful when a bereaved family member experiences guilt and regret related to the patient's illness, medical decision-making, or circumstances of death or when there is unfinished business with the patient.

Grief interventions theoretically grounded in meaning reconstruction can involve providing psychoeducation about the impact of beliefs on grief reactions and facilitate construction of a meaningful narrative about the death, the deceased's life, and the meaning of the surviving family member's life through directed journaling and reflection prompts. While reconstructing a narrative may not eliminate the pain of grief, this approach can support bereaved individuals in coexisting with their grief and finding significance in it.

Meaning-Centered Grief Therapy

MCGT is a structured, time-limited, cognitive-behavioral-existential intervention grounded in meaning reconstruction theory and developed initially specifically for bereaved parents to decrease the intensity of debilitating grief symptoms by paradoxically helping them to coexist with their grief.[14] Using psychoeducation, structured reflection questions, and experiential exercises, this 16-session therapy highlights four core concepts with grieving parents, including their ability to (1) choose their attitude in the face of suffering; (2) use sources of meaning as "lighthouses" in the distance to transcend the suffering they experience; (3) construct meaning of events, their lives, and their emotional reactions and to author their and the deceased's stories; and (4) maintain a meaningful connection to the deceased. Clinicians systematically unpack available sources of meaning to help grievers connect to their "why's" (i.e., their reasons for living, to help them to coexist with their painful grief). MCGT supports parents' continued connection with their child through mindfulness-based guided imagery, imaginal conversations, and letter writing. A pilot trial of MCGT found improvements in prolonged grief, depression, and sense of meaning in life.[14] Continued research on MCGT and the development of adaptations for other bereaved populations is under way.

Prolonged Grief Disorder Therapy

PGDT, previously referred to as *complicated grief treatment*, is a 16-session therapy that incorporates the dual process model of coping, attachment theory, interpersonal psychotherapy (IPT), and cognitive-behavioral approaches like prolonged exposure.[19,21] PGDT is organized around seven core themes, including understanding and accepting grief, telling the story of the death, and learning to live with reminders of the deceased. Activities that employ these core themes include audiotaping the bereaved individual retelling the story of the death and replaying the audiotape while the therapist provides a supportive presence. When compared to IPT, PGDT has demonstrated greater efficacy and quicker decreases in PGD symptoms than IPT,[19] and individuals who receive PGDT show significant improvement in global functioning related to their grief.[21]

Cognitive Behavioral Therapy

CBT in bereavement focuses on examining unhelpful cognitions and behaviors that may be playing a role in maintaining depression, anxiety, and prolonged grief symptoms.[22] Clinicians offer psychoeducation about the bidirectional relationship between thoughts, feelings, and behaviors and may invite alternative perspectives on cognitions related to feelings of regret, guilt, and anger. To address the common avoidance of distressing feelings and thoughts related to the loss, gradual or prolonged in vivo and imaginal exposure exercises can be used. Behavioral activation, which involves setting behavioral goals and engagement in pleasurable activities, may also be helpful for grieving individuals, particularly those with more depressive symptoms and older adults. Trials of CBT have demonstrated promising results, especially when exposure to memories of the death is incorporated, with reductions PGD symptoms maintained even 2 years after the completion of therapy.[22]

Interpersonal Psychotherapy

IPT focuses on an individual's relationships and how difficulties within those relationships may relate or contribute to depressive symptoms.[19] Clinicians choose a specific problem area that is believed to be contributing to depression, including "grief or complicated bereavement." The therapy is time-limited and can be anywhere from 8 to 16 sessions. Based on the decided length of therapy, clinicians move through beginning, middle, and end phases of treatment that include assessment and efforts to address the selected problem area. IPT has a strong evidence base in treating depression.[19] For PGD, a comparison of IPT and PGDT showed that both interventions led to a reduction in symptoms, though, as noted above, PGDT was superior.[19]

Family-Focused Grief Therapy

Though primarily a preventative intervention, FFGT is designed to facilitate continuity of care for families by being delivered before and after a patient's death. In bereavement, FFGT focuses on supporting family members in expressing and communicating about their grief to create a shared experience and scaffold the family in supporting one another.[15] FFGT in bereavement continues its focus on prevention with the idea of promoting adaptive adjustment but not necessarily targeting psychological symptoms. FFGT has demonstrated efficacy in reducing PGD symptoms in bereaved family members.[15]

Group Interventions

Group grief interventions may be helpful to increase grievers' sense of permission to express their feelings and receive validation and advice about helpful coping strategies from individuals who "get it."[4] They also can reduce isolation and provide opportunities to increase the bereaved individual's support network outside of the group.[4] Various psychotherapeutic approaches can be delivered in a group format. For example, a group format can also be used to deliver general supportive counseling or more specific psychotherapy approaches, such as CBT.[22]

Psychopharmacological Interventions

In some cases, it may be appropriate to use psychopharmacological interventions to address mental health challenges in bereavement in conjunction with psychotherapy. During the acute bereavement phase, anxiolytics and sleep aids may be useful to manage symptoms. Among individuals who present with clinically concerning depressive symptoms—beyond the expected sadness and surges of low mood that is reflective of acute grief—selective serotonin reuptake inhibitors (SSRIs) and serotine and noradrenergic reuptake inhibitors may be recommended and prescribed as appropriate.[23] The presence of bereavement risk factors and suicidality can guide such clinical decisions. However, prescribing clinicians should be careful to, in parallel, provide psychoeducation about grief in order to avoid unintentionally suggesting that the family member is "not grieving well." Psychoeducation about distinctions between normative grief and depressive symptoms may be helpful (see Chapter 17).

Medical treatment for PGD may be considered as well. Although there is a paucity of high-quality evidence, a number of medications have been tested, including SSRIs, tricyclic antidepressants (TCAs), and benzodiazepines.[23] Researchers have shown SSRIs to be only moderately effective in abating grief symptoms in the setting of methodological limitations (e.g., lack of randomization and blinding, small sample size, comorbid mental health diagnoses).[23] One trial examining the combination of PGDT and citalopram found that the addition of the SSRI did not lead to incremental improvements in PGD symptoms but did improve comorbid depressive symptoms.[21] The projected time for SSRIs to achieve full efficacy (e.g., weeks to months) must be weighed in tandem with grief symptom severity. To date, TCAs and benzodiazepines have not been shown as effective psychopharmacological interventions for PGD symptom management. A trial examining the effects of naltrexone on PGD is under way based on its hypothesized reward-based etiology.[24]

Special Considerations

Supporting Bereaved Parents

Although continuity of care is critical for any bereaved kin, it is all the more important to extend support to parents who have lost a child. Bereaved parents not only face the profound and often enduringly painful loss of their child, but also may experience a secondary loss of the treatment team. They may struggle with challenges to their sense of identity as a parent and caregiver and may grapple with guilt around decisions made related to their child's treatment.[16] Palliative care psychiatrists can offer their continued support and answers to questions parents have about their child's end-of-life experience. When providing bereavement support to parents, it is important to treat parents as experts in their own experience, avoid pathologizing protracted grief responses, and make space to honor their child's life. Meaning-centered approaches may be particularly helpful.[14] The offering of resources such as bereaved parent support groups, memorials honoring their child, and remembrance of their child at birthdays and their death anniversary is also valued.

Supporting Staff After Patient Loss

Though grief interventions are generally focused on bereaved family members, patient deaths also inevitably impact palliative care psychiatry clinicians. They often are in the position of facilitating difficult end-of-life discussions and providing intimate emotional support to patients, all while witnessing innumerable deaths and suffering in those family members left behind. Burnout, moral injury, and secondary trauma are thus challenges frequently experienced by palliative care clinicians, and these have only become exacerbated in the wake of the COVID-19 pandemic.[25] The worldwide burden of suffering amid COVID-19 has caused mass bereavement and suffering for professionals across the disciplinary spectrum.[25] See Chapter 17 for additional details.

Interventions are needed to support health professionals experiencing multiple patient losses, and the need has become all the more urgent since the pandemic. Both individual coping strategies (e.g., seeking social support, problem-solving) and workplace action (e.g., staff support and recognition, clear communication) should be promoted to support health professionals' psychological well-being.[25] Meaning-centered approaches may help professionals connect with what is most meaningful about their job as a way of buoying them in times of increased distress. In addition, peer support offered through group and individual sessions, as well as town halls, may be valuable for sustaining the psychological health and resilience of the workforce. Communication strategies that employ an empathic and staff-centered coaching approach to support staff debriefing and processing may also provide health professionals the critical space to navigate their grief in work cultures that demonstrate care for their employees.[25]

Future Directions

Though advances have been made in the development of evidence-based grief interventions, there remains a significant need for methodologically rigorous research on not only the efficacy of grief interventions, but also on their implementation and adaptation for different types of loss. For example, very few grief interventions have been developed for parents who have lost a child to life-limiting illness despite this being considered one of the most devastating forms of loss. Additional research on grief interventions for bereaved older adults is also sorely needed with the increased isolation, rates of bereavement, and health vulnerabilities experienced by this cohort in the wake of the COVID-19 pandemic.[3] Additional research on and institutional commitment to bereavement services in palliative care more broadly is critical to providing the care grieving families need.

Systematically providing condolence calls and conducting bereavement risk screening before and/or after a patient's death are two interventions to which psychiatrists in palliative care are well-suited. Nevertheless, and despite clinicians themselves recognizing the need for such bereavement care, there are ongoing systemic issues that hinder such support from being provided consistently across bereaved families and institutions. These include a lack of clarity about who is responsible for bereavement care, need for staff and financial resources, lack of evidence-based training in grief, and lack of support for the clinicians who already do so much and suffer from their own grief. The provision of grief support requires a multilevel, persistent approach and a rededication of the palliative care field to its duty to deliver continuity of care through bereavement.[1]

Key Points

- Grief interventions in palliative care may be delivered either or both pre- and post-loss to mitigate poor bereavement outcomes.
- Cognitive behavioral, meaning-centered, and family-focused interventions appear to have the most promise.
- The limited research on pharmacological approaches suggests their efficacy in treating depressive symptoms but less promise in treating prolonged grief symptoms.

- Interventions are useful not only for bereaved family members, but also for palliative care clinicians as they face carrying the grief of others while they experience multiple losses themselves.

References

1. National Consensus Project for Quality Palliative Care. *Clinical Practice Guidelines for Quality Palliative Care*, 4th ed. Richmond, VA: National Coalition for Hospice and Palliative Care; 2018.
2. Worden J. *Grief Counseling and Grief Therapy: A Handbook for the Mental Health Practitioner*. New York: Springer; 2018.
3. Lichtenthal WG, Roberts KE, Prigerson HG. Bereavement care in the wake of COVID-19: Offering condolences and referrals. *Ann Intern Med*. 2020;173:833–835.
4. Neimeyer RA. *Techniques of Grief Therapy: Creative Practices for Counseling the Bereaved*. New York: Routledge; 2012.
5. Currier JM, Neimeyer RA, Berman JS. The effectiveness of psychotherapeutic interventions for bereaved persons: A comprehensive quantitative review. *Psychol Bull*. 2008;134:648–661.
6. Prigerson HG, Boelen PA, Xu J, Smith KV, Maciejewski PK. Validation of the new DSM-5-TR criteria for prolonged grief disorder and the PG-13-Revised (PG-13-R) scale. *World Psychiatry*. 2021;20:96–106.
7. Maass U, Hofmann L, Perlinger J, Wagner B. Effects of bereavement groups: A systematic review and meta-analysis. *Death Stud*. 2022;46(3):708–718.
8. Johannsen M, Damholdt MF, Zachariae R, Lundorff M, Farver-Vestergaard I, O'Connor M. Psychological interventions for grief in adults: A systematic review and meta-analysis of randomized controlled trials. *J Affect Disord*. 2019;253:69–86.
9. Burke LA, Clark KA, Ali KS, Gibson BW, Smigelsky MA, Neimeyer RA. Risk factors for anticipatory grief in family members of terminally ill veterans receiving palliative care services. *J Soc Work End Life Palliat Care*. 2015;11:244–266.
10. Hudson P, Hall C, Boughey A, Roulston A. Bereavement support standards and bereavement care pathway for quality palliative care. *Palliat Support Care*. 2018;16:375–387.
11. Applebaum A, Breitbart W. Care for the cancer caregiver: A systematic review. *Palliat Support Care*. 2013;11:231–252.
12. Chi NC, Demiris G. A systematic review of telehealth tools and interventions to support family caregivers. *J Telemed Telecare*. 2015;21:37–44.
13. Lichtenthal WG, Viola M, Rogers M, Roberts KE, Lief L, Cox CE, et al. Development and preliminary evaluation of EMPOWER for surrogate decision-makers of critically ill patients. *Palliat Support Care*. 2022;20(2):167–177.
14. Lichtenthal WG, Catarozoli C, Masterson M, Slivjak E, Schofield E, Roberts KE, et al. An open trial of meaning-centered grief therapy: Rationale and preliminary evaluation. *Palliat Support Care*. 2019;17:2–12.
15. Kissane DW Zaider TI, Li Y, Hichenberg S, Schuler T, Lederberg M, et al. Randomized controlled trial of family therapy in advanced cancer continued into bereavement. *J Clin Oncol*. 2016;34:1921–1927.
16. Lichtenthal WG, Roberts KE, Catarozoli C, Schofield E, Holland JM, Fogarty JJ, et al. Regret and unfinished business in parents bereaved by cancer: A mixed methods study. *Palliat Med*. 2020;34:367–377.
17. Roberts KE, ankauskaite G, Slivjak E, Rubin L, Schachter S, Stabler S, et al. Bereavement risk screening: A pathway to psychosocial oncology care. *Psycho-Oncology*. 2020;29(12):2041–2047.
18. Waller A, Turon H, Mansfield E, Clark K, Hobden B, Sanson-Fisher R. Assisting the bereaved: A systematic review of the evidence for grief counselling. *Palliat Med*. 2016;30:132–148.
19. Shear MK, Frank E, Houck PR. Treatment of complicated grief: A randomized controlled trial. *JAMA*. 2005;293:2601–2608.
20. Neimeyer RA. Meaning reconstruction in bereavement: Development of a research program. *Death Stud*. 2019;43:79–91.

21. Shear MK, Reynolds CF 3rd, Simon NM, Zisook S, Wang Y, Mauro C, et al. Optimizing treatment of complicated grief: A randomized clinical trial. *JAMA Psychiatry.* 2016;73:685–694.
22. Bryant RA, Kenny L, Joscelyne A, Rawson N, Maccallum F, Cahill C, et al. Treating prolonged grief disorder: A 2-year follow-up of a randomized controlled trial. *J Clin Psychiatry.* 2017;78:1363–1368.
23. Bui E, Nadal-Vicens M, Simon NM. Pharmacological approaches to the treatment of complicated grief: Rationale and a brief review of the literature. *Dialogues Clin Neurosci.* 2012;14:149–157.
24. Gang J, Kocsis J, Avery J, Maciejewski PK, Prigerson HG. Naltrexone treatment for prolonged grief disorder: Study protocol for a randomized, triple-blinded, placebo-controlled trial. *Trials.* 2021;22:110.
25. Rosa WE, Ferrell BR, Applebaum AJ. The alleviation of suffering during the COVID-19 pandemic. *Palliat Support Care.* 2020;18:376–378.

42

Psilocybin-Assisted Psychotherapy in Palliative Care

Stephen Ross and Anthony P. Bossis

Introduction

For the person diagnosed with cancer or other life-threatening illnesses, the prospect of facing the end of life is often fraught with emotional distress and marked elevations in depression and anxiety, with prevalence rates as high as one-third or more,[1] which are associated with poor outcomes such as increased mortality[2] and up to four-fold increase in suicide.[3] Treatment of depressive and anxiety spectrum disorders in cancer by pharmacologic and psychosocial interventions is common, but effectiveness is limited and mixed. Medications are prescribed for daily use over a period of months to years, and significant side effects adversely affect adherence. Clinical response to antidepressants is slow, relapse rates are high, and meta-analyses of placebo-controlled trials of antidepressants for cancer-related depression found no clear superiority of antidepressants over placebo.[4]

The World Health Organization and the Institute of Medicine have identified the domains of spiritual and existential distress as integral to the emotional well-being of the palliative care patient, and these are now understood to be important determinants of quality-of-life in persons contending with advanced or end-of-life illness. Spirituality has been defined in palliative care as that "aspect of humanity that refers to the way individuals seek and express meaning and purpose and the way they experience their connectedness to the moment, to self, to others, to nature, and to the significant or sacred."[5] Clinical symptoms of existential distress are common in palliative care settings, as high as approximately 20% in persons with advanced cancer or other progressive medical disorders,[6] and are associated with increased anxiety and depression, desire for hastened death

(DHD), suicidal ideation and behaviors, and pain sensitivity, along with more healthcare visits and decreased quality of life.[7] A manifestation of existential distress, the demoralization syndrome is characterized by hopelessness, helplessness, and loss of meaning and hope in the face of serious life-threatening medical illnesses.[8] While demoralization shares common symptomatology with depression, such as increased symptom burden, it has been hypothesized to be clinically distinct from depression and less likely to respond to conventional psychopharmacologic treatments and more responsive to meaning-centered therapeutic modalities.[9] Differentiating depression from demoralization in part is the loss of meaning and hope forming the central symptoms of demoralization[6] and highlighting the need for emerging effective meaning-making and novel therapies to treat this cohort of patients. This is consistent with a growing literature on the efficacy of manualized existential psychotherapies, specifically targeting loss of meaning in advanced cancer, in decreasing existential distress (e.g., desire for a hastened death [DHD]).[10,11] There are currently no medications or evidence-based combined pharmacologic-psychosocial interventions to improve the psychological, emotional, and existential status of people with serious medical illnesses such as cancer. This chapter will review the rationale of researching and developing psilocybin-assisted psychotherapy (PAP) as a novel pharmacologic-psychotherapeutic intervention to treat psychiatric and existential in palliative care. We discuss the history, anthropology, ethnobotany, neuropharmacology, safety, efficacy data from first and second waves of psychedelic research, putative mechanisms of action, and future directions.

History, Anthropology, and Ethnobotany

Psilocybin mushrooms are a type of Basidiomycota fungi, with more than 200 species, that contain psychedelic alkaloids (psilocybin, psilocin); they can be found on all continents with a predominance in Latin America.[12] Throughout history, there is a record of several civilizations having consumed psilocybin mushrooms, especially in Mexico where psilocybin mushrooms were ingested as visionary sacraments used as part of indigenous spiritual and therapeutic practices, including use in death and dying.[12] Following suppression of Indigenous use during the Spanish Inquisition, the historical existence of psychedelic mushrooms was rediscovered by the renowned Harvard ethnobotanist Richard Evan Schultes and amateur mycologists R. Gordon Wasson and Dr. Valentina Wasson. This led to Albert Hofmann, famed chemist at Sandoz laboratories who serendipitously discovered the psychedelic properties of lysergic acid diethylamide (LSD) in 1943, identifying psilocybin in 1958 as the psychedelic component in the fungi samples.[13] Sandoz then began manufacturing and distributing pure synthetic psilocybin capsules (brand name *Indocybin*) to interested researchers and physicians worldwide.

Promising early-phase clinical research with classic or serotonergic psychedelics (e.g., 5-HT2a agonists) was conducted from the late 1950s through the mid-1970s in the United States and Europe on more than 40,000 research participants, mostly with LSD and, to a much lesser degree, psilocybin, yielding more than a thousand scientific papers.[13] In 1959, the first publications of psilocybin administration in animals, normal human participants, and clinical populations ("convulsive neurosis") appeared in the medical literature. From 1959 to 1977, open-label high-dose ("psychedelic therapy") psilocybin was studied to treat a variety of clinical populations in psychiatry, with some data suggesting positive effects in neurotic spectrum disorders as well as schizophrenia and childhood treatment-resistant autism.[13] Lower-dose psilocybin was utilized clinically as a means of facilitating psychotherapy ("psycholytic therapy"), especially combined with psychoanalytically oriented approaches to treat somatoform, depressive, and anxiety spectrum disorders. Approximately 2,000 participants received psilocybin during this first phase of clinical research.[13]

In reaction to public health concerns about an increase in recreational use and associated harmful effects (i.e., psychosis, reckless behavior), the United States began to restrict the use of psilocybin, LSD, and all serotonergic psychedelics by the general public starting in the mid-1960s. In 1966, the United States passed laws that prohibited the production, trade, and consumption of psychedelic drugs, and, in that same year, Sandoz terminated production of LSD and psilocybin. Further backlash occurred against psychedelics, culminating in Richard Nixon declaring war on drugs and labeling Timothy Leary "the most dangerous man in America." In 1970, Congress passed the Controlled Substance Act and all classical psychedelics (including psilocybin) were classified in the most restrictive category as Drug Enforcement Agency (DEA) schedule I drugs, defined as having high addictive liability and no known medical utility. Due to stigma and legal restrictions, federal funding (mostly through the National Institutes of Mental Health [NIMH], which had spent several million dollars funding psychedelic research in this first wave of research) ended for clinical research with psychedelics. Following this, clinical researchers working in this area were marginalized and had to abandon their programs of research. The research was halted before any definitive conclusions could be reached concerning the clinical efficacy of psychedelic therapy for any psychiatric disorder. However, clinical research conducted in that era, in addition to establishing a very good safety profile, strongly suggested therapeutic signals of psychedelic-assisted psychotherapy, with the most robust data in treating alcoholism, followed by end-of-life cancer-related psychiatric and existential distress.[14]

Pharmacology, Molecular Effects, and Neural Correlates

Psilocybin (4-phosphoryloxy-N,N-dimethyltryptamine) is a substituted indolealkylamine and belongs to the chemical family of hallucinogenic tryptamines. Psilocybin, a pro-drug, is rapidly dephosphorylated to psilocin in the intestinal mucosa and liver, by alkaline phosphatase and a nonspecific esterase, before entering the systemic circulation and penetrating into the central nervous system where it exerts its psychoactive effects. Competitive blockade of the dephosphorylation of psilocybin to psilocin abolishes the psychedelic effects of psilocybin, confirming that psilocin (N,N-dimetyltryptamine) is the main psychoactive metabolite and psychedelic substance in hallucinogenic mushrooms.[15] Psilocin is glucuronidated by endoplasmic enzymes UDP-glucuronosyltransferase (UGTs) to psilocin-O-glucuronide (the main urinary metabolite), as well as undergoing oxidative metabolism with demethylation and deamination to 4-hydroxyindole-3-yl-acetaldehyde (4-H1A), followed by oxidation to 4-hydroxyindole-3-acetic-acid (4-HIAA) and 4-hydroxytryptophol (4-HT).[15] Psilocin has a half-life of 2.5 hours in plasma, and, following oral administration of psilocybin in humans, onset of psychoactive/psychedelic effects begin within 20–40 minutes (coinciding with detectable plasma levels of psilocin). peak concentration and effects occur between 60 and 90 minutes, followed by an approximate 60-minute plateau before decreasing concentration; within 6–8 hours, the main effects have mostly disappeared.[15] The elimination of psilocin (mostly glucuronidated metabolites) as well as unaltered psilocybin (3–10%) occurs through the kidneys, with most of the psilocybin excreted within the first 3 hours following oral intake and completely within approximately 24 hours.[15]

Psilocin, like all of the classical psychedelics, has a high affinity for serotonin receptors in the brain. It has predominant agonist activity on serotonin 5-HT2A, 5-HT2C and 5-HT1A receptors. Pre-administration of ketanserin, a 5-HT2A receptor antagonist, abolishes almost all of the psilocin-induced psychedelic effects, supporting the primacy of 5-HT2A receptor activation in mediating its subjective effects.[14] Interactions with non-serotonergic receptors also contribute to the subjective and behavioral effects of psilocybin. Psilocybin indirectly increases dopamine transmission in striatal brain regions, although it fails to significantly activate the nucleus accumbens in positron emission tomography (PET) imaging studies, consistent with the lack of evidence linking classical psychedelics with addiction.[14] Psilocybin also appears to have neuroplastic effects mediated through glutamatergic mechanisms of action, with activation of postsynaptic 5-HT2A receptors located on a subpopulation of pyramidal cells in the deep layers of the prefrontal cortex leading to an increase in glutamatergic recurrent network activity, in turn activating AMPA and NMDA receptors on cortical pyramidal neurons and leading to increased expression of brain-derived neurotrophic factor (BDNF) involved in synaptic plasticity and neurogenesis.[16]

Data from functional magnetic resonance imaging (fMRI), electroencephalography (EEG), and magnetoencephalography (MEG) research with psilocybin conducted in normal volunteers and clinical populations (i.e., major depressive disorder) suggests that psilocybin acutely reduces overall brain activity within (modularity) brain networks, including the prefrontal cortex, and between (integration) brain networks with evidence of deactivation of the default mode network (i.e., precuneus, medial PFC [mPFC], posterior cingulate cortex [PCC]), a brain network implicated in the pathophysiology of a variety of neuropsychiatric disorders.[17] In addition, following "disintegration" of brain networks, there is evidence to suggest a reorganization into new local-range networks and an increase in transient, distinct brain patterns compared to waking consciousness (i.e., increased plasticity).[18]

Physiological and Psychological Effects: Safety Data

Psilocybin is a very safe drug from the perspective of physiological toxicity when administered to humans and is not associated with major organ system damage (i.e., cardiac, neurologic, hepatic, renal), carcinogenicity, teratogenicity, enduring neuropsychological deficits, or overdose deaths.[13] The psychological and experiential effects of psilocybin include significant alterations in perception (i.e., visual and auditory illusions or hallucinations; synesthesia), cognition (i.e., tangential thought process, dissociative phenomenon), and affect (i.e., mood fluctuations ranging from euphoria to extreme anxiety). Acute adverse psychological experiences ("bad trips") remain the biggest concern in psilocybin administration and typically include anxiety, panic (i.e., fear that the experience will never end or fear of losing one's mind), dysphoria, depersonalization, psychotic-like phenomenon (i.e., paranoid ideation, hallucinations), and agitation. Psilocybin can also occasion subjective often profound and memorable experiences of ego dissolution, mystical-type, or "peak" experiences involving the loss of a coherent, consistent set of narratives about oneself that defines both whom one thinks oneself to be at any given time and across time and the psychological boundaries separating oneself from others.[13]

Psilocybin administration to adult participants in clinical trials has an excellent clinical safety record, from both the perspective of psychological and physiological treatment-related adverse effects. These trials, enrolling 275 adult participants, included open-label, dose-escalating studies as well as randomized, double-blind trials, and enrolled both healthy volunteers and various subpopulations with differing therapeutic indications.[19] Of the 275 participants enrolled across these studies, 264 received at least one dose of oral psilocybin, 180 participants received two doses, 71 participants received three doses, and 14 participants received four doses. In total, 529 oral psilocybin doses were administered with doses ranging from "very low dose" (45 µg/kg) to "high dose" (600 µg/kg; 0.6 mg/kg). A subset ($n = 92$) of the 275 participants were participants with life-threatening, advanced, or terminal cancer who received single-dose psilocybin ranging from 0.2 mg/kg to approximately 0.3 mg/kg. For all 275 adult participants, there were no reports of any psilocybin-related serious adverse events (SAEs), including no reports of serious medical toxicity and no reported cases of addiction, prolonged psychosis, or hallucinogen persisting perception disorder (HPPD).[19] The key commonality among all these studies, from the perspective of risk reduction and safety, was the careful attention to screening (i.e., screening out individuals with psychotic spectrum illnesses or unstable medical conditions), optimal setting for dosing sessions, and careful psychological preparation before dosing sessions and psychological integration following dosing sessions.

First Wave of Psychedelic-Assisted Psychotherapy Research in Psycho-Oncology and Palliative Care (1964–1977)

Kast research. The first research studies to explore the therapeutic effects of serotonergic psychedelics in advanced medical illness were conducted in the early 1960s by Eric Kast at Chicago Medical School, initially investigating the efficacy of LSD to treat the physical pain of terminally ill cancer patients in an inpatient medical setting. In a comparative efficacy trial assessing the analgesic effects of single-dose LSD 100 µg compared to single-dose conventional opioid medications (hydromorphone 2 mg; meperidine 100 mg) in 50 severely ill end-of-life patients (most with cancer diagnoses) with refractory pain syndromes, the LSD group was found to have better short-term sustained (i.e., several weeks) analgesic effects than the opioid groups, and, surprisingly, Kast also reported on decreased depression and improvements in attitudes toward death and dying, suggesting for the first time the potential of psychedelic compounds in treating cancer-related psychiatric and existential distress.[20] In accounting for the potential analgesic effects of LSD, Kast hypothesized that the subjective perception of cancer pain could be reduced through the "attenuation of anticipation" experienced through temporary altered states of consciousness generated by the drug action. Based on these findings, Kast went on to treat 128 terminally ill cancer patients with refractory pain syndromes with an open-label design using single-dose LSD 100 µg and reported on acute and sustained (i.e., several weeks) analgesic effects, decreased depressive symptoms and fear associated with the advancement of cancer and impending death, and improvements in sleep.[21] No serious medical complications were reported despite Kast's mostly being a chemotherapeutic model without preparation, psychological support during dosing sessions, and post-dose integrative psychotherapy.

Spring Grove Studies (psychedelic-assisted psychotherapy model). Following this research, a watershed development in the history of psychedelic therapy in treating end-of-life distress occurred at Spring Grove State Hospital in Maryland, beginning in 1967. In administering the psychedelic compounds LSD and DPT (*N,N*-dipropyltryptamine) to terminally ill cancer patients over a 10-year period in an outpatient setting, this pioneering group developed a novel therapeutic model tailored specifically for the profound changes in consciousness generated by psychedelic compounds.[22] This psychedelic treatment model established guidelines for therapeutic optimization and safety while minimizing adverse effects. This approach was also used in the psychedelic treatment of alcohol use disorder in the mid-20th century and is still currently the dominant therapeutic model used in contemporary psilocybin trials in cancer distress and other clinical applications such as alcohol use disorder and major depressive disorder.[13]

Unlike in Kast's prior research, the research at Spring Grove established the therapeutic concept of "set and setting" based on the theory and observation that the subjective effects and non-ordinary states of consciousness generated by LSD and other psychedelic compounds are largely dependent on variables associated with the individual and the environment. The model was that the psychedelic medication would be delivered in conjunction with a psychotherapeutic platform and, as such, can optimally be described as *psychedelic-assisted psychotherapy. Set* refers to the mindset of the person taking the drug, their personal history, and expectations regarding the session. *Setting* describes the social and physical environment in which the psychedelic is taken. Following careful medical and psychiatric screening, this treatment model consists of three phases delivered by a dyadic therapeutic team: (1) a preparatory phase prior to the experimental drug session, (2) the experimental drug session, and (3) a post-drug session integration period. The preparatory phase consists of typically 2–4 weeks of meetings with two trained therapists to review the patient's emotional and existential reaction to cancer or other life-threatening illness, a life review including developmental and psychosocial factors and intention for entering the study. Central to minimizing potential adverse effects occurring during the drug session (notably, fear and anxiety) is the development of trust and rapport between the therapists and participant during this period of preparation. Following the preparatory phase is an all-day experimental drug session which takes place in a living-room like setting within the hospital, with the intention to evoke the feeling of a nonmedical atmosphere. The patient, lying on a couch supine, is encouraged to wear eyeshades and headphones playing preselected music to encourage attention inward to the unfolding changes in consciousness and to distract from environmental stimuli during the medication sessions (approximately 6–8 hours with psilocybin and approximately 8–12 hours with LSD). Interpersonal support and assurance are provided throughout the session by the therapists with recommendations to accept, trust, and be open to the changes in consciousness. Typically, there is minimal conversation with the therapists during the medication session, with the period of follow-up therapeutic integration sessions in the days and weeks after the psychedelic administration allowing for discussion and exploration of the psychological and often spiritual material that emerged during the experimental session day. A core feature of this treatment model was the administration of moderate to high doses of the psychedelic compound to purposely generate a mystical or peak experience which was hypothesized to mediate reductions in psychiatric and existential distress.[22,23] Key subjective and phenomenological features of mystical/peak experiences include *Unity*, a strong sense of the interconnectedness of all people and things—all is one—an awareness being part of a dimension greater than oneself; *Transcendence*, a sense of timelessness with past, present, and future collapsed into the present moment; *Sacredness*, a strong feelings of awe, wonder, reverence, humility; *Noetic quality*, a sense of encountering ultimate reality or knowledge, *Deeply felt positive mood*, love, blessedness, joy, peace; and *Ineffability*, an experience felt to be beyond words, that cannot be adequately described.[23]

The findings from the open-label Spring Grove studies, conducted from 1967 to 1977, supported Kast's findings suggesting efficacy of LSD-assisted psychotherapy in treating psychiatric and existential distress as well as pain in end-of-life cancer. The first publication of the Spring Grove group was a case series study conducted by Walter Pahnke that included 22 participants who were treated open-label with single to repeated dosing sessions of LSD (200–300 μg). The group reported on decreases in pain, opioid medication use, depression, anxiety, and fear of death.[23] In linking the LSD-occasioned mystical experience to therapeutic outcomes, Pahnke noted, "The most dramatic effects came in the wake of a psychedelic mystical experience. There was a decrease in fear, anxiety, worry, and depression. Sometimes the need for pain medications was lessened, but mainly because the patient was able to tolerate what pain he had more easily. There was an increase in serenity, peace, and calmness. Most striking was a decrease in the fear of death."[23] In another study led by Stanislav Grof, of 44 participants with terminal cancer who received open-label single-dose LSD (200–500 μg)-assisted psychotherapy, a systematic analysis including 31 participants reported on significant pre-post within-group differences relative to baseline regarding decreased pain severity and pain catastrophizing, decreased depression and anxiety, and decreased fear of death.[22]

Second Wave: Scientific Findings of Recent Contemporary Trials (2011–Current)

After a quiescence of about two decades, human research with classic psychedelics resumed in the early 1990s. Shortly after the turn of the 21st century, psilocybin once again entered therapeutic clinical trials, reigniting this promising area of research. In the past decade, clinical trials have resumed investigating the effects of psilocybin in the treatment of a spectrum of neuropsychiatric illnesses (i.e., cancer-related psychiatric and existential disorders, major depressive disorder, obsessive compulsive disorder) and addictive disorders (i.e., alcohol, nicotine, cocaine). The studies that have been completed to date are open-label or randomized controlled trials (RCTs) with small sample sizes, and, although the results have been very promising, they are not sufficient to definitively establish treatment efficacy. The most studied indication and the one with the most robust data from phase II RCTs is the use of PAP to treat advanced cancer-related psychiatric and existential distress. A recent systematic review[4] of clinical trials in which participants with advanced cancer and related psychiatric and existential distress were treated with LSD, psilocybin, or dipropyltryptamine (DPT) identified six open-label trials published between 1964 and 1980, and four RCTs ($n = 104$) published between 2011 and 2016. Four of these used LSD ($n = 244$), three psilocybin ($n = 92$), and one DPT ($n = 30$).

Three RCT studies[24–26] conducted since 2011 have examined the efficacy of PAP in patients with advanced cancer-related psychiatric and existential distress. At the University of California Los Angeles Harbor Medical Center, 12 participants with late-stage cancer and related significant psychiatric distress (a Diagnostic and Statistical Manual of Mental Disorders [DSM-IV] diagnosis of adjustment disorder with anxiety, generalized anxiety disorder, acute stress disorder, or anxiety disorder due to cancer) were treated in a randomized, crossover study using single "moderate" dose (0.2 mg/kg) psilocybin versus single-dose active placebo (niacin), with both arms delivered with a "set and setting" psychotherapeutic platform.[24] The trial demonstrated safety and feasibility of recruitment with no serious psilocybin-related psychiatric or medical SAEs. Although it failed to find significant differences between groups, prior to crossover at 2 weeks, in reducing anxiety and depression, there were trends for acute reductions in anxiety and depression in the psilocybin-first group over the niacin-first group, prior to crossover, as well as significant reductions in anxiety (at 1 and 3 months) and depression (at 6 months), collapsed across groups, measured relative to medication administration.[24] This pilot study, enrolling only patients with advanced cancer, was limited by a lack of gender diversity (11 women), a small sample size, and a low dose of psilocybin.

Johns Hopkins University (JHU) Medical Center conducted a randomized, double-blind, active-placebo controlled, crossover (at 5 weeks post dose 1) trial that included 51 participants with life-threatening cancer and compared single "high" dose of psilocybin (0.31 mg/kg) with single "very low" dose psilocybin active control (1 or 3 mg/70 kg [.014 or 0.043 mg/kg]), both delivered in conjunction with a psychotherapy platform, to treat cancer-related depression, anxiety, and existential distress.[25] Patients were treated for adjustment disorder with anxiety or depression (44%), major depressive disorder (27%), and generalized anxiety disorder (10%). Primary endpoints for depression and anxiety were scores on the clinician-rated GRID-Hamilton Depression Scale-17 (GRID-HAMD- 17) and clinician-rated GRID-Hamilton Anxiety (GRID-HAM-A) scale. There were no medical or psychiatric SAEs attributable to psilocybin. High-dose PAP produced large and sustained (up to 5 weeks) post single-dose improvements in cancer-related depressive/anxiety symptoms. For example, at 5 weeks post-session 1, 92% of the high-dose-first group demonstrated 50% or greater improvement in depression on the GRID-HAM-D-17 versus the low-dose-first group's 32% response rate. Similarly, 76% of high-dose-first participants met criteria for a clinically significant anxiolytic response rate versus 24% in the low-dose-first group. Compared to the placebo group, PAP produced mystical type experiences that correlated with and partially mediated anxiolytic and antidepressant effects (at 5 weeks post-dosing of psilocybin).[25] Limitations included a crossover design, a heterogeneous sample of cancer patients (early- and late-stage disease), little ethnic diversity, and too small a sample to optimally examine potential psycho-spiritual mechanisms of action.

Another RCT examining the use of PAP to treat advanced cancer-related psychiatric and existential distress was conducted at NYU Langone Health (NYULH) and NYU College of Dentistry's Bluestone Center for Clinical Research.[26] The trial included 29 randomized individuals (90% White; 62% female) with a mix of early- (38%) and advanced-stage (62%) cancer and the following primary psychiatric diagnoses: adjustment disorder with anxiety ($n = 18$, 62%), adjustment disorder with anxiety and depression ($n = 8$, 28%), and generalized anxiety disorder ($n = 3$, 10%). This RCT, with crossover at 7 weeks (after dose 1) and a final outcome assessment 6.5 months after dose 2, compared single high-dose psilocybin (0.3 mg/kg) to single-dose niacin (250 mg), with both arms delivered in conjunction with a psychotherapeutic platform consisting of elements of supportive and existential psychotherapies (i.e., meaning-centered psychotherapy). Primary endpoints measuring cancer-related anxiety and depression were the Hospital Anxiety and Depression Scale (HADS), Beck Depression Inventory (BDI), and State-Trait Anxiety Inventory (STAI). Consistent with prior clinical research, no psychiatric or medical SAEs were attributable to psilocybin. Robust, rigorous findings were demonstrated prior to crossover comparing psilocybin-first to niacin-first groups: PAP produced rapid (1 day prior to the psilocybin session to 1 day post-dose), substantial (between-groups effect sizes ~0.8 to 1.7), sustained (up to 7 weeks post single-dosing), and significant clinical improvements in cancer-related anxiety and depressive symptoms (Figure 42.1a). For instance, at 1 day post-psilocybin session 1, 82% of psilocybin-first subjects met criteria for antidepressant remission (e.g., ≥50% reduction plus a HADS ≤7 or BDI ≤12) versus 24% in the niacin-first group. At 7 weeks post psilocybin session 1, 81% of psilocybin-first subjects met criteria for antidepressant remission versus 12% in the niacin-first group. This trial found sustained anxiolytic/antidepressant response rates of 60–80% at the 6.5-month follow-up (Figure 42.1a). Complementing the primary outcomes, prior to crossover (2 weeks after dose 1), PAP was associated with significant improvements in cancer-related hopelessness, demoralization, quality of life, and spiritual well-being. At the 6.5-month follow-up, in addition to sustained improvements in quality of life, existential distress, and spiritual well-being, patients improved on a measure of attitudes toward death and dying, although there were no acute or longer-term

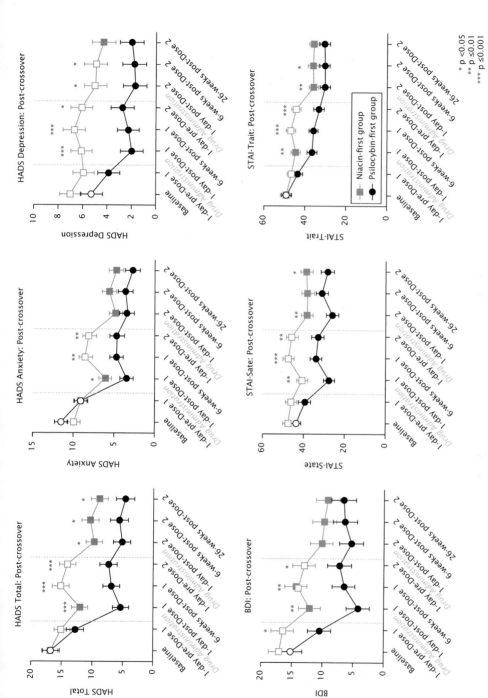

FIGURE 42.1A Anxiety and depression (post-crossover). Means (±SE) for primary outcome measures are shown in the two treatment groups at the following time points: baseline (psilocybin first $n = 14$, niacin first $n = 15$), 1-day pre dose-1 (psilocybin first $n = 14$, niacin first $n = 15$), 1 day post-dose 1 (psilocybin first $n = 14$, niacin first $n = 14$), 7 weeks post-dose 1, 1 day pre-dose 2 (psilocybin first $n = 14$, niacin first $n = 12$, niacin first $n = 14$), 1 day post-dose 2 (psilocybin first $n = 12$, niacin first $n = 11$), 26 weeks post-dose 2 (psilocybin first $n = 11$, niacin first $n = 12$). Asterisks indicate significance level of between-group t-tests. Closed points represent significant within-group differences relative to scores at baseline.

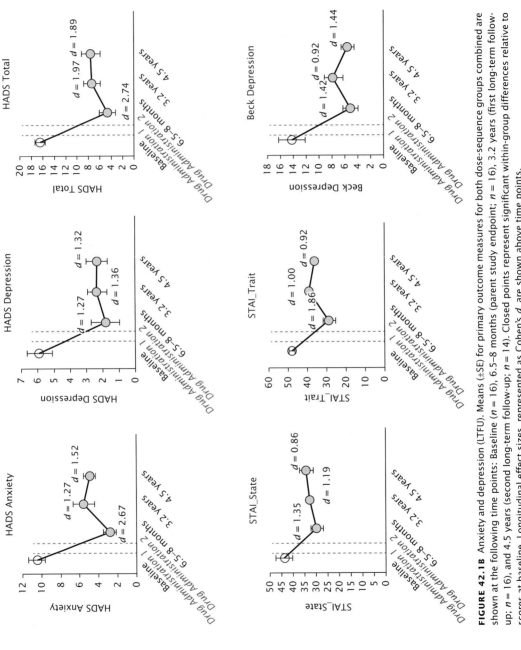

FIGURE 42.1B Anxiety and depression (LTFU). Means (±SE) for primary outcome measures for both dose-sequence groups combined are shown at the following time points: Baseline ($n = 16$), 6.5–8 months (parent study endpoint; $n = 16$), 3.2 years (first long-term follow-up; $n = 16$), and 4.5 years (second long-term follow-up; $n = 14$). Closed points represent significant within-group differences relative to scores at baseline. Longitudinal effect sizes, represented as Cohen's *d*, are shown above time points.

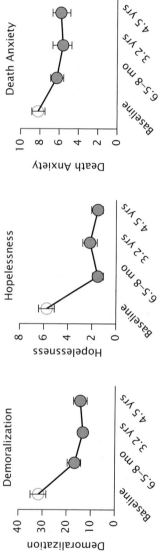

FIGURE 42.1C Existential distress (LTFU). Means (±SE) for secondary outcome measures for participants (in both dose-sequence groups combined) are shown at the following time points: Baseline (*n* = 16), 6.5–8 months (parent study end-point; *n* = 16), 3.2 years (first long-term follow-up; *n* = 16), and 4.5 years (second long-term follow-up; *n* = 14.) Closed points represent significant within-group differences relative to scores at baseline.

improvements on a death anxiety measure. As in the JHU trial, psilocybin-induced mystical experience intensity correlated with and suggested a role in mediating anxiolytic and antidepressant effects of psilocybin at 7 weeks post-dose.[26]

A long-term follow-up trial of the NYULH pilot RCT was conducted with two follow-ups at means of 3.2 and 4.5 years after subjects' PAP sessions, using the same measures.[27] Sixteen of the original cohort of 29 participants who were still alive were contacted for the long-term follow-up study and 14 provided data at the later (4.5 year) follow-up assessment. Significant within-group improvement relative to baseline was found at 4.5-year follow-up; effect sizes for reductions in anxiety and depression ranged from 0.86 to 1.89 (Figure 42.1b). Anxiolytic/antidepressant response rates were ~60–80%; depression remission rates were ~50–80%. Existential distress (including demoralization and death anxiety) was improved at 4.5-year follow-up compared to baseline (Figure 42.1c). Participants (71–100%) attributed positive life changes to the psilocybin experience at the second follow-up and rated it among the most spiritually significant and personally meaningful experiences of their lives.

Patients with advanced cancer are at elevated risk of DHD, suicidal ideation, and completed suicide.[3,28] Loss of meaning, a component of the demoralization syndrome, can be increased in advanced cancer and predicts DHD and suicidal ideation. In a secondary analysis from the NYULH RCT of PAP in advanced cancer, among participants with elevated suicidal ideation at baseline, PAP was associated with rapid (i.e., within 8 hours) within-group reductions in suicidal ideation that persisted for 6.5 months post-dosing.[29] PAP also produced large reductions in loss of meaning measured from baseline to 2 weeks after medication administration, and this remained significant and substantial at 6.5-month, 3.2-year, and 4.5-year follow-up. Exploratory analyses suggested that PAP may mediate anti-suicidal effects due to its therapeutic impact on hopelessness and demoralization and its effects on meaning-making in particular. These preliminary results support the potential of utilizing PAP as an intervention in treating DHD and suicidal ideation in patients with advanced cancer or other life-threatening or end-of-life conditions, and these warrant further investigation.

With demoralization emerging as an important clinical concept in palliative care, there are also promising signs of PAP being effective in treating this indication in persons with AIDS. Consistent with findings of acute and long-term sustained (i.e., months to years) reductions in demoralization found with PAP in advanced cancer-associated existential distress,[26,27] an open-label study investigating the safety and preliminary efficacy of PAP among long-term male AIDS survivors (a population with a high degree of demoralization and traumatic loss) reported a 50% reduction in demoralization following psilocybin administration.[30]

Potential Mechanisms of Action: Causal Model of Change

If PAP is found to produce acute/rapid and long-term sustained reductions in psychiatric distress (e.g., depression, anxiety, suicidality) and existential distress (e.g., demoralization, hopelessness, death anxiety) in patients at the end of life, it would be important to explore causal mechanisms of action. The potential mechanism of therapeutic action is likely complex, multifactorial, and not just a drug effect per se, but rather a drug plus psychotherapy interaction of an intervention delivered by a dyad therapeutic team within a set and setting framework (i.e., preparation, support during medication sessions, integration followed sessions). The optimal psychotherapeutic platform utilized in conjunction with psilocybin administration would have an evidence base supporting efficacy and have the potential to work synergistically with the hypothesized mechanisms of action of psilocybin. Treatment models based on the principles of *supportive psychotherapy* and *existentially oriented* psychotherapies appear to be ideal for this context. This therapeutic model contrasts with conventional pharmacotherapies, where medicine is taken daily to achieve desired effects, and there can be often weeks before onset of clinical change. In psychedelic therapies, the medication is taken typically for one or two sessions.

A conceptual model of causality, supported by evidence in published literature, could be broken down into neurobiological and psycho-spiritual pathways leading to persisting effects and change mechanisms, further narrowing to final common change mechanisms and, ultimately, a reduction in target symptoms. An example of such a model could be the exploration of how PAP might improve DHD and suicidality in palliative care patients such as those with advanced cancer, keeping in mind the main drivers of DHD and suicidal ideation in cancer patients: depression, demoralization, hopelessness, and chronic pain[29] (see Figure 42.2). To assess causal mechanisms of action, a trial would need to be optimally designed and powered to interrogate each potential mechanism of action in accounting for improvement in long-term clinical outcomes and could include measures to assess for the various psychological change mechanisms (i.e., mystical experience, cognitive flexibility, structural personality assessment, challenging experiences, emotional breakthrough) as well as potential neurobiological mechanisms of action (i.e., neuroimaging to assess sustained changes in brain network connectivity, neuro-inflammatory biomarkers such as tumor necrosis factor [TNF-α], and neuroplasticity biomarkers such as brain-derived neurotrophic factor [BDNF]).

Regarding potential psycho-spiritual mechanisms of action, a key finding spanning from the first wave of research from the mid-20th century to the recent clinical trials utilizing psilocybin has been the emergence and clinical significance of the mystical or peak experience. The NYULH and JHU trials both found that the intensity of the mystical experience during the dosing session partially mediated antidepressant and anxiolytic effects approximately 1–2 months post dosing.[25,26] The subjective human experience of self-transcendence is a potentially powerful one. It can provide the opportunity for radical shifts in consciousness, allowing novel insights and perspectives on the nature of self, suffering, death, and consciousness.[31,32] The ability, through self-transcendence, to subjectively identify with something more enduring than the ill or failing body allows for the possibility of transformative and therapeutic insight and improved existential and spiritual well-being. Furthermore, the phenomenology of psychedelic-generated states of consciousness offers the palliative care or advanced-illness patient the potential to cultivate personal meaning amid the challenging and often existentially distressed period following diagnosis and throughout the arc of illness up until end of life.[32] Meaning and transcendence are cited as among the most potentially beneficial variables at the end of life. In both the NYULH and

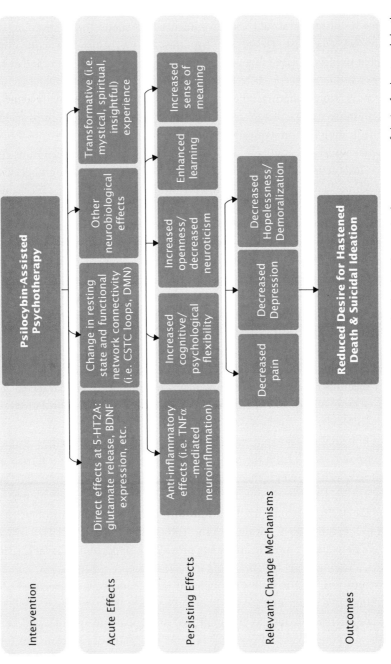

FIGURE 42.2 Proposed theoretical causal model. Therapeutic effects of psilocybin therapy in the treatment of desire for hastened death (DHD) and suicidal ideation (SI) following a cancer diagnosis.

5-HT2A, serotonin 2A receptor; BDNF, brain-derived neurotrophic factor; CSTC, cortico-striato-thalamo-cortical; DMN, default mode network; TNFα: tumor necrosis factor-α.

JHU pilot RCTs, the psilocybin experience was rated as among the most meaningful and spiritually significant events of participants' entire lives. For example, 70% (NYULH) and 67% (JHU) of participants rated the psilocybin experience as among the five most meaningful experience of their lives, including the single most meaningful experience.[25,26]

Qualitative analyses from the NYULH pilot RCT also support the hypothesis that psycho-spiritual mechanisms may underlie the therapeutic action of psilocybin and reported themes of self-forgiveness, improved relational functioning, revised life priorities, transition from separateness to interconnectedness, lasting changes to sense of identity, acknowledgment of cancer's place in life, emotional uncoupling from cancer, reconnection to life, greater confidence in the face of cancer recurrence, and reconciliation with death.[33,34] A heuristic model of potential psycho-spiritual mechanisms of action of PAP in treating existential distress in advanced cancer or other serious medical disorders could include (1) increased sense of meaning and purpose; (2) ability to cognitively or emotionally reframe the meaning of cancer in one's life; (3) increased capacity for appreciation of time living and to commit to living life as fully as possible until death; (4) improved interpersonal relationships with loved ones, family, and friends with enhanced capacity for expressions of love, intimacy, and forgiveness; (5) increased appreciation and experience of interconnectedness beyond the self (i.e., nature, the cosmos); (6) ability to attend to unfinished business or unresolved conflicts; and (7) the possibility to reconceptualize the process of death and dying in a positivistic framework (i.e., not the end but a transition of some manner in continuation of consciousness) and achieve increased acceptance and peace with death.[31]

In addition to the transpersonal realm of mystical or peak experience, reports from the first wave of psychedelic research in palliative care suggested the importance of psychodynamically oriented or autobiographical-type experiences where traumatic memories, unresolved interpersonal conflicts, and unresolved grief or mourning were revisited and resolved, often leading to insight and feelings of forgiveness and love toward others and self.[22,23]

Future Directions

In summary, the three FDA phase II trials in the United States that examined single-dose PAP for advanced cancer-related psychiatric distress included a total cohort of 92 participants.[24-26] Combined, these trials strongly suggest that psilocybin-assisted therapy for patients with cancer-related psychiatric and existential illness produces rapid, robust (e.g., large effect sizes, large antidepressant and anxiolytic response and remission rates), and sustained improvements (e.g., several months to several years) in cancer-related anxiety, depression, and suicidal ideation, as well as improvements in existential distress (e.g., demoralization, hopelessness, death and dying-related distress) and quality of life. In addition, psilocybin occasioned mystical-type experiences, experienced as highly meaningful and spiritual, partially mediated anxiolytic and antidepressant effects assessed longitudinally (i.e., 5 to 7 weeks) post psilocybin administration, suggesting a potential psychological mechanism of action.

Given that these trials had relatively small sample sizes and lacked ethnic diversity, they are liable to various biases (i.e., selection), the possibility of type I errors, and lack of external validity. It is therefore important as a next step to proceed to larger clinical trials with the goal of replicating the findings.[4] Given the implications of this intervention in end-of-life care, it would be important to focus on a population of patients with end-stage cancer. Such a trial would likely be a multicenter one that would include a nationally representative sample of patients with advanced cancer-related psychiatric and existential distress. It would be important to optimally design the trial to replicate some of the most novel and interesting findings from the phase 2 trials (i.e., rapidity of onset of psilocybin and sustained clinical benefits). One approach could be parallel design without a cross-over, single-dose psilocybin at 25 mg versus active placebo, both delivered in conjunction with a psychotherapeutic platform consisting of a mix of supportive and existential psychotherapy components to treat anxiety, depression, and demoralization associated with end-of-life cancer. It should be designed and sufficiently powered (i.e., $N = 200$) to interrogate potential mechanisms of action including psycho-spiritual change mechanisms and neurobiological mechanisms of action. Such multicenter trials could be funded through a public–private partnership such as a combination of funding from National Institutes of Health (NIH) and National Cancer Institute (NCI), plus private philanthropy or through biotech/pharma. If co-sponsored by a pharma entity for the purpose of drug development, these pivotal phase 3 trials could be used as part of a new drug application (NDA) to the FDA that could go toward rescheduling of psilocybin for advanced cancer-related psychiatric and existential distress. At NYULH, there is an active attempt to conduct multicenter phase 3 pivotal trials of single-dose PAP to treat advanced cancer-related psychiatric and existential distress with funding from NCI and biotech (S. Ross, personal communication, June 14, 2021).

The availability of psilocybin-assisted therapy could provide a novel treatment model for patients with end-of life cancer-related psychiatric and existential distress[4] in several ways.

1. *Rapidity of therapeutic effect.* A medication that can work immediately for cancer-related depression and suicidality would have considerable benefits for patients with a limited life span, especially in contrast to the delay (e.g., weeks) for typical antidepressants to exert their effects and their relative lack of efficacy in treating cancer-related depression.
2. *Sustained anxiolytic and antidepressant clinical benefits from single dosing (i.e., months).* The benefits could include minimization of side effects related to having to take an antidepressant or anxiolytic (i.e., benzodiazepine) on an ongoing basis. Further research is needed to establish the length of therapeutic benefit of single-dose psilocybin and examine the necessity for repeated dosing regimens.
3. *Providing a pharmacologic-psychotherapeutic intervention for existential distress at the end of life.* Existential distress is underrecognized and undertreated in cancer patients within Western medicine: there are no established medications with efficacy or effectiveness for this typology of distress, and having an intervention that can reduce the fear associated with the dying process could have enormous clinical and quality-of-life benefits for patients with end-of-life cancer as they approach death.

It is important to extend research utilizing PAP to treat psychiatric and existential distress beyond advanced cancer to other end-of-life medical illnesses (i.e., cardiac, pulmonary, renal, neurodegenerative disorders). At present, there are several protocols in development to explore the safety and efficacy of PAP in treating psychiatric (i.e., anxiety, depression) and existential (i.e., demoralization, DHD, death anxiety) distress in a palliative care cohort at the Lundquist Institute at Harbor-UCLA and NYU Langone Medical Center (multicenter RCT; C. Grob and A. Bossis, personal communication, June 14, 2021), Emory Winship Cancer Institute (open-label; A. Zarrabi, personal communication, November 10, 2020), and Dana-Farber Cancer Institute (open-label; Y. Beaussant, personal communication, May 3, 2021). A group at the Aquilino Cancer Center in Maryland is nearing completion of an open-label psilocybin-assisted group therapy trial with cancer-associated distress with demoralization as an exploratory end point (NCT 04593563). Also, given the promising historical data suggesting acute and short-term sustained (e.g., several weeks) analgesic effects of single-dose LSD 100 μg in patients with terminal cancer refractory pain syndromes,[20,21] it would be important to study LSD and psilocybin as novel pain therapeutics in advanced cancer pain syndromes. One such study is a funded RCT, in development at the NYULH Center for Psychedelic Medicine, of LSD-assisted psychotherapy in advanced cancer pain syndromes on chronic opioid therapy with pain as the primary outcome and secondary outcomes including opioid sparing, psychiatric distress (e.g., anxiety, depression), existential distress (e.g., demoralization, death anxiety, DHD), quality of life, and spirituality (S. Ross, personal communication, June 14, 2021).

With a paucity of pharmacologic-psychotherapeutic interventions to effectively treat the emotional and existential distress in palliative care patients and a call for novel modalities to emerge, PAP potentially provides a promising approach. If larger scale trials can demonstrate the efficacy of PAP in treating psychiatric and existential distress in end-of-life conditions (cancer and other serious medical illnesses), the dissemination and utilization of this intervention could be especially useful for patients in outpatient or inpatient hospice settings. It could aid the process of dying with dignity to help facilitate a "good" death and help patients approach death with improved psychological, emotional, and spiritual well-being.

Key Points

- Psychiatric (e.g., anxiety, depression) and existential distress (e.g., demoralization, DHD, death anxiety) are common in palliative care settings and are associated with poor psychiatric and medical outcomes.
- Current pharmacologic and psychotherapeutic treatments for end-of-life psychiatric and existential distress are of limited efficacy, and there is a need to develop novel therapeutics in this clinical population.
- From the 1960s to 1970s, extensive open-label research, mostly with LSD, suggested efficacy of psychedelic-assisted psychotherapy in treating psychiatric and existential distress in end-of-life cancer.
- From 2011 to the present, three pilot RCTs of single-dose PAP strongly suggested that this intervention produces rapid, clinically meaningful, and sustained (e.g., several

months to several years) improvements in advanced cancer-related anxiety, depression, and suicidal ideation, as well as improvements in existential distress (e.g., demoralization, hopelessness, death and dying-related distress) and quality of life.

- There are active efforts to conduct larger trials of PAP in advanced cancer-related psychiatric and existential distress to attempt to replicate efficacy findings from the pilot trials and determine potential causal mechanisms of action.
- There are efforts to extend research of PAP as a novel treatment approach in palliative care for anxiety, depression, and existential distress in serious medical conditions beyond cancer.

References

1. Mitchell AJ, Chan M, Bhatti H, Halton M, Grassi L, Johansen C, Meader N. Prevalence of depression, anxiety, and adjustment disorder in oncological, haematological, and palliative-care settings: A meta-analysis of 94 interview-based studies. *Lancet Oncol*. Feb 2011;12(2):160–174. doi:10.1016/s1470-2045(11)70002-x

2. Satin JR, Linden W, Phillips MJ. Depression as a predictor of disease progression and mortality in cancer patients: A meta-analysis. *Cancer*. Nov 15 2009;115(22):5349–5361. doi:10.1002/cncr.24561

3. Zaorsky NG, Zhang Y, Tuanquin L, Bluethmann SM, Park HS, Chinchilli VM. Suicide among cancer patients. *Nature Comm*. Jan 14 2019;10(1):207. doi:10.1038/s41467-018-08170-1

4. Ross S. Therapeutic use of classic psychedelics to treat cancer-related psychiatric distress. *Int Rev Psychiatry (Abingdon, England)*. Aug 2018;30(4):317–330. doi:10.1080/09540261.2018.1482261

5. Puchalski C, Ferrell B, Virani R, et al. Improving the quality of spiritual care as a dimension of palliative care: The report of the Consensus Conference. *J Palliat Med*. Oct 2009;12(10):885–904. doi:10.1089/jpm.2009.0142

6. Robinson S, Kissane DW, Brooker J, Burney S. A systematic review of the demoralization syndrome in individuals with progressive disease and cancer: A decade of research. *J Pain Sympt Manage*. Mar 2015;49(3):595–610. doi:10.1016/j.jpainsymman.2014.07.008

7. LeMay K, Wilson KG. Treatment of existential distress in life threatening illness: A review of manualized interventions. *Clin Psychol Rev*. Mar 2008;28(3):472–493. doi:10.1016/j.cpr.2007.07.013

8. Kissane DW, Clarke DM, Street AF. Demoralization syndrome: A relevant psychiatric diagnosis for palliative care. *J Palliat Care*. Spring 2001;17(1):12–21.

9. Ignatius J, De La Garza R, 2nd. Frequency of demoralization and depression in cancer patients. *Gen Hospital Psychiatry*. Sep-Oct 2019;60:137–140. doi:10.1016/j.genhosppsych.2019.04.013

10. Breitbart W, Rosenfeld B, Pessin H, Applebaum A, Kulikowski J, Lichtenthal WG. Meaning-centered group psychotherapy: An effective intervention for improving psychological well-being in patients with advanced cancer. *J Clin Oncol*. Mar 1 2015;33(7):749–54. doi:10.1200/jco.2014.57.2198

11. Breitbart W, Pessin H, Rosenfeld B, Applebaum AJ, Lichtenthal WG, Li Y, Saracino RM, et al. Individual meaning-centered psychotherapy for the treatment of psychological and existential distress: A randomized controlled trial in patients with advanced cancer. 2018;124(15):3231–3239.

12. Stamets P. *Psilocybin Mushrooms of the World: An Identification Guide*. Berkeley, CA: Ten Speed Press; 1996.

13. Ross S, Franco Corso S, Reiff C, Agin-Liebes G. Psilocybin. In: Grob CS, Grigsby J, eds. *Handbook of Medical Hallucinogens*. New York: Guilford Press; 2021:181–214.

14. Bogenschutz MP, Ross S. Therapeutic applications of classic hallucinogens. *Curr Topics Behav Neurosci*. 2018;36:361–391. doi:10.1007/7854_2016_464

15. Tyls F, Palenicek T, Horacek J. Psilocybin--summary of knowledge and new perspectives. *Eur Neuropsychopharmacol*. Mar 2014;24(3):342–356. doi:10.1016/j.euroneuro.2013.12.006

16. Ly C, Greb AC, Cameron LP, Wong JM, Barragan EV, Wilson PC, et al. Psychedelics promote structural and functional neurcal plasticity. *Cell Rep.* Jun 12 2018;23(11):3170–3182. doi:10.1016/j.celrep.2018.05.022

17. Carhart-Harris RL, Leech R, Hellyer PJ, Shanahan M, Feilding A, Tagliazucchi E, et al. The entropic brain: A theory of conscious states informed by neuroimaging research with psychedelic drugs. *Front Hum Neurosci.* 2014;8:20. doi:10.3389/fnhum.2014.00020

18. Tagliazucchi E, Roseman L, Kaelen M, Orban C, Muthukumaraswamy SD, Murphy K, et al. Increased global functional connectivity correlates with LSD-induced ego dissolution. *Curr Biol.* Apr 25 2016;26(8):1043–1050. doi:10.1016/j.cub.2016.02.010

19. Usona Institute. Psilocybin Investigator Brochure (Version 4). 2021. https://www.usonainstitute.org/wp-content/uploads/2018/12/psilocybin-ib-v4.pdf

20. Kast EC, Collins VJ. Study of lysergic acid diethylamide as an analgesic agent. *Anesth Analg.* May-Jun 1964;43:285–291.

21. Kast E. Attenuation of anticipation: A therapeutic use of lysergic acid diethylamide. *Psychiatric Q.* Oct 1967;41(4):646–657.

22. Grof S, Goodman LE, Richards WA, Kurland AA. LSD-assisted psychotherapy in patients with terminal cancer. *Int Pharmacopsychiatry.* 1973;8(3):129–144.

23. Pahnke WN, Kurland AA, Goodman LE, Richards WA. LSD-assisted psychotherapy with terminal cancer patients. *Curr Psychiatric Ther.* 1969;9:144–152.

24. Grob CS, Danforth AL, Chopra GS, Hagerty M, McKay CR, Halberstadt AL, et al. Pilot study of psilocybin treatment for anxiety in patients with advanced-stage cancer. *Arch Gen Psychiatry.* Jan 2011;68(1):71–78. doi:10.1001/archgenpsychiatry.2010.116

25. Griffiths RR, Johnson MW, Carducci MA, Umbricht A, Richards WA, Richards BD, et al. Psilocybin produces substantial and sustained decreases in depression and anxiety in patients with life-threatening cancer: A randomized double-blind trial. *J Psychopharmacol (Oxford, England).* Dec 2016;30(12):1181–1197. doi:10.1177/0269881116675513

26. Ross S, Bossis A, Guss J, Agin-Liebes G, Malone T, Cohen B, et al. Rapid and sustained symptom reduction following psilocybin treatment for anxiety and depression in patients with life-threatening cancer: A randomized controlled trial. *J Psychopharmacology (Oxford, England).* Dec 2016;30(12):1165–1180. doi:10.1177/0269881116675512

27. Agin-Liebes GI Malone T, Yalch MM, Mennenga SE, Ponté KL, Guss J, et al. Long-term follow-up of psilocybin-assisted psychotherapy for psychiatric and existential distress in patients with life-threatening cancer. *J Psychopharmacology (Oxford, England).* Feb 2020;34(2):155–166. doi:10.1177/0269881119897615

28. Chochinov HM, Wilson KG, Enns M, Lander S. Depression, hopelessness, and suicidal ideation in the terminally ill. *Psychosomatics.* Jul-Aug 1998;39(4):366–370. doi:10.1016/s0033-3182(98)71325-8

29. Ross S, Agin-Liebes G, Lo S, Zeifman RJ, Ghazal L, Benville J, et al. Acute and sustained reductions in loss of meaning and suicidal ideation following psilocybin-assisted psychotherapy for psychiatric and existential distress in life-threatening cancer. *ACS Pharmacol Translat Sci.* Mar 18, 2021. doi:10.1021/acsptsci.1c00020

30. Anderson BT, Danforth A, Daroff PR, Stauffer C, Ekman E, Agin-Liebes G, et al. Psilocybin-assisted group therapy for demoralized older long-term AIDS survivor men: An open-label safety and feasibility pilot study. *EClinicalMedicine.* 2020;27:100538–100538. doi:10.1016/j.eclinm.2020.100538

31. Grob CS, Bossis AP, Griffiths RR. Use of the classic hallucinogen psilocybin for treatment of existential distress associated with cancer. *Psychol Aspects Cancer.* 2013:291–308.

32. Bossis A. *Utility of Psychedelics in the Treatment of Psycho-Spiritual and Existential Distress in Palliative Care: Handbook of Medical Hallucinogens.* New York: Guilford; 2021.

33. Belser AB, Agin-Liebes G, Swift TC, Terrana S, Devenot N, Friedman HL, et al. Patient experiences of psilocybin-assisted psychotherapy: An interpretative phenomenological analysis. *J Humanistic Psychol.* 2017/07/01 2017;57(4):354–388. doi:10.1177/0022167817706884

34. Swift TC, Belser AB, Agin-Liebes G, Devenot N, Terrana S, Friedman HL, et al. Cancer at the dinner table: Experiences of psilocybin-assisted psychotherapy for the treatment of cancer-related distress. *J Humanistic Psychol.* 2017/09/01 2017;57(5):488–519. doi:10.1177/0022167817715966

PART VII

Life Cycle Considerations in Palliative Care

43

Human Development and Personal Well-Being in Life-Threatening Conditions

Therapeutic Insights and Strategies Derived from Positive Experiences of Individuals and Families

Ira Byock

Introduction

Suffering rightly commands the attention of clinicians. Responding to people in distress constitutes the historical roots and moral underpinnings of the caring professions. An innate drive to care was the impetus for the caring professions and motivates individuals to become clinicians today. Western medicine, particularly, focuses on the problems of illness and injury and the suffering they cause. The predominant goals of medicine are cure, extending survival with chronic illness, restoration of functional independence, adaptation to life with special needs, and alleviation of symptoms and suffering. Each specialty within medicine contributes a distinct set of diagnostic approaches and therapeutic interventions to these collective goals.

This problem-based orientation is demonstrably effective but has inherent limitations.[1] In palliative medical practice, problem-oriented assessments, diagnostic procedures, and therapeutic interventions provide a means of addressing most manifestations of illness, including physical symptoms, functional disability, and psychiatric conditions. While equipping clinicians to address discrete problems, such as pulmonary edema, cancer pain, or anti-cholinergic delirium, problem-based approaches are insufficient to understand or respond to a range of lived experiences of patients who would benefit from broader guidance. Importantly, problem-bound frameworks foreclose understanding of and opportunities to foster positive personal experiences and growth that are not rooted in responses to diagnoses.

Consider two hypothetical patients followed by a palliative care service.

Case 1

Mr. K, a towering 78-year-old executive recently diagnosed with metastatic esophageal cancer, expresses regrets for not having retired years sooner and the opportunities he missed to spend time with his family. He says "an undertow of sadness" pulls at him because he is leaving his recently widowed 42-year-old daughter and her two young sons and daughter, his grandchildren. His emotional pain does not meet requirements for a psychiatric diagnosis, yet Mr. K's palliative care clinicians strive to alleviate his sadness and improve his quality of life. They wonder if it is possible for someone in Mr. K's circumstances to achieve a sense of well-being.

Case 2

Mrs. V is a 63-year-old Mexican American woman with heart failure and advanced respiratory insufficiency due to pneumonia with bacteria resistant to multiple antibiotics. After 15 days in the ICU she remains ventilator dependent. Mrs. V is alert and interactive. She is fully oriented and reports her pain as 2 or 3 on a 0–10 scale. She breathes through a recently placed tracheostomy with assist-control ventilator settings. She is receiving several IV antibiotics. Mrs. V has always been the caregiver for others in her large family. "She is our rock," one daughter says during a family meeting. Her four siblings nod in agreement. Mrs. V has never been depressed during her life, but now evinces a somber mood and at times seems emotionally distant. She shows less interest in communicating, which she does through facial expressions and gestures to her family and, when needed, an alphabet board on her bedside stand. She has told a nurse she is close to and a Catholic chaplain that she worries about being a burden to her children. A psychiatry consultant recommended an antidepressant that is being administered through her percutaneous gastrostomy tube.

Mrs. V's intensive care and palliative care teams hold a care planning meeting to consider ways of addressing her sense of being a burden and depressed mood. How can they respond to her children's pleas to give the best care possible to their ailing mother? How can their family maintain a sense of coherence and well-being even as they acknowledge and begin to grieve their mother's dying?

Health and Quality of Life in the Context of Life-Threatening Conditions

Questions about the nature of health, quality of life, and well-being underlie the purpose and practice of palliative care.

The World Health Organization's definition of health, adopted in 1948, reads: "Health is a state of complete physical, mental and social well-being and not merely the absence of disease or infirmity."[2] While presumably intending to escape the constraints of disease and infirmity, the definition's wording instead *requires* absence of diagnosable pathology as a precondition for health. This deep-rooted assumption influences healthcare systems and operations in myriad ways. Therapeutic plans are constrained by assuming that health and well-being are precluded by injury, disease, and associated distress. Dominant research paradigms and tools perpetuate these assumptions and constraints.

Palliative care expands beyond the problem-based goals of medicine by explicitly striving to improve quality of life for persons with serious illness or injury. This raises important issues about how "quality of life" is defined and measured. Answers to these questions operationally define the scope of palliative care practice and research.[3-5]

Consensus is lacking on these matters. Neil Aronson, a leading quality of life researcher, opined,

> Undoubtedly, such issues as happiness and life satisfaction factor heavily into an individual's judgment of his or her quality of life. Yet, these issues are so distal to the goals and objectives of healthcare that it would seem inappropriate to apply them as criteria against which to judge the efficacy of medical interventions.[6]

Palliative care tacitly rejects this assertion, operating from an assumption that a patient's subjective quality of life has intrinsic validity. Definitions of health, quality of life, and the proper scope of healthcare may seem abstract or academic, but they carry far-reaching implications for palliative medical practice and research.

Several commonly used quality of life assessment tools assume that a person's lived experience is determined by physical symptoms and functional capacity. An ill person who has daily pain and becomes progressively less able to engage in activities and gradually dependent on others for daily needs, including eating, dressing, personal grooming, and toileting, is expected to experience declining quality of life. When that occurs, such quality of life tools function adequately. However, problem-based assessment scales are effectively blind to the experiences of persons who describe themselves as "well" despite the discomforts and dependencies of late-stage illness. In this manner, measurement tools appear to affirm—and thereby perpetuate—cultural assumptions about health and well-being that constrict the very scope of healthcare.

Oncologist Kenneth Calman observed that a key determinant of subjective quality of life for people living with progressive illness with physical symptoms and functional limitations was the gap between their expectations and current, experienced reality.[7] *Calman's gap*, the discrepancy between expectations and experience, can explain the occasional, seemingly paradoxical improvements in people's quality of life in the face of far advanced illness and impending death. By expecting some degree of physical comfort and functional dependence, and shifting emphasis to emotional, relational, internal, and spiritual realms of experience, an ill person may maintain his or her baseline quality of life. Some may even express feeling more well than before their physical illness. This phenomenon is recognized as a methodological challenge, termed "response shift," by researchers studying quality of life in populations of patients with cancer and other serious diseases.[8]

In 1983, palliative medicine clinician-researchers Balfour Mount and John Scott pointed out the limitations of measurement methodologies in a commentary of an early study of hospice care that reported no measurable differences between the outcomes of patients who died in an urban Veterans hospital and those who died at home with hospice care.[9,10]

> I shall long remember the young patient who in dying commented that his final months (which had been characterized by relentless physical deterioration and considerable suffering) had been "the best year of my life." The day he made that comment this young athlete, scholar, and executive who had measured 10/10 on the [Spitzer] QL throughout his life, measured 2/10. Clearly he was referring to something not embraced by the scales measuring activities of daily living and not reflected in the Spitzer QL.[9]

The authors asserted that to have detected such differences,

> the study would have had to measure an increased sense of personhood and an enhanced context of meaning, improved communication within the family and between family members and healthcare workers, lessened uncertainty and fear of the unknown, greater acceptance of the reality facing them, greater ability to express fears, doubts, guilts, and anger, and the significance of being able to pray together, alongside the hospice physician and nurses.[9]

With the exception of people who die suddenly while enjoying subjectively good health, the experiences of physical decline, illness, and dying are universal. To encompass the full range of human experience, social and clinical sciences require a concept of health that encompasses physical disabilities and discomforts related to serious medical conditions, including life-threatening conditions. Understanding psychological adjustments and adaptations which underlie healthy human responses to terminal illness is necessary for specificity in clinical assessments and corresponding plans of care within geriatrics and palliative care.

Empirically, it is common for people with advanced illness to consider themselves to be healthy. In Marjorie Kagawa-Singer's study of cancer patients from both Anglo-American and Japanese American ethnic backgrounds, 49 of 50 subjects expressed a sense of being healthy. One subject, a 59-year-old woman living with metastatic breast cancer who described that she had needed to "move with a walker with both hands to steady myself," just 10 days earlier, said

> I washed and ironed ten shirts yesterday! I don't consider myself sick. I just have this problem, but it doesn't necessarily make you sick. I just can't get around like everyone else, and I'd like to. Otherwise, I think of myself as healthy![11]

Kagawa-Singer determined that "health" for these patients involved a sense of self-integrity that they were able to maintain within the physical and social context of their life situation. She observed, "Their physical condition did not destroy their sense of self. Their lives made a difference, and they could die 'healthy.'"[11]

A rich and expanding literature of illness narratives make clear that an individual's quality of life is dynamic and affected by environmental and external circumstances as well as by physical symptoms, their personal attitude, and expectations. Although the risk of suffering caused by illness and pain is high, a physically ill individual's quality of life may range from persistent suffering to profound well-being. Depressed mood, demoralization, and true clinical depression are all too common; however, instances of joy and even exhilaration occur.[12-15] It is, therefore, essential for the conceptual and clinical frameworks of palliative medicine and the knowledge base of the field to incorporate the phenomenology of positive experiences. Clinical assessment tools and quality of life surveys used in research must also encompass the potential for subjectively positive experiences.

A series of categorical questions confront clinicians and researchers striving to understand the nature and variety of elevated quality of life and expressions of well-being among medically ill individuals and their families. Are there commonalties and themes within these experiences? What comprises a sense of being "well" in the context of life-threatening conditions? How should subjectively positive quality of life be measured? What counseling approaches or other therapeutic modalities can help people maintain or achieve a sense of well-being in the face of a poor prognosis and difficult circumstances?

Building on Foundations Within Psychology and Psychiatry

As noted, contemporary psychiatry and clinical psychology are almost exclusively problem-focused and rarely consider health in the face of advanced illness. Clinical guidelines address treatment and care of individuals who are experiencing discomfort or dysfunction of sufficient severity to meet criteria for a diagnosis, such as anxiety or depression. Correspondingly, reimbursement systems and insurance policies typically require a diagnosis to pay for a clinical encounter. In the prevailing sociocultural and regulatory milieu, pathology legitimizes care. Particularly in adult medicine, preventive healthcare is limited. Patient-level preventive counseling or treatments are rare in the contemporary clinical psychology and psychiatry practice.

Existential psychology and developmental psychology are exceptions which challenge these conceptual assumptions and the constraints they impose. Existential psychology acknowledges the reality of an individual's circumstances and recognizes negative and positive poles of personal experience, represented by suffering and subjective well-being. Ultimate concerns or major themes of life include death, freedom and responsibility, isolation and meaninglessness. While existential psychotherapy recognizes no absolute answers to these ultimate life concerns, counselors help people identify and work toward achievable goals.[16,17]

Eric Cassell's concept of personhood is widely cited in palliative medicine literature and complements an experiential understanding of life with serious physical illness.[18]

Cassell conceptualized personhood as a dynamic interactive matrix of an individual's attributes and spheres of experience that collectively comprise the individual's sense of self. Personhood is comprised of bodily and physical attributes, mind, and mental gifts and limitations and the unique imprints and influences of a person's past on their present experiences. Although each person is an individual, their relationships—with relatives and friends, co-workers and colleagues, neighbors, and even casual acquaintances—occupy a key dimension of their personhood.

Persons have formal and informal roles. Most people can identify multiple simultaneous roles they hold in their work, within their families, and in a variety of social networks and communities. Persons have ethnic or regional cultures in which they grew up and of which they retain some level of traits. Many also have a religious culture that, to greater or lesser extent, influences their values, customs, and preferences. Persons have spiritual beliefs and disbeliefs which range broadly in depth and fervency and may or may not be consistent with their religious upbringing. Persons have opinions on social and political matters, habits, and partialities (and aversions) regarding their entertainment, relaxation, and food. Importantly, each person has a sense of the future, a dimension which for seriously ill people is threatened.[19]

These attributes are contained within a whole person who, by human nature, is motivated by inherent drives for meaning and connection.[16,20] A quest for meaning is a defining characteristic of *Homo sapiens*.

The drive to make meaning is not a choice or yearning but a trait embedded within the physical and psychological human substrate.[21] It can be viewed as a blessing or a curse. Meaning is to a person's emotional and spiritual well-being what nourishment and sleep are to physical health. The need for meaning, when unmet, can cause a person to suffer no less than can hunger or exhaustion. Even in absence of physical pain, profound suffering may result when illness or injury robs a person of the ability to fulfill valued, long-held responsibilities, engage in accustomed activities, or maintain vocational or social roles. In acknowledging the irreversibility and finality of aggregate and ultimate losses, a dying person may experience the dread of impending personal, existential annihilation. In Cassell's terms, this suffering arises from threats to the integrity or intactness of the person.[19]

The clinical challenge and opportunity is illustrated by the hypothetical case of Mrs. M.

Mrs. M is a 68-year-old woman who has been fiercely independent and proud of her appearance. She becomes deeply distressed when a sudden stroke and exacerbation of heart failure force her to stop driving, require that she use a urinary catheter, and make grooming her hair and nails nearly impossible. In order to emerge from suffering resulting from these assaults to her personhood, Mrs. M must somehow accept and adapt to these unwanted circumstances and re-establish a sense of intactness.

Carl Jung's observations acknowledge the existential concerns and reflect a developmental therapeutic perspective.

> all the greatest and most important problems of life are fundamentally insoluble. They must be so, for they express the necessary polarity inherent in every self-regulating system. They can never be solved, but only outgrown.[22]

Developmental psychology examines the critical events in a person's life and brings a wellness-based framework for preparing for predictable crises. Twentieth-century developmental psychologists, among them Erik Erickson, Jean Piaget, and Abraham Maslow, focused mostly on childhood development yet recognized human development to be a life-long process. In seeing living with advanced disease as predictably difficult and risk prone, but also inherently normal, palliative care reflects a similar perspective. Within a developmental framework, functional decline and dependencies associated with physical illness share features of age-defined stages of life. Developmental landmarks during infancy, childhood, adolescence, adulthood, and advanced age are often preceded by a period in which a person's self-concept, assumptions, aspirations, relationships, and sense of stability are threatened. Incurable illness demands that an individual either adjust to a new unwanted personal reality and situation or suffer the consequences—an impending sense of disintegration—of clinging to one's past sense of self, circumstances, and expectations.

Developmental landmarks and corresponding task work pertinent to meeting the challenges of this waning stage of life can be discerned (e.g., Table 43.1).[21] The specific characteristics of personal experience with advanced illness, dying, and grieving vary from person to person, as do the particular tasks that a person feels a need to do. Despite individual differences common personal and relational opportunities can be identified.

A developmental approach to the experience of people living with advanced illness is derived from clinical observations and counseling experience and offers a framework for psycho-social research.

In a single week, a hypothetical palliative care service based in an urban academic medical center cares for a 55-year-old Jewish American man recently diagnosed with rapidly progressing amyotrophic lateral sclerosis (ALS), a 32-year-old Chinese American mother of two living with stage IV breast cancer, and a 75-year-old African American grandfather slowly dying from congestive heart failure. Each individual is at a different point in the trajectory of their illness. Despite markedly different demographics, cultural backgrounds, personal styles, tastes, and politics, when asked by a member of their care team if there are important things left undone, each person expresses a desire to choose what property and cherished possessions to leave to others. In his or her own words, each says that the thought of leaving their loved ones is the hardest aspect of dying. Each feels that there are things he or she wants to say to important people in their life. Furthermore, in the context of the palliative care team's supportive counseling, each person accepts the idea of spending time

TABLE 43.1 Developmental landmarks and taskwork

Landmarks	Taskwork
Sense of completion with worldly affairs	Transfer of fiscal, legal, and formal social responsibilities.
Sense of completion in relationships with community	Closure of multiple social relationships (employment, commerce, organizational, congregational). Components include expressions of regret, expressions of forgiveness, acceptance of gratitude and appreciation; leave taking; the saying of goodbye.
Sense of meaning about one's individual life	Life review. The telling of "one's stories." Transmission of knowledge and wisdom
Experienced love of self	Self-acknowledgment. Self-forgiveness.
Experienced love of others	Acceptance of worthiness.
Sense of completion in relationships with family and friends	Reconciliation, fullness of communication, and closure in each of one's important relationships. Component tasks include expressions of regret, expressions of forgiveness and acceptance, expressions of gratitude and appreciation, acceptance of gratitude and appreciation, expressions of affection. Leave-taking; the saying of goodbye.
Acceptance of the finality of life, of one's existence as an individual	Acknowledgment of the totality of personal loss represented by one's dying and experience of personal pain of existential loss. Expression of the depth of personal tragedy that dying represents. Decathexis (emotional withdrawal) from worldly affairs and cathexis (emotional connection) with an enduring construct. Acceptance of dependency.
Sense of a new self (personhood) beyond personal loss	Developing self-awareness in the present.
Sense of meaning about life in general	Achieving a sense of awe. Recognition of a transcendent realm. Developing/achieving a sense of comfort with chaos.
Surrender to the transcendent, to the unknown: "letting go"	Note: In pursuit of this landmark, the doer and "taskwork" are one. Here, little remains of the ego except the volition to surrender.

Adapted from Ira Byock, The nature of suffering and the nature of opportunity at the end of life, *Clin Geriatr Med.*, 1996;12(2):237–251.

recording stories of their early life to leave for their families. Although only one belongs to a religious congregation, each person expresses a sense of being a spiritual person.

This amalgam of existential and developmental approaches is well-suited to predicting personal challenges that those with incurable conditions may confront, thereby enhancing specificity of clinical assessments and counseling. Importantly, in addition to treating psychosocial and spiritual distress, this growth-based perspective may identify personal opportunities that patients and their families value. This opens therapeutic opportunities for clinicians to explore that may help people avoid suffering and experience a degree of well-being.

While clinicians or researchers working from either a problem-based or existential-developmental framework would likely use similar measurement tools to assess a patient's pain intensity and functional status, they would almost certainly respond to the full impact of disease on the individual in importantly different ways. Within a problem-based approach the effects of disease diminish and threaten to disintegrate an individual's sense of self. In contrast, while acknowledging the potential for disintegration, an existential-developmental perspective recognizes opportunities for the person to adapt to unwanted circumstances through a process of personal development, maturation, and expansion of the self.[23-27]

Marie de Hennezel, a French psychotherapist working with HIV and cancer patients, observed,

> Life has taught me three things: The first is that I cannot escape my own death or the deaths of the people I love. The second is that no human being can be reduced to what we see, or think we see. Any person is infinitely larger, and deeper, than our narrow judgments can discern. And third: He or she can never be considered to have uttered the final word on anything, is always developing, always has the power of self-fulfillment, and a capacity for self-transformation through all the crises and trials of life.[28]

A developmental framework that encompasses a taxonomy and terminology of growth does not diminish the significance of a person's suffering or romanticize their experience of dying. Developmental landmarks come unbidden and can be experienced as burdens. The personal tasks of life completion and closure can be sources of distress as well as (albeit unwanted) opportunities for growth.

Fear of death has been considered the taproot of human anxieties.[29] The developmental crisis of incurable illness entails a need to adjust to the reality of one's life coming to an end, grieve the impending losses of everyone and everything one values in life, complete one's practical affairs, and complete interpersonal, social, and spiritual aspects of one's life. These tasks are inherently difficult, often heart-wrenching, and may seem insurmountable. From the perspectives of existential and developmental psychologies, they are not optional. When people willfully ignore the personal challenges that serious, life-threatening conditions impose, suffering predictably results.

Carl Jung wrote

> I have observed that a directed life is in general better, richer and healthier than an aimless one, and that it is better to go forward with the stream of time than backward against it. To a psychotherapist, an old man who cannot bid farewell to life appears as feeble and sickly as a young man who is unable to embrace it. . . . As a physician I am convinced that it is hygienic—if I may use the word—to discover in death a goal toward which one can strive; and that shrinking away from it robs the second half of life of its purpose.[30]

Personal development tends to be arduous at any stage of life. A dying person may find value and sense of enhanced meaning and well-being despite—and concomitant with—considerable suffering. Commenting on a case report of a person approaching death, Zinker and Fink concluded, the psychology of death is a psychology of life because it concerns human needs, human hopes, human motivations, human satisfactions, and human frustrations. Human beings remain human beings when they are dying, and death brings out in humanity its goodness (with its capacity to love, transcend, grow) and its capacity to hate, to destroy, and to deteriorate psychologically.[27]

While a person who successfully accomplishes pressing developmental tasks may experience an improved mood, personal growth is not synonymous with being happy. Expressions of well-being in circumstances of incurable illness or the progressive frailty of age are consistent with Kagawa-Singer's formulation of enhanced personal integrity.

Evidence in support for this conceptual framework comes from a number of primary and clinical studies. Karen Steinhauser and associates conducted an interview study with patients with advanced illness and their families. Qualitative content analysis of transcripts revealed that people assign importance to domains of preparation for death, a sense of completion, and feeling that they are contributing or have contributed to others.[31] In an in-depth ethnographic study of nine terminally ill individuals and their primary caregivers, Janice Staton, Roger Shuy, and I demonstrated the relevance of this construct and specific developmental landmarks for people who are aware that they have only a few months to live.[32]

Therapeutic Opportunities

In assisting people in accomplishing tasks of life completion, palliative care extends beyond management of symptoms to focus on the personal priorities of individuals and their families. These conceptual underpinnings carry pragmatic applications to clinical care.

A number of well-studied and common therapeutic practices can be understood in developmental terms. Life review has been long utilized in counseling people living with advanced age or life-threatening conditions. Myrna Lewis and Robert Butler observed,

> The therapeutic possibilities of the life review are complex. There is the opportunity to reexamine the whole of one's life and to make sense of it, both on its own terms and in comparison with the lives of others. Identity may be reexamined and restructured. There is the chance to resolve old problems, to make amends and restore harmony with friends and relatives.[33]

Life review offers a means of transmitting special knowledge and wisdom from one generation to another. Victoria Fitch commented,

> The fruit of life review for the elderly is the accomplishment of transmission, or handing on to others the essence of their knowledge of the world around them: how to do things; how to think about things; how to simply be.[34]

Ethical wills, derived from ancient Judaic tradition, offer a formal means of leaving a legacy of knowledge and wisdom. The writing of an ethical will has been used in counseling with people with cancer and may be useful in diminishing emotional distress caused by concern for others, unfinished business, and fear of the future.[35,36]

Building from the insights of Viktor Frankl,[19] psycho-oncologist William Breitbart and colleagues developed meaning-centered psychotherapy as an improved alternative to supportive counseling for cancer patients. The modality has been manualized to an eight-session protocol and has shown promise in alleviating anxiety, enhancing the sense of meaning and spiritual well-being.[37,38]

Dignity therapy, described by Harvey Chochinov, shares features of ethical wills and includes a prominent role for life review. Dignity therapy assists individuals in addressing their own priorities in psychosocial and spiritual aspects of life. It has demonstrated effectiveness in reducing depressive symptoms and suffering and in fostering a sense of purpose, a sense of meaning, and will to live.[39-41]

Steinhauser, Alexander, and research colleagues (including myself) developed the OUTLOOK intervention, a three-session series of semi-structured interviews as a practical, standardized way of assisting patients to identify unfinished business. OUTLOOK guides people in addressing important relationships, offering or receiving forgiveness, and expressing gratitude and love. In common with dignity therapy, OUTLOOK is designed to help people develop or strengthen a sense of meaning in life.[42,43]

In developmental terminology, activities of this nature represent ways to assist people with tasks of life completion. Clinicians can help people to identify what matters most to them during this phase of their life. The process may begin by gently asking a person to consider whether there would be important practical or business affairs that would be left undone if he or she were to suddenly suffer a serious complication of their illness, such as a stroke or overwhelming infection?

Absent such a sudden functional deterioration, if the person is currently able to travel, are there places he or she would want to visit? Are there important things that would feel incomplete in their work or social roles? Are there important things that feel unsaid between them and people they love? Such inquiries frequently identify tangible goals people feel worth achieving and corresponding tasks worth undertaking.

This perspective and conceptual framework offer ways for clinicians to integrate the inevitable losses of illness with a recognition that human suffering is not immutable. As categorical spheres of a person's life are completed through a developmental process, individuals can come to feel more settled and better able to allow aspects of life to diminish in importance or fall away. Consistent with Cassel's multidimensional framework of personhood, an individual can release spheres of his or her personhood while maintaining a sense of personal integration and well-being.

Nature of Wellness

Just as the loss of meaning can cause profound suffering, even in absence of physical illness or injury, human resilience relies in large part on people's capacity to make meaning in the face of arguably senseless adversity of their own injuries, disease, or impending death or their grief at the illness or death of others. Similarly, while a sense of isolation can predictably cause physically healthy people to suffer, a sense of being connected to and supported by others reliably comforts people during times of devastating illness and tragic loss. It is not surprising, therefore, that themes of connection and meaning are common in instances in which people express feelings of well-being despite living with advanced, incurable disease.

Mr. S was a successful businessman, well-educated and well-traveled, who, at age 39, was forced by progressive HIV disease to confront his approaching death. He wrote a last letter to his mother, so that she would never doubt that he lived fully and joyfully through the last stage of his life. The following excerpts are from that letter.

> Dear Mom,
> This last part of my life could have been very unpleasant, but it wasn't. In fact, in many ways, it has been the best part of my life. I've had the opportunity to get to know my family again, a chance very few people have or take advantage of. . . . I probably never would have slowed up enough to really appreciate all of you if it hadn't been for my illness. That's the silver lining in this very dark cloud.
>
> When you get down to it, I'd have to live several hundred years to fulfill all the dreams I've had. . . . I feel sorry for people who die (at whatever age) who haven't had the chance in life to fulfill some of their dreams, as I have. That is a real tragedy.
>
> If anyone ever asks you if I went to heaven, tell them this: I just came from there.[44]

Themes of meaning and connection carry spiritual connotations, and the prevalence of their importance to people who are facing the end of life underlies spiritual aspects of palliative care. While there is no consensus regarding any single definition of spirituality within the fields of psychiatry and palliative medicine, meaning and connection are common characteristics of the many definitions in use. An existential-developmental approach enables clear, dispassionate explorations of both distress and subjective well-being that are based in these realms of experience. Within existential and developmental constructs, spirituality can be thought of as the human response to the mystery of life, which many people faced with a life-threatening condition acutely feel.[45] When the human drives for meaning and connection confront the mystery of life—including its finite nature of mortal life—the resulting experience can be awe-inspiring or terrifying and evoke well-being or suffering.

The ability to retain or develop a sense of meaning in the face of serious, likely terminal illness may seem philosophical or esoteric, but sources of meaning that most people identify tend to be tangible and uncomplicated. While sources of meaning are deeply personal, common features and attributes can be discerned. Older people with advanced illness tend to say that seeing their children and grandchildren well and generally happy are among the things that matter most. It is also common for people to assign importance to feeling that they have been a good spouse and parent and to having been a good child to their parents. Those with a strong religious faith commonly say they find comfort in their confidence of God's love.

Finding Happiness

Mr. G was an outpatient seen in a hospital-based palliative care practice.

I asked Mr. G if he considered himself a spiritual person. The gruff New England farmer said "No," shook his head and grinned, revealing his few remaining teeth. I returned his smile and asked if he had a sense of what comes after this life. He chuckled sarcastically and replied, "The worms go in; the worms go out," with an undulating motion of his hand.

Half-expecting such a response, I asked. "And where will the worms go in and out of your bones?"

"Oh, we have a family cemetery on a hill in Thetford. We G's have been buried there for over a century and I suspect my grandchildren and their grandchildren will be there, too."[46]

Mr. G was not religious. He didn't believe in God or pray, but he possessed a visceral connection to the land and to his family stretching back to distant ancestors and forward to generations to come. Although Mr. G may not have considered himself to be spiritual, the meaning and value he derived from being part of something larger and more enduring than his own life can be fairly considered attributes of spiritual experience.

Suffering and Well-Being Within Relationships

In its core principle of approaching each patient *with his or her family* as the focus of care, palliative medicine draws on evidence from ethology, anthropology, and psychology that human beings are inherently social animals.[47-49] The most important fact to recognize about relationships is the most obvious: people intrinsically matter to one another. When asked, "What is most important in your life now?" a 78-year-old man facing major heart surgery, a 43-year-old woman starting whole-brain radiation for metastatic cancer, and a 22-year-old hoping for a lung transplant for cystic fibrosis all prominently include in their answers the names of people they love. Whether satisfying or strained, those relationships intrinsically matter. This characteristic of personal experience transcends age, ethnicity, and demographics. People's relationships with family, beginning with their mothers and fathers, siblings, closest relatives, and friends are primal sources of gratification in life as well as common sources of emotional suffering.

Measuring Relational Experience Within Quality of Life

Quality of life is conceptually defined as an attribute of individuals. In clinical practice and research, however, measured quality of life is artifactually influenced by the methodologies used to assess it. Quality of life for individuals and the people for whom they matter is inextricably linked. Because whenever one person receives a serious diagnosis, everyone who loves that person shares in the illness. The multiple impacts of disease-related pain and disability, and the shifts in roles, responsibilities, and plans, flow in both directions. Within families, emotions often behave as if they were contagious. Suffering is almost always shared, although suffering manifests in individual ways. The husband of a critically ill woman may suffer with anxiety and depressive symptoms in watching his wife's distress and reflecting on the losses they've already sustained. He fears her impending death. From her hospital bed, the woman's anxiety and depression may deepen as she witnesses her husband's suffering despite his best efforts to put on a brave face for her.

For purposes of measurement and quality of life survey design, a person's relationships can be considered to be a discrete domain of experience. While methodologically sound, this design feature yields approximations of people's subjective reality. In lived experience, the influences of close relationships are interwoven within multiple domains of personhood. Rather than being confined to a discrete category of experience, the emotional tenor of important relationships pervades a person's experience in a manner somewhat analogous to the physical influences of weather on a community or the temperature and lighting on the environment of a room.

Palliative medicine clinicians recognize the rich pleomorphism and diversity of human families. Although it is often useful to consider a person's family as a discrete subset of the domain of relationships, here again, this construct is a simplification. In reality, people often experience themselves as having multiple families. Mr. Y, a 69-year-old engineer who is hospitalized with left-sided weakness from a glioblastoma, talks about the family he grew up in, the family he lived with during college and with whom he stays in close touch, and the families he generated through two marriages, as well as the friends he identifies as informal family. Similarly, it is common for a person to have concurrent family relationships of child, parent, sibling, spouse, in-law, cousin, niece or nephew, uncle or aunt. All of these relationships and familial roles contribute to a person's sense of self and, by extension, contribute to a person's sense of well-being or dis-ease.

Hospital-based palliative teams are well-positioned to address the suffering of family members and contribute to the concurrent family support provided by oncology, surgery, cardiology, and critical care teams. The depth of tragedy, and the severity and complexity of suffering families experience, can be intense, leading many clinicians to conclude that it is untouchable. Yet palliative care teams draw from their clinical experiences with families who describe meaningful interactions, events, and positive feelings, at times concurrent with sadness and suffering (Box 43.1).

In recognizing the inextricable connections between individuals and their close relatives and friends, palliative care extends a developmental perspective to families of people who are seriously ill. As with individuals, although each family is unique, a set of emotional and relational needs and opportunities can be discerned that are common to many families.

Predictably, families want to know that their ill member is receiving optimal care, including the right treatments for the disease or injury as well as their comfort. The best care extends to meeting the person's basic needs for hygiene, grooming, privacy, and dignity.

BOX 43.1 Illustrative Case

Mrs. N was just 36, the mother of a 14-month-old daughter, when she was diagnosed with esophageal carcinoma. It first appeared to be localized, but a positron emission tomography (PET) scan revealed involvement of multiple thoracic nodes. She developed mediastinitis following placement of a stent to alleviate dysphagia, became hypotensive and underwent emergency esophagectomy, and subsequently required vasopressor and ventilatory support.

The diagnosis of cancer had been a shock to her husband and their closely knit family of her two sisters and their mother and father. Now, the news that the cancer could not be treated as they had hoped and that Mrs. N's condition was precarious—including the possibility that she might not survive her ICU stay—was emotionally devastating.

During the 3 weeks Mrs. N survived in the ICU, family meetings were regularly convened, and Mrs. N and her family were frequently updated by the critical care and surgery teams and by the consulting palliative care team. Analgesics and anxiolytics were carefully titrated to keep her comfortable. Her family spent hours together in the ICU and at Mrs. N's bedside. Through long days and nights, they shared the news of her condition, expressed sadness, and spent time just visiting. They mostly sat in quiet or talked about mundane matters. Every day they read to Mrs. N words of support that various relatives and friends had written. In the middle of those weeks there were a few good days when her energy allowed Mrs. N to visit with her daughter.

Unfortunately, the relative stability proved brief; within days another infection overwhelmed her cardiovascular and hepato-renal systems. After 48 hours of high-dose vasopressor infusions and rapidly escalating ventilator settings, Mrs. N's family requested that life support be withdrawn. The palliative care team coordinated and oversaw the withdrawal of life support. Led by the team's Spiritual Care Coordinator, they conducted an informal service of readings within the family's faith tradition and expressed love for her and one another.

After her death, Mrs. N's family wrote a note of thanks to the palliative care team in which they described her death as "beautiful." They said that as sad as they felt, they were as close as they had ever been as a family and would cherish the memory of Mrs. N's final days.

Families value knowing that the person's stated or perceived preferences for care are being honored to the full extent possible. It is not the details of an advance directive as much as the spirit of the person's and family's values that are important. Families who know that time with a loved one is limited value opportunities to say the things "that matter most." Expressing love for the person who is dying is a normal component of healthy family grieving and can begin prior to death. Finally, members of a dying patient's family often feel a need or value opportunities to honor and celebrate the ill person and, in the process, comfort one another in their shared loss (Box 43.2).

Direct and secondary effects of physical illness can strain relationships. Serious medical conditions and their treatments are inevitably disruptive. Necessities may arise which force changes to schedules and daily plans, sometimes without notice. These disruptions challenge people's ability to fulfill usual interpersonal and social expectations and maintain roles and responsibilities. A life-threatening disease commonly assaults an individual's self-image and self-confidence, contributing to anxieties and darkening the person's mood. In these and other pragmatic and emotional ways, being seriously ill can sap a person's energy and engagement in close personal relationships.

Palliative care clinicians witness a variety of patterns of communication and coping with difficult feelings that potentially terminal conditions evoke. Common maladaptive responses include conspiracies of silence. A person who receives a serious diagnosis may keep the information secret to avoid worrying others. Such well-meaning decisions tend to backfire because deception is erosive to relationships. Eventually, with cancer, motor-neuron disorders, Alzheimer's disease, or other progressive conditions, signs of illness make disclosures unavoidable, leaving family members feeling excluded or distrusted. Late in the course of incurable illness, conspiracies of silence may involve an ill person avoiding any acknowledgment or discussion of dying with a spouse, adult child, or close friends. People's conscious motive is to protect those they love from the emotional pain the discussion would cause. All the while, a person's relatives and friends pretend the individual is getting better, despite obvious progressive decline, ostensibly to avoid destroying hope. In wanting to protect each other, they unwittingly collaborate in emotionally distancing themselves from one another.

Fortunately, pretentions of this nature predictably dissolve in the tender warmth of a guided, honest conversation. Counseling can occur privately with an ill person, separately with members of the person's family, or together. Such conversations typically begin with the clinician openly acknowledging and normalizing the emotionally straining situation the person and family are in and the good intentions of all involved. It may help for the

---

BOX 43.2 Family Needs and Opportunities in Situations of Life-Threatening Conditions

- To feel the person receives the "best care possible" for their medical condition and comfort
- To feel that the person's or their family's preferences for care are followed
- To feel the person is treated in a dignified manner
- To say and do things "that matter most" and would be left unsaid or undone in event of a sudden death
- To honor and celebrate the person
- To grieve together

clinician to say aloud that the love and concern that people have for one another is apparent. Naturally, personal information is shared only with permission, and clinicians find it prudent to ask how much medical information the patient or family wants to know. Frequently, one need only ask the ill person what they understand about their condition and treatments to evoke their concerns about the possibility of not getting better. Similarly, asking a close relative or friend what they understand about a person's condition often reveals their recognition and concerns about its progressive, incurable nature. By conveying information about people's shared concerns, the fears that form the bases for conspiracies of silence often dissipate.

Skillful clinicians may respectfully assert that it is impossible within families to protect people from vicarious suffering when another is hurting or facing the end of life. The unwanted truth is that a person's family already owns the pain of a beloved person's illness. The choices a seriously ill person makes about sharing information, expressing feelings, and deciding where, how, and by whom they will be cared for cannot fully protect others from the illness. It can only lessen or heighten the impacts his or her illness has on others.

It is common for progressively ill and physically disabled patients to express worry about being or becoming a burden to their family. Counseling directed toward reframing their situation can contextualize caring within human history and family lifecycles. Since the dawn of humankind, families have borne responsibility of caring for one another at the beginning and through the end of life. Every individual is dependent on others for basic biological and personal needs during infancy and early childhood. So, too, the large majority of people become dependent on others during the final phase of life, whether that phase lasts several years, months, or only a few days.

This analogy to early childhood extends to an observation that most families want to care—or *feel a need to care*—for their ill member during the waning phase of life. When a clinician is confident of a family's desire and ability to provide care for a seriously ill person, it may help to invite them to voice their feelings to the person who feels themself to be a burden. Despite the ongoing practical and emotional challenges of caring, such reframing may help a person to allow themself to be cared for in ways that contribute to their own and their family's well-being.

Completing Troubled Relationships

Not all relationships that seriously ill people have would be described as intact, warm, or satisfying. As psychiatric and clinical psychologists well know, distress and dysfunction within relationships between people who love—*or once loved*—one another are all-too-common. Most families and parents are protective and nurturing of their children. Yet abuse during childhood—whether emotional, physical, or sexual—seems an endless source of life-long distress. The diagnosis of a life-threatening condition does not resolve any of these hard emotions, personal traumas, or relational strains. On the contrary, physical illness often complicates already complex interpersonal dynamics.

In clinical psychology and psychiatric practice, the work of unraveling such complexities and steps toward rebuilding trust can require many months and even years of therapy. Palliative care clinicians often must work at an accelerated pace. Progressive illness challenges counselors to find ways of helping those who are running out of time and want to complete fractured relationships with important people in their lives.

Yet empiric experience demonstrates that, at least for some people, even when relational healing seems daunting, it is possible. Clinicians working in palliative realms of care can draw from innumerable instances in clinical and biographic literature in which life-limiting illness has catalyzed healing of deeply fractured relationships.[15,42,48] When a long-strained or deeply fractured relationship involving a person who is dying does reconcile or otherwise heal, it is welcomed as a minor miracle. The dynamics of naturally occurring healing within relationships can inform counselors' ability to guide families living through life-limiting circumstances.

Reconciliation and Forgiveness

Although medical illness often complicates interpersonal dynamics, at times the destabilizing impact of an illness expands possibilities for healing. Awareness that death may be nearing can raise questions of whether relationships can be mended between an adult child, or siblings, close friends, and current—or former—lovers. If some degree of reconciliation were possible, would those involved want to reconnect? Forgiveness, gratitude, and love are common themes in instances of strained relationships that end well.

Counseling can proceed from a basic truth: human beings are imperfect. Even emotionally healthy individuals experience episodes and degrees of anger, rage, jealousy, anxiety, sadness, and depression. And even the wisest and the most psychologically robust people occasionally make bad decisions, say things they later regret, or otherwise hurt someone else's feelings.

The facts of human imperfection and fallibility can be shared with patients and open a range of therapeutically rich opportunities for soothing strained relationships, even those which are acrimonious and deeply fractured. The relational dynamics involve a proportion of reconciliation and forgiveness, which represent related, deliberate emotional adjustments.

Forgiveness is frequently misunderstood. It may be equated with forgetting or acting as if hurtful things were never said or transgressions never occurred. People may think of forgiveness in terms exonerating a person of responsibility or guilt for misdeeds. In reality, it involves none of this. Psychiatrist Thomas S. Szasz observed, "The stupid neither forgive nor forget; the naive forgive and forget; the wise forgive but do not forget."[50]

The maxim, "forgiveness means giving up all hope for a better past" (probably attributable to psychiatrist Gerald Jampolsky) can provide a context and opening for counseling.[51] Reconciliation does not require anyone to deny the past, but only accept the realities of imperfect people living in an imperfect world. Although the past cannot be changed, people need not allow their pasts to control their futures.

Often the person one most needs to forgive is one's self. People find it hard to forgive themselves for mistakes they have made, failures they have had, opportunities they missed, dreams they never fulfilled, people they hurt or let down. It may be useful and non-threatening to ask the person to think of her life as a long biographical novel. "As a reader, would you have mercy for this person? Would you recognize the protagonist's good intentions, the traumas and challenges she encountered, and the suffering that she has endured? If so, can you find it within you to extend similar mercy to yourself? You are not perfect; you have made mistakes, but after all, you're only human."

A similar approach applies to relationship counseling. Since individuals are imperfect, it is not surprising that human relationships tend to be less than perfect. Even a healthy, loving relationship may include past misunderstandings, indiscretions, and inadvertent—or intentional—misdeeds.

Forgiveness can be a deliberate strategy for freeing a person from damaging patterns of feelings and behaviors that erode their own quality of life. Anger is an entirely legitimate, healthy emotional response to hateful, hurtful, callous, or irresponsible acts. But it is not the only legitimate response to being the victim of malintent and offences. The problem with anger is that it extracts its own emotional toll.

There is a frequently told story from Buddhism about anger and forgiveness. Two monks meet years after being released from a prison in which they'd been tortured. Referring to their jailers, one monk asks the other, "Have you forgiven them?" "I will never forgive them! Never!" the second monk replies. "Well," says the first, "I guess they still have you in prison, don't they?"[52]

An economic analogy may help explain the potential of forgiving another person for the sake of one's own well-being. If someone buys something on time from you but never fully pays for it or borrows money or a tool and doesn't return it, a debt results. This financial debt accrues interest and grows from month to month. In a similar way, anger over wrongs and transgressions can grow within a person over time.

Accounting practices allow business owners to accept a loss, thereby zeroing out the balance on their ledger or spreadsheet. They need not forget the unpaid debt, nor act in the future as if it never occurred. A prudent businessperson does not readily re-extend credit to someone who has failed to pay their debts. But the process clears the books, frees the business from carrying the debt, and provides an accurate accounting of the current financial status. A similar process can free a person from even the most justifiable and longstanding anger, whether or not they choose to reconnect or renew a relationship with an individual who harmed them.

Counseling that fosters and supports forgiveness and healing between people is among the most exciting therapeutic work of palliative care. At times experiences of progressive illness and dying provoke healing that might otherwise have seemed impossible. When instances in which people restore long-held friendships or love relationships after years of anger and acrimony occur, the story of the relationship—and at times the history of a family—may be transformed. All the pain, anger, and separation become prelude to a better ending. An ongoing relationship may be considered "complete" when there is nothing important that has been left unsaid. When one member of a relationship is living with a progressive illness, subsequent time together is likely to feel lighter, more genuine and satisfying, even with the sadness of impending death (Box 43.3).

BOX 43.3 Steve's Story

Steve Morris was dying hard. When the hospice team met him, Steve was struggling for every breath, unable to walk without gasping for air, yet unable to sit still because of the anxiety that defined his life. He was scared of dying and suffered through every waking moment.

By vocation Steve had been a lineman for the phone company before a heart attack and emphysema forced his retirement. By avocation, he was a real Montana cowboy, living for his horses, winning numerous riding competitions and the affections of many for his willingness to teach horsemanship to any child eager to learn. In appearance and in his life-long smoking habit, Steve was also the prototypical Marlboro Man. He was a man's man, not one to express emotions or even admit to having them. Often, work and his horses had come before relationships and family.

Now he was at the end of his rope. Specialists had exhausted every hope, including the lung transplant he had desperately sought. Steve was the one dying, but he was not the only victim. His wife Dot was his constant companion, nurse, handmaiden, and co-sufferer. If she was out of sight for more than a minute, he would ring his bell or shout in his panicked, muffled voice, "Dot. Dot!"

It took our hospice team 2 weeks to gain Steve's confidence through a combination of pharmacy, counseling, and pragmatism. This included meticulous medication management, carefully selected relaxation tapes, practical suggestions regarding placement of his recliner, and volunteers to spell Dot so she could shop for groceries, see her own doctor, and get a few moments of rest. These efforts, drawing on the experience and resources of palliative care, helped diminish—at least slightly—Steve's breathlessness and paralyzing fear.

As we learned more of Steve's personal history, we realized that his anxiety stemmed in part from the fractured nature of several key relationships and from his complex, conflicted family life.

One Thursday, while I was visiting Steve and Dot at home, I told them that over the years I'd observed that, "People often value saying four things to one another before they say goodbye. Please forgive me. I forgive you—because if this was a significant relationship there will always be some history of hurt. Thank you. And, I love you"

"Those are really good, doc," Steve responded with unexpected enthusiasm. "Write those down for me, will ya?"

At my next scheduled home visit, Steve was sitting up, awaiting my arrival. He and Dot excitedly related the events of the past weekend. On Sunday their children and grandchildren had come over for dinner. At the table, Steve had announced he had some things he needed to say. He began, "You know the doctors tell me that this emphysema is finally going to get me. And I know I haven't always been the best father, or husband," he paused, gathering breath and confidence, "but I love you all and there are some things I want to say." With his eyes on my handwritten list, one-by-one he recited the four things in his own words.

The effect was remarkable. Although his anxiety did not disappear, in the wake of his remarks, its grip weakened. Tenderness and affection that had not been present for years, if ever, were now evident in the family's interactions. Steve's life didn't become easy, but it did become less anguished. The quality of Dot's life and their family life certainly improved.

Ironically, as he faced life's end, Steve said he was more happy with himself than he could ever remember being. Paradoxically, in the process of dying, he was becoming well within himself and helping his family to become closer and more openly loving.

Adapted from Ira Byock, *The Four Things That Matter Most*, New York: Free Press; 2004.

Opportunity, Love, and Celebration Within Families

Positive experiences can occur naturally but can also be engendered in therapeutic ways. Psychiatrist Verena Kast suggests conducting life review with people by guiding them in constructing personal histories of joy through their lives. In the process of recalling times of joy in years gone by—which often include cherished interactions with a parent or close friend, but may also include episodes of childhood mischief or misadventure—it is fairly common for the person in the present to smile, chuckle, or laugh aloud.[53]

When there is nothing left undone, the interactions between people may assume characteristics associated with celebration. Within a hospital room or a home where an ill person is being cared for, people tend to touch and hug one another. They commonly reminisce and retell stories, and often share food and drink.

In common with formal celebrations, such as weddings, first communions, and memorial services, in circumstances of serious illness people more readily tend to express love to one another. Expressing and receiving expressions of love are elements of human well-being. Human beings have an intrinsic need to love and to feel loved. The capacity to love and feel loved can engender satisfaction and a sense of well-being even in the midst of disease, physical distress, and impending death.

Love is rarely considered in medical therapeutics, except in the context of elaborating professional boundaries and warning clinicians against having sexual relations with patients. Yet in Western culture the phrase, "tender, loving care" connotes excellence in the manner in which care is delivered. Nurses recognize that, when performed in a loving manner, mundane tasks of patient care, such as bathing and grooming, can enhance the comfort and well-being of the person. In palliative practice, loving care can be thought of as interactions that convey positive regard, improve comfort and quality of life, and promote a sense of well-being. This includes fostering loving connections between people. Loving care extends to evoking pleasure when possible. This opens therapeutic opportunities to nurture and pamper a patient which are foreclosed by a problem-based approach. A number of complementary therapies can be understood in this light, such as music played for or sung with a person; keeping company, perhaps in silence or with music; massage; therapeutic touch; aroma therapy; aesthetic grooming; pet therapy; prayer; or meditation.[54]

Research into psychedelic-assisted therapies in caring for people with serious medical conditions began in the mid-20th century and has undergone a major renewal. Psychedelic medications are administered within a counseling framework of trust that extends from preparatory sessions, guiding of the 6- to 8-hour experience and subsequent integration sessions. Psychedelics may reset long-standing cognitive and emotional patterns of thought and feelings. Psychedelic-assisted therapies can help a person reframe their ongoing life experience in ways that advance developmental landmarks. Medically ill patients in clinical trials of psychedelic-assisted therapies commonly express feelings of profound meaning, deep connection to nature, and love for other people.[55]

A woman living in fear of cancer recurrence who participated in a clinical trial of psilocybin-assisted psychotherapy described feeling, "Just overcome with love and all the love that I have for my family and my friends. I felt that it was coming from them . . . if I were religious it definitely would have been a religious experience. I would have said bathed in God's love. And I don't think English really has a way to say this without using that word 'God'. . . Bathed in universal love."[56]

Love can be healing. A person who is able to love and feel loved may express a sense of well-being despite the pain of being sick, fears of the future, and rigors of treatments. An oft-cited definition for mental health attributed to Sigmund Freud is the ability to love and to work. When frailty forces a person to relinquish expectations of work, capacities to love and feel loved become the predominant determinants of personal well-being.

Clinician Self-Knowledge

Assessment tools and algorithms are essential but ultimately insufficient in supporting people during these intensely personal and poignant times of life. Clinicians require a degree of self-knowledge to effectively counsel seriously ill patients who are confronting the end of life or families living with an anticipated death. At very least, clinicians benefit from identifying their own death anxieties. Cultivating a level of comfort can enable clinicians to approach and stay present with a medically ill patient or grieving family. James Kemp suggested that,

> For those who choose the rewards and sorrows of working with older persons, it is important to accept death, generally and personally. It is useful to know that giving up life is a process, a series of events, images, feelings, ideas, and fantasies. The counselor who is unwilling or unable to place his or her death in a in a meaningful perspective will find it impossible to be successful with clients who are frail and dying.[57]

By emotionally meeting people who are suffering where they are, counseling clinicians can draw on their "receptive imagination."[58] Because one person cannot fully know the personal experience of another, the assertion, "I know what you're going through," while well-intended, can sound callous. However, if a clinician invests the emotional energy and discomfort to make the statement true, saying, "I can only imagine how difficult this must be for you," communicates genuine empathy.

This process of "putting oneself in the other's place" may be emotionally uncomfortable for the clinician for it requires imagining not only the person's physical pains and personal losses, but also the fears and dread about the collective losses to come. This is the essence of compassion, a word derived from the Latin, "to suffer with." It demands that the clinician be willing to become open and vulnerable toward these feelings in service of a patient's well-being.

Authentic compassion advances tangible therapeutic goals. A counselor or palliative care clinician who comes into imaginative alignment with a patient—listening to the patient's story as if he or she were the teller and seeing the world as if through the patient's eyes—can recruit their "generative imagination" to envision what meaningful experiences or interactions may remain. Are there are any achievable goals that are worth hoping for and working toward? From this depth of therapeutic alliance, a counseling clinician can gently explore whether well-being is still possible from the ill person's perspective.

As mentioned in the discussion of forgiveness, a clinician may invite a patient to imagine their experience as a late chapter in a poignant biography. "What would be left undone if the hero or heroine of the story died suddenly, today?" Given the protagonist's history, personality, yearnings, and current medical condition, "What would success look like, even now?" or "How might the story unfold in a way that feels meaningful to the hero or heroine?"

This use of generative imagination can maintain or evoke a re-emergence of hope. Within a problem-based mindset of medicine, when there is no realistic expectation of cure, hope is confined to the potential for comfort. This is tantamount to saying that best that terminally ill people can hope for is to avoid suffering. If the potential for personal development does exist at the end of life, hope expands.

Learning from and Being Enriched by Those We Serve

It is not mere rhetoric or platitude to note that therapeutic encounters benefit both giver and receiver of care. Palliative care clinicians commonly express the sense of learning from and feeling enriched by relationships with the people they serve. Palliative care clinicians bring skills and experience to the care and counseling they offer, but, perhaps most importantly, they accompany people with progressive, ultimately fatal, conditions.

Deborah Fahnestock, a 52-year-old medical social worker, who had undergone surgery, chemotherapy, and radiation treatments for metastatic lung cancer wrote,

When curing is no longer possible and this message is communicated to or intuited by the patient, a pregnant moment for healing arises for both physician and patient. The focus and fight for life can give way to a new alliance based on sharing the inevitabilities of the human contract. . . . Herein lies the opportunity for physicians to go beyond their conventional model of relating to patients. This is when the conventional therapeutic tools can be set aside in favor of the most powerful contribution of all: the physician's caring itself. The only requirement is a willingness to extend conscious listening and basic humanity to the dying patient. The simple act of visitation, of presence, of taking the trouble to witness the patient's process can be in itself a potent healing affirmation, a sacramental gesture received by the dying person who may be feeling helpless, diminished, and fearful that they have little to offer others.

How meaningful it is to be told by my physicians that they are learning from me! I feel honored and joined by my physicians as we participate in these human, vulnerable, and mysterious moments at the end of my life.

The willingness to extend to the patient with freshness, innocence, and sincere concern far outweighs any technique or expertise. . . . Practice and exposure hone these skills and deepen one's personal awareness, which in itself is the fertile soil for end-of-life completion work for both parties.[59]

Future Directions

Existential and developmental psychologies provide important frameworks for clinically assessing and caring for seriously ill patients and their families. By incorporating the potential for subjective well-being within its knowledge base and scope of research and practice, palliative medicine can improve the quality of caring and contribute to the psychological sciences and clinical disciplines.

The evidence base for counseling directed toward existential and developmental goals, including dignity therapy and logotherapy, continues to expand. Psychedelic-assisted therapies, such as those discussed in Chapter 42, may become important adjuncts to counseling related to life completion, the drive for meaning, and love in human life.

Key Points

- Subjectively positive and meaningful personal experiences occasionally occur during serious illness and dying.
- Western medicine, including palliative care and psychiatry, are based on conceptual frameworks that respond to health problems—illnesses and injuries—which do not encompass the phenomenology of health and well-being during illness and dying.

- Commonly used quality of life indices and assessment tools, as well as mainstream counseling modalities, tend to assume baseline (pre-illness or injury) quality of life and emotional and spiritual health as therapeutic goals.
- Existential psychology and developmental psychology encompass experiences of personal growth and well-being that palliative care can integrate to expand clinical assessments and therapeutic modalities to enhance its response to suffering and foster well-being.
- Dignity therapy, meaning-centered psychotherapy, and the OUTLOOK intervention represent modalities that facilitate human development and promote well-being for people with life-limiting medical conditions.
- Integrating the potential for human growth and well-being through illness and dying can expand and enhance specificity in assessing and clinically caring for people living with serious medical conditions and facing death.

References

1. Byock IR. Conceptual models and the outcomes of caring. *J Pain Symptom Manage*. Feb 1999;17(2):83–92.
2. World Health Organization. Preamble to the Constitution of the World Health Organization as adopted by the International Health Conference, New York, 19–22 June, 1946; signed on 22 July 1946 by the representatives of 61 States (Official Records of the World Health Organization, no. 2, p. 100) and entered into force on 7 April 1948. Geneva: WHO; 1948.
3. National Consensus Project for Quality Palliative Care. Clinical Practice Guidelines for quality palliative care, executive summary. *J Palliat Med*. Oct 2004;7(5):611–627.
4. Last Acts. Precepts of palliative care. *J Palliat Med*. 1998(2):109–112.
5. Byock I. Principles of palliative care. In: Walsh D, ed., *Palliative Medicine*. Philadelphia, PA: Elsevier; 2006: 33–41.
6. Aaronson N. Quality of Life Research in Cancer Clinical Trials: A need for common rules and language. *Oncology*. 1990;4(5):59–66.
7. Calman KC. Quality of life in cancer patients: An hypothesis. *J Med Ethics*. Sep 1984;10(3):124–127.
8. Sprangers MA, Schwartz CE. The challenge of response shift for quality-of-life-based clinical oncology research. *Ann Oncol*. Jul 1999;10(7):747–749.
9. Mount BM, Scott JF. Whither hospice evaluation. *J Chronic Dis*. 1983;36(11):731–736.
10. Greer DS, Mor V, Morris JN, Sherwood S, Kidder D, Birnbaum H. An alternative in terminal care: results of the National Hospice Study. *J Chronic Dis*. 1986;39(1):9–26.
11. Kagawa-Singer M. Redefining health: living with cancer. *Soc Sci Med*. Aug 1993;37(3):295–304.
12. Trillin C. *About Alice*. New York: Random House; 2006.
13. Broyard A. *Intoxicated by My Illness*. New York: Ballantine Books; 1993.
14. Buchwald A. *Too Soon to Say Goodbye*. New York: Random House; 2006.
15. Byock IR. *Dying Well: The Prospect for Growth at the End of Life*. New York: Riverhead, Putnam; 1997.
16. Yalom ID. *Existential Psychotherapy*. New York: Basic Books; 1980.
17. Yalom ID. *Love's Executioner: & Other Tales of Psychotherapy*. New York: Harper Perennial Modern Classics; 2000.
18. Penfield W. *The Mystery of the Mind: A Critical Study of Consciousness and the Human Brain*. Princeton, NJ: Princeton University Press; 1975.
19. Cassell EJ. The nature of suffering: physical, psychological, social, and spiritual aspects. *NLN Publ*. Mar 1992(15-2461):1–10.

20. Frankl VE. *Man's Search for Meaning.* New York: Washington Square Press; October 1984.

21. Byock IR. The nature of suffering and the nature of opportunity at the end of life. *Clin Geriatr Med.* May 1996;12(2):237–252.

22. Wilhem R, Young CG, Lü T-p. *The Secret of the Golden Flower: A Chinese Book of Life.* New York: Harcourt; 1935.

23. Block SD. Perspectives on care at the close of life: Psychological considerations, growth, and transcendence at the end of life: The art of the possible. *JAMA.* Jun 13 2001;285(22):2898–2905.

24. Byock IR. Growth: the essence of hospice. From a physician's point of view. *Am J Hosp Care.* Nov–Dec 1986;3(6):16–21.

25. Byock I. Five minutes with Ira Byock. Interview by Yvonne Parsons. *Contemp Longterm Care.* May 1997;20(5):88.

26. Zinker JC, Hallenbeck CE. Notes on loss, crisis, and growth. *J Gen Psychol.* Oct 1965;73(2d Half):347–354.

27. Zinker J, Fink S. The possibility for psychological growth in a dying person. *J Gen Psychol.* 1966(74):185–199.

28. de Hennezel M. *Intimate Death.* New York: Knopf; 1997.

29. Becker E. *The Denial of Death.* New York: Free Press Paperbacks; 1973.

30. Jung CG. *Modern Man in Search of A Soul.* London: Routledge; 1933.

31. Steinhauser KE, Christakis NA, Clipp EC, McNeilly M, McIntyre L, Tulsky JA. Factors considered important at the end of life by patients, family, physicians, and other care providers. *JAMA.* Nov 15 2000;284(19):2476–2482.

32. Staton J SR, Byock I. *A Few Months to Live.* Washington, DC: Georgetown University Press; 2001.

33. Lewis MI, Butler RN. Life-review therapy: Putting memories to work in individual and group psychotherapy. *Geriatrics.* Nov 1974;29(11):165–173.

34. Fitch VT. The psychological tasks of old age. *Naropa Institute J Psychol.* 3:90–106 1988.

35. Baines BK. Writing an ethical will. *Minn Med.* Jan 2004;87(1):26–28.

36. Gessert CE, Baines BK, Kuross SA, Clark C, Haller IV. Ethical wills and suffering in patients with cancer: a pilot study. *J Palliat Med.* Aug 2004;7(4):517–526.

37. Breitbart, W, Rosenfeld B, Gibson C, et al, Meaning-centered group psychotherapy for patients with advanced cancer: A pilot randomized controlled trial. *Psycho-Oncology.* 2020; 19 (1): 21–28.

38. Montross Thomas LP, Meier EA, Irwin SA. Meaning-centered psychotherapy: A form of psychotherapy for patients with cancer. *Curr Psychiatry Rep.* 2014; 16(10): 488.

39. Chochinov HM. Dying, dignity, and new horizons in palliative end-of-life care. *CA Cancer J Clin.* Mar-Apr 2006;56(2):84–103; quiz 104–105.

40. Chochinov HM, Hack T, Hassard T, Kristjanson LJ, McClement S, Harlos M. Dignity therapy: A novel psychotherapeutic intervention for patients near the end of life. *J Clin Oncol.* Aug 20 2005;23(24):5520–5525.

41. Chochinov HM, Krisjanson LJ, Hack TF, Hassard T, McClement S, Harlos M. Dignity in the terminally ill: Revisited. *J Palliat Med.* Jun 2006;9(3):666–672.

42. Steinhauser KE, Byock I, George L, Tulsky JA. *OUTLOOK: An Intervention to Improve Quality of Life for Patients at End-of-Life.* Charleston, SC: International Conference on Communication in Healthcare; October 2007.

43. Alexander SC, Tulsky JA, Byock I, George L, Steinhauser KE. *Development of a Semi-Structured Interview to Assist Life Competition Tasks for Patients Approaching End-of-Life.* Charleston, SC: Conference on Communication in Healthcare; 2007.

44. Byock I. *The Four Things That Matter Most: A Book About Living.* New York: Free Press; 2004.

45. Byock I. Notes of a hospice physician. *WJM.* 1996;164(4):367–368.

46. Byock IR. To life! Reflections on spirituality, palliative practice, and politics. *Am J Hosp Palliat Care.* Dec-2007 Jan 2006;23(6):436–438.

47. Vanderpool HY. The ethics of terminal care. *JAMA.* Feb 27 1978;239(9):850–852.

48. Zoloth L. First, make meaning: An ethics of encounter for healthcare reform. *Tikkun.* July 1993 1993;8(4):133–135.

49. Goleman D. *Emotional Intelligence: Why It Can Matter More Than IQ.* New York: Bantam; 1997.

50. Szasz T. *The Second Sin: "Personal Conflict."* Garden City, NJ: Anchor Press/Doubleday; 1973.
51. Varady AN. Aharon's Omphalos. Tracking down the author of the popular quote: Forgiveness means giving up all hope for a better past. 2016. https://aharon.varady.net/omphalos/2016/04/first-said-forg iveness-giving-hope-better-past accessed May 15, 2021.
52. Moffitt P. Forgiving the unforgivable. *Yoga J.* 2002(Jan/Feb):59–65.
53. Kast V. *Joy, Inspiration, and Hope.* Paperback ed. College Station: Texas A&M University Press; 1994.
54. Byock I. The ethics of loving care. *Health Prog.* Jul–Aug 2004;85(4):12–19, 57.
55. Byock I. Taking psychedelics seriously. *J Palliat Med.* Apr 21, 2018;4:417–421.
56. Swift TC, Bossis A, Ross S, et. al. Cancer at the dinner table: Experiences of psilocybin-assisted psycho-therapy for the treatment of cancer-related *Distress J Humanistic Psychol* 2017;57(5):488–519.
57. Kemp JT. Learning from clients: Counseling the frail and dying elderly. *Personnel Guidance J.* 1984;62(5):270–272.
58. Byock IR. When suffering persists. *J Palliat Care.* Summer 1994;10(2):8–13.
59. Fahnestock DT. A piece of my mind: Partnership for good dying. *JAMA.* Aug 18 1999;282(7):615–616.

Psychiatry in Multidisciplinary Pediatric Palliative Care

Julia A. Kearney and Megan Gilman

The field of pediatric palliative care (PPC) has evolved significantly after initially lagging behind adult palliative care, with well-developed care delivery models and published standards of care based on a growing body of evidence.[1] Beyond the common association with hospice care and end of life, modern PPC teams espouse the World Health Organization model, defining palliative care as *total care of the whole child—body, mind and spirit*, with care that begins at diagnosis and continues through end of life or survivorship.[2]

The role of psychiatry in PPC can be defined broadly as addressing the psychological, cognitive, and emotional needs of the child or adolescent and family during illness and through end of life. More specifically, the psychiatrist is tasked with diagnosing psychopathology while recognizing and addressing nonpathologic emotions and behaviors that veer from how the child was prior to the illness. Psychotherapies are tailored to provide developmentally appropriate opportunities for expression and navigation of a patient's and family's intense thoughts and feelings, address traumatic experiences and cognitive distortions, and facilitate communication among patients, families, and teams. Psychopharmacology offers additional tools for managing the patient's symptoms that interfere with important functions like sleep or participation in medical care, or with important relationships with parents and siblings, friends, or the medical treatment team.

The centrality of the family in children's care and well-being is a tenet of pediatrics. The pediatric patient is simultaneously viewed as an individual with their own hopes, fears, and goals of care and as a part of an interdependent family unit whose dynamics are critical to understanding the individual. The scope of PPC considers the profound impact a child's illness has on family dynamics and functioning, integrates family roles and relationships in treatment planning, and addresses family members' distress. Approaches to assessment and therapy with the child may differ outside of and in the presence of parents and other caregivers. For example, a young patient may project optimism and hope for the benefit of their family while harboring fear and worry. Only when engaged in an individual therapeutic exercise might the patient share their fear of dying or distress related to the grief of parents and siblings. Pediatric mental health clinicians can bring a nuanced understanding of children's and adolescents' developing autonomy and the skills needed to develop the therapeutic relationships with parents and children within which sensitive conversations can occur.

This chapter covers the unique developmental and psychiatric needs of children, adolescents, and their families facing life-threatening illness and special considerations for treatment. It will also highlight fundamentals of pediatric palliative communication and the role of the pediatric psychiatric practitioner (child and adolescent psychiatrists, psychiatric nurse practitioners, and nurses) in multidisciplinary PPC settings. Any pediatric behavioral health clinician (e.g., psychologist, social worker, or child life therapist) can benefit from this chapter's guidance in understanding and providing psychoeducation about the role of psychiatry in PPC.

Developmental Considerations for Psychosocial Assessment and Intervention in PPC

The child's understanding of illness and death changes across the developmental stages of childhood and is not fully realized until adolescence. Death is defined by four concepts: non-functionality, universality, irreversibility, and causality. *Non-functionality* means that all physiologic and physical functions stop with death. *Universality* and *irreversibility* mean, respectively, that death comes to all living things and that, once someone or something has died, death is forever. *Causality*, the concept grasped last by the developing child, relates to what events or behaviors can lead to death.[3]

- *Infancy (0–18 months)*. In infancy, the child seeks comfort from pain, hunger, discomfort, and aloneness. Erik Erikson, in *Eight Ages of Man*, described successful completion of the developmental task of infancy as achievement of basic trust, meaning that the infant trusts that the caregiver will provide comfort and that the infant can tolerate urges until comfort is provided.[4] Illness challenges basic trust by introducing previously unencountered needs and unfamiliar care providers. For infants with serious illness, their needs are practical, and their fears are concrete. There is an immediacy to the child's concerns at this stage, rather than a preoccupation with what might happen and what is to come, which can be protective. Maintaining bonds with familiar caregivers is a primary comfort for infants, while memory-making and addressing parent and family grief are often primary tasks for psychiatric providers.
- *Toddler (18 months–3 years)*. Through early experiences and exposures from media, games, and stories, toddlers may have some idea of death but often have a misperception of death as an impermanent, transitory absence. John Bowlby emphasized that, in these early years of development, the child understands and experiences the death of another

as a separation only, suggesting the possibility of a reunion.[5] As the child approaches 3 years of age, separation anxiety is consistently experienced as part of normal development. Erikson explained that, at this stage, the child's "environment encourages him to stand on his own two feet" as the child grows to develop a sense of autonomy.[4] While the ill toddler is not yet able to comprehend or prepare for death, many aspects of serious illness can result in an exacerbation of separation anxiety. Illness, pain, fatigue, cognitive changes, and hospitalizations deny the patient opportunities for self-expression and control and are barriers between the child and those they depend upon, as well as from the self they know. Therapeutic interventions can focus on continuity, predictability, and simple anticipatory guidance.

- *Early childhood (3–5 years).* Erikson defined initiative—"the quality of undertaking, planning, and 'attacking' a task for the sake of being active and on the move"—as evidence of growth in preschool aged children. Initiative is demonstrated through cooperative play or games that involve sharing of ideas and working toward a shared goal.[4] Illness disrupts initiative through normal regression and dependency on caregivers, so children need support and explanations around loss of milestones (e.g., needing assistance to walk or eat or having to wear diapers again). Imagination and curiosity become increasingly important, and the child asks questions about things seen or heard about as well as things the child has only thought about. For the pediatric patient of preschool age, the medical setting stimulates curiosity and leads to questions. Support and developmentally informed education can bolster a child's sense of mastery and help improve self-esteem and a sense of control even in the face of symptoms and functional declines. Young children benefit from play therapy, and drawing has been shown to be a powerful outlet for expression of distress related to the child's experience of medical illness.[6] While the concepts of universality, irreversibility, non-functionality, and causality continue to evade the child's understanding, the child is beginning to wonder about death and associating death with sadness. They are already aware of taboos of talking about death and, even when aware of their own impending death, may not ask directly.[7] Euphemisms should be avoided when answering questions about death as the young child's concrete thought process can lead to confusion. When a child asks about death, particularly when illness has personalized the question, Elisabeth Kubler-Ross emphasized that it is important to "be honest with them because they are aware of your pains and worries. Shared sorrow is much easier to bear than leaving them with feelings of guilt and fear that they are the cause of all your anxiety." Many children's book authors have created gentle and imaginative story books to give children language and permission to talk about death in a safe, slightly removed, hypothetical way.[8] The works of psychologist Barbara Sourkes and anthropologist Myra Bluebond-Langner stand out as classic manuals to the therapist learning to tread lightly into the clinical interactions with young children about death and dying, always with the goal of alleviating emotional suffering of children and their families.[7,9]

- *Late childhood (5–12 years).* A more complete understanding of death develops in school-aged children. Children of this age, according to Erikson, are motivated to prove themselves industrious and useful, with a sense of inferiority if they do not.[4] The medically ill child is limited physically and cognitively by the effects of disease and treatment, unable to keep pace with peers, and can feel inadequate as a result. As the child struggles to understand these limitations, questions may shift to the physical and biological aspects of death and dying. By age 12, children understand death as a final and permanent absence of all function, but children in this age group may still blame themselves for their own illness and feel guilty for causing sadness and burden to their families. Starting with open-ended inquiries about what children understand about their illness and about their hopes and fears, psychosocial and palliative providers can partner with parents to identify what information will be useful to the child and what words to use. Conversations around a child's preferences for quality of life, symptom management, and even death and dying can help children and parents feel aligned and close during this difficult time, preventing guilt, loneliness, and worry, even if sadness remains. Therapeutic tools, including a specialized board game[10] and a pediatric advance care planning document (My Wishes by Aging with Dignity: https://fivewishes.org/shop/order/product/pediatric-my-wishes) can foster age-appropriate communication around difficult subjects.

- *Adolescence (12–18 years).* In adolescence, the primary developmental task described by Erikson is the establishment of a distinct identity. The adolescent tries on different representations of self, changing physical appearance and taste in music, circles of friends, and future goals, in what Erikson called a requestioning of "all samenesses and continuities" previously adhered to in a "search for a new sense of sameness and continuity."[4] Adolescence is a time for exploration and growth. For the adolescent with a serious illness, the search for one's identity occurs against a backdrop of fear, pain, and the specter of death. Rather than choosing how to present oneself, the patient's appearance is altered by disease and treatment side effects. When the adolescent should be growing their group of friends, the patient's support network is shrinking to rely on parental support. At a time when the adolescent should be exploring independence, the patient is forced to regress into a role of having basic needs met by a care provider. The more unique the individual sees oneself, the more there is to lose in illness and death; the more plans one makes for the future, the more there is to grieve should that future be lost.

The adolescent understands death: that it is non-functional, universal, and irreversible. When faced with an illness that could cause death, identity development is made more challenging by this existential reality. Even after full awareness that they are dying, it is common for children and adolescents to talk about the future, going to college, getting married, or travel and career plans. It is not usually a sign of pervasive "denial" as much as a sign of the normalcy of looking to the future, exploring what "could be" (or "could have been") and living in the "fluctuating awareness" of dying that makes living tolerable.[9] Younger children and adolescents may achieve the "double awareness" described in adults facing terminal illness, where one can be engaged in an existential dialectic, living in the world while preparing for impending death. If psychotherapy is established with a good therapeutic alliance with parents and patients, sensitive timing may allow for exploration of different states of awareness of death and more synthesis toward an open acknowledgment of living and dying at the same time.[11] However, sometimes a child or adolescent copes using less "mature" defenses, more compartmentalization, suppression, and denial which may provide a sense of control, good emotional quality of life, and can be normalized and supported.

Additionally, an adolescent may experience existential guilt, a state of regret for not living to one's fullest potential due to an early death. Meaning-centered approaches in psychotherapy have been found useful in adult patients with advanced cancer and may be adapted for adolescents who express a loss of meaning in life or existential distress (see Chapter 35).

Affording the adolescent patient opportunities to participate in their own care with a role in medical decision-making helps to restore a sense of independence and future-orientation. Interventions tailored for advance care planning and support for adolescents and young adults (AYAs) facing end of life (like Voicing My Choices available online by Aging with Dignity: https://fivewishes.org/shop/order/product/voicing-my-choices) have growing evidence of improved communication, quality of life, and trust between the patient and their caregivers.[12,13] It is important, when possible, to time these conversations when the patient and family are not in crisis; earlier introduction of palliative care and related concepts is highly recommended. Close coordination of care with primary pediatric teams regarding language used in discussions around scan results and treatments, how palliative options are introduced and presented, or when clinical information is changing allows for iterative conversations that permit the adolescent time to process and respond to news, seek support, and approach the next stage of conversation with a greater sense of autonomy and control. Zadeh et al. include a three-point readiness assessment for adolescents prior to end-of-life conversations that includes three yes/no questions: "(1) whether talking about what would happen if treatments were no longer effective would be helpful, (2) whether talking about medical care plans ahead of time would be upsetting, and (3) whether they would be comfortable writing down/discussing what would happen if treatments were no longer effective."[13] They suggest an approach that aligns with the patient's hope and yet introduces the need for preparing "in case" things do not go as hoped, in order to address assignment of proxies and expression of preferences for end-of-life care and other existential and practical concerns.

Disconnection from important peer and other relationships may detract from quality of life for children and adolescents engaged in palliative care. When goals of care have shifted to quality of life over more potentially toxic treatments, patients may experience improved functioning and a freer schedule that allows them to return for a time to meaningful school or social activities if desired. Barriers to inclusion in these activities may be addressed in multidisciplinary fashion, targeting symptoms that interrupt the school day, preserving energy, reducing treatment interruptions of school, or arranging check-ups around special social events. Psychosocial staff may guide parents and the patient's school team in preparing and supporting classmates and friends for changes in appearance or the possibility that the patient may die. If school is not an option, or as an added support, age-matched group therapy (even conducted over telemedicine) allows pediatric patients to discuss shared experiences and alleviates some sense of isolation that medical illness can cause.

The care of a child or adolescent during acute suffering and at end of life requires balancing the anticipatory grief of the child or adolescent and the grief of the caregivers, celebrating the accomplishments and meaning in a young life and recognizing the great losses in a foreshortened one, accepting impending absences and acknowledging the injustices that accompany the premature death of a young person.

Psychiatric Diagnosis and Symptom Management in PPC

The emotional state of the child or adolescent diagnosed with an illness may be rich and layered or blunted by physical and cognitive symptoms of the disease. Psychopathology is differentiated from normal emotional and behavioral responses to the situation by considering possible psychiatric syndromes, family history, and corroborative history of baseline emotional functioning, as well as illness and treatment factors. It is important to become familiar with the typical behavioral and systemic effects of pediatric illness and treatment through collaboration with the primary team and through continuity of care. Even terminally ill children may demonstrate transient "illness behaviors" of regression, clinginess, irritability, low energy, and appetite, which resolve partially or fully when treatment toxicities improve (e.g., from chemotherapy), infections are treated (e.g., *C. Difficile* or urinary tract infection), or fluid and electrolyte abnormalities are repleted.

Psychiatric medications may be used in pediatric patients when symptoms (1) result in the patient presenting a danger to themselves or others, (2) create an obstacle to medical treatment, or (3) cause suffering. Weight-based pediatric dosing is available and appropriate in end-of-life settings.[14] Off-label use of psychotropics in pediatrics is common and should be discussed with patients and parents for consent.

- *Depression*: The criteria for diagnosing depressive disorders in pediatric patients, including adjustment disorder with depressed mood and major depressive disorder, are the same *Diagnostic and Statistical Manual of Mental Disorders* (DSM-5) criteria used to identify these diagnoses in the adult population. Symptoms of medical disease and side effects of medical treatment can mask or mimic depressive symptoms, and psychological symptoms like anhedonia, irrational guilt, and hopelessness may need to be given more weight than somatic and neurovegetative symptoms when making a diagnosis.[15] In children and adolescents, uncharacteristic irritability is a prominent symptom of depressive disorders. Expression of sadness or frustration at challenging points in a child's illness are expected and, when appropriate, should be validated and normalized. Persistent joylessness or retreat from friends and activities previously enjoyed indicates the need for a psychiatric treatment plan to address depression. If prognosis is expected to be weeks to months, selective serotonin reuptake inhibitors (SSRIs) may be warranted, but contraindications often apply due to bleeding risk or QTc prolongation with polypharmacy. Otherwise, low-dose stimulants, flexibly dosed around desired experiences and times of day, can be helpful to combat fatigue and depressive symptoms.

- *Anxiety*: Although it is common for children to be fearful of things and to worry at times, the severity of these fears and whether they interfere with functioning in social, familial, or academic domains can suggest a diagnosis of anxiety. Anxiety disorders in the pediatric population include specific phobias, separation anxiety, social anxiety, panic disorder, and generalized anxiety disorder. Specific phobias and separation anxiety are especially significant in the medical setting, where fear of needles or of separation from a parent can cause significant distress and potentially impede assessment, treatment, and quality of life. Exposure to frightening experiences or painful stimuli can lead to an adjustment disorder with anxiety or posttraumatic stress symptoms that complicate the need for regular medical visits and repeat procedures. Pediatric patients benefit from clear explanations of aspects of treatment with the support of Child Life specialists as well as opportunities to explore and identify ways to cope with their anxieties in individual and group therapies. Short-acting anxiolytics, like benzodiazepines, and long-acting anxiolytics, like SSRIs may also have roles.

- *Delirium*: Infants, children, and adolescents experience delirium as a consequence of systemic illness and pharmacologic interventions, as well as multisystem failure at end of life (terminal delirium). Assessment should be standardized and developmentally informed (using tools such as the Preschool Confusion Assessment Method,[16] Pediatric Confusion Assessment Method,[17] and Cornell Assessment of Pediatric Delirium[18]). Interventions should be multimodal, such as removing offending medications and addressing sleep deficits and other environmental factors. Low-dose atypical antipsychotics or intravenous haloperidol or chlorpromazine may be useful for providing anxiolysis, sedation, and antiemetic relief, sparing more deliriogenic medications like benzodiazepines.

- *Other symptom management*: Familiarity with the use of psychotropics for other symptom management can be helpful for psychiatrists working in PPC. Intractable nausea often requires multimodal pharmacologic regimens, which may include intravenous haloperidol or chlorpromazine, or oral olanzapine. Severe pain may be treated with opiates in conjunction with neuropathic agents including antidepressants or duloxetine or amitriptyline, and with intravenous ketamine when available (with appropriate oversight and safety protocols). Sedation at end of life with lorazepam or another benzodiazepine or sedative may be a compassionate option directed by palliative teams.[14]

Palliative Communication in Pediatrics

Palliative communication refers to the skills needed for creating a shared understanding among teams, patients, and their families about the meaning of and planning for a person's illness, death, and dying. It encompasses conversations around diagnosis, prognosis, quality of life, goals of care, end-of-life preferences, resuscitation choices, and anticipatory guidance for patients and caregivers about the dying process. It is also inclusive of emotional, psychological, and spiritual aspects of care like love, hope, faith, grief, and bereavement. Good pediatric palliative communication is child- and family-centered, culturally competent, and developmentally informed. There is strong evidence linking quality of communication to improved physical and emotional quality of life for dying children and improved bereavement outcomes for parents after the death of a child.[19-21] Some of the main tenets of PPC communication are listed here, but practitioners are encouraged to pursue further reading at the references cited and consider advanced certifications in pediatric palliative communication skills through programs like Northwestern University's Education in Palliative and End of Life Care (EPEC) (https://www.bioethics.northwestern.edu/programs/epec/) or Harvard University's Palliative Care Education and Practice (https://pallcare.hms.harvard.edu/courses/pcep).

- *Communication with children about their own diagnosis and ongoing disease information is a standard of care in pediatrics and should be supported and facilitated by all team members.* Parents need support and psychoeducation by all members of the team when they resist efforts to communicate with children in developmentally appropriate ways about their disease. Parents' wish to protect children is normal, and they may fear that telling their child their diagnosis or disease-related information would be too frightening or take away hope. However, children who do not have adequate information or preparation may have increased levels of maladjustment, anxiety, and depressive symptoms.[22] While children do not need the same level of detail or extent of information (see below on prognosis) as their adult caregivers and proxies, there is ample evidence that children do need enough information to (1) be prepared for what treatment they will undergo (e.g., preparation and rationale for procedures, side effects), (2) maintain trust in important adults in their life as valid sources of truth about their illness (e.g., not overhearing or learning from a hospital playmate that they have cancer), and (3) establish a dialogue about the illness as a place for their own fears, concerns, and wishes to be expressed.
- *Disclosure to children about their own prognosis, particularly about dying, should be sensitive to parent and child wishes and informed by child development.* Based on a child's age, developmental maturity, and burden of symptoms, sometimes it is appropriate and compassionate to be protective of children and not explicit about the fact of their own dying. In other cases, parents or staff may suspect that the child knows they are dying, or would want to know, and want to support them by addressing this explicitly. Even so, they often struggle for language and the emotional composure to have the conversation with their child.[23] Psychosocial clinicians can assess a child's understanding of their predicament, and clarify the child's wishes for information, reassurance, or support. They can help set up the conversation(s) and provide sample language to parents as well as in-person or behind the scenes support for parents to address their child's fears or wishes in a way that is iterative and child-led. As children develop into adolescents it is increasingly important to include them in a fuller understanding of their illness and prognosis, as well as treatment decisions using tools discussed above.[6,20]
- *Hope can coexist with an accurate understanding of prognosis and terminal illness.* Family members' expressions of hope may be seen as unrealistic signs of denial or misunderstanding. Medical teams who feel responsible for communicating prognostic information may be anxious that they have not done their job because the family still has "hope" despite the increasing certainty of death. Studies have shown that families can hold both

realistic medical understanding of the terminal nature of disease and hold out hope, bringing meaning and purpose to daily life. Psychosocial and palliative clinicians often lead conversations with open-ended questions such as "What are your fears for your child?" and "What are your hopes for your child?" which can support conversations that lead to a broader understanding of the context of hopes that may change over time, from hope for miracle cures (acknowledging it would take a higher power to render a cure), to hope for more time with their child, to hope for resilience in the face of the tragedy. Expert palliative communicators can both embrace and share families' hopes while simultaneously helping to prepare them for the dying process.[20]

• *Expert PPC means supporting parents' choices regarding goals of care and end-of-life preferences.* Obtaining patient or parent consent for a do not resuscitate (DNR) order cannot be the optimal quality marker for good palliative care. Family preferences that prioritize religious or cultural beliefs or survivors' psychological needs may be ethically appropriate even if they differ from the medical team's recommendations for DNR. If, after adequate communication around prognosis, risks and benefits of DNR, and possible strategies for palliation of symptoms around end of life, a family declines DNR and wants "full code" for resuscitation, their wishes should be respected nonjudgmentally and not revisited unless the clinical information changes. If medical team members are struggling to accept parent's wishes for full code for their child, a pediatric ethics consultation can be a useful mechanism for objective exploration of the case and clarification of parents' rights, as well as support for staff members' personal moral distress.[20]

• *Expertise in PPC communication greatly impacts how parents experience their child's dying and bereavement after the death.* Feeling understood, respected, and supported matters greatly to all parents and families. They remember interactions that did not provide these considerations as traumatic and adding to their grief.[21,24] Reinforcing that "good parents" may choose different things for their children and understanding what each parent values by being the "good parent" for their child can be supportive and comforting to parents and clarifying for staff. Good PPC is preventive medicine.[1,25]

Interdisciplinary Collaboration in PPC

The interdisciplinary nature of PPC is paramount. PPC teams are ideally comprised of multidisciplinary practitioners who bring a range of expertise to the care of a child and family. Emotional support of the child and family is a shared task of all clinicians as families face the heartbreaking daily challenges of caring for medically ill children. Defining the boundaries and scope of the specific roles for each discipline can help provide the integrated, collaborative experience that benefits patients and families and makes the work sustainable and meaningful for team members.[26]

The roles of PPC physicians and child psychiatrists can be visualized as a Venn diagram with some overlapping skills and other distinct ones, as seen in Figure 44.1.[26] The role of the individual psychiatrist in a particular PPC setting may vary, reflecting their training and experience and depending on the resources available in the unit and hospital. While

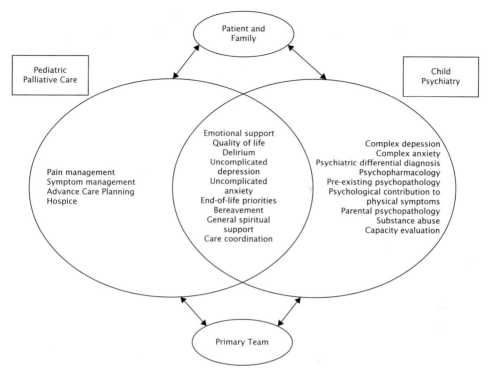

FIGURE 44.1 Overlapping and distinct expertise. Reproduced with permission from Muriel AC, Wolfe J, Block SD. Pediatric palliative care and child psychiatry: A model for enhancing practice and collaboration. *J Palliat Med.* Oct 2016;19(10):1032–1038; permission conveyed through Copyright Clearance Center, Inc.

many pediatric centers have developed both PPC teams and inpatient child and adolescent psychiatry consultation liaison services, these can be underresourced and roles may need to be expanded or negotiated in individual centers to meet clinical needs. Child and adolescent psychiatrists' expertise in the assessment and management of the biological, psychological, and social factors contributing to the child's psychiatric symptoms can help the team realize each unique patient's palliative goals. Subspecialty training in a child and adolescent psychiatry fellowship includes aspects of neuropsychology, child development, and family systems as well as rotations in consultation liaison psychiatry (care of the medically ill pediatric patient).

A child and adolescent psychiatry consultation can provide much needed parenting support, psychoeducation, and reassurance for families in these tragic circumstances, benefitting patient, family, and staff. Pediatric consultation liaison teams should be flexible in their approach to requests for help and collaboration from pediatric staff caring for terminally ill children and their families, even if the child patient presents as well-adjusted and supported.[27,28] A child psychiatric assessment and successful engagement of patient, family, and staff can reassure and guide, shift a pattern of interactions, reduce trauma, and improve communication.

Consulting psychiatrists (and other psychosocial clinicians), as team members with formal training in the recognition and management of countertransference, may recognize pediatric staff distress as contributing to a larger picture in the case of a dying child or adolescent. Multidisciplinary treatment team meetings, debriefing meetings, and individual "curbside" consults can be appropriate places to normalize and support staff frustration with patient's and families' choices, guilt for one's own health, professional boundary concerns, sadness, helplessness, horror, and grief.

The psychiatric clinician in PPC must also be aware of their own countertransference and how they process their own grief, loss, and other reactions to witnessing the suffering of children. Barbara Sourkes suggests that clinicians in PPC must always reassess their own "capacity for repeated cycles of attachment and loss."[9] With vulnerable children, adolescents, and families, one must be present and authentic to be effective, which is difficult if one is physically or emotionally exhausted. Furthermore, the truths encountered at the bedside in PPC may lead to self-examination of one's own sense of meaning and peace in the face of existential realities. For PPC clinicians, including psychiatrists, individual psychotherapy can be a substantial commitment toward self-care and a deeper understanding of one's relationship to this work. Participation in professional societies and conferences on PPC is also an invaluable support, source of inspiration, and further enrichment of palliative skills.

Future Directions

Child psychiatry training programs should include specific competencies in the multidisciplinary role of psychiatry in PPC. Additional research is needed into best practices in resource-poor areas without access to PPC or child psychiatry, such as the democratization of primary palliative skills for all pediatric teams and the use of online interventions and telepsychiatry in home-based hospice care and inpatient pediatric units. More evidence-based interventions are needed to address communication challenges with pediatric illness and end of life. Additional research is also needed to clarify the safety and role of psychotropics in PPC.

Key Points

- PPC is multidisciplinary, child- and family-centered, developmentally informed, holistic care for children, adolescents, and their families when facing life-threatening illness. It aims to relieve physical, emotional, and spiritual suffering of the child and family through illness, dying, and death and into bereavement.
- Child and adolescent psychiatrists in PPC contribute valuable skills in assessment of emotional and behavioral symptoms, diagnosis of psychiatric syndromes, understanding family dynamics, participating in nuanced communication, and tailoring psychological interventions. Symptom management with psychotropic medications is appropriate to provide comfort and relief from physical or emotional distress.
- Communication with children and adolescents about their own death and dying should be done in conjunction with parent psychoeducation and support in the context of a

therapeutic relationship, and it should be developmentally informed, iterative, individualized, and child-led. Adolescents and young adults should be increasingly included in goals-of-care discussions, as appropriate.

- Evidence-based therapeutic interventions and communication tools such as advance care planning guides and therapeutic games are invaluable tools at the bedside in PPC.
- Expertise in palliative communication is shown to be closely correlated with child quality of life and parent bereavement outcomes after the death of a child. The scope of PPC includes the overall well-being of the family, which should be evaluated and supported by the multidisciplinary team to serve the shared goals of comfort, meaning, and wholeness in the face of trauma, loss, and tragedy.

References

1. Weaver MS, Heinze KE, Bell CJ, Wiener L, Garee AM, Kelly KP, et al. Establishing psychosocial palliative care standards for children and adolescents with cancer and their families: An integrative review. *Palliat Med.* Mar 2016;30(3):212–223. doi:10.1177/0269216315583446
2. WHO. Definition of palliative care. 2020. Accessed September 13, 2021. https://www.who.int/health-topics/palliative-care
3. Bates AT, Kearney JA. Understanding death with limited experience in life: Dying children's and adolescents' understanding of their own terminal illness and death. *Curr Opin Support Palliat Care.* Mar 2015;9(1):40–45. doi:10.1097/SPC.0000000000000118
4. Erikson EH. *Childhood and Society.* 1st ed. New York: Norton; 1950.
5. Terr L. *Too Scared to Cry: Psychic Trauma in Childhood.* 1st ed. New York: Harper & Row; 1990:xii.
6. Sourkes BM. Children's artwork: Its value in psychotherapy in pediatric palliative care. *Child Adolesc Psychiatr Clin N Am.* Oct 2018;27(4):551–565. doi:10.1016/j.chc.2018.05.004
7. Bluebond-Langner M. *The Private Worlds of Dying Children.* Princeton, NJ: Princeton University Press; 1978:xv.
8. Arruda-Colli MNF, Weaver MS, Wiener L. Communication about dying, death, and bereavement: A systematic review of children's literature. *J Palliat Med.* May 2017;20(5):548–559. doi:10.1089/jpm.2016.0494
9. Sourkes BM. *Armfuls of Time: The Psychological Experience of the Child with a Life-Threatening Illness.* Pittsburgh, PA: University of Pittsburgh Press; 1995:xiv.
10. Wiener L, Battles H, Mamalian C, Zadeh S. ShopTalk: A pilot study of the feasibility and utility of a therapeutic board game for youth living with cancer. *Support Care Cancer.* Jul 2011;19(7):1049–1054. doi:10.1007/s00520-011-1130-z
11. Colosimo K, Nissim R, Pos AE, Hales S, Zimmermann C, Rodin G. "Double awareness" in psychotherapy for patients living with advanced cancer. *J Psychother Integr.* Jun 2018;28(2):125–140. doi:10.1037/int0000078
12. Lyon ME, Jacobs S, Briggs L, Cheng YI, Wang J. Family-centered advance care planning for teens with cancer. *JAMA Pediatr.* May 2013;167(5):460–467. doi:10.1001/jamapediatrics.2013.943
13. Zadeh S, Pao M, Wiener L. Opening end-of-life discussions: How to introduce Voicing My CHOiCES, an advance care planning guide for adolescents and young adults. *Palliat Support Care.* Jun 2015;13(3):591–599. doi:10.1017/S1478951514000054
14. Kearney JA BA, Pao M. Psychiatric issues in pediatric oncology: Diagnosis and management. In: Abrams AN, Muriel AC, Wiener L, eds., *Pediatric Psychosocial Oncology: Textbook for Multidisciplinary Care.* New York: Springer; 2016:119–141.
15. Shemesh E, Bartell A, Newcorn JH. Assessment and treatment of depression in medically ill children. *Curr Psychiatry Rep.* Apr 2002;4(2):88–92. doi:10.1007/s11920-002-0040-7

16. Smith HA, Gangopadhyay M, Goben CM, et al. The preschool confusion assessment method for the ICU: Valid and reliable delirium monitoring for critically ill infants and children. *Crit Care Med*. Mar 2016;44(3):592–600. doi:10.1097/CCM.0000000000001428

17. Smith HA, Boyd J, Fuchs DC, et al. Diagnosing delirium in critically ill children: Validity and reliability of the Pediatric Confusion Assessment Method for the Intensive Care Unit. *Crit Care Med*. Jan 2011;39(1):150–157. doi:10.1097/CCM.0b013e3181feb489

18. Traube C, Silver G, Kearney J, et al. Cornell Assessment of Pediatric Delirium: A valid, rapid, observational tool for screening delirium in the PICU. *Crit Care Med*. Mar 2014;42(3):656–63. doi:10.1097/CCM.0b013e3182a66b76

19. DeCourcey DD, Silverman M, Oladunjoye A, Wolfe J. Advance care planning and parent-reported end-of-life outcomes in children, adolescents, and young adults with complex chronic conditions. *Crit Care Med*. Jan 2019;47(1):101–108. doi:10.1097/CCM.0000000000003472

20. Wolfe J, Hinds PS, Sourkes BM. *Interdisciplinary Pediatric Palliative Care*. 2nd ed. New York: Oxford University Press; 2021.

21. Mack JW, Hilden JM, Watterson J, et al. Parent and physician perspectives on quality of care at the end of life in children with cancer. *J Clin Oncol*. Dec 20 2005;23(36):9155–9161. doi:10.1200/JCO.2005.04.010

22. Thompson AL, Young-Saleme TK. Anticipatory guidance and psychoeducation as a standard of care in pediatric oncology. *Pediatr Blood Cancer*. Dec 2015;62 Suppl 5:S684–693. doi:10.1002/pbc.25721

23. Davies DE. Talking about death with dying children. *N Engl J Med*. Jan 6 2005;352(1):91–92; author reply 91–92. doi:10.1056/NEJM200501063520117

24. Sisk BA, Zavadil JA, Blazin LJ, Baker JN, Mack JW, DuBois JM. Assume it will break: Parental perspectives on negative communication experiences in pediatric oncology. *JCO Oncol Pract*. Jun 2021;17(6):e859-e871. doi:10.1200/OP.20.01038

25. Weaver MS, October T, Feudtner C, Hinds PS. "Good-parent beliefs": Research, concept, and clinical practice. *Pediatrics*. Jun 2020;145(6):e20194018. doi:10.1542/peds.2019-4018. OMID: 32439815; PMCID: PMC7263052

26. Muriel AC, Wolfe J, Block SD. Pediatric palliative care and child psychiatry: A model for enhancing practice and collaboration. *J Palliat Med*. Oct 2016;19(10):1032–1038. doi:10.1089/jpm.2015.0354

27. Kearney JA, Salley CG, Muriel AC. Standards of psychosocial care for parents of children with cancer. *Pediatr Blood Cancer*. Dec 2015;62 Suppl 5:S632–683. doi:10.1002/pbc.25761

28. Jones BL, Contro N, Koch KD. The duty of the physician to care for the family in pediatric palliative care: Context, communication, and caring. *Pediatrics*. Feb 2014;133 Suppl 1: S8–15. doi:10.1542/peds.2013-3608C

Special Care Considerations for the Seriously Ill Older Adult

Ayla Pelleg, R. Sean Morrison, and Diane E. Meier

Introduction

The majority of patients with serious illness are older adults. As palliative care is now the gold standard of care for those with serious illness, knowledge of how age influences pathophysiology, pharmacology, function, cognition, and comorbid illness is essential. This knowledge will maximize the benefit and minimize the harm of what medical providers do in an effort to provide care that improves quality of life and function, which are the highest priorities to patients. In this chapter, older adults will be defined as those older than 65 years of age. Palliative care and symptom management research often exclude older adults in studies, which is an important caveat in assessing the applicability of studies to seriously ill older adults. This chapter focuses on how aging impacts delivery of care during serious illness by looking at aging biology, the demographics of older adults, common geriatric syndromes and their implications during serious illness, and the applicability of the 4M's framework in all care settings. The Age Friendly Health Systems initiative, led by the Institute for Healthcare Improvement (IHI) and the John A. Hartford Foundation in partnership with the American Hospital Association (AHA) and the Catholic Health Association of the United States (CHA), emphasizes 4M's (Mobility, Mentation, Medication, and what Matters) as a framework for improving care for older adults that is evidenced-based in high-quality care.[1]

Biology of Aging

The aging process varies greatly among older adults. The physiologic reserves that in younger adults allow for the maintenance of homeostasis when faced with environmental, emotional, and physiological stressors diminish in a linear manner with increasing age, resulting in reduced physiologic reserve and resilience in response to stressors. Disruption of homeostasis under stress from an acute illness or a chronic illness exacerbation is thus more likely to lead to a decrease in functional capacity, progression of chronic disease(s), and death in older adults. There are many age-related physiological changes that influence clinical management. For example, as one ages, there is a decrease in nephron, gastrointestinal, and hepatic function and therefore a reduction in renal and liver metabolism. Decreases in renal and liver metabolism require medication adjustments (e.g., titrating medications slowly, spacing out dosing internals). Additionally, bone tissue, bone density, and muscle mass and strength decrease as part of normal aging, resulting in increase in fractures with minimal movement and a higher prevalence of osteopenia and osteoporosis.

Demographics of Aging

While increases in aging populations are occurring worldwide, this chapter focus on the aging demographics within the United States. By 2030, one of five Americans will be over the age of 65.[2] According to the US Census Bureau, the 2012 US population (43.1 million) is expected to nearly double by 2050 (83.7 million).[3] Despite the recent drop in life expectancy in the past few years attributed both to COVID-19 and the rise in so-called deaths of despair,[4] the US aging paradigm has shifted. The leading causes of death, unlike at the turn of the 20th century when infectious diseases topped the list, are now due to chronic medical illnesses such as heart disease, stroke, cancer, chronic obstructive pulmonary disease, and dementia.[5]

In the US, location of deaths is shifting toward the home, assisted living facilities, and nursing homes instead of hospitals. Between 2003 and 2017, hospital deaths for those with chronic illnesses have decreased in the United States, specifically from 56% to 35.6% for chronic kidney disease (CKD) and end-stage kidney disease (ESKD), from 44.4% to 28.3% for chronic lung disease (CLD), and from 12.7% to 8% for Alzheimer's disease-related dementias (ADRD).[6-8] Compared to other illness, older adults with cancer were more likely to die at home or in a hospice facility and have the lowest odds of dying in a nursing facility.[9] While hospitals remain the most common place of death for those with end-stage renal disease and chronic liver disease, the proportion of deaths at home and hospice facilities has increased. Health disparities exist across chronic diseases in regard to location of death, with persons of color being more likely to die in a hospital setting. Decisions about where a patient dies are complex and can be related to housing, family availability and ability, and ethnic and cultural beliefs, as well as finances and insurance coverage, which often dictate where patients can get needed care.

Access to Palliative Care in the United States

Ensuring access to palliative care is crucial to improving the needs of older adults with serious illness. Access to palliative care is variable among older adults geographically and depending on the care setting (e.g., hospitals, nursing homes, assisted living facilities, home). Geographically speaking, palliative care services are more available in states that are less racially diverse, that have higher socioeconomic status, and that have higher openness (i.e., trying new things, hearing new ideas).[10] Access to palliative care services, primarily received in a hospital setting, has increased in the past two decades. Although 72% of US hospitals with more than 50 beds have some form of a palliative care team, only 17% of hospitals with more than 50 beds in rural areas have a palliative care program. Hospitals that are nonprofit, geographically based in the northeast and mountain regions, and in urban areas are more likely to have palliative care teams.[11] With telemedicine (i.e., telephone and video visit clinical services) growing over the past few decades and acutely accelerated by the COVID-19 pandemic, access to palliative telemedicine can still remain a challenge for older adults due to lack of access to technology, low technology literacy, and sensory deficits such as hearing and vision impairments.[12,13] By addressing these challenges, telemedicine can help improve access to palliative care access in a sustainable and scalable manner for patients currently unable receive palliative care services.

While palliative care is increasingly available in hospitals and at the end of life through hospice within the United States, the great majority of those with serious illness are at home (including nursing homes and assisted living facilities) where there is little or variable access to palliative care. The limited data available suggest that the prevalence of hospice and palliative care services is increasing in nursing homes and assisted living facilities. Simultaneously, facilities with palliative care services showed decreases in both hospitalized deaths and hospitalizations in the last 30 days of life.[14] Community-based palliative care (CPC) models have been proposed to increase palliative care access across care settings and entire illness trajectories, allowing for palliative care services in both inpatient and outpatient settings.[15] Additionally, partnering with community service agencies for older adults creates opportunities to expand palliative care by generating palliative care champions within agencies, training staff in core palliative care skills, and partnering with hospital palliative care teams to complete in-person or telehealth comprehensive assessments.[16]

Functional Impairment and Caregiving

Given increased life expectancies, people are living longer with multiple chronic conditions. In a 2014 report, about 80% of Medicare beneficiaries had at least two chronic conditions.[17] Over time, the burden of these illnesses begins to compromise ability to function independently, requiring assistance with activities of daily living (ADLs) and instrumental ADLs (IADLs) (Table 45.1). Among people 65 years old or older with multiple chronic conditions, 45% are dependent in one or more ADLs and require another person to help them get through the day.[18] Most of this care is provided by unpaid and untrained family members. Based on the 2011 National Health and Aging Trends Study (NHATS) and the National Study of Caregiving (NSOC), 14.7 million family and unpaid caregivers helped 7.7 million older adults; of those 7.7 million older adults, 6.5 million (44.1%) needed substantial support, often leading to increased emotional and financial distress and decreased

TABLE 45.1 List of activities of daily living (ADLs) and instrumental ADLs (IADLS)

6 Activities of daily living (ADLs)	7 Instrumental activities of daily living (IADLs)
Ambulating	Cleaning and home maintenance
Bathing	Cooking or meal preparation
Dressing and Grooming	Managing communication (e.g., telephone)
Feeding	Managing finances
Transferring (positions)	Managing medications
Toileting	Managing transportation
	Shopping

This table lists ADLs and IADLs that older adults with serious illness may need increasing help with as diseases progress.

productivity among caregivers.[19] If family members are not available, are unable, or are unwilling to provide this care, personal care services must be paid for out of pocket as they are not covered by Medicare and are only minimally supported for those in poverty by Medicaid. Variation in caregiving can depend on socioeconomic status and gender. Most unpaid caregivers are women and family members. Caregivers who provide substantial help with healthcare have increased emotional, physical, and financial difficulties.[19] Less family support also correlates inversely with hospice enrollment.[20,21]

Chapter 19 goes into detail about cancer caregivers; nonetheless, it is important to mention the importance of providing support for and educating and training paid and unpaid caregivers who take care of older adults with serious illness. Imminent and projected deficits of the caregiving workforce will have major implications for care of older people with serious illness, which may lead to increased healthcare costs (with a smaller tax base to support such costs), healthcare utilization (e.g., hospitalizations, emergency department visits), nursing home placement, and morbidity and mortality among older adults.[22] Within the next decade, as the US birthrate falls and more women enter in the workforce, there will be a shortage of formal and informal caregivers available to care for functionally impaired patients due to demographic changes.[23] According to an American Association of Retired Persons (AARP) 2013 report on caregivers within the United States, in 2010 there were 7 possible caregivers to every person older than 80 years; this ratio is supposed to decrease to 4 possible caregivers to every person older than 80 years in 2030, and down to 2.9 possible caregivers to every person older than 80 in 2050.[23] Understanding the availability, willingness, and ability of family and others to provide assistance is an essential element of care for patients with any serious illness.

Geriatric Syndromes

A number of phenomena become increasingly common with age, though they are far from universal. These include frailty, falls, mobility problems, memory loss, altered level of consciousness (delirium), incontinence, vision and hearing loss, and dental problems. Frailty, associated with cognitive decline, fatigue, low activity, muscle weakness and muscle loss, slowed performance, and appetite and weight loss, is a clinical syndrome related to chronic inflammation and correlated with adverse health outcomes.[24] Frail older adults are at higher risk for geriatric syndromes that cause a cumulative adverse effect on the health of older adults.[25] Common geriatric syndromes include chronic inflammation, cognitive impairment, delirium, disability, falls, frailty, impaired homeostasis, incontinence, malnutrition, and multiple comorbidities (>3–4 chronic illnesses).[26] Geriatric conditions complicate a patients' ability to tolerate the impact of a serious illness and its treatments, often leading to functional decline from acute insults or a steady decline over time from chronic illnesses. Symptoms may have atypical presentations and go unrecognized and/or untreated. For example, the presenting symptom for COVID in many older adults is delirium or a fall, as opposed to the dyspnea and fatigue common in younger people. To mitigate symptom burden in older adults with serious illness, especially prior to death, awareness of atypical presentations and nonverbal signs of distress as a marker of uncontrolled symptoms is imperative. For instance, vocalization and resistance to care among older adults with cognitive impairment is often mistakenly assumed to be a consequence of the underlying dementia when in fact it can be an expression of unrecognized and untreated pain or other discomfort that the patient can no longer articulate verbally.

The 4M's Framework

Developed by the John A. Hartford Foundation, Institute for Healthcare Improvement and with the input of leading geriatricians, the 4M's Framework is a standardized approach to care for vulnerable older adults intended to maximize the benefits and minimize the harms of encounters with our healthcare system. This is achieved by focusing on four actionable and critical areas: Mobility, Mentation, Medication, and what Matters.

Mobility

Within the 4M's framework, emphasis on mobility encourages older adults to keep moving safely in order to maintain function. Serious illness can impair mobility due to increased fatigue (e.g., chronic heart failure [CHF], chronic obstructive pulmonary disease [COPD], cancer), pain, or progressive weakness and loss of coordination (e.g., amyotrophic lateral sclerosis [ALS], Parkinson's disease, history of cerebrovascular accident [CVA], dementia). Impaired mobility, particularly when in the hospital or a nursing facility, can lead to serious health consequences (e.g., reduced nutritional status, pressure injuries, decreased muscle mass). On average, muscle strength declines by around 3–4% for men and 2–3% for woman eash year;[27] however, with bedrest for older adults, muscle strength can decrease by ~5% per day (compared to 1–1.5% per day for young adults).[28] Deconditioning happens rapidly, while reconditioning can take much longer and often leads to a new functional baseline. Even a single day of bedrest leads to loss of reserve and mobility and becomes irreversible over time. Compared to functional status on admission, up to 30–40% of hospitalized older adults lose one or more ADLs at the time of discharge, resulting in a condition called *hospital acquired disability* and increased dependence on others for help.[29] Older adults who have a decline in mobility can lose their independence, confidence, and become dependent on daily assistance from another person. Hence, ensuring daily mobility, including sitting upright in a chair and walking, is critical for seriously ill hospitalized adults when their condition permits.

Falls are the leading cause of injury among older adults, resulting in 35.6 million falls and 8.4 million fall-related injuries in the United States in 2018, which constitutes 27.5% and 10.2%, respectively, of the US population 65 years old and older.[30] Falls are sentinel events for older adults. In 2018, falls led to 3 million US emergency department visits, 950,000 hospitalizations, and 32,000 deaths.[30] Falls are preventable and often require addressing multiple risk factors.[31] Fall prevention strategies include assessing for polypharmacy and deprescribing medications (e.g., sedative hypnotics, anticholinergic medications, excess diuresis, antihypertensive regimens), optimizing pain management to increase mobility, doing a home safety evaluation, and prescribing physical and occupational therapy to improve strength, flexibility, and balance.

Once patients leave the hospital, insurance benefits may limit access to rehabilitation therapies within the United States. When it comes to physical therapy (PT) and occupational therapy (OT), Medicare Part B will cover outpatient PT/OT sessions, though patients may have to pay a premium for these services (unless patients have supplemental coverage plans [e.g., Medigap, Medicaid, Employer insurance]). For patients going to skilled nursing facilities (SNF) or subacute rehabilitation facilities (SAR), PT/OT services will be provided as long as patients are making active progress in set rehabilitation goals. If an older adult has Medicare Part A benefits, patients pay $0 for the first 20 days in a SNF/SAR, then a co-insurance amount (which can be around $185.50/day in 2021) for days 21–100, and subsequently all costs beyond day 101 in a SNF/SAR.[32] For older adults in a long-term care (LTC) nursing facility (where patients typically need assistance with >2 ADLs), PT/OT services are provided if there is an acute change in clinical status and typically for a short period of time until functional goals are met or functional status improvement plateaus. LTC is paid predominantly by Medicaid (which is means-tested and only available to those meeting or spending down to meet the required levels of poverty), followed by out-of-pocket, followed by LTC insurance. For those getting home healthcare, PT/OT services are provided by Certified Home Health Agencies (CHHA) who teach patients and caregivers home exercise routines often 1–3 times a week for a few weeks. For older adults with serious illnesses enrolled in home hospice, which is covered by Medicare Part A, PT/OT services are covered and can be helpful for assisting in educating caregivers on passive range of movement exercises and transfers (e.g., from the bed to a chair, from the commode to the bed) to decrease symptoms, improve comfort, and maximize remaining functional activity.[33]

Mentation

The focus on mentation in the 4M's Framework acknowledges the critical role of cognition on function, quality of life, and medical outcomes and encourages clinical attention to the range of factors that can influence mentation. Syndromes affecting cognition include altered level of consciousness (delirium), psychiatric disorders like depression and anxiety, and various forms and stages of dementia.

Delirium

Often unrecognized and misdiagnosed, delirium, an altered level of consciousness, is the most common adverse consequence of hospitalization in older adults. Delirium is a medical emergency because it results in life-altering and serious complications (Box 45.1). Delirium is common in emergency departments, hospitals, and nursing facilities and can lead to permanent cognitive impairment, presumably due to irreversible neuronal damage.[34] Those with underlying cognitive impairment and those with a previous history of delirium are at significantly higher risk for getting hospital- or nursing facility-acquired delirium.

As described in Chapter 6, delirium can present as hyperactive delirium (i.e., combative, shouting, groaning, agitated), hypoactive delirium (i.e., withdrawn, somnolent, "out of it"), or a mixed hyper- and hypoactive delirium. Delirium typically waxes and wanes and is often undiagnosed, especially in instances of hypoactive delirium where somnolent or apathetic patients are not interfering with their medical care and therefore evading the attention of clinicians. Daily screening for delirium is best practice; using the Confusion Assessment Method (CAM) at the same time as vital signs are checked is an effective method of detecting delirium.[35] Because delirium is seen commonly in older adults with serious illness who are not terminally ill and is a red flag marker of increased risk for developing dementia requiring long-term institutionalization and hospital complications or adverse events, screening and prevention are essential.

Delirium etiology is usually multifactorial (Box 45.2). Prevention is essential because once delirium occurs it is hard to treat. The best intervention for delirium is to be proactive and prevent delirium using a multifaceted approach (Box 45.3). Delirium is preventable

---

BOX 45.1 Delirium consequences in older adults with serious illness

Decreased independence
Higher institutionalization rates
Higher readmission rates
Increased healthcare costs
Increased immobility (leading to impaired ADLs/IADLs)
Increased morbidity and mortality
Increased risk for future delirium
Permanent cognitive impairment
Prolonged hospitalizations

This list identifies delirium consequences, impacting health outcomes, quality of life, and health care utilization.

BOX 45.2 Delirium causes in older adults with serious illness

Change in physical environment

Constipation

Dehydration or reduced oral intake

Infection

Immobility

Interrupted sleep wake patterns

Medications (especially sedative hypnotics and drugs with anticholinergic effects)

Physical or chemical restraints

Sensory impairments (vision, hearing)

Stress (physical, mental, emotional)

Uncontrolled pain

Underlying cognitive impairment

Urinary retention

This list highlights the many causes of delirium in older adults with serious illness.

through avoidance of polypharmacy, especially sedative-hypnotics and anticholinergic agents; identification and prevention of constipation and or urinary retention; management of pain (pain is a risk factor for delirium[36]); identification and management of infection; and recognition that in older adult patients delirium may represent an atypical presentation of many illnesses (e.g., myocardial infarction, COVID, stroke, pneumonia, sepsis). It is unclear whether delirium is a marker or is itself a causal precipitant of subsequent dementia,

BOX 45.3 Delirium precautions in older adults with serious illness

Avoid anticholinergic medications, antihistamines, and benzodiazepines

Bowel and bladder management

Early mobility

Frequent reorientation

Maintain sleep wake cycle

Pain management

Reduce tethers when appropriate (avoid catheters and restraints)

This lists interventions to proactively take to prevent delirium in older adults with serious illness.

functional impairment, and need for institutionalization. Though healthcare systems may view a live discharge from a hospital (albeit with delirium or new-onset cognitive impairment) to a LTC facility as a "successful outcome," this is a dreaded and unacceptable outcome for many patients. Avoidance of nursing homes and maintaining independence are among the highest priorities of older adults.

Depression

Depression is not "normal" in old age and is common in the context of comorbid serious illness.[37] Coexisting depression is an independent predictor of mortality in many serious illnesses, including cancer, heart failure, stroke, and end-stage renal disease.[38] It is unknown whether depression in this context is due to an underlying disease, an inflammatory syndrome, or is a consequence of the quality-of-life limitations imposed by a serious illness. Moreover, it can be challenging to differentiate grief due to a serious illness from depression in all patients, including older adults. Grief, a normal reaction, results from a particular loss where feeling numb and being in disbelief can be normal while still being able to plan for the future and find pleasure in life.[39] Depression in serious illness is a clinical diagnosis and often associated with feelings of worthlessness, guilt, and impaired functioning.[39] Untreated depression results in increased mortality, decreased quality of life, and increased economic burden.[40] Regardless, depression is safely treatable, hence routine screening for and treatment of depression when found is a core responsibility of any health professional caring for patients with serious illness.[41] Brief validated screening tools, such as asking the single question, "Are you feeling down, depressed, or hopeless most of the time over the past 2 weeks?"[42] followed by the Patient Health Questionnaire-9 (PHQ-9) screening tool are recommended for older adults with serious illness. Details on these validated screening tools can be found in the Center to Advance Palliative Care [CAPC]'s online curriculum, in its module titled "Depression in Serious Illness."

For older adults, loss of purpose and meaning, loneliness, and irritability are common manifestations of depression while among younger cancer patients, tearfulness, social withdrawal, and apathy are more indicative symptoms of depression.[43] Due to overlapping symptoms of serious illness and depression (e.g., weight loss, anorexia, difficulty concentrating, fatigue, insomnia), alternative diagnostic criteria have been suggested for depression in cancer and other seriously ill patients, including those developed by Cavanaugh et al. (1983), Endicott (1984), and Zimmerman et al. (2010).[43] Endicott criteria for depression in cancer patients emphasize that the physical signs of depression are replaced by psychological or affective features of depression such as brooding, guilt, hopelessness, self-pity, and pessimism (Table 45.2).[44] For patients with serious illness, the question, "Are you feeling down, depressed, or hopeless most of the time over the past 2 weeks?" yielded the highest sensitivity, specificity, and positive predictive value for depression.[45]

Dementia

Like depression, cognitive impairment and dementia are not normal in older adults but are manifestations of a disease process. That said, the rate of cognitive impairment increases steadily with age, reaching approximately 50% of people older than 85 in the United States.

TABLE 45.2 Depression screening in older adults with serious illness

Physical/Somatic symptoms	Affective/Psychological symptoms
Change in appetite/weight	Brooding, self-pity, pessimism
Decreased concentration	Feelings of hopelessness, helplessness worthlessness, guilt, thoughts of death
Fatigue, loss of energy	Lack of reactivity, blunting
Sleep disturbances	Social withdrawal, decreased talkativeness
	Tearfulness, depressed appearance

This table outlines the Endicott Criteria for depression, substituting physical criterial for phycological criteria when assessing a patient with serious illness for depression.

The dominant cause of dementia is Alzheimer's disease, followed by vascular dementia (due to multiple small strokes) and mixed dementia (Alzheimer's disease plus vascular dementia). Less common forms of dementia that are important to recognize include dementia associated with Parkinson's disease, frontotemporal dementia, Lewy body dementia, and Creutzfeldt-Jakob disease.

It is important to screen for and identify dementia in early stages because it allows patients and families to plan and prepare for financial and caregiving challenges to come (Box 45.4). In addition, in the early stages of dementia, patients are usually able to articulate what is most important to them, appoint a healthcare proxy or healthcare power of attorney (important for future healthcare decision-making), and indicate what treatments they would want if they got to a point where they were no longer able to recognize and interact with loved ones. Despite decades of intensive research efforts, there are no effective pharmacologic treatments to meaningfully prevent or slow the progression of Alzheimer's disease. In contrast, the course of vascular dementia can be halted or slowed via meticulous risk factor management (e.g., blood pressure control, lipid-lowering agents, weight loss, exercise, smoking cessation, diabetes management).

Medication

More than a third of people over age 65 take five or more medications every day, a number that is associated with at least one significant drug problem (e.g., toxicity, drug interactions).[46] Fall rate rises with the number of medications, as does mortality.[47] The high prevalence of multimorbidity often requires medications for each problem, resulting in additional medications to manage side effects of other drugs, leading to a so-called *prescribing cascade*. Polypharmacy is defined as multiple (≥5 regularly prescribed medications) and inappropriate medication use (taking more medications than indicated). Besides the sheer number of pills an older adult with serious illness may need to remember to take, it is important to think about the logistics of taking these medications, including obtaining medications (e.g., costs, insurance coverage, picking them up at a pharmacy), taking medications (e.g., organizing them, remembering to take them, being able to swallow large pills, being

---

BOX 45.4 Dementia screening tools

7-Minute Screen (7MS)

Abbreviated Mental Test Score (AMTS)

AD8 Dementia Screening

Addenbrooke's Cognitive Examination Revised (ACE-R)

Clock Drawing Test (CDT)

General Practitioner Assessment of Cognition (GPCOG)

Memory Impairment Screen (MIS)

Mini-Cog Test

Mini-Mental State Examination (MMSE)

Montreal Cognitive Assessment (MoCA)

Six-Item Cognitive Impairment Test (6CIT)

Test Your Memory test (TYM)

Verbal or category fluency tests

This lists commonly used dementia screening tools for older adults with serious illness. Screening tools should assess various cognitive domains that are impacted by dementia, including learning and memory, language, executive function, complex attention, perceptual-motor, and social cognition.

---

able to open pill bottles), and medication side effects and effectiveness.[48] There are many guidelines for starting medications; there are few guidelines on when to stop medications or when harms outweigh the benefits of taking a medication.[49] Before prescribing a new medicine for a new symptom or a potential side effect, consider whether one or more drugs may account for the problem and whether the benefit of the offending agent outweighs its risks.

Polypharmacy is compounded by the widespread use of dangerous over-the-counter medications which patients assume are safe. A classic example is the high prevalence of the antihistamine diphenhydramine (Benadryl) in sleep and cold aids in drug stores. Diphenhydramine is a potent anticholinergic agent, markedly increasing the risk for confusion, delirium, falls, dry mouth, and constipation among older adults. Other frequently used over-the-counter medicines include acetaminophen, which in doses higher than 3 g per day for older adults is associated with substantial risks of hepatotoxicity, and nonsteroidal anti-inflammatory drugs (NSAIDs; e.g., ibuprofen and naproxen), which are associated with increased risk of renal failure, gastritis, and bleeding. Herbal and dietary supplements, associated with risky drug interactions and other toxicities, are used by the majority of older adults who often do not inform their clinicians about these agents. Age-related changes in pharmacokinetics and pharmacodynamics lead to increased plasma concentrations and greater sensitivity to drug effects and side effects.

Identifying polypharmacy and medications that are high risk for adverse drug effects (ADEs) for older adults are important. Equally essential is *deprescribing*, which is reducing or stopping medications that may be causing harm or are no longer providing benefit. Deprescribing entails patient-centered care, involves shared decision-making to decide which medications to stop taking, and can lead to decreases in healthcare expenses and unnecessary side effects. Deprescribing is important in older adults with serious illness especially near end of life as often the benefits of medications for primary or secondary prevention will not be seen at that stage of life (e.g., statins for coronary artery disease or antidiabetic medications if a hemoglobin A1C is <8%). Medical provider inertia is a common reason for continuing medications that are no longer appropriate, so engaging patients, pharmacists, nurses, and community organizations to help with deprescribing efforts is important.[50] Deprescribing and reducing polypharmacy results in decreased mortality and more manageable drug regimens with fewer side effects, achieving true patient-centered care.[51]

As a result of ADEs, hospitalizations occur at a greater frequency in older adults compared to younger patients. In one study of 168,000 Medicare beneficiaries with hip, shoulder, or wrist fractures, 75% had been taking non-opioid drugs associated with falls and fractures (e.g., sedatives, atypical antipsychotics, or excess antihypertensives) in the 4 months prior to the fracture.[52] ADEs lead to increased morbidity and mortality, with death rates higher than many common cancers.[49] To help clinicians avoid ADEs, medical providers should refer to the Beer's Criteria Medication List to identify and avoid potentially harmful medications for older adults.[53] Many potentially inappropriate medications prescribed for patients with serious illness are on the Beer's Criteria Medication List, including NSAIDS, muscle relaxants, benzodiazepines, opioids, anticholinergic agents, and antihistamines. If these classes of medications are necessary in older adults with serious illness to manage symptoms, starting with the lowest possible dose, titrating up slowly, and monitoring for side effects are important.

Anticholinergic drugs are especially harmful in older adults. Adverse drug reactions associated with anticholinergic agents include dry eyes, urinary retention, constipation, fecal impaction, dizziness, delirium, cognitive impairment, and falls. Many commonly prescribed medications have anticholinergic properties, including anti-allergy or antihistamines, antihypertensives, benzodiazepines, antipsychotics, tricyclic antidepressants, oxybutynin and tolterodine for urinary frequency, and diuretics. To assess the additive anticholinergic effects of patients' drug regimens, medical providers can use the free anticholinergic burden calculator ACB Calculator (accessed at http://www.acbcalc.com/) to add up the combined anticholinergic burden of specific medications.

A stepwise approach to prescribing begins with a routine medical reconciliation of current prescribed and unprescribed medications (Box 45.5). A comprehensive medical reconciliation should happen at all outpatient visits, hospitalizations, and especially at any transition of care phase (e.g., a post-hospital discharge clinic visit or a discharge to a nursing home). Rather than rely on memory, clinicians should ask patients to bring in all medications, including prescribed medications, vitamins, supplements, over-the-counter medications, eye drops, non-oral medications (e.g., injections, patches, oils or creams, suppositories) to determine what patients are actually taking. This thorough

---

BOX 45.5 Medication management in older adults with serious illness

Review all medication, including over the counter medications and topical agents.

Ask how patients are taking each medication (dose and frequency may differ from prescription instructions)

Assess changes in health status (e.g., renal function, liver function, oropharyngeal dysphagia)

If changes in health status are noted, adjust medication dosing and routes of administration.

Deprescribe medications that are no longer necessary, fail to achieve patient goals, or cause harm exceeding benefit.

If starting a new medication, assess value of medication and ensure medication is not treating a side effect of another medication, preventing a medication prescribing cascade.

This box highlights what steps to include as part of a comprehensive medication reconciliation done at any clinical encounter (e.g., clinic, hospital, subacute rehab, long-term acute care hospital) that can help mitigate adverse drug events.

---

medication reconciliation often identifies duplicative agents with different names from different prescribers, new medicines prescribed in a hospital or by other clinicians, or inadvertent discontinuation of needed medications. A comprehensive medication reconciliation should also include asking patients or caregivers about substance use (e.g., alcohol, drug, tobacco, prescription drug misuse). Asking about substance use is important to assess for drug-drug interactions impacting metabolism and to determine risks for certain medications (e.g., opioids, benzodiazepines) to prevent drug misuse or substance use disorder. Older adults are less likely to be screened for substance use disorders compared to younger adults.[54]

Identification of redundant, harmful, or unnecessary medication should lead to deprescribing accompanied by a clear explanation about why something a patient may have been taking for years or a prescription from a trusted medical provider no longer provides benefit and may cause harm. Drug discontinuation should be done one at a time in order to assess for adverse consequences, and many agents should be tapered before discontinuation (e.g., β-blockers, antidepressants, corticosteroids, gabapentin, opioids). Always use the lowest possible effective dose of any medication. Be aware of how age-related declines in renal function, liver function, and volume of distribution change dosing and frequency. Finally, every medication should have a clear goal (e.g., bringing blood pressure to a safer level, reducing low-density lipoprotein [LDL] cholesterol levels, improving pain enough to walk outside). If a medication is not achieving a desired goal, consider dose adjustment, switching to a potentially more effective agent, or stopping that medication.

What Matters

Clinicians may assume that patients' highest priority is living as long as possible, regardless of the quality of that life. A qualitative study asked 357 older adults attending a senior center to rank in terms of their importance living longer, relief from pain and symptoms, and remaining independent; more than 75% of respondents ranked remining independent as their highest priority, followed by relief from symptoms, followed in last place by living longer.[55] Life in a nursing home is widely feared and considered by many people to be a fate worse than death.[56]

Hence, when informing patients and caregivers about the risks of procedures and treatments, mortality risk is not the only important consideration. In order to align care with what is most important, patients and caregivers should also be informed about the risk of permanent cognitive impairment, functional dependence, and discharge to a LTC facility.

Precisely for this reason, What Matters in the 4M's Framework focuses on knowing and aligning care with health outcome goals and care preferences to achieve goal-concordant care.[57] Patient Priority Care (https://patientprioritiescare.org/) is a program, created in 2018, to guide clinician conversations to help ensure patients received goal-concordant care.[57,58] Personalizing approaches to medical care can reduce unwanted outcomes. Before deciding about any medical intervention or procedure, patients and their loved ones should be aware of important potential negative outcomes and think through benefits, risks, and alternatives to help guide decisions. This is applicable no matter how big the decision is—from going to the emergency department after a fall to getting a preventative colonoscopy with anesthesia to getting emergent surgery for an acute abdomen. When assessing what matters, it is important to remember that often what hospitals measure as a quality success or failure (e.g., mortality) is in contradiction to what patients measure as a success or failure (e.g., remaining independent). Medical providers taking care of older adults with serious illness should share what short- and long-term consequences of a medical decision may be to help patients make informed decisions about their health. For example, independence is usually the most important thing that matters to older adults.[59] Some patients may opt out of various treatments if they know there would be a high likelihood of cognitive or functional impairment.[60]

By better understanding what matters to patients most, medical providers can help guide patients in making the best decision for each clinical scenario. Prognostic tools (e.g., ePrognosis, Geriatric Trauma Outcome Score [GTOS], Walter Prognostic Index) and functional scoring tools (e.g., Eastern Cooperative Oncology Group [EGOC], Palliative Performance Scale [PPS], Karnofsky Performance Status Scale [KPS]) can help assess morbidity or mortality rates in patients and help align treatment to what matters most to patients. Once potential consequences of an intervention are shared and the patient chooses to move forward, it is imperative to optimize preoperative status (e.g., through physical therapy) and mitigate peri- and postoperative complications (e.g., hospital-acquired delirium) as much as possible by looking at medications that can be modified or stopped prior to an intervention. According to a study by Ernst et al., a pre-, peri-, and postoperative palliative care consult reduced 180-day mortality rate by 33% whether the patient opted for surgery or chose not to have surgery.[61] Yefimova et al. found that decedents of patients within the Veterans Affairs (VA) system who had high-risk operations and received a palliative care consult between 2012 and 2015 were more likely to rate the care their loved one received as excellent, specifically in regard to end-of-life communication and support.[62]

To ensure what matters most is achieved for older adults with a serious illness, mitigating hospital complications and having a safe transitions of care plan is imperative (e.g., hospital to subacute rehabilitation, nursing facility to hospital, hospital to an LTC facility). Some studies suggest that complications of hospitalization may be the third leading cause of death in the United States.[63,64] The safety challenges associated with hospitalization of older adults with serious illness are many and include medical errors, infection, delirium, restricted visiting hours leading to loneliness and social isolation (themselves independent predictors of mortality), declines in functional status and mobility, pressure injury, adverse medication effects, poor nutrition, loss of social support as needs escalate, and difficulty ensuring a safe discharge location and home safety. These potential hospitalization challenges need to be considered when creating a patient-centered care plan. Clinicians across all healthcare settings can help determine what matters most to older adults with serious illnesses through honest conversations about the reality of their illness(es) and likely outcomes of potential treatments.

Future Directions

Most serious illness occurs in older adults. Any clinician caring for patients in this age group needs to gain the knowledge and skill necessary to optimize quality of care, quality of life, and the experience of receiving medical care. Operationalizing the 4M's Framework (Mobility, Mentation, Medication, and what Matters) for older adults has the potential to both reduce harm and increase the likelihood of successful treatment. To ensure that palliative care access for older adults with serious illness improves, educational efforts, policy changes, and expanding research are necessary. Additionally, innovative models are needed to help support older adults with serious illness across all care settings.

Key Points

- Given the increase in patients living with chronic medical conditions and the rise in life expectancy, medical providers would benefit from a standardized and consistent approach to taking care of older adults with serious illness.
- When approaching older adults with serious illness, it is imperative to recognize normal aging versus pathology.
- Approaching older adults with serious illness using the 4M's framework (Mobility, Mentation, Medications, and what Matters) will increase safety and patient-centered and goal-concordant care.

References

1. Institute for Healthcare Improvement. What is an age-friendly health system? 2012. Accessed February 23, 2021. http://www.ihi.org/Engage/Initiatives/Age-Friendly-Health-Systems/Pages/default.aspx

2. United States Census Bureau. Older people projected to outnumber children for first time in U.S. history. 2018. Accessed March 13, 2021, https://www.census.gov/newsroom/press-releases/2018/cb18-41-population-projections.html

3. Ortman JM VV, Hogan H. An aging nation: The older population in the United States population estimates and projections. May 2014. Accessed March 12, 2021. https://www.census.gov/content/dam/Census/library/publications/2014/demo/p25-1140.pdf

4. Arias E, Tejada-Vera B, Ahmad F. Provisional life expectancy estimates for January through June, 2020. February 2021. Vital statistics rapid release. Accessed March 12, 2021. https://www.cdc.gov/nchs/data/vsrr/VSRR10-508.pdf

5. Ahmad FB, Anderson RN. The leading causes of death in the US for 2020. *JAMA*. May 2021;325(18):1829–1830. doi:10.1001/jama.2021.5469

6. Cross SH, Ely EW, Kavalieratos D, Tulsky JA, Warraich HJ. Place of death for individuals with chronic lung disease: Trends and associated factors from 2003 to 2017 in the United States. *Chest*. 2020;158(2):670–680. doi:10.1016/j.chest.2020.02.062

7. Cross SH, Lakin JR, Mendu M, Mandel EI, Warraich HJ. Trends in place of death for individuals with deaths attributed to advanced chronic or end-stage kidney disease in the United States. *J Pain Symptom Manage*. 2021;61(1):112–120.e1. doi:10.1016/j.jpainsymman.2020.08.001

8. Cross SH, Kaufman BG, Taylor DH, Kamal AH, Warraich HJ. Trends and factors associated with place of death for individuals with dementia in the United States. *J Am Geriatr Soc*. 2020;68(2):250–255. doi:10.1111/jgs.16200

9. Cross SH, Warraich HJ. Changes in the place of death in the United States. *N Engl J Med*. 2019;381(24):2369–2370. doi:10.1056/NEJMc1911892

10. Hoerger M, Perry LM, Korotkin BD, Walsh LE, Kazan AS, Rogers JL, et al. Statewide differences in personality associated with geographic disparities in access to palliative care: Findings on openness. *J Palliat Med*. 2019;22(6):628–634. doi:10.1089/jpm.2018.0206

11. Center to Advance Palliative Care and National Palliative Care Research Center America's care of serious illness: At state-by-state report card on access to palliative care in our nation's hospitals 2019. 2019. Accessed May 1, 2021. https://reportcard.capc.org/

12. Calton B, Abedini N, Fratkin M. Telemedicine in the time of coronavirus. *J Pain Symptom Manage*. 2020;60(1):e12–e14. doi:10.1016/j.jpainsymman.2020.03.019

13. Calton BA, Rabow MW, Branagan L, et al. Top ten tips palliative care clinicians should know about telepalliative care. *J Palliat Med*. 2019;22(8):981–985. doi:10.1089/jpm.2019.0278

14. Miller SC, Dahal R, Lima JC, et al. Palliative care consultations in nursing homes and end-of-life hospitalizations. *J Pain Symptom Manage*. 2016;52(6):878–883. doi:10.1016/j.jpainsymman.2016.05.017

15. Kamal AH, Currow DC, Ritchie CS, Bull J, Abernethy AP. Community-based palliative care: The natural evolution for palliative care delivery in the U.S. *J Pain Symptom Manage*. 2013;46(2):254–264. doi:10.1016/j.jpainsymman.2012.07.018

16. Reid MC, Ghesquiere A, Kenien C, Capezuti E, Gardner D. Expanding palliative care's reach in the community via the elder service agency network. *Ann Palliat Med*. 2017;6(Suppl 1):S104–S107. doi:10.21037/apm.2017.03.10

17. Fabbri E, Zoli M, Gonzalez-Freire M, Salive ME, Studenski SA, Ferrucci L. Aging and multimorbidity: New tasks, priorities, and frontiers for integrated gerontological and clinical research. *J Am Med Dir Asso* 2015;16(8):640–647. doi:10.1016/j.jamda.2015.03.013

18. Jindai K, Nelson CM, Vorderstrasse BA, Quiñones AR. Multimorbidity and functional limitations among adults 65 or older, NHANES 2005–2012. *Prev Chronic Dis*. 2016;3(23):E151. doi:10.5888/pcd13.160174.

19. Wolff JL, Spillman BC, Freedman VA, Kasper JD. A national profile of family and unpaid caregivers who assist older adults with health care activities. *JAMA Intern Med*. 2016;176(3):372–379. doi:10.1001/jamainternmed.2015.7664

20. Kumar V, Ankuda CK, Aldridge MD, Husain M, Ornstein KA. Family caregiving at the end of life and hospice use: A national study of Medicare beneficiaries. *J Am Geriatr Soc*. 2020;68(10):2288–2296. doi:10.1111/jgs.16648

21. Ornstein KA, Kelley AS, Bollens-Lund E, Wolff JL. A national profile of end-of-life caregiving in the United States. *Health Aff (Millwood)*. 2017;36(7):1184–1192. doi:10.1377/hlthaff.2017.0134

22. National Academies of Sciences, Engineering, and Medicine. *Families Caring for an Aging America*. Washington, DC: The National Academies Press; 2016. doi:10.17226/23606

23. Redfoot D, Feinberg L, Houser A. The aging of the baby boom and the growing care gap: A look at future declines in the availability of family caregivers. AARP. 2021. Accessed July 1, 2021. https://www.aarp.org/content/dam/aarp/research/public_policy_institute/ltc/2013/baby-boom-and-the-growing-care-gap-insight-AARP-ppi-ltc.pdf

24. Lazris A. Geriatric palliative care. *Prim Care*. 2019;46(3):447–459. doi:10.1016/j.pop.2019.05.007

25. Tinetti ME, Inouye SK, Gill TM, Doucette JT. Shared risk factors for falls, incontinence, and functional dependence: Unifying the approach to geriatric syndromes. *JAMA*. 1995;273(17):1348–1353.

26. Kane RL, Shamliyan T, Talley K, Pacala J. The association between geriatric syndromes and survival. *J Am Geriatr Soc*. 2012;60(5):896–904. doi:10.1111/j.1532-5415.2012.03942.x

27. Goodpaster BH, Park SW, Harris TB, et al. The loss of skeletal muscle strength, mass, and quality in older adults: The health, aging and body composition study. *J Gerontol A Biol Sci Med Sci*. 2006;61(10):1059–1064. doi:10.1093/gerona/61.10.1059

28. Creditor MC. Hazards of hospitalization of the elderly. *Ann Intern Med*. 1993;118(3):219–223. doi:10.7326/0003-4819-118-3-199302010-00011

29. Covinsky KE, Pierluissi E, Johnston CB. Hospitalization-associated disability: "She was probably able to ambulate, but I'm not sure". *JAMA*. 2011;306(16):1782–1793. doi:10.1001/jama.2011.1556

30. Moreland B, Kakara R, Henry A. Trends in nonfatal falls and fall-related injuries among adults aged ≥65 years — United States, 2012–2018. *MMWR Morb Mortal Wkly Rep*. 2020;69(27):875–881.

31. Tinetti ME, Kumar C. The patient who falls: "It's always a trade-off". *JAMA*. 2010;303(3):258–266. doi:10.1001/jama.2009.2024

32. Medicare. Skilled nursing facility (SNF) care. 2021. Accessed July 5, 2021. https://www.medicare.gov/coverage/skilled-nursing-facility-snf-care

33. Putt K, Faville KA, Lewis D, McAllister K, Pietro M, Radwan A. Role of physical therapy intervention in patients with life-threatening illnesses. *Am J Hosp Palliat Care*. 2017;34(2):186–196. doi:10.1177/1049909115623246

34. Witlox J, Eurelings LS, de Jonghe JF, Kalisvaart KJ, Eikelenboom P, van Gool WA. Delirium in elderly patients and the risk of postdischarge mortality, institutionalization, and dementia: A meta-analysis. *JAMA*. 2010;304(4):443–451. doi:10.1001/jama.2010.1013

35. Wei LA, Fearing MA, Sternberg EJ, Inouye SK. The Confusion Assessment Method: A systematic review of current usage. *J Am Geriatr Soc*. 2008;56(5):823–30. doi:10.1111/j.1532-5415.2008.01674.x

36. Feast AR, White N, Lord K, Kupeli N, Vickerstaff V, Sampson EL. Pain and delirium in people with dementia in the acute general hospital setting. *Age Ageing*. 2018;47(6):841–846. doi:10.1093/ageing/afy112

37. National Institutes of Health: National Institute on Aging. Depression and older adults. US Department of Health & Human Services. 2021. Accessed July 5, 2021. https://www.nia.nih.gov/health/depression-and-older-adults

38. Benton T, Staab J, Evans DL. Medical co-morbidity in depressive disorders. *Ann Clin Psychiatry*. 2007 Oct–Dec 2007;19(4):289–303. doi:10.1080/10401230701653542

39. McKee KY, Kelly A. Management of grief, depression, and suicidal thoughts in serious illness. *Med Clin North Am*. 2020;104(3):503–524. doi:10.1016/j.mcna.2020.01.003

40. Lloyd-Williams M, Shiels C, Taylor F, Dennis M. Depression: An independent predictor of early death in patients with advanced cancer. *J Affect Disord*. 2009;113(1-2):127–132. doi:10.1016/j.jad.2008.04.002

41. Nezu AM, Nezu CM, Felgoise SH, McClure KS, Houts PS. Project Genesis: Assessing the efficacy of problem-solving therapy for distressed adult cancer patients. *J Consult Clin Psychol*. 2003;71(6):1036–1048. doi:10.1037/0022-006X.71.6.1036

42. Chochinov HM, Wilson KG, Enns M, Lander S. "Are you depressed?" Screening for depression in the terminally ill. *Am J Psychiatry*. 1997;154(5):674–676. doi:10.1176/ajp.154.5.674

43. Saracino RM, Rosenfeld B, Nelson CJ. Towards a new conceptualization of depression in older adult cancer patients: A review of the literature. *Aging Ment Health*. 2016;20(12):1230–1242. doi:10.1080/13607863.2015.1078278

44. Endicott J. Measurement of depression in patients with cancer. *Cancer*. 1984;53(10 Suppl):2243–2249. doi:10.1002/cncr.1984.53.s10.2243

45. Lloyd-Williams M, Spiller J, Ward J. Which depression screening tools should be used in palliative care? *Palliat Med*. 2003;17(1):40–43. doi:10.1191/0269216303pm664oa

46. Qato DM, Wilder J, Schumm LP, Gillet V, Alexander GC. Changes in prescription and over-the-counter medication and dietary supplement use among older adults in the United States, 2005 vs. 2011. *JAMA Intern Med*. 2016;176(4):473–482. doi:10.1001/jamainternmed.2015.8581

47. Leelakanok N, Holcombe AL, Lund BC, Gu X, Schweizer ML. Association between polypharmacy and death: A systematic review and meta-analysis. *J Am Pharm Assoc (2003)*. 2017 Nov–Dec 2017;57(6):729–738.e10. doi:10.1016/j.japh.2017.06.002

48. Nicosia FM, Spar MJ, Stebbins M, et al. What is a medication-related problem? A qualitative study of older adults and primary care clinicians. *J Gen Intern Med*. 2020;35(3):724–731. doi:10.1007/s11606-019-05463-z

49. Farrell B, Mangin D. Deprescribing is an essential part of good prescribing. *Am Fam Physician*. 2019;99(1):7–9.

50. Steinman MA, Landefeld CS. Overcoming inertia to improve medication use and deprescribing. *JAMA*. 2018;320(18):1867–1869. doi:10.1001/jama.2018.16473

51. Sawan M, Reeve E, Turner J, et al. A systems approach to identifying the challenges of implementing deprescribing in older adults across different health-care settings and countries: A narrative review. *Expert Rev Clin Pharmacol*. 2020;13(3):233–245. doi:10.1080/17512433.2020.1730812

52. Munson JC, Bynum JP, Bell JE, et al. Patterns of prescription drug use before and after fragility fracture. *JAMA Intern Med*. 2016;176(10):1531–1538. doi:10.1001/jamainternmed.2016.4814

53. American Geriatrics Society. 2019 Updated AGS Beers Criteria® for potentially inappropriate medication use in older adults. *J Am Geriatr Soc*. 2019;67(4):674–694. doi:10.1111/jgs.15767

54. Han BH, Moore AA. Prevention and screening of unhealthy substance use by older adults. *Clin Geriatr Med*. 2018;34(1):117–129. doi:10.1016/j.cger.2017.08.005

55. Fried TR, Tinetti ME, Iannone L, O'Leary JR, Towle V, Van Ness PH. Health outcome prioritization as a tool for decision making among older persons with multiple chronic conditions. *Arch Intern Med*. 2011;171(20):1854–1856. doi:10.1001/archinternmed.2011.424

56. Positive Aging Sourcebook. Research study: Aging in place in America. 2020. Accessed July 1, 2021. https://www.retirementlivingsourcebook.com/articles/research-study-%E2%80%9Caging-in-place-in-america-%E2%80%9D%C2%9D

57. Tinetti M, Dindo L, Smith CD, et al. Challenges and strategies in patients' health priorities-aligned decision-making for older adults with multiple chronic conditions. *PLoS One*. 2019;14(6):e0218249. doi:10.1371/journal.pone.0218249

58. Tinetti ME, Naik AD, Dindo L, Costello DM, Esterson J, Geda M, et al. Association of patient priorities-aligned decision-making with patient outcomes and ambulatory health care burden among older adults with multiple chronic conditions: A nonrandomized clinical trial. *JAMA Intern Med*. 2019;179(12):1688–1697. doi:10.1001/jamainternmed.2019.4235

59. Fried TR, Street RL, Cohen AB. Chronic disease decision making and "what matters most." *J Am Geriatr Soc*. 2020;68(3):474–477. doi:10.1111/jgs.16371

60. Fried TR, Bradley EH, Towle VR, Allore H. Understanding the treatment preferences of seriously ill patients. *N Engl J Med*. 2002;346(14):1061–1066. doi:10.1056/NEJMsa012528

61. Ernst KF, Hall DE, Schmid KK, et al. Surgical palliative care consultations over time in relationship to systemwide frailty screening. *JAMA Surg.* 2014;149(11):1121–1126. doi:10.1001/jamasurg.2014.1393

62. Yefimova M, Aslakson RA, Yang L, et al. Palliative care and end-of-life outcomes following high-risk surgery. *JAMA Surg.* 2020;155(2):138–146. doi:10.1001/jamasurg.2019.5083

63. James JT. A new, evidence-based estimate of patient harms associated with hospital care. *J Patient Saf.* 2013;9(3):122–128. doi:10.1097/PTS.0b013e3182948a69

64. Leapfrog Group. *Hospital Errors Are the Third Leading Cause of Death in the US, and the New Hospital Safety Scores Show Improvements Are Too Slow.* Washington, DC: Leapfrog Group; 2013.https://leapfroggroup.org

Index